Handbook of Experimental Pharmacology

Continuation of Handbuch der experimentellen Pharmakologie

Vol. 73

Radiocontrast Agents

Contributors

T. Almén · J. L. Barnhart · P. B. Dean · S. El-Antably · H. W. Fischer
K. Golman · C. B. Higgins · G. B. Hoey · E. C. Lasser · G. P. Murphy
J. A. Nelson · D. B. Plewes · K. R. Smith · M. Sovak · M. R. Violante

Editor

M. Sovak

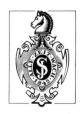

Springer-Verlag
Berlin Heidelberg New York Tokyo 1984

Professor Dr. MILOS SOVAK

University of California in San Diego
School of Medicine
Department of Radiology, S-009
La Jolla, CA 92093/USA
and
Biophysica Foundation
3333 Torrey Pines Ct.
La Jolla, CA 92037/USA

With 189 Figures

ISBN 3-540-13107-8 Springer-Verlag Berlin Heidelberg New York Tokyo
ISBN 0-387-13107-8 Springer-Verlag New York Heidelberg Berlin Tokyo

Library of Congress Cataloging in Publication Data. Main entry under title: Radiocontrast agents. (Handbook of experimental pharmacology; vol. 73) Includes bibliographies and index. 1. Diagnosis, Radiography. 2. Contrast media. I. Almén, T. (Torsten) II. Sovak, Milos. III. Series: Handbook of experimental pharmacology; v. 73. [DNLM: 1. Contrast Media. W1 HA51L v. 73/WN 160 R1285] QP905.H3 vol. 73 [RC78] 615'.1s [616.07'572] 84-5448 ISBN 0-387-13107-8 (U.S.)

© by Springer-Verlag Berlin Heidelberg 1984
Printed in Germany

The use of registered names, trademarks, etc. in this publication does not imply, even in the absence of a specific statement, that such names are exempt from the relevant protective laws and regulations and therefore free for general use.

Product liability: The publisher can give no guarantee for information about drug dosage and application thereof contained in this book. In every individual case the respective user must check its accuracy by consulting other pharmaceutical literature.

Typesetting, printing and bookbinding: Brühlsche Universitätsdruckerei, Giessen
2122/3130-543210

List of Contributors

T. ALMÉN, Department of Radiology, Malmö General Hospital, 21401 Malmö, Sweden

J. L. BARNHART, University of California in San Diego, School of Medicine, Department of Radiology, H-755, San Diego, CA 92103/USA

P. B. DEAN, University of Turku, School of Medicine, Department of Radiology, 20520 Turku 52, Finland

S. EL-ANTABLY, Research Department, Medical Products Group, Mallinckrodt, Inc., P.O. Box 5439, St. Louis, MO 63147/USA

H. W. FISCHER, University of Rochester, School of Medicine, Department of Radiology, Rochester, NY 14642/USA

K. GOLMAN, University of Lund, Department of Experimental Research, Malmö General Hospital, 21401 Malmö, Sweden

C. B. HIGGINS, University of California in San Francisco, School of Medicine, Department of Radiology, San Francisco, CA 94143/USA

G. B. HOEY, Research Department, Medical Products Group, Mallinckrodt, Inc., P.O. Box 5439, St. Louis, MO 63147/USA

E. C. LASSER, University of California in San Diego, School of Medicine, Department of Radiology, S-004, La Jolla, CA 92093/USA

G. P. MURPHY, Research Department, Medical Products Group, Mallinckrodt, Inc., P.O. Box 5439, St. Louis, MO 63147/USA

J. A. NELSON, University of Utah, College of Medicine, Department of Radiology, 1A71 Medical Center, Salt Lake City, UT 84132/USA

D. B. PLEWES, Radiology Department, University of Rochester, Medical Center, Box 648, Rochester, NY 14642/USA

K. R. SMITH, Research Department, Medical Products Group, Mallinckrodt, Inc., P.O. Box 5439, St. Louis, MO 63147/USA

M. Sovak, University of California in San Diego, School of Medicine, Department of Radiology, S-009, La Jolla, CA 92093/USA and Biophysica Foundation, 3333 N. Torrey Pines Ct., La Jolla, CA 92037/USA

M. R. Violante, University of Rochester, School of Medicine, Department of Radiology, Rochester, NY 14642/USA

Preface

Contrast media are drugs by default. Had there been no default, there would be no need for a related pharmacology, and thus no need for this book. Radiographic contrast media (CM) are substances whose primary purpose is to enhance diagnostic information of medical imaging systems. The position of CM in pharmacology is unique. First, there is the unusual requirement of biological inertness. An ideal CM should be completely biologically inert, i.e., stable, not pharmacologically active, and efficiently and innocuously excretable. Because they fail to meet these requirements, CM must be considered drugs.

The second unusual aspect of CM is that they are used in large quantities, their annual production being measured in tens of tons. It is not in spite of, but because of, the increased use of new radiographic systems, computed tomography, digital radiography, etc., that consumption is on the rise. And, it is not likely that the other emerging imaging modalities – NMR, ultrasonography, etc. – will displace radiographic CM soon; it is quite probable that these remarkable compounds will continue to play an active role in diagnostic imaging in the foreseeable future.

Following some 20 years of relative stagnation, the early seventies saw a major improvement with the first nonionic CM, metrizamide. Recently, a second generation of nonionic CM, compounds of low toxicity and high stability, was introduced. It seems only logical to assume that future developmental efforts will be directed toward design of compounds of equally good properties, but of lower cost. Expenditures for medical care are rising excessively, and their containment is rapidly becoming an important issue in most countries. Since the currently used ionic CM are almost acceptable for most general applications, the new generation of improved CM will not only have to be qualitatively superior to justify their introduction, but will also have to be economically feasible. By reviewing past experience in the design of improved CM, defining the state of the art, and presenting the basic methodology of CM research, the aim of this book is to inspire further progress in the important field of radiopharmacology and medical imaging.

I should like to express my thanks to Minerva Kunzel and William Shufflebotham, who helped me edit the manuscripts, and to Carol King and Mary Seeberger, who patiently typed and retyped the ever-changing text. Further, I wish to thank Sterling-Winthrop and Mallinckrodt Companies for their support, and the Editorial Board of the Handbook and the Publisher for the care that made this book possible.

La Jolla   M. Sovak

Contents

Introduction: State of the Art and Design Principles of Contrast Media.
M. Sovak. With 9 Figures 1
References 19

CHAPTER 1

Chemistry of X-Ray Contrast Media. G. B. Hoey and K. R. Smith
in collaboration with S. El-Antably and G. P. Murphy. With 38 Figures

A. Introduction and Scope 23
B. Biological Requirements 23
    I. Physicochemical Properties 24
        1. Water Solubility 24
        2. Viscosity 25
        3. Osmolality 25
    II. Chemical Stability 26
    III. Biological Safety 28
C. Ionic Contrast Media 31
    I. Synthesis 31
    II. Evolution of Structural Types 32
        1. Improving the Functional Groups 34
        2. Reduction of Hypertonicity 51
D. Nonionic Contrast Media 54
    I. Solubility Aspects of Nonionic Media 76
    II. Viscosity Considerations 77
    III. Osmolality 78
    IV. Stability 79
        1. Deiodination 80
        2. Instability of the Polyhydroxylalkyl Group 80
        3. Hydrolysis of the Coupler Group 83
    V. Synthesis of Nonionic Compounds 85
        1. Synthetic Approaches 85
        2. Manufacturing Costs 92
    VI. Stereochemical Aspects of Contrast Media 95
        1. Isomers Resulting from Restricted Rotation 96
    VII. High-Pressure Liquid Chromatography 99
    VIII. Water-Insoluble Nonionic Contrast Media 101
        1. Oily Contrast Media 102

    2. Benzoate Esters 103
    3. Perfluoroalkyl Halides 106
E. Oral Cholecystographic Agents 107
References 114

CHAPTER 2

Urographic Contrast Media and Methods of Investigative Uroradiology
K. GOLMAN and T. ALMÉN. With 35 Figures

A. Introduction 127
B. Historical Remarks 128
C. Attenuation of X-Rays 132
   I. Contrast Medium Concentration in Different Regions of the
     Urinary Tract; Factors Influencing the Nephrogram and Pyelogram 133
    1. Effects of Plasma Iodine Concentration 135
    2. Effects of Urine Iodine Concentration 138
  II. Urinary Tract Volume Changes 146
    1. Urine Flow 146
    2. Theoretical Effects of Changes 146
    3. Experimental Effects of Changes 148
D. Pharmacodynamics 149
   I. Intravenous Lethal Dose 149
  II. Causes of Death 151
    1. Lung Edema and Red Blood Cell Changes 151
    2. Nephrotoxicity 153
  III. Other Adverse Reactions 158
  IV. Advantages of Ratio-3 Media 158
E. Methods of Investigative Uroradiology 158
   I. Introduction 158
    1. Choice of Species 159
    2. Anesthesia 159
    3. Surgical Procedures 160
  II. Assays for Contrast Media 160
  III. Methods for the Measurement of the Depth of the X-Ray
     Attenuating Layer 163
    1. Planimetry 163
    2. Urine Flow 164
  IV. Methods for Studying Excretion Mechanisms 166
    1. Clearance of Contrast Media 166
    2. Tubular Micropuncture and Microperfusion 170
    3. Cell Culture 171
   V. Methods for Studying Renal Pharmacodynamics 171
    1. Urine Osmolality 171
    2. Ability to Concentrate Urine 171
    3. Urine Flow 172
    4. Vascular Changes 172
    5. Glomerular Damage 175

6. Tubular Damage 176
References 180

CHAPTER 3

Contrast Media in the Cardiovascular System. C. B. HIGGINS.
With 10 Figures

A. Introduction 193
B. Classification of Cardiovascular Actions of Contrast Media 193
C. Importance of Experimental Conditions 195
   I. Influence of the Experimental Model Used for Studying
     Cardiovascular Effects of Contrast Media 195
   II. Influence of the Site of Injection of Contrast Media 196
D. Specific Effects 199
   I. Electrophysiologic Cardiac Effects 199
     1. Impulse Generation 200
     2. Impulse Conduction 202
     3. Arrhythmias 204
     4. Electrocardiographic Changes 208
   II. Hemodynamic Cardiac Effects 210
     1. Hemodynamic Changes During Contrast Ventriculography . . 210
     2. Use of Contrast Media as a Stress Test in Coronary Artery
       Disease 212
   III. Direct Myocardial Effects 213
     1. Isolated Heart and Isolated Cardiac Tissue 213
     2. Intracoronary Administration in the Intact Heart 216
     3. Effects on Ischemic Myocardium and Failing Myocardium . . 224
     4. Mechanism of Action of Direct Cardiac Effects 224
     5. Clinical Evaluation of Contrast Media Used for Coronary
       Arteriography 227
   IV. Reflex or Neurally Mediated Circulatory Effects 228
     1. Vascular Effects 231
     2. General Circulation and Limb Circulation 231
     3. Renal Circulation 233
     4. Splanchnic Circulation 236
     5. Carotid Circulation 237
     6. Coronary Circulation 238
     7. Microcirculation and Vascular Endothelium 240
E. Summary 243
References 243

CHAPTER 4

Basic Methods of Investigative Cardiovascular Radiology
M. SOVAK and C. B. HIGGINS. With 7 Figures

A. Introduction 253
B. Contrast Media 253
   I. Pharmacological Evaluation of Radiographic Contrast Media . . 254

C. Experimental Cardioradiographic Visualization 259
D. Choice of Experimental Animals 260
    I. Infrahuman Primates 260
    II. Cats. 261
    III. Calves. 261
    IV. Rabbits 261
    V. Pigs. 262
        1. Catheterization: Implantation of Chronic Catheters 263
        2. Acute Catheterization 263
    VI. Dogs 263
E. The Laboratory for Cardiovascular Contrast Media Research 267
F. Cardiovascular Catheterization 272
G. Animal Models of Cardiovascular Pathological States 276
References. 287

CHAPTER 5

Contrast Media for Imaging of the Central Nervous System. M. SOVAK

A. Introduction 295
B. Angiographic Contrast Media in Neuroradiology 296
    I. Current Ionic Contrast Media 297
        1. Cranial Angiography 297
        2. Spinal Cord Angiography 301
    II. Newer Nonionic Monomers and Monovalent Dimer in
        Neurovascular Use 302
C. Intrathecal Contrast Media 304
    I. Intrathecal Visualization 306
    II. New Developments in Intrathecal Contrast Media 320
References. 326

CHAPTER 6

Basic Methods of Investigative Neuroradiology
M. SOVAK. With 1 Figure

A. Introduction 341
B. Anesthesia 341
    I. Premedication 342
    II. Injectable Anesthetics 342
    III. Volatile Anesthetics 344
C. Neurovascular Experimental Methods 344
D. Experimental Methods for the Subarachnoid Space 349
        1. Choice of Animal. 349
        2. Methods of Access to the Subarachnoid Space 350
E. Toxicity Screening of Experimental Compounds 355
        1. Aversion Conditioning 355
        2. Electrophysiological Methods 356
References. 361

CHAPTER 7

Hepatic Disposition and Elimination of Biliary Contrast Media
J. L. BARNHART. With 25 Figures

A. Introduction 367
B. Anatomic Considerations 367
    I. Liver Anatomy 367
    II. Liver Blood Flow 367
    III. Classic Liver Lobule 368
    IV. Hepatic Cellular Anatomy 368
    V. Gallbladder Anatomy 373
C. Biliary Physiology 374
    I. Composition of Bile 374
    II. Bile Formation 376
        1. Canalicular Bile Flow 376
        2. Ductular Bile Flow 378
    III. Hepatocyte Cytoskeleton and Bile Flow 379
D. Pharmacokinetic Principles 380
E. Cholecystographic and Cholangiographic Contrast Media . . 383
    I. Physicochemical Properties 384
    II. Intestinal Absorption 387
    III. Transport in Blood 391
    IV. First-Pass Effect 391
    V. Hepatic Uptake 392
    VI. Biotransformation 393
    VII. Biliary Excretion 394
F. Concentration of Contrast Media 398
    I. Choleresis 398
    II. Biliary Concentration 400
    III. Electrolyte Composition 402
G. Gallbladder Function 403
H. Enterohepatic Circulation 404
J. Renal Excretion 405
K. Toxicity 406
L. Future for Biliary Contrast Media 407
References 408

CHAPTER 8

Laboratory Techniques for Studying Biliary Contrast Media
J. L. BARNHART. With 28 Figures

A. Introduction 419
B. Choice of Animal Species 420
C. Anesthesia 424
D. Holding and Restraint 426
E. Administration of Anesthetic 428
F. Cannulation of Veins 431

G. In Vivo Animal Preparation 434
H. In Vitro Liver Preparations 442
J. Instrumental Methods of Analysis 451
    I. Spectrophotometer 451
    II. Fluorescent Excitation Analysis 452
    III. Chromatographic Analysis 454
K. Methods of Analysis 456
    I. Bilirubin 456
    II. Iodine (Chemical) 457
    III. Bile Salts 458
    IV. Protein 459
References 460

CHAPTER 9

Contrast Media in Lymphography. M. SOVAK

A. Introduction 463
B. Methods of Lymphography 464
C. Physiology and Pharmacology of Lymphokinetics 466
D. Animal Models in Investigative Lymphangiology 470
E. Experimental Contrast Media for Lymphography 471
References 473

CHAPTER 10

Contrast Media in Computed Tomography. P. B. DEAN and D. B. PLEWES.
With 20 Figures

A. Introduction 479
B. Basic Aspects of Computed Tomography Relevant to Contrast
   Enhancement 479
C. Measurement of Contrast Enhancement with Computed Tomography 482
    I. Contrast Enhancement from Iodine 482
    II. Contrast Enhancement from Other High Atomic Number
       Absorbers 484
D. Image Manipulation 485
    I. Subtraction 486
    II. Multiple Energy Methods 486
    III. High Atomic Number Absorbers and Dual-Energy Computed
       Tomography 490
E. Dynamic Scanning 492
    I. Conventional Computed Tomography Equipment 492
    II. Artifacts 493
    III. Very High Speed Scanners 496
F. Pharmacokinetics of Contrast Enhancement 497
    I. Body Compartments 497
    II. Diffusion of Contrast Media 497
    III. Nonequilibrium Kinetics 499
    IV. Dynamic Aspects of Contrast Enhancement 499

    V. Dynamic Computed Tomography 500
   VI. Functional Imaging 506
  VII. Distribution Volume 506
 VIII. Adverse Effects of Contrast Media in Computed Tomography 507
   IX. Intraarterial Contrast Media Administration 507
    X. Intracavitary Contrast Enhancement 507
   XI. Noble Gases 508
  XII. Reticuloendothelial System Contrast Enhancement 508
G. Practical Applications of Contrast Enhancement 508
    I. To Enhance or Not To Enhance? 508
   II. Basic Problems of Contrast Enhancement 509
  III. Contrast Enhancement in Cranial Computed Tomography . . 509
      1. Detection of Lesions 510
      2. Differentiation of Cranial Lesions with CT Contrast
         Enhancement 510
      3. Xenon Enhancement 511
   IV. Contrast Enhancement in Body Computed Tomography . . . 511
      1. Maximizing Enhancement 511
      2. Cardiac Computed Tomography 512
      3. Chest, Lung, and Mediastinal Computed Tomography . . . 513
      4. Hepatic and Splenic Computed Tomography 513
      5. Pancreatic Computed Tomography 513
      6. Renal and Adrenal Computed Tomography 514
      7. Computed Tomography of Abdominal Blood Vessels . . . 514
      8. Computed Tomography of the Pelvic Organs 514
      9. Intracavitary Enhancement 514
    V. Choice of Intravascular Contrast Medium 514
References 515

CHAPTER 11

Adverse Systemic Reactions to Contrast Media. E. C. Lasser.
With 1 Figure

A. General Considerations 525
B. Pathogenesis 526
C. Pretesting 529
References 530

CHAPTER 12

Are Contrast Media Mutagenic? J. A. Nelson. With 5 Figures

A. Introduction 533
B. Methods 534
C. Results 536
D. Discussion 540
References 541

CHAPTER 13

Particulate Suspensions as Contrast Media.
M. R. VIOLANTE and H. W. FISCHER. With 10 Figures

A. Introduction 543
    I. Definition and Scope 544
B. Particulate Contrast Media 544
    I. Formulation 544
    II. Interactions with Blood Components 556
    III. Phagocytosis 550
        1. Reticuloendothelial System-Species Differences 550
        2. Particle Size 552
        3. Particle Surface Charge 552
        4. Dose 554
        5. Reticuloendothelial System Blockade 556
C. Emulsions 558
D. Computed Tomography Enhancement 560
E. Other Potential Applications 568
    I. Lymphography 568
    II. Angiography 569
References 571

CHAPTER 14

Appendix: Basics of Anesthesia for Experimental Animals. M. SOVAK

A. Introduction 577
B. Anesthesia for Cardiovascular Experiments 577
C. Intravenous Anesthesia 580
    I. Barbiturates 580
    II. Chloralose 581
    III. Urethane 581
    IV. Chloral Hydrate 581
    V. Ketamine HCl 582
D. Volatile Anesthetics 582
E. Short-term Reversible Hypotension 583
F. Blood Transfusion 583
G. Euthanasia 583
    I. Anesthesia in Dogs 584
    II. Anesthesia in Pigs 584
    III. Anesthesia in Rabbits 585
References 586

Subject Index 589

Introduction: State of the Art and Design Principles of Contrast Media

M. SOVAK

The concept of contrast media (CM) emerged shortly after Roentgen's discovery. A large number of radiopaque compounds were tested in vivo; of these, only barium sulfate has survived to the present day, while many simple organic and inorganic compounds were soon abandoned after their high toxicity became obvious. The quest for a safe CM followed a tortuous path which began by trial and error. Later, as the correlation between drug toxicity and structure became better understood, development proceeded by working toward a rational design. The historical events surrounding the development of the first clinically usable urographic CM have been discussed in an excellent review [1].

The first CM emerged as by-products of large-scale programs of industrial chemical synthesis. It was only later, when their diagnostic value and toxicity manifestations became recognized, that rational design of CM became an intellectual game played by both chemists and physicians. Unlike most other drugs, a unique relationship with radiology guaranted CM the undivided attention of an entire medical specialty. The CM toxicity mechanisms were gradually elucidated also by interdisciplinary efforts, first at the physiological and morphological, and later at molecular, levels.

Development of CM chemistry and pharmacology from their inception until the late 1960s has been well reviewed in two volumes assembled by KNOEFEL, and published in the *International Encyclopedia of Pharmacology and Therapeutics* in 1971 [2]. The purpose of this volume is to review events since 1971 and, at the same time, provide a compendium of basic methodology and physiological aspects of investigative work with CM. Certain CM, or areas of CM applications, have been purposely omitted either because of stagnating or disappearing use, or because they have been reviewed extensively in other publications. Thus, methodology of arthrography, hysterosalpingography, and bronchography, and use of CM in gastrointestinal radiology have been thoroughly dealt with by MILLER and SKUCAS in *Radiographic Contrast Agents* [3]. Other important publications are *Contrast Media in Radiology* by AMIEL [4] and the very recent containing comparative studies of the latest nonionic and ionic media edited by TAENZER and ZEITLER [5].

The emphasis of this volume is on the experimental aspects of CM development. Therefore, only a section of the most relevant and/or illustrative clinical literature has been included. Also, to make the text more readable, cited literature is referenced not by name but by numbers only, and the formulas of the various compounds discussed throughout the entire volume are shown only in this "Introduction" and in Chap. 1.

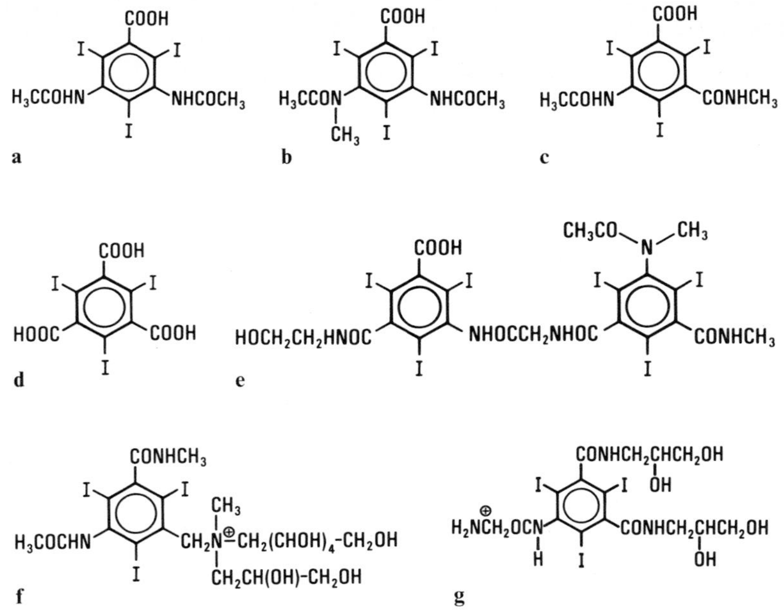

Fig. 1 a–g. Ionic media:
1. Radiopaque anions, monomeric, monovalent: **a** diatrizoic acid (Schering AG, Sterling-Winthrop, Squibb); **b** metrizoic acid (Nyegaard); **c** iothalamic acid (Mallinckrodt) (derivatives obtained by variation of the C-3 position: ioxithalamic acid [with –CONHCH₂CH₂OH (Guerbet)], ioglycic acid [with –CONHCH₂CONHCH₃ (Schering AG)]
2. Radiopaque anions, monomeric, trivalent: **d** trimesic acid (precursor for nonionic nd ionic CM) (Schering AG)
3. Radiopaque anions, dimeric, monovalent: **e** ioxaglic acid (Guerbet)
4. Radiopaque cations, monomeric, monovalent: **f** cp 11 (Sovak et al.); **g** cp III (Schering AG)

Until the late 1960s, the ionic character of iodobenzene derivatives was accepted as an immutable state of the art. Only minor toxicity improvements were achieved by oligomerization of the ionic monomers and/or by introduction of more hydrophilic substituents into the basic moieties. There is some justification to what, in retrospect, appears as stagnation. In spite of their numerous vices, ionic triiodo monomeric salts of diatrizoic, metrizoic, iothalamic, ioglucinic, ioxithalamic, and similar acids (Fig. 1 a–c) have a remarkably low toxicity for drugs which are delivered in large quantities at rapid rates. It is therefore understandable that the clinical community has found these compounds almost acceptable for most applications, and certainly acceptable economically.

A truly quantitative leap forward was made with the nonionic, water-soluble contrast medium, metrizamide (Fig. 2a), developed by Almen working with Nyegaard Co., Oslo, Norway. This feat demonstrated that the inherent toxicity of triiodinated benzene can be decreased dramatically, and it gave birth to a new generation of CM. In designing new compounds, the basic concept of metrizamide has been followed by both academia and industry, with researchers striving for transposition of the theoretical drug structure-activity relationships into the practice of chemical synthesis and pharmaceutics.

Efforts to develop an even better CM than metrizamide, of improved toxicity and cost, have led to a number of so-called second-generation compounds, some of which are currently being introduced into clinical practice. Undoubtedly, further improvements will be attempted. Therefore, it seems appropriate to review whatever cues we have to the solution of the often enigmatic relationship between the molecular structure of CM and their biological effects.

What is the present state of the art, and what remains to be done? The current CM make opacification of practically any vascular and parenchymatic structure possible, and they have a relatively low toxicity. Nevertheless, further improvements are desirable. The current nonionic monomers cause patient discomfort in a number of applications, and occasionally they induce more serious side effects [6]. With the large i.v. dose of these media needed for contrast enhancement in fast proliferating computed tomography (CT), the absolute numbers of patients suffering from side effects of current CM also tend to increase. Yet, these problems should be carefully balanced in clinical practice against the benefits of the current CM whenever they are suspected of being more harmful than they actually are; Nelson's chapter in this volume (Chap. 13) addresses the question of alleged CM teratogenicity.

In contrast to angiographic and urographic use, the incidence of side effects of ionic CM in the intrathecal space has been much higher. In this respect, nonionic CM have made a major contribution to the safety of the neuroradiologist's patient. The dramatic decrease of epileptogenicity and chronic inflammatory reactions in both the central nervous tissue and its envelopes makes the nonionic CM not only qualitatively superior to the ionic CM, but also to the oily opaque substances. Most of one chapter (Chap. 5, Sect. C) has been dedicated to the description of these developments.

Cholecystographic media occupy a firm place in the radiodiagnostic process. Cholecystography remains a well-established procedure, which, however, could be ameliorated by using less toxic CM with the ultimate goal of opacifying the bile excretory pathways with an oral agent.

There are a number of physiological safeguards which limit more efficient transport of cholecystographic CM from blood to bile. The complexity of the hepatic physiology and its impact on future developments of cholecystography is a subject of Barnhardt's chapters (Chaps. 7, 8).

Opacification of the liver and spleen parenchyma has been achieved by a number of compounds used in conjunction with CT. Some i.v. water-soluble CM binding strongly to the proteins have shown promise, as well as iodinated oil emulsions and particulate CM which are entrapped by the RES of the liver and spleen. Such CM nevertheless are biologically active.

Although CT and the fast-improving digital radiography have made great contributions toward parenchymal visualization of a number of organs and their pathological states, the search continues for an organ-specific CM. Intravenous agents which would selectively depict pancreatic, myocardial, and central nervous structures, and perhaps reflect the metabolic state of the tissues as well as altered morphology, would be a boon to radiology. So far, only isotope techniques with their inherently low resolution have had some success in this regard, the greatest promise being shown by nuclear magnetic resonance (NMR).

The search for identification of the causes of CM toxicity has been an important theme in radiology research, which, after a long period of descriptive and documental work, is on the verge of elucidating the mechanisms of adverse reactions to CM. It became obvious that adverse reactions cannot be attributed to a single cause but rather to a composite of immunological, cardiovascular, and neurological perturbances. The complexity of the mechanisms behind the adverse reactions is a subject of Lasser's chapter (Chap. 11).

If carefully looked at, CM can be shown to interfere virtually with any physiological system, given sufficient time, dose, and setting. Behind each of the altered physiological parameters measured in the laboratory is a long chain of causes and effects, intertwined and retrolinked by feedback loops and amplification systems. Many segments of this labyrinth have been researched and many conjunctions identified, but what appears to be the very initiating factor of the adverse reactions is the capacity of CM to damage the body cells mechanically by the osmotic strength of their solution and/or, at the molecular level, to perturb the functions of the biomacromolecules.

In all areas of radiology, the common denominator of an ideal CM should be complete biological inertness. In addition to the search for an organ-specific CM, further development in the field should consider biological inertness a primary goal and take into consideration the requirements of physicochemical stability and economical feasibility. In this respect, the new generations of nonionic CM represent an important achievement not only of pharmacology, but especially of chemical synthesis. This is because most demands on an ideal compound seem mutually exclusive: nonionicity and water solubility; high hydrophilicity and high iodine content; and low osmolality and low viscosity. In the following, we will consider relationships between the molecular structure and its physical and biological effects.

1. Hypertonicity. For clinical usefulness, solutions of CM must have a certain concentration which is proportional to their iodine content. The current ionic monomers must be so highly concentrated that the osmolality of their solutions is six to seven times higher than that of the body milieu. When a hyperosmolal solution is injected intravenously, blood is drawn from the cells. By this mechanism, the exposed endothelial cells are irreversibly damaged and new endothelial cells grow into their place. In normal vessels, such repair is accomplished rapidly. Since the junctions between the endothelial cells are often the main site of the so-called barriers protecting various organs, a barrier breakdown potentiates the chemotoxicity of the injected compound.

Hypertonic CM solutions deform the erythrocytes and thus affect the blood rheology. Hyperosmolality activates the baroreceptors in the heart and the great vessels, leading to a sequence of reflectoric responses resulting in cardiovascular disturbances. These aspects are considered in more detail in several chapters.

Osmolality of an aqueous solution is proportional to the number of the dissolved particles. The higher the number of particles, the higher the osmotic pressure of the solution. If osmotic pressure of CM is to be reduced, the number of solvated particles must be smaller while the iodine content must remain the same. There are a number of ways to achieve this goal: first, we shall consider the possibility of CM consisting of microparticles suspended in a water carrier.

The remarkable lack of acute toxicity of one of the first CM, Thorotrast, was largely attributable to both the osmotic and chemical inertness of that compound. Had it not been for its lack of biodegradability which led to the compound being entrapped in the reticuloendothelial system, and were it not for its radioactivity, Thorotrast would have possibly survived to the present.

As an alternative to Thorotrast, a colloidal preparation of tin oxide has been tested experimentally [7]. This material was also rapidly taken up by the liver and spleen. Other inorganic colloids, based on rare earth oxides were also tested [8]. The latter materials, while being extremely expensive, showed no substantial difference from the previously tested inorganic colloids. The subject lay dormant for many years, but with the increasing availability of newer methods, digital radiography, dynamic CT, and scanned projection radiography, it became apparent that a particulate CM would not only have the toxicological advantage of decreasing the solution osmolality drastically, but by remaining in the blood pool, i.e., in the vascular compartment, it would reduce the dose and extend the diagnostic information. Current ionic or nonionic monomers leak from the capillary bed readily into the interstitium of the overlying tissues, which degrades the image contrast. Because of the rapid diffusion, the duration of contrast enhancement is limited. To compensate, large amounts of CM must be injected, with a concomitant increase in the frequency of adverse reactions. These aspects of CM use are discussed in Dean's chapter (Chap. 10). A truly inert blood pool CM would probably increase the diagnostic capabilities of the newer imaging techniques in detection and differential diagnosis of tumors, and might perhaps assist the often frustrating task of finding the source of intermittent gastrointestinal bleeding. The vascular imaging, too, could attain new dimensions as well as the visualization of parenchyma of a number of organs. A blood pool CM would further eliminate the interference of the extravascular opacity in digital angiography.

To that end, a number of nonbiodegradable colloids have been tested. Long polymers of the ionic CM were synthesized but the toxicity and viscosity of these CM were too high and, in many cases, water solubility was too low. Theoretically, a blood pool CM based on a water-soluble, nontoxic molecule large enough to remain in the vascular bed could be synthesized and, even if the problem of high viscosity could be overcome, the molecules would have to be engineered to become rapidly biodegradable in order to be excreted.

The concept was further tested using partially soluble organic microparticles of iodine-bearing molecules [9]. These developments are described in detail in the chapter by Violante and Fischer (Chap. 13). Another approach is based on iodinating starch particles [10], or using emulsion of iodinated oils [11]. As the iodinated oils are also rapidly removed from the circulation by the reticuloendothelial system, the medium was explored in clinical trials as an intravenous liposoluble CM for CT of the liver and spleen [12]. It can be expected that, also in the future, efforts to develop a safe blood pool agent will inadvertently result in CM with hepatolienographic potential.

An alternative way toward a truly inert particulate CM which would not be rapidly filtered from the blood pool could be to encapsulate water-soluble CM into liposomes. This approach has been explored using the currently available liposomic materials [11, 13, 14]. Such liposomes, nevertheless, are thermodynamically unstable and the instability is further potentiated by the hyperosmolality of the encapsulated water-soluble CM. As a result, liposomes cannot be sterilized by industrially acceptable means and, furthermore, their life "on the shelf" and in circulation is impractically short. Some improvement has been achieved with brominated liposomes. Attempts have been made to polymerize the liposomic layers for the purpose of a more predictable drug delivery, but such polymers lacked biodegradability. Furthermore, the surface of current liposomes is relatively hydrophobic when in the blood milieu and, as a result, liposomes are rapidly removed by the reticuloendothelial system, especially of the liver and spleen. Hopefully, future developments will bring liposomic materials which will be truly inert and biodegradable. This could be accomplished with highly hydrophilic surfaces and polymerization with biodegradable links. Indeed, liposomes coated with a hydrophilic protein were shown to be less prone to be retained by the macrophages than the uncoated lipophilic liposomes [16]. One can further envision that the stability of such liposomes would be enhanced if they incorporated water-soluble CM of high iodine content, but of low osmolality.

If truly stable and inert microparticles could be developed, not only radiographic CM but also inert gases could be encapsulated to yield CM for imaging with ultrasound technology. Microparticles of standardized diameter, made of gelatin, have been shown to be useful in microvascular imaging with ultrasound. This work supported the concept of echogenic CM, useful not only in the diagnosis of pathological morphology, but also in the measurement of hemodynamic parameters [17]. Recently, emulsions of various perfluorocarbons were shown to be echogenic in an experimental lapine hepatic tumor [18].

Other alternatives for reduction of osmolality of water-soluble CM can be considered. One way of diminishing the number of solvated particles in water, and thus reducing osmotic pressure, would be to make every such particle contain iodine. Theoretically, this could be accomplished by combining the tri- or hexaiodinated anions with radiopaque cations by nonionic monomers or nonionic oligomers, or by anionic molecules containing at least six iodines and only one carboxyl group.

A number of radiopaque cations have been synthesized and tested, but found to have low tolerance (Fig. 1f) [19]. Recently, new biologically acceptable radiopaque cations were reported (Fig. 1g) With the current ionic monomeric or dimeric anions, the new cations form salts of low viscosity and low osmolality [20].

Another way of reducing osmolality is to increase the iodine content of a single anion. This has been accomplished in the synthesis of hexaiodinated compounds carrying one charge. A number of monovalent dimers have been synthesized and the concept thoroughly researched at the Guerbet Laboratories, culminating in the development of sodium meglumine salts of ioxaglic acid (Hexabrix) (Fig. 1e) (see Chaps. 1, 4). The osmolality of Hexabrix is about one-half that of the ionic monomers, but its hydrophobicity is similar. Since vascular pain has been shown to correlate with hyperosmolality [21, 22], Hexabrix has found its primary application in angiography. It has been shown previously that vascular pain can, at least to some extent, be mitigated with intraarterial anesthetics [23, 24], but direct clinical comparison of sodium meglumine ioxaglate with meglumine diatrizoate has shown that with no anesthetic Hexabrix elicited no pain [25, 26]. One study found that Hexabrix produced less heat sensation than iopamidol in cerebral angiography [27]. Hexabrix is formulated as a 19.65 w/v sodium and 39.3 w/v meglumine ioxaglate mixture. This is considerably less than in conventional ionic monomers, in which excessive sodium load presented problems in renal, hepatic, or congestive cardiac failures and in infants [28].

Substantial reduction of osmolality can be achieved with nonionic compounds, i.e., molecules which, although without charge, are water soluble per se and thus do not require formulation as salts. When compared with ionic monomers of approximately the same iodine content, for the same osmotic pressure, twice the number of molecules of a nonionic monomer would theoretically be needed. In practice, however, nonionic molecules transiently aggregate in solution, forming larger particles. Inasmuch as solution osmolality is determined by the number of particles in solution, such aggregation decreases the solution's tonicity beyond the value theoretically expected on the basis of the chemical formula. In metrizamide, which is solubilized by a covalently attached sugar moiety, the sugar's hydroxyl groups avidly form hydrogen bonds not only with water, but also with each other. The conceptual analog of metrizamide, the reverse amide Ioglunide (Fig. 2 b) (Guerbet Labs), also forms solutions of low osmolality. Compounds of the second generation of nonionic monomers aggregate to a lesser degree since, instead of sugar residues, aminoalkanols such as serinol in iopamidol (Fig. 2 c), aminopropanediol in iohexol (Fig. 2 d), iopromide (Fig. 2 e), MP-328 (Fig. 2 g), and JI-1 (Fig. 2 h), or aminotetritols in VA-7-88 (Fig. 2 i) or ZK 38593 (Fig. 2 j) are utilized. Consequently, for the same iodine content, osmolality of these CM is higher than that of metrizamide or ioglunide.

At present, three nonionic monomers are in incipient clinical use: iopamidol, iohexol, and iopromide. The development of iopamidol resulted from totally novel chemistry introduced by Felder and Pitrè (for details see Chap. 1). Not only did these authors demonstrate that small aminoalcohols can replace sugar in a nonionic triiodinated moiety, they also showed that the water solubility of such molecules can often depend on the isomerism of the substituent [29, 50].

Iohexol is one of the numerous compounds synthesized by Nyegaard Co., in an effort to replace the relatively expensive aminoalkanol serinol used in iopamidol with the cheaper 2,3-aminopropanediol (aminoglycerol). (References to preclinical and clinical testing of iohexol can be found throughout this volume.)

Development of iopromide by Schering AG [30] took the chemistry of the aminoglycerol-based compounds one step further. N-methylated aminoalcohol was introduced in an effort to further water solubility while utilizing a low molecular weight substituent, methoxyacetic acid, at the C-5 position. Compared with iohexol, this strategy resulted in a slight decrease in hydrophilicity, while the osmolality of iopromide is lower (Table 1). The pharmacokinetic profile of iopromide indicates considerable similarity to the other nonionic monomers [5, 31]. The first clinical experience has also been reported, indicating systemic toxicity similar to the other nonionic contrast media, except that pain in angiography oc-

Abb. 2 a—j

Table 1. Basic properties of newer contrast materials

	Mol. wt.	%I	Osmolality at 37 °C, 300 mg I/ml (mOsm/kg)	Viscosity at 37 °C, 300 mg I/ml (cps)	i.v. LD_{50} mice (g I/kg)	i.v. LD_{50} rats (g I/kg)	Hydrophilicity (relative activity I_{50} of serum complement activation) (mg I/ml)
Metrizamide	789	48.2	485	6.2	17.5–18.7 12–13 [a,b] 12.1 [a]	12.1(m) 10.9(f) 10.3 [a] 13 [a]	95 [a], 101 [a]
Iohexol	821	46.4	690	6.1	23.4(m) 25.1(f) 16–18 [a] 16.5–19.5 [b]	12.3(f) 15(m) 11.5–12.1 [b]	245 [a] (95)
Iopamidol	777	49.0	619	4.5	21.8 16.4(12.1) [a] 17–20 [b]	13.8 11.3(10.3) [a]	233 [a](95)
Iopromide	791	48.1	607	4.8	16.5(12.1)	11.4(10.3) 12.9(13)	176 [a](101)
MP-328	807	47.2	716	8.7	20	–	–
Iodecol	1,565.4	48.6	320	7.2	14	38	
Iogulamide	881.4	43.2	1,040 [c]	9.6	19.5	18	–
Ioglunide	807	47.2					
Iotrol	1,626	46.8	300	9.1	26–29(12.8)	12.7(9.6)	447(95)
Iotasul	1,608	100.0	Extra low	~24.0	>14 [d]	>11 [d]	
Hexabrix [e] (Sodium meglumine, 1:2 salt of ioxaglic acid)	1,269	60.0	600	7.5			

All data are from the laboratories of origin except where indicated. CM authors: metrizamide, iohexol, Nyegaard Co.; iopamidol, Bracco Ind. Chem. SA; Iopromide, Iodecol, Iotasul, Schering AG; MP-328, Iogulamide, Mallinckrodt Inc.; Hexabrix, Ioglunide, Guerbet Lab.; iotrol, University of California, San Diego Numbers in parentheses are values for metrizamide when used in the same experiment as a control. All i.v. LD_{50} data are based on a 1:1 male/female ratio except where indicated; (m) male; (f) female. Other data for a concentration of 320 mg I/ml

[a] Data from Schering AG
[b] Data from University of California, San Diego
[c] At 25 °C
[d] Intracutaneous. At these doses, no mortality was observed
[e] Mol.-wt. and %I for ioxaglic acid only

Fig. 2 a–j. Nonionic monomers (triiodinated compounds):
1. In clinical use/testing: **a** metrizamide (Nyegaard/Sterling Winthrop); **b** ioglunide (Guerbet); **c** iopamidol (Bracco/Squibb); **d** iohexol (Nyegaard/Sterling Winthrop); **e** iopromide (Schering AG); **f** iogulamide (Mallinckrodt)
2. Nonionic compounds in development: **g** MP-328 (Mallinckrodt); **h** JI-1 (Sovak, Ranganathan); **i** VA-7-88 (Sovak, Ranganathan); **j** ZK 38593 (Schering AG/Sovak, Ranganathan)

curs with a lesser frequency than with iohexol, and similar to iopamidol [5]. From clinical studies comparing the new nonionic agents and on the basis of preclinical experience, it is possible to conclude tentatively that systemic toxicity of the nonionic monomers iopamidol, iohexol, and iopromide is very close and similar to that of metrizamide, and clearly superior to that of ionic agents including ioxaglate. The only clinically significant difference appears to be vascular pain. While arteriography with ioxaglate, iopamidol, and, to a greater extent, iopromide, is virtually painless, higher frequency of pain has been reported with iohexol [32–39]. It has been shown previously that vascular pain is attributable not to hydrophobicity, but primarily to osmolality of CM solutions [40]. A review of the first clinical experience suggests that the critical pain threshold in arteriography lies approximately between 650 and 800 mOsm, in most patients.

Iopamidol and iohexol are also being considered for myelography; the toxicity of these agents in the intrathecal space is reviewed in Chap. 5, Sect. C.

Nephrotoxicity of all current CM is dealt with by GOLMAN and ALMEN in Chapt. 2. One of the most important aspects of contrast media toxicity, anaphylactoid reactions, has previously been reported to be greatly reduced with metrizamide. Although the numbers of preclinical studies at this time are too small to permit a final conclusion, there are many indications that the rate of such reactions will be considerably lower and perhaps eliminated altogether with the highly hydrophilic, nonionic media [5, 32, 41].

To reduce the osmolality of the nonionic monomers further, investigators have tried to condense them into oligomers. Any oligomers larger than dimers would, however, increase viscosity to intolerable levels, and the compounds would form solutions of osmolality lower than that of body fluid. Research, therefore, has concentrated on synthesis of hexaiodinated larger molecules containing two benzene rings. Such a structure, popularly called a "dimer", is a chemical misnomer; however, inasmuch as the expression "dimer" has attained a colloquial level, it will be employed in this text. Experimental, nonionic dimers were explored by several investigators, but so far only three compounds have been developed [E. FELDER and D. PITRE 1982, personal communication; 42–46].

Iotasul (Schering AG) (Fig. 3 a) is a dimer containing sulfur in the bridge, aggregating to a high degree and thus transiently forming high molecular particles, giving solutions of extremely low osmolality. In the milieu of body fluid, this dimer forms two-phase solutions, a property which makes it useful for indirect lymphography (Chap. 9).

Iodecol (Fig. 3 b), a dimer using a short (malonyl) bridge, contains ten hydroxyls and has low osmolality (Table 1). In a 10-ml dose of 350 mg I/ml, it has been shown to induce fewer spasms in the intracranial arteries following vertebral angiography in rabbits than the nonionic monomers iopromide and iopamidol. Although in this study the toxicity of iodecol was greater, the author concluded that this could have been attributable to the minimal effect of iodecol on the intracranial vessels. In contrast to iodecol, the nonionic monomers were shown to induce vasospasm, resulting in shunting some CM away from the cerebral into the extracranial arteries [47].

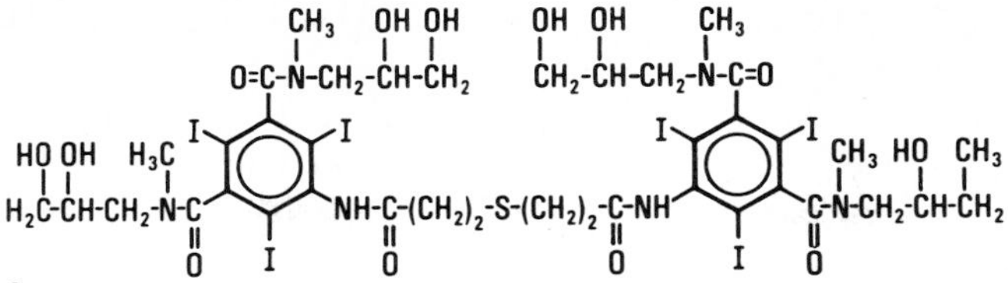

Fig. 3 a–c. Nonionic "dimers" (hexaiodinated compounds): **a** iotasul (Schering AG); **b** iodecol (Schering AG); **c** iotrol (Sovak, Ranganathan/Schering AG)

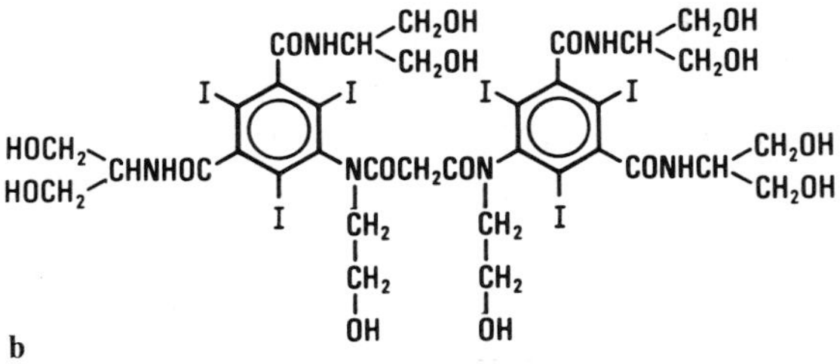

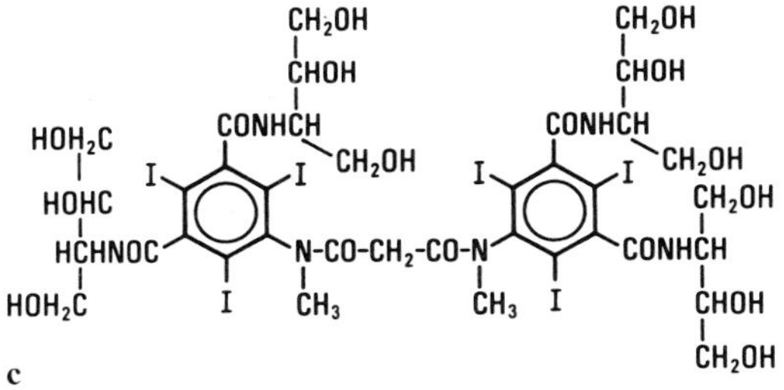

A nonionic dimer, iotrol (M. SOVAK and R. RANGANATHAN) (Fig. 3c), with twelve hydroxyls, is the most hydrophilic CM known. It makes stable solutions and has an osmolality equal to the body milieu at 300 mg I/ml. This CM contains new substituents, D,L-aminothreitol, which confer on the molecule not only high water solubility, but also exceptionally low systemic and neural toxicity. Iotrol is currently being clinically introduced as a myelographic CM (Chap. 5, Sect. C).

Because of its isotonicity with synovial fluid, as recent arthrographic studies indicate, iotrol does not rapidly dilute and degrade radiographic detail as the hypertonic CM all do [48].

The dimers which form solutions of low osmolality are consequently slowly excreted by the kidneys. It is imperative therefore that such compounds, to be useful as angiographic agents, must have low renal toxicity. In this conjunction, a very important observation has been reported recently: certain nonionic dimers, which show extremely slow renal excretion in mice, rats, and rabbits, and consequently considerable renal toxicity, have been found to be excreted rapidly in nonhuman primates [49]. It is conceivable that rapid renal excretion of compounds of low osmolality could also be achieved by incorporating a potentially ionic group into the molecule.

There is one obvious limit to the polymeric concept of nonionic CM. With higher molecular size and larger and more branched molecules, viscosity increases dramatically. A potential area for exploration is the design of a polyiodo molecule of approximately globular form.

2. Water Solubility. Water solubility of CM is relatively easy to achieve in ionic compounds. At biological pH levels, salts of triiodobenzoic acid derivatives are generally water soluble thanks to the ionic group. In nonionic compounds, solubility is achieved by covalently attaching hydrophilic substituents to the iodinated aromatic moiety. Such substituents contain hydroxyl groups. Under six and beyond seven hydroxyls per triiodinated benzene ring, the degree of hydrophilicity does not necessarily parallel solubility. Water solubility is a largely unpredictable interplay of molecular steric conditions and hydrogen-bonding capabilities which determine the degree of molecule integration into the molecular network of water. Hydroxyls and amides increase water solubility. Other solubility-promoting factors are optical isomerism and asymmetricity which, by inducing entropy through nonuniformity, usually prevent coordination of the parent molecule into the lattice of a crystalline structure. Therefore, most isomeric, hydrophilic mixtures prefer the aqueous milieu to the crystalline form. In CM synthesis, only one exception to this rule has been found. While careful studies of optical purity were conducted, an analog of iopamidol containing a racemic mixture of lactic acid was found less water soluble than iopamidol containing the L-enantiomer of the same substituent [50]. The chemical aspects of water solubility are discussed in more detail in Chap. 1.

3. Chemotoxicity. Chemotoxicity is a result of interaction between the molecules of CM and of the biological system. At the molecular level, the nature of CM chemotoxicity has been identified by the pioneering work of LASSER and LANG [51] and LEVITAN and RAPOPORT [52] as binding of CM to the biomacromolecules, resulting in perturbance of their function. Such binding directly interferes with the organization of living matter by disturbing the function of an important organizing factor in living organisms, the so-called hydrophobic effect. Responsible for the three-dimensional structure of complicated molecules and folding of the proteins, the hydrophobic effect makes it possible for the "toxic" segments of important biomacromolecules to avoid interaction with other molecules. In biological systems, the hydrophobic effect is responsible for assembling certain molecular regions by excluding the water rather than by forming polar bonds [53]. The molecules of CM are relatively rigid and are constantly exposing areas of high hydrophobicity; therefore, they bind to the organism's proteins [51]. A compound with a character opposite to hydrophobic is hydrophilic; it is known that toxicity is inversely related to hydrophilicity. A hydrophilic CM extensively forms hydrogen bonds in aqueous solutions. If a part of the compound cannot be fully integrated into the network of the water hydrogen bonds, the intersurface remains unsolvated, i.e., dry and hydrophobic. Once water is excluded from that region, a hydrophobic area capable of biological interaction is formed.

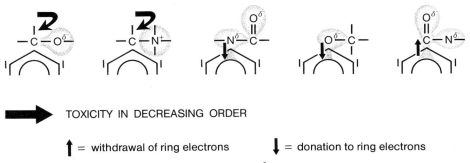

TOXICITY IN DECREASING ORDER

↑ = withdrawal of ring electrons   ↓ = donation to ring electrons

Fig. 4. Effects of various ring substituents on the withdrawal of ring electrons and toxicity of contrast media. The curved arrow indicates areas unable to form hydrogen bonds with water.

An ideal CM should be completely hydrophilic. In practice this is hardly possible to achieve due to the inherently highly hydrophobic character of the iodine atoms. Even in compounds where iodines are masked by hydrophilic substituents, some effects of iodine hydrophobicity must be expected.

The advent of the structure/activity relationship rules discovered by HANSCH [54] promised to put the strategy of drug design on a rational basis. It seemed that CM could be designed with substituting groups which now could be chosen on the basis of their hydrophobicity/philicity determined by partition of model compounds between highly hydrophilic (aqueous) or hydrophobic (oily) milieu. The partition method is but one of a number of ways of measuring the hydrophobic effect in vitro. It is useful only for initial screening of the compounds since it reflects the *total* hydrophobicity of the molecule, in physicochemical terms. Studies of interference with enzyme kinetics in the presence of CM are more relevant for pharmacology, since they reflect effects of any region of the CM molecule [51].

When we examine the structure/effect relationship in a series of CM, a correlation between low toxicity and presence of substituting groups known to withdraw the ring (pi) electrons was found. In a series of model compounds, the toxicity decreased with the presence of substituent groups in the following order: oxymethylene, aminomethylene, carboxamido, alkoxy, carbamoyl (Fig. 4) [55]. The reduction to practice of the second generation of nonionic monomers has vindicated this observation. Amides, either as carboxamides ($-N-\overset{\overset{O}{\|}}{C}-O$) or carbamoyls ($-\overset{\overset{O}{\|}}{C}-N-$) proved to be the most useful linkages due to their stability and high capacity to form transient bonds with hydrogens of the aqueous milieu. As for the second point, concerning the detoxification of the benzene ring by pi electron withdrawal, the least toxic compound was expected to contain several carboxyls. This expectation has been confirmed by GRIES, who synthesized triiodotrimesic acid (Fig. 1 d) and a number of its derivatives. When experimental ionic CM, derived from triiodotrimesic acids, were compared with their analogs based on triiodoiothalamic and diatrizoic acids, decreasing toxicity in that order was found

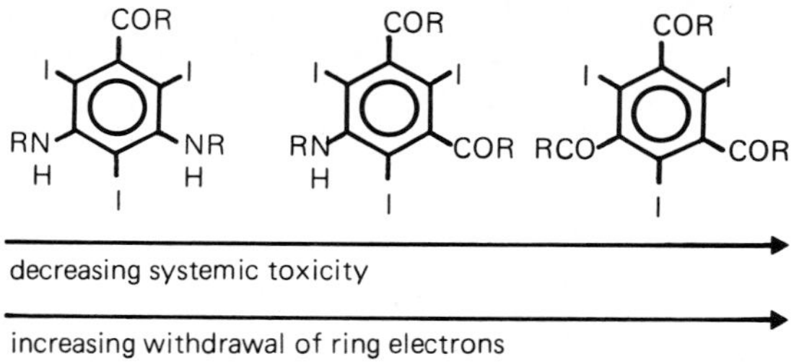

decreasing systemic toxicity

increasing withdrawal of ring electrons

Fig. 5. Toxicity-structure relationship of various triiodobenzene derivatives

(Fig. 5) [56]. Even better evidence for the validity of the pi electron withdrawal theory was provided when the experimental trimesic-based compound, ZK 38593 (Schering AG) (Fig. 2j), was compared with its isophthalic analog, VA-7-88 (Sovak and Ranganathan) (Fig. 2i). The murine i.v. LD_{50} of the former indicated a tolerance about 40% better than that of the latter; both compounds were found, in the same experiment, toxicologically superior to iohexol, iopamidol, and metrizamide.

The new nonionic compounds have confirmed that the hydrophilic character of the substituents and their even distribution on the ring are prerequisites for low chemotoxicity. This point of the design theory can, however, be extended to include the importance of steric conformations of the substituents inasmuch as their significance seems to exceed the previously considered viscosity. The less globular a shape a particle has, independent of its size, the more viscous a solution it is likely to form [57]. When molecular models of iohexol and iopamidol are compared (Figs. 6, 7), it is obvious that the 2,3-aminopropanediol residue in the former protrudes to a greater extent beyond the average molecular parameter than the serinol residue in the latter (Fig. 7). This may explain in part why iohexol is more viscous than iopamidol (Table 1). One additional factor which can be gleaned from these models is the "crowding effect", i.e., masking of the iodines by the substituents. It can be seen from the model of iotrol (Fig. 8) that the substituents containing three OH groups (as D,L-aminothreitols) mask the iodines to a greater extent than the two-hydroxyl-containing propanediols. It can also be seen that masking of iodines is affected by alkylation of carbamoyls or carboxamides. In iohexol, the 5-position is occupied by an alkylated carboxamide $(CH_3-CO-N-CH_2-CH_2-OH)$, which masks the neighboring iodines to a greater extent than the unsubstituted carbamoyls. An experimental compound, JI-1 (Sovak and Ranganathan) (Figs. 2 h, 9), containing two alkylated carboxamides and one alkylated carbamoyl, has shown a high degree of biological tolerance [58, 59], thus demonstrating that the masking effects of iodines can mitigate the lesser pi electron withdrawal by carboxamides than by carbamoyls.

The alkylated substituents should also induce formation of isomeric mixtures which, as mentioned above, should promote water solubility in most cases. The N-alkylation of carbamoyls and carboxamides is but an example of a practical approach to iodine masking, but it should suggest extension of the design theory:

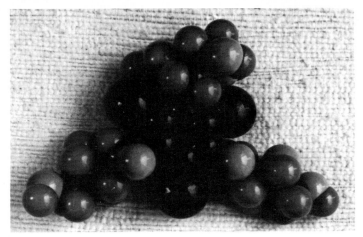

Fig. 6. Molecular model of iohexol

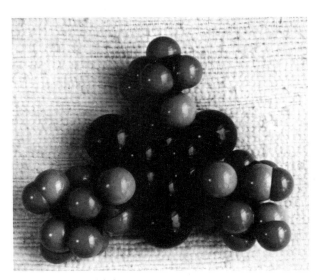

Fig. 7. Molecular model of iopamidol

The substituents should mask iodines sterically; they should be compact, not exceeding the average parameter of the molecule, which should be nearly globular; they should induce isomerism in the substituted, triiodinated moiety.

4. Charge. The presence of charged groups increases the total hydrophilicity of the molecule and its water solubility dramatically, but it also almost invariably increases the toxicity. By disturbing the electrolytic balance and increasing the conductivity of the body fluids, the exogenous ions, by disturbing the ionic milieu,

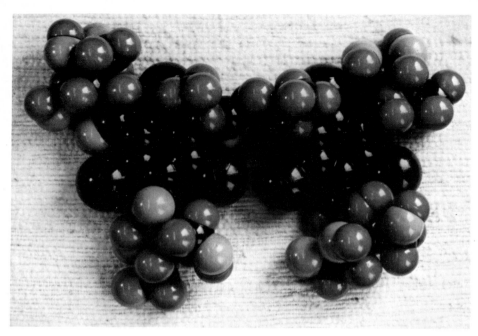

Fig. 8. Molecular model of iotrol

affect the bioprocesses, especially those of the neural tissue. Epileptogenicity encountered with CM brought into contact with neurons by a damaged blood-brain barrier, or via the subarachnoid space, is attributable also to chemotoxicity but it is the charge that plays the predominant role. The rational design of compounds of minimal toxicity must include elimination and/or limitation of charged groups. For myelographic media, nonionicity must be considered indispensable.

5. *Stability.* An extremely important requirement for radiographic CM is stability, i.e., a capability to withstand sterilization by autoclaving. The major drawback of metrizamide is its hydrolytic lability, which necessitates dispensing the compound in lyophilized form and preparing fresh solutions just prior to their use. A systematic investigation of the mechanisms of the decomposition of the first generation of nonionic CM in water found that in metrizamide the sugar residue, although remaining on the ring, rearranges and consequently decomposes, while, in ioglunide, the sugar residue is cleaved off to yield a triiodoaniline moiety [60]. The nonionic compounds containing aminoalcohols attached as amides show no decomposition under the conditions of industrial sterilization. Since the ability to sterilize the final product by autoclaving, rather than ultrafiltration, is a major cost-containing factor, polyhydroxyalkylamides should preferably be used, although they confer less hydrophilicity, molecule for molecule, than the sugars on the triiodinated moiety. Although a way of attaching stable sugars to the ring in a stable fashion could be found [61], economic considerations favor the use of aminoalkanol substitutes.

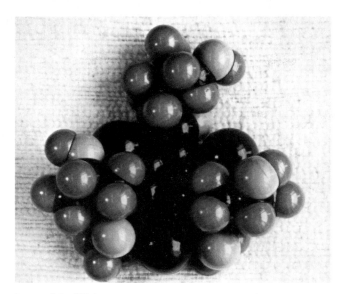

Fig. 9. Molecular model of JI-1

One of the reasons that this book is being published is to stimulate interest in the development of improved CM. In the following, we will consider possible perspectives of such development.

Several times in the past it has been questioned whether some other element besides iodine could be used as a source of opacity. In the late 1950s, cesium, lead, bismuth, and other metals, chelated by complexing agents still in use today, were tested [62–64]. Although acute toxicity of some of the complexes was low, invariably some heavy metal toxicity was encountered. This can be expected to happen since, no matter how high the metal-binding constant is, two disintegrating forces are at play in vivo: competition between the injected and the organism's own metals, as well as chelating systems. Although application of Le Chatelier's principle – injecting an excess of the chelating agents to favor chelate formation – results in nearly quantitative excretion, the concept has failed to provide clinically safe compounds.

Bromine was considered in both early and recent developments. Although stable, aliphatic and aromatic bromine compounds, due to the physical characteristics of the element, would result in unacceptable radiation at maximum opacifying levels.

The opacifying characteristics of iodine, on the other hand, are optimal due to the proximity of K-edge to the average energy levels generated by standard X-ray equipment. The aliphatic iodine compounds are insufficiently stable for CM purposes, but the aromatic carbon-iodine bond withstands even the most adverse conditions in vivo.

With iodine in aromatic structures accepted as fundamental, possibilities of innovations are limited. Unless a radically new concept emerges, synthetic chemistry of the polyiodinated aromatic structures will remain restricted to only those variations which can be made around the basic design principles. There is still some room for maneuver. Not all permutations have been played out, and some new compounds can still by synthesized. Can such new endeavors induce dramatic changes in general clinical radiology?

The toxicity of the first generation of nonionic CM (represented by metrizamide and ioglunide) is dramatically superior to that of the ionic CM. For intrathecal use, the first nonionic CM were far from the ideal of biological inertness, but for cardiovascular/urographic applications, their low toxicity is a quantitative improvement. Unfortunately, general use of these compounds is not feasible not only because of the previously mentioned lack of hydrolytical stability, but also because of the prohibitive cost.

During the past decade, almost every CM research laboratory has worked hard on developing a new generation of nonionic CM. These efforts have resulted in a number of new compounds. All are based on the same principles, and all show similarity of design and synthetic technology, such as iohexol, iopamidol, iopromide, and MP-238. It is tempting to speculate what the next, third generation of nonionics will be like. Ironically, the problem of the second generation of nonionic CM is their toxicological excellence in the cardiovascular system. The ongoing clinical trials suggest that these CM may not leave much to be desired, at least in terms of general systemic toxicity, if not the patient's discomfort. Under the pressure of legal and marketing requirements, and stronger competition, manufacturers of the second-generation CM are understandably subjecting their new compounds to complex toxicity evaluation. The variability of the new compounds in vivo is likely to show some differences in one of the many tests. Many tests often encounter the problem of reproducibility caused by such imponderable variables as interference with the biological rhythms of the experimental animals, kind of species, weather, and temperature. These variables, which are outside the investigator's control, may even affect such basic toxicity parameters as i.v. murine LD_{50} [65]. Throughout this volume and the reference literature the reader will find sometimes large differences in the values reported from different laboratories for the same compounds and seemingly identical tests. Many investigators attempted to alleviate the problem by employing comparative compounds as "standards", but even there the value of conclusions extrapolated from such data is not always certain. What matters ultimately is clinical experience. Results of the first cardiovascular studies of iohexol, iopamidol, and iopromide are cited in Chaps. 3 and 5, Sect. C, throughout the volume, and in Ref. [5]. What can be gleaned from the composite testing picture is the impression that the systemic toxicity of the second generation of nonionic CM may be different in detail, but not in principle, and that the levels of their biological tolerance approach the ideal of inertness more closely than any other previous compounds. It is thus not only questionable whether further improvements are possible in this area, but whether they would be needed. In angiography, media of low osmolality are clearly less prone to elicit vascular pain, and improvements in this area are therefore justifiable.

Containment of cost will in all probability be a major topic of medical care in the immediate future. In that regard, second-generation CM are caught in a double bind: unless produced in very large quantities they cannot be cheaper; if not economically feasible, they cannot be used extensively. What contributes mainly to the high cost of this second generation is the complicated synthesis carried out in five to seven steps (see Chap. 1). Second, there is the need for expensive aminoalcohols and the necessity for purification of the final products by large-scale chromatography. Attempts to improve on these factors were recently reported [58]. The new technology employs a single-unit process and inexpensive industrial reagents in a three-step synthesis. With this approach, nonionic CM can be made very economically. Hopefully, new, previously synthetically inaccessible compounds, a "second generation of nonionic CM," will emerge.

In the immediate future, the ionic monomers will continue to play their important role in medical imaging and provide a point of reference for further endeavors. It will thus, as in the past, be extremely important to develop further accurate and simple method of screening the general patient population for potential candidates for anaphylactoid reactions. Anaphylactoid catastrophes can be minimized by appropriate premedication and/or utilization of the nonionic, highly hydrophilic media [66].

There is a need for an extension of our imaging capabilities. The explosive development of imaging technologies calls for organ-specific CM which would depict not only morphology, but also the dynamic factors of organ pathology. Efforts should be made to develop materials which, by reflecting the metabolism of the organs, could detect defective functions. With CT competing with NMR for imaging of the CNS, radiographic CM will be sought which, while excreted into the CSF from the blood, would obviate the need for puncturing the intrathecal space. Blood pool CM should permit the use of smaller doses while producing higher diagnostic yields, not only in dynamic CT, but also in digital radiography and scan-projection radiography.

References

1. Grainger RG (1982) Intravascular contrast media – the past, the present and the future. Br J Radiol 55:1–18
2. Knoefel PK (ed) (1971) Radiocontrast agents. In: International encyclopedia of pharmacology and therapeutics, Sect. 76. Pergamon, Oxford
3. Miller Re, Skucas J (1977) Radiographic contrast agents. University Park Press, Baltimore
4. Amiel M (ed) (1982) Contrast media in radiology. Springer, Berlin Heidelberg New York
5. Taenzer V, Zeitler E (eds) (1983) Contrast media in urography, angiography and computerized tomography. Thieme, New York
6. Ansell G (1970) Adverse reactions to contrast agents – scope of problem. Invest Radiol 5:374–391
7. Fischer HW (1957) Colloidal stannic oxide: animal studies on a new hepatolienographic agent. Radiology 68:488–498
8. Seltzer SE, Adams DF, Davis MA, Hessel SJ, Hurlburg A, Havron A (1979) Development of selective hepatic contrast agents for CT scanning. Invest Radiol 14:356
9. Fischer HW, Barbaric ZL, Violante MR, Stein G, Shapiro BA (1979) Iothalamate ethyl ester as hepatolienographic agent. Invest Radiol 12:96–100

10. Cohen Z, Seltzer SE, Davis MA, Hanson RN (1981) Iodinated starch particles: new contrast material for computed tomography of the liver. J Comput Assist Tomogr 5:843–846
11. Cassel DM, Young SW, Brody WR, Muller HH, Hall AL (1982) Radiographic blood pool contrast agents for vascular and tumor imaging with projection radiography and computed tomography. J Comput Assist Tomogr 6:141–146
12. Vermess M, Doppman JC, Sugarbaker P, Fisher RI, Chatterji DC, Lutzeler J (1980) Clinical trials with a new intravenous liposoluble contrast material for computed tomography of the liver and spleen. Radiology 137:217–222
13. Gottlob R, Solutions of X-ray contrast agents. European Patent Application 12,926
14. MacKaness GB, Hon JP, Contrast media containing liposomes as carriers. US Patent 4,192,859
15. Caride VJ, Sostman HD, Twickler J, Zacharis H, Stelios CO, Jaffe CC (1982) Brominated radiopaque liposomes: contrast agent for computed tomography of liver and spleen. Invest Radiol 17:381–385
16. Torchilin VP, Berdichevsky VR, Barsukov AA, Smirnov VN (1980) Coating liposomes with protein decreases their capture by macrophages. FEBS Lett 111:184–188
17. Carroll BA, Turner RJ, Tickner EG, Boyle DB, Young SW (1980) Gelatin encapsulated nitrogen microbubbles as ultrasonic contrast agents. Invest Radiol 15:260–266
18. Mattrey RF, Leopold GR, van Sonnenberg E, Gosink BB, Scheible W, Long DM (1983) Perfluorochemicals as liver- and spleen-seeking ultrasound contrast agents. J Ultrasound Med 2:173–176
19. Sovak M, Weitl FL, Lang JH, Higgins CB (1979) Development of a radiopaque cation: toxicity of the benzylammonium group. Eur J Med Chem 14:257–260
20. Speck U, Klieger E, Mutzel W (1981) Triiodinated aminoacetamido isophthalamide X-Ray contrast agents. US Patent 4,283,381 (August 11, 1981)
21. Grainger GR (1979) A clinical trial of a new low osmolality contrast medium. Br J Radiol 52:791–796
22. Holder JC, Dalrymple GJ (1981) Pain and aortal femoral arteriography: the importance of chemical structure and osmolality of contrast agents. Invest Radiol 16:508–513
23. Eisenberg RL, Mani RL, Hedgecock MW (1978) Pain associated with peripheral angiography: is Lidocaine effective? Radiology 127:109–111
24. Guthaner DF, Silverman JF, Hayden WG, Wexler L (1977) Intraarterial analgesia in peripheral arteriography. Am J Roent 128:737–739
25. Heystraten FMJ, van den Berg FG, Mulderije ED (1983) Comparison of pain and heat sensation of contrast media in aortofemoral angiography: meglumine-amidotrizoate (Angiographin) mixed with Lidocaine versus sodium-meglumine-ioxaglate (Hexabrix). Diagnostic Imaging 52:141–144
26. Hagen B, Clauss W (1982) Kontrastmittel und Schmerz bei der peripheren Arteriographie. Radiologe 22:470–475
27. Molyneux AJ, Sheldon PWE (1982) A randomized blind trial of Iopamidol and meglumine calcium metrizoate (Triosil 280, Isopaque Cerebral) in cerebral angiography. Br J Radiol 55:117–119
28. Dawson P, Pitfield J, Britton J (1983) Contrast media and bronchospasm: a study with Iopamidol. Clin Radiol 34:227–230
29. Pitre D, Felder E (1980) Development of chemistry and physical properties of iopamidol and its analogs. Invest Radiol 15:S301–S309
30. Speck U, Blaszkiewicz P, Seidelmann D, Klieger (1979) German Patent DOS 2909439
31. Mutzel W, Speck U (1983) Pharmacochemical profile of iopromide. AJNR 4:350–352
32. Bryan RN, Miller SL, Roehm JOF Jr, Weatherall PT (1983) Neuroangiography with Iohexol. ANJR 4:344–346
33. Hindmarsh T, Bergstrand G, Ericson K, Olivecrona H (1983) Comparative double-blind investigation of meglumine metrizoate, metrizamide and Iohexol in carotid angiography. AJNR 4:347–349

34. Mancini GB, Bloomquist JN, Bhargava V, Stein JB, Lew W, Slutsky RA, Shabetai R, Higgins CB (1983) Hemodynamic and electricardiographic effects in man of a new nonionic contrast agent (Iohexol): advantages over standard ionic agents. Am J Cardiol 51:1218–1222

35. Mills SR, Wertman DE, Heaston DK, Moore AV Jr, Bates M, Allen S, Rommel AJ, Thompson WM (1982) Study of safety and tolerance of Iopamidol in peripheral angiography. Radiology 145:57–58

36. Widrich WC, Beckman CF, Robbins AH, Scholz FJ, Srinivasan MK, Hayes EJ, Kellum CD, Newman T (1983) Iopamidol and meglumine diatrizoate: comparison of effects on patient discomfort during aortofemoral arteriography. Radiology 141:61–64

37. Fletcher EWL (1982) A comparison of iopamidol and diatrizoate in peripheral angiography. Br J Radiol 55:36–38

38. Whitehouse GH, Snowdon SL (1982) An assessment of Iopamidol, a non-ionic contrast medium, in aorto-femoral angiography. Clin Radiol 33:231–234

39. Hacking PM, Soppitt D (1983) A comparative study of two non-ionic contrast media, iopamidol and metrizamide, in translumbar aortography. Clin Radiol 34:87–90

40. Speck U, Siefert HM, Klinik G (1980) Contrast media and pain in peripheral arteriography. Invest Radiol 15:335–339

41. Littner MR, Ulreich S, Putman CE, Rosenfield AT, Meadows G (1981) Bronchospasm during excretory urography: lack of specificity for the methylglucamine cation. AJR 137:477–481

42. Jacobson T (1984) The preclinical development of iohexol. Invest Radiol 19: S142–S143

43. Pfeiffer H, Speck U (1978) German Patent DOS 2628517 (January 5, 1978)

44. Sovak M, Ranganathan R (1982) US Patent 4,341,756 (July 27, 1982)

45. Schering AG (1983) US Patent 4,367,216 (January 4, 1983)

46. Speck U, Muetzel W, Mannesmann G, Siefert HM (1980) Pharmacology of nonionic dimers. Invest Radiol [Suppl] 15:317–320

47. Skalpe IO (1983) The toxicity of nonionic water soluble monomeric and dimeric contrast media in selective vertebral angiography: an experimental study in rabbits. Neuroradiology 24:219–223

48. Guerra J, Resnick DL, Haghighi P, Sovak M, Cone R (1984) Investigation of a new arthrographic CM: Iotrol. Invest Radiol 19:228–234

49. Speck U, Muetzel W, Press WR (1984) Kidney toxicity testing in animals. Invest Radiol 19:S123

50. Felder E, Pitre D, Grandi M (1982) Radiopaque contrast media: determination of the optical purity of iopamidol. Il Farmaco 37:3–8

51. Lang JG, Lasser EC (1971) Nonspecific inhibition of enzymes by organic contrast media. J Med Chem 14:233–236

52. Levitan H, Rapoport SI (1975) Contrast media: quantitative criteria for designing compounds with low toxicity. Acta Radiol [Diagn] (Stockh) 17:81–92

53. Tanford C (1978) The hydrophobic effect and the organization of living matter. Science 200:1012–1018

54. Hansch C (1968) The use of substituent constants in drug modification. Farmaco [Sci] 23:293–320

55. Sovak M, Ranganathan R, Lang JH, Lasser EC (1978) Concepts in design of improved intravascular contrast agents. Ann Radiol 21:283–289

56. Speck U, Gries H, Klieger E, Muetzel W, Press WR, Heinmann HJ (1984) New contrast media developed at Schering AG: first experience. Invest Radiol 19:S144

57. Almen T (1969) Contrast agent design. J Theoret Biol 24:216–222

58. Sovak M, Ranganathan R, Douglass J, Gallagher J, Nagarajan G (1984) Low cost nonionic media: new synthetic concepts. Invest Radiol 19:S145

59. Sovak M, Ranganathan R (1983) US Patent Application 544,308

60. Sovak M, Ranganathan R (1980) Stability of nonionic water-soluble contrast media: implications for their design. Invest Radiol 15:S323–S328

61. Sovak M, Ranganathan R (1980) Syntheses of new nonionic radiographic contrast media: acylamino-triiodophenyl ethers of sugars. Invest Radiol 15:S296. US Patent 4,243,653
62. Shapiro R, Papa D (1959) Heavy-metal chelates and cesium salts for contrast radiology. Ann NY Acad Sci 78:756–763
63. Rubin M, Di Chiro G (1959) Chelates as possible contrast media. Ann NY Acad Sci 78:764–778
64. Nalbandian RM, Rice WT, Nickel WO (1959) A new category of contrast media: water-soluble radiopaque polyvalent chelates. Ann NY Acad Sci 78:779–792
65. Sovak M, Lang JH, Rosen L (1977) Toxicity of metrizamide. Radiology 123:242–243
66. Rapoport S, Bookstein JJ, Higgins CB, Carey PH, Sovak M, Lasser EC (1982) Experience with metrizamide in patients with previous severe anaphylactoid reactions to ionic contrast agents. Radiology 143:321–325

CHAPTER 1

Chemistry of X-Ray Contrast Media

G. B. Hoey and K. R. Smith
in collaboration with S. El-Antably and G. P. Murphy

A. Introduction and Scope

X-ray contrast media (CM) have been used since the first discovery of X-rays by
Roentgen in 1895. The function of such media is to opacify an organ or portion
of the body to X-rays, providing thereby greater diagnostic information to the
physician. Many opaque atoms have been studied in many chemical forms; for
example, bismuth, barium, tantalum, strontium, and bromine have all been used
in a variety of compounds. Although many water-soluble compounds have been
evaluated, by 1980 only two atoms, iodine and bromine, have been found to be
of significant diagnostic use. This chapter will devote itself to iodinated organic
compounds, since they are by far the most diagnostically useful, in particular, we
shall discuss mainly water-soluble compounds. The pertinent literature has been
surveyed through mid-1980.

This discussion will not attempt to evaluate all reported iodine-containing X-
ray CM but will rather concentrate on general chemical principles, reviewing only
"model" compounds within a given structural class. There are several excellent
summaries of early work [1–6]. Interested readers should consult these for the early history and development of X-ray CM.

B. Biological Requirements

Translating the biological requirements of contrast media into chemical/pharma-
cological terms, compounds are needed which can be administered in aqueous solution, which are stable both in vitro and in vivo, which are nontoxic, and which
are concentrated and/or excreted by a desired pathway. Historically, iodinated
CM have evolved from water-insoluble, highly toxic substances into water-soluble, reasonably safe compounds. Safety became of increasing importance as the
radiologist recognized that higher and higher doses led to better diagnostic information. Salts of 3-amino-2,4,6-triiodobenzoic acid derivatives were found most
useful and versatile in most applications. Since this first work, many ionic compounds have been made in an attempt to improve biological safety. The upper
limit of safety now appears to have been approached with ionic CM, as the subsequent discussion will show. This limitation is reflected by the chemical nature
of these compounds wherein as ions they exert electrical and osmotic effects
which lead to more or less pronounced toxicity manifestations.

The development of nonionic CM provided even safer compounds (see below). Since these compounds do not exert electrical effects and their solutions have improved osmotic properties, they are in general toxicologically superior to the ionic CM.

Today, the criteria for a diagnostically useful radiocontrast medium are as follows: [1]

1. Opacity to X-rays
2. High water solubility at high iodine concentration, low viscosity, and low osmolality as close as possible to those of body fluids
3. Chemical stability
4. Biological safety.

I. Physicochemical Properties

1. Water Solubility

Water solubility of ionic compounds arises from a salt formation with an appropriate cation, generally sodium or N-methylglucamine (meglumine). Such salts can give highly concentrated solutions of up to 40%–50% w/v iodine. Meglumine salts, in general, are more water soluble than sodium salts, but in solutions of comparable iodine content meglumine salts are generally more viscous. Water solubility is not conferred solely by salt formation alone as shown in Table 4, where the sodium and meglumine salt solubility of the "parent" triiodobenzoic acid are compared with a series of substituted triiodobenzoic acids. Thus, for example, the addition of an acetamido or methylcarbamyl function to the triiodobenzoic acid can improve substantially both water solubility and biological safety. The acetamido or another acylamido group is common to almost all CM.

In general terms, water solubility is enhanced by polar functional groups, e.g., acetamido and carbamyl functions. Water solubility is likewise conferred by the introduction of hydroxyalkyl functions. Such compounds are somewhat more lengthy to prepare and provide solutions which are generally of higher viscosity than those containing simple amide groups. Hydroxyl groups attached to the benzene ring (phenols) likewise can confer water solubility but may also provide a strong degree of protein binding due to their acidic nature [8]. This, in turn, results in toxic manifestations in vivo. Ether functions (methoxy 1,2-dihydroxypropoxy) likewise may enhance water solubility. (See Tables 4, 6–9, 11 for examples.)

$$CH_3-\overset{\overset{\textstyle O}{\|}}{C}-NH- \qquad\qquad CH_3O-$$

Acetamido   Methoxy

$$CH_3-NH-\overset{\overset{\textstyle O}{\|}}{C}- \qquad\qquad HOCH_2-CHOH-CH_2O-$$

N-Methylcarbamyl   Dihydroxypropoxy

---

1 To the researcher who wants to develop a compound suitable for successful commercial development, considerations of patentability and manufacturing cost are also important.

2. Viscosity

Viscosity has a great influence on clinical tolerance. It is a function of the shape, number, and charge of the solute particles as well as the solvent viscosity. A low viscosity is needed for rapid transit through the capillary beds and for rapid injection rates.

The iodine content and viscosity of a formulation suit the clinical use. Thus, intravenous urographic agents are formulated to contain between 28% and 40% iodine (280–400 mg I/ml) and are administered in doses of 50–150 ml. Rapid injection is often employed, although infusions are also used. For angiographic use, solutions containing up to 37% iodine (370 mg I/ml) are required of a relatively low-viscosity agent so that a sufficiently large bolus can be injected rapidly. For intrathecal administration, lower concentrations are used (170–280 mg I/ml). As the dose is small (10–20 ml) and administered slowly, high viscosity is not a hindrance; indeed, high viscosity of water-soluble myelographic media can provide a better diagnostic yield. The primary consideration is one of low toxicity.

Table 1. Viscosity and osmolality of ionic X-ray CM

Medium [a]	Conc. (mg I/ml)	Viscosity		Osmolality (mOsm/kg)
		25 °C	35 °C	
Iothalamate [b]	282	6.1	4.0	1,485
Diatrizoate [b]	282	6.2	4.1	1,520
Metrizoate [c]	280	2.7	4.0	1,460
Ioxitalamate [d]	280	–	4.4	–
Iocarmate [c]	280	–	7.2	1,040
Ioxaglate [e]	320	15.7 [f]	7.5	580
Human blood	–	–	2.40–2.90	300
CSF	–	–	1.02–1.03	300

[a] Meglumine salts
[b] Ref. [9]
[c] Ref. [10]
[d] Ref. [11]
[e] Ref. [12]
[f] 20 °C

3. Osmolality

The osmotic pressure of an aqueous solution is defined as the force that must be applied to counterbalance the force arising from the flow of water across a semipermeable membrane [13].

In vivo osmotic effects of high concentrations of CM result in hypertonicity causing intracellular water to pass from the interior of a cell to the surrounding fluid.

The osmolality of a solution is proportional to the sum of the concentrations of the different molecular or ionic species present. For an ionic CM (which contains both anion and cation), the total ionic concentration is twice that of the un-ionized species. For nonionic agents, the osmolality is proportional to the concen-

Table 2. Amount of iodine available per molecule of dissolved substance

Contrast medium	No. of iodine atoms/molecule	No. of ions/ particles	Ratio of atoms of iodine to ions or particles
Ionic monomer	3	2	1.5
Ionic bis compound (dimer)	6	3	2.0
Ionic tris compound (trimer)	9	4	2.25
Mono-acidic bis compound [a]	6	2	3.0
Nonionic monomer	3	1	3.0
Nonionic bis compound (dimer)	6	1	6.0

[a] e.g., ioxaglate

tration of the compound, which is theoretically half the value of the salt of an analogous ionic compound which has two ionic species.

Originally, hypertonicity of CM solutions was considered insignificant [14]. Later osmolality was found to contribute to endothelial injuries [15, 16], and to be the prime cause of vascular permeability alteration [17, 18].

The hyperosmolality of CM solutions transfers water and electrolytes between intracellular and extracellular spaces [19–24]. For adequate visualization in most clinical applications a high dose of a highly concentrated solution of the agent is required. The high osmolality of such a solution plays an important role in producing side effects such as pain, decrease in blood pressure, and vascular damage. Attempts to reduce the osmolality were made by increasing the number of iodine atoms per particle through the synthesis fo dimers, trimers, and nonionic agents. Table 2 illustrates the amount of iodine available per molecule of dissolved substance.

The effect of some CM on the endothelium has been compared to that of equiosmolal sodium chloride solution [25]. For the same iodine content nonionic media cause less endothelial damage than the ionic agents. Endothelial damage ascribed to the solution hypertonicity is known to occur when CM are injected rapidly in angiography [26]. Such damage may result in electrolytic imbalance [27] and partial breakdown of a blood-organ barrier [28].

Damage to the blood-brain barrier, however, is due not only to the hyperosmolality of CM solutions but also to the chemical nature of the agent [28]. From a study on long-chain monocarboxylic acids, it has been suggested that organic electrolytes, even if almost completely dissociated, can cross the blood-brain barrier if highly lipid soluble [29, 32].

Convulsions induced by intrathecal injection of a CM are not even related to its hyperosmolality but to its chemotoxic properties [30]. An increase in cerebrospinal fluid osmolality following intrathecal injection of a hypertonic saline solution or a CM canot alone explain the incidence of arachnoiditis [31].

II. Chemical Stability

The compound must be chemically stable in aquaeous solution so that it can be sterilized and so that it will have a reasonable shelf life (2–3 years).

From the early days of iodinated, water-soluble organic CM, chemists have recognized that most types of carbon-iodine bonds are not sufficiently thermally stable for autoclaving. Thus, the work of BINZ and others with the iodopyridones was the first attempt to provide vinylic carbon-iodine linkages [33]. These were known to be chemically more stable than aliphatic carbon-iodine bonds. The most stable of the vinylic carbon iodine-bonds, however, is that in an aromatic nucleus. Their suitability was first shown by LONG and BURGER in 1941 [34] but received the first practical refinement by WALLINGFORD in 1948 [7], with the synthesis of aminotriiodobenzoic acid and its N-acetyl derivative. Thus salts of these compounds can be formulated in water solution and subjected to sterilization at 121 °C for 20 min with only negligible decomposition as shown by very sensitive analytical methods. In his early work, WALLINGFORD discovered that trace (ppm) quantities of certain cations (e.g., Fe, Cu) could catalyze the deiodination of these compounds during the formulation and sterilization process. He corrected for this by the addition of very small quantities of calcium disodium edetate as a se- questering agent to prevent catalytic deiodination. Addition of small quantities of buffer proved an aid in the formulation and sterilization processes and in pro- viding a useful shelf life.

More recently studies on the deiodination kinetics of iodobenzoic acids have emphasized the importance of preventing catalysis of deiodination by Cu(II) [35]. It should also be noted that certain CM formulations may require the addition of sulfite or bisulfite as an antioxidant (e.g., meglumine iocarmate) for optimum stability.

While in general the use of small amounts of chelating agents, buffers, etc. as stabilizers has no effect on the biological safety of a CM, some investigators feel that citrate ion or tetrasodium edetate may be deleterious in vivo by depleting cal- cium ion in the heart [36].

In theory, ionic iodinated CM in water solution can degrade by several mech- anisms. These include decarboxylation, deiodination, and hydrolysis (deacetyla- tion) of the molecule. Consequently, one must conduct long-term stability studies to show the absence of these effects with time. A properly formulated CM should remain stable in water solution at room temperature for at least 5 years *if pro- tected from light*. All organic carbon iodine bonds undergo cleavage by photoly- sis, the rate of which is dependent on the structure of the molecule, its concentra- tion, and radiation intensity.

The stability of CM can be monitored in several ways. Ordinarily stability studies are conducted by evaluating changes in pH and color, and by the appear- ance of iodide ion and any hydrolysis product (amino compound). In more recent years, stability-indicating assays for the iodinated acid [usually by high-perfor- mance liquid chromatography (HPLC)] have been developed [37]. Figure 1 illus- trates the possible pathways of decomposition, and the ways in which the stability parameters monitor each pathway are as follows:

Decomposition by	*Parameter changed*
Decarboxylation	pH, color, assay
Deiodination	Iodide, color, pH
Hydrolysis	pH, color, amine content, assay

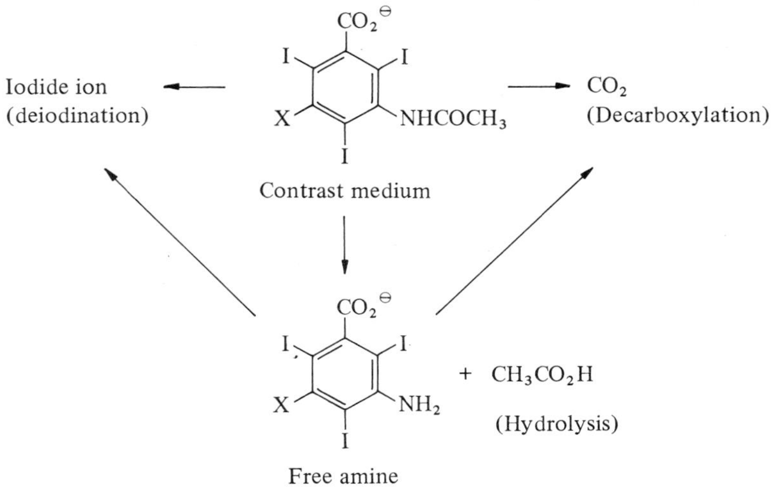

Fig. 1. Possible routes of decomposition of CM

Tables 40 and 41 give the results of long-term stability studies with both typical sodium and meglumine salt formulations.

If other sensitive functional groups are present in the molecule, then a suitable test must be developed to detect any changes possibly due to their degradation. Calcium disodium edetate has been found to be stable in a variety of formulations (see Table 40).

Stability studies are generally conducted at several temperatures, often as high as 50 °C. At this higher temperature, CM solutions will degrade over a period of 6 months or more depending on the conditions employed. Generally, the parameters of iodine and pH, as well as color, will change.

Sodium triiodobenzoates per se are not unstable in water solutions. On the other hand, it has been shown that a meglumine triiodobenzoate, if heated for extended periods at high temperature, will decompose (MALLINCKRODT, Research Department, St. Louis, unpublished results).

In summary, CM are formulated in water solution to be sterile and pyrogen free and with a degree of chemical stability such that no toxic degradation products are produced during the shelf life of the material. CM must be protected from light; they are then chemically quite stable.

III. Biological Safety

In contradistinction to therapeutic agents, diagnostic agents such as X-ray CM should be totally pharmacologically inert. Such pharmacological inertness in terms of chemical and biochemical stability means the CM are not metabolized in vivo. Theoretically, metabolic processes would include deiodination, hydrolysis of amide linkages, and decarboxylation. (Conjugation in the liver is precluded by the fact that triiodobenzoic acids are all strong acids, highly hydrophilic, and usually weakly protein bound.) None of these have ever been observed in animals

Table 3. Preclinical pharmacology and toxicology evaluation for diagnostic X-ray CM. [45]

A. Studies prior to phase I/II clinical trials (IND)

    I. Acute pharmacodynamics
        1. Anesthetized dogs
        2. Intravenous and clinical route if not intravascular
        3. Determine after two to three elevated dosage levels:
            a) Direct cardiovascular effects
            b) Indirect autonomic effects

    II. Acute pharmacokinetics
        1. Two species, usually rat and dog
        2. Intravenous and clinical route if not intravascular
        3. Determine after clinical dose level:
            a) Absorption (if not intravascular)
            b) Tissue distribution
            c) Metabolism
            d) Excretion route, degree, and rate

    III. Acute Toxicity
        1. LD_{50} determination in mice and rats, and estimation in rabbits and dogs
            a) Intravenous if water soluble
            b) Relevant clinical route(s) if nonvascular and feasible
            c) Usually includes necropsy of delayed mortalities (24 h) and histopathology
               of suspected drug-related lesions
        2. Special determinations at sublethal doses dependent upon clinical use, e.g.,
            a) Blood-brain barrier toxicity (rat and dogs)
            b) Intrathecal neurotoxicity (dogs and monkeys)
            c) Direct nephrotoxicity (dogs)
            d) Direct coronary cardiotoxicity (dogs), etc.

    IV. Subacute toxicity (repeat dose)
        1. Two weeks in two species, usually rat and dog
        2. Clinical route if feasible, i.v. employed if not
        3. Three elevated dosage levels with negative control
        4. Parameters include:
            a) Behavior, food consumption, and body weights
            b) Hematology (include prothrombin time for dogs)
            c) Clinical chemistry profile [include protein-bound iodine (PBI) and thyroid
               function]
            d) Ophthalmological examination
            e) Urinalysis
            f) Gross and microscopic examination:
               α) All major organs in control and high-dose groups
               β) Target organs in low- and mid-dose groups

    V. Special studies
        1. To characterize primary potential toxicity
        2. Directed toward clinical utility, e.g.,
            a) Blood and/or CSF compatibility
            b) Venous irritation
            c) Direct arterial vascular effects
            d) In vitro studies, etc.

B. Studies prior to phase III clinical trials (NDA)

    I. Teratological study
        1. Two species, usually rat and rabbit
        2. Clinical route if feasible, i.v. if not
        3. Two dose levels and negative control

Table 3 (continued)

II. Special studies
   1. Dictated by expected clinical use
   2. May include:
      a) Acute toxicity in neonates
      b) Drug interaction studies
      c) Long-term tissue irritation studies
      d) Efficacy studies, etc.

III. Supplement studies
   1. Dictated by previous test results
   2. May include:
      a) Additional LD_{50} determinations
      b) Pharmacokinetics in different species
      c) Adverse effect reversal studies
      d) Repeated studies to verify original results, etc.

---

or in humans. Pharmacological activity of CM can be a function of protein binding and osmolality [38, 39].

The subject of biological safety and toxicological methodology will be reviewed in detail in other sections of this book, but it is instructive to outline here the primary pharmacological evaluation of all candidate CM whether ionic or nonionic.

Following determination of a new compound's water solubility and chemical stability, the next stage is to evaluate the safety of the compound in mice and rats. To this end, intravenous, intracerebral, and intracisternal toxicity testing is conducted in mice and rats using the standard protocols. Several of these protocols have been published [40–43], and methods of testing the neurotoxicity summarized [44].

Assessment of systemic toxicity by intravenous administration in mice requires a concentration of 28%–37% iodine and an injection rate of around 1 ml/min. With such standard protocols, quite reproducible and reliable values of LD_{50} can be obtained. An early screen of central nervous system toxicity is intracisternal injection in rats [4]. Solutions in the range of 4%–14% iodine have been employed depending on the toxicity of the compound.

Following these early and somewhat approximate screens, the investigator can proceed to more specialized studies such as in the isolated rabbit heart and administration in higher animal species, depending on the interest and formulation desired.

The toxic potential of the compound is of prime importance, especially in the anticipated clinical route of administration. Since CM usually are intended for single-dose administration, long-term animal studies are not necessary except for unique situations, like inflammatory effects of myelographic agents. The clinical indications should be closely simulated by animal experiments, and the relationship between toxic doses in animals and intended clinical doses should be established. The anticipated patient population may require additional or more extensive studies in specific areas, e.g., pediatrics or pregnancy. Table 3 summarizes the types of studies which may be required.

C. Ionic Contrast Media

I. Synthesis

Ionic monomers are synthesized as shown in Fig. 2.

The starting materials are the readily available nitro aromatic compounds, which can be manipulated in many ways. Thus the nitro compound is reduced to the amino compound which provides the needed activation of the benzene ring for substitution by iodine. Iodination generally is accomplished with iodine monochloride or with sodium or potassium iododichloride under acid conditions.

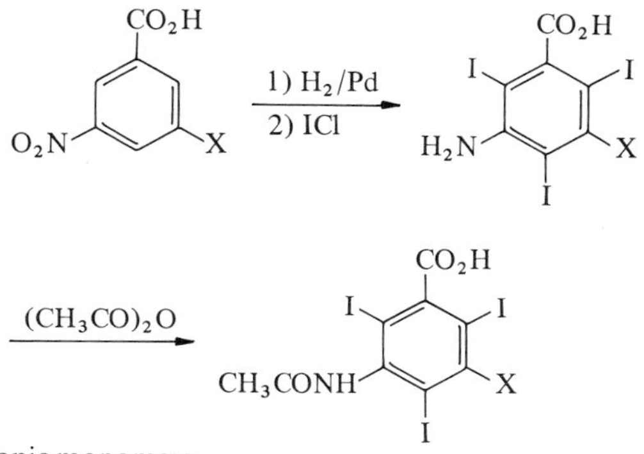

Fig. 2. Synthesis of ionic monomers

The iodination goes smoothly to give the triiodinated compound, which is water insoluble and, therefore, easily isolated and purified. Following this, the amino group can be acylated to "lock" the iodine into the ring. This part of the reaction sequence provides the triiodophenyl structure as well as the acetamido (acyl) linkage. The remaining position (X) on the benzene ring can be manipulated to provide the desired final structure – either before or after hydrogenation and iodination as required by the chemistry of the compound desired. The resulting triiodobenzoic acid derivative is subjected to very careful purification prior to its formulation as a CM salt solution. Purification can involve reprecipitation, treatment with ion exchange resins, charcoal, etc. Analysis of the final product is thorough and the absence of byproducts and degradation products is rigidly established. Manipulation of the other functional groups on the triiodophenyl ring involves relatively simple chemistry, e.g., esterification, selective hydrolysis, acylation, and alkylation. Achievement of maximum yields and minimum production costs requires extensive organic and analytical chemical knowledge. Manufacturing costs are a function both of the synthesis yields as well as of the number of steps which affect the labor cost. Since these compounds are quite highly water soluble in salt form but extremely water insoluble as free acids, purification can be quite efficiently and thoroughly carried out by a reprecipitation process. To be fully practical, the acid compound should be synthesized in three to eight steps. Syntheses requiring any greater effort may result in compounds too costly to be of commercial significance. Exceptions to this would, of course, be any compounds with substantially improved safety. (An example is ioxaglic acid.)

II. Evolution of Structural Types

Efforts to improve ionic media have been directed primarily toward discovering substituted triiodobenzoic acids with improved water solubility and biological safety. The substituents in the 3- and 5-positions on the aromatic nucleus represent groups which can both solubilize and detoxify the basic triiodobenzoic acid moiety; thus, the search has been directed primarily toward more efficient solubilizing and detoxifying groups in these positions. Table 4 attempts to trace evolution of improved CM; thus from 3-acetamido, 2,4,6-triiodobenzoic acid, chemists proceeded to add an additional 5-acetamido function (diatrizoate) followed shortly by a 5-N-methylcarbamyl function (iothalamate), 5-N-methylacetamido function (metrizoate), and 5-acetamidomethyl function (iodamide).

Three general combinations of amide side chains or functional groups are now available. They are acyl/acyl, carbamyl/acyl, and acylamidomethyl/acyl (Table 5). Recently Gries and co-workers have described the synthesis of carbamyl/carbamyl compounds (Table 5) [46, 46a].

In the early evolution of these compounds, it was learned that the coupling of the two acyl triiodobenzoic acids via an aliphatic chain resulted in compounds that remained, in spite of their high molecular weight, highly water soluble and, by virtue of their protein binding, excreted by the biliary rather than renal system. These bis compounds (or as they are more often described, "dimers") provided an additional class of improved CM [47, 48].

The first CM were strongly protein bound and thus excreted via the biliary rather than the renal system (e.g., iodipamide). Subsequently, additional highly water soluble compounds were synthesized which did not bind to the protein, e.g., iocarmate. In both the bis and mono series toxicity is a function of protein binding, decreasing from acetrizoate to the iothalamate/diatrizoate type in the mono series and from iodipamide to iocarmate in the bis series.

The next extension of the concept, namely tris compounds ("trimers"), was described later by Wiegert [49, 50].

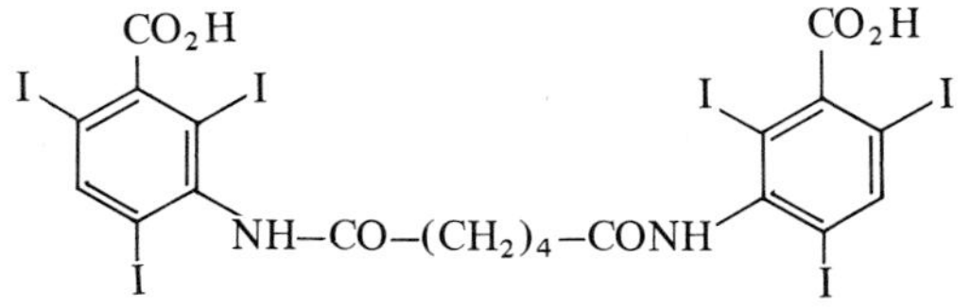

Bis compound
(iodipamide)

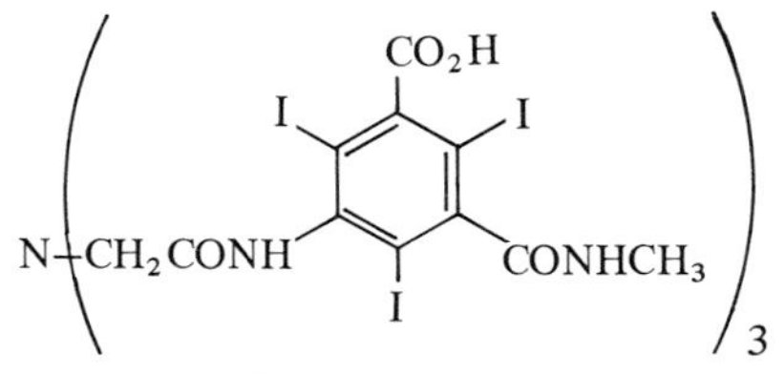

Tris compound

Table 4. Substituted triiodobenzoic acids

X	Y	H_2O solubility (% w/v)	Toxicity[a] (mg I/kg)			Ref.
			i.v.	i. cereb.	i. cis.	
H–	–H	9 (Na); 5 (M)	455	–	22.5	c
CH_3CONH-	–H	94 (Na)	5,400	–	–	[7], c
CH_3CONH-	$-NHCOCH_3$	60 (Na); 89 (M)	5,400	–	4	[174]
$-NHCOCH_3$	$CH_3CON(CH_3)-$	80 (Na); > 65 (M)	8,700	130	–	[175]
CH_3CONH-	$-CONHCH_3$	> 80 (Na); > 100 (M)	6,000	300	73	c
CH_3CONH-	$-CONHCH_2CH_2OH$	> 80 (Na); > 60 (M)	8,800	120	–	[11]
CH_3CONH-	$-CH_2NHCOCH_3$		7,000	97	20^b	[176]
CH_3CONH-	$-N(CH_2CH_2OH)COCH_3$		9,500	425	–	[175]
CH_3CONH-	$-CO_2CH_3$	30	7,744	–	< 5	c
CH_3CONH-	$-NHCONHCH_3$	60	–	–	–	[177]
CH_3CONH-	$-OCH_3$	35 (Na)	>9,000	–	–	c
CH_3OCH_2CONH-	$-CONHCH_3$	65	6,000	480	40	[178]
$CH_3CON(CH_3)-$	$-CONHCH_3$		–	350	–	[179]
$CH_3CON(CH_2CH_2OH)-$	$-CONHCH_3$		–	400	–	[180]
$CH_3CON(CH_3)-$	$-CONHCH_2CH_2OH$		–	350	–	[179]

a Meglumine salt   b Rabbit   c Mallinckrodt, Research Department, St. Louis (unpublished data)

Table 5. Combinations of acyl side chains

	X	Y	Example	X; Y type
	CH$_3$CONH−	−NHCOCH$_3$	Diatrizoic acid	Acyl/acyl
	CH$_3$CONH−	−CONHCH$_3$	Iothalamic acid	Acyl/carbamyl
	CH$_3$CONH−	−CH$_2$NHCOCH$_3$	Iodamide	Acyl/acylmethyl
	CH$_3$CONH−	−N(CH$_3$)COCH$_3$	Metrizoic acid	Acyl/acyl
	CH$_3$CONH−	−CONHCH$_2$CH$_2$OH	Ioxitalamic acid	Acyl/carbamyl
	CH$_3$NHCO−	−CONHCH$_3$	−	Carbamyl/carbamyl

In summary, capitalizing on the general utility of the acyltriiodobenzoic acid structure, research efforts have been directed toward improving safety. Keys to greater safety were established as:

1. High iodine content at comparable toxicity (Lower dose)
2. Reduction of hypertonicity of the CM solutions by bis or tris compounds
3. Improved viscosity (by adjusting the ratio of sodium to meglumine salt)

1. Improving the Functional Groups

Since the early discoveries of acetamido, carbamyl, and acylamidomethyl as acceptable side chains, numerous compounds have been synthesized and screened. Tables 6–9, 11–16, 19 summarize the structural types evaluated recently and provide a summary of representative compounds.

(a) Mono Type

(α) *Acyl/Acyl Series* (Table 6). Novel side chains proposed in recent years are:

Acyl type	*Examples*
Alkylureido-	CH$_3$NH−CO−NH−
Alkoxyacylamido-	CH$_3$O−CH$_2$CONH−
Hydroxyacetamido	HOCH$_2$CONH−
Butyrolactamido-	CH$_2$−CH$_2$−CH$_2$−N− (with −CO− bridge)
Succinimido-	CH$_2$−CH$_2$−CO−N− (with −CO− bridge)
Trifluoroacetamido-	CF$_3$CONH−

In addition, the acetamido function has been modified by alkylation with groups such as hydroxyethyl and dihydroxypropyl. These side chains are relatively simple to prepare chemically and be advantageous in terms of either toxicity and/or water solubility.

Table 6. Substituted triiodobenzoic acids: acyl/acyl series

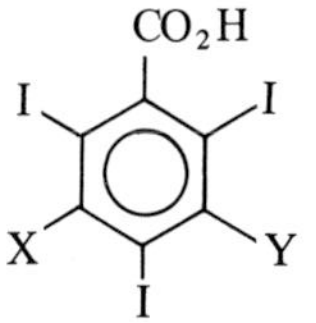

X	Y	Water solubility[a] (% w/v)	Toxicity[b] i.v.	i. cereb.	i. cis	Ref.
CH_3CONH-	$-NHCOCH_3$[c]	60 (Na), 89 (M)	5.4 g I/kg	–	4	f
$CH_3CON(CH_3)-$	$-NHCOCH_3$[d]	80 (Na), 65 (M)	8.7 g I/kg	130	–	[174, 175, f]
CH_3CONH-	$-N(CH_3CH_2OH)COCH_3$		9.5 g I/kg	425	–	[175]
$CH_3CON(CH_3)-$	$-N(CH_2CH_2OH)COCH_3$	>80 (M)	8.3 g I/kg	425	–	[175]
CH_3CONH-	$-NHCOCH_2OH$		8.5 g/kg (salt)	–	–	[182]
CH_3CONH-	$-NHCOC(CH_2OH)_3$	64	6.0 g I/kg	150	<20	[183]
CH_3CONH-	$-NRCONHCH_3$	60				[177]
$CH_3NHCONH-$	$-NHCONHCH_3$[e]					[177]
CH_3CONH-	$-N\begin{smallmatrix}CO-CH_2\\CO-CH_2\end{smallmatrix}$[e]		2.5–20.0 g/kg (salt)	–	–	[184]
CF_3CONH-	$-NHCOCF_3$	–	13.1 g/kg (salt)	–	–	[185, 186]

a Na, sodium salt; M, meglumine salt

b In mice [intravenous (i. v.) or intracerebral (i. cereb.)] or rats [intra-cisternal (i. cis.)] as meglumine salt unless otherwise noted; results in mg I/kg unless otherwise noted

c Diatrizoic acid

d Metrizoic acid

e Example of structural type – many related compounds in the reference given

f Mallinckrodt, Research Department, St. Louis (unpublished data)

Table 7. Substituted triiodobenzoic acids: carbamyl/acyl series

X	Y	Water solubility[a] (w/v)	Toxicity[b] (mg I/kg) i.v.	i. cereb.	i. cis	Ref.
CH₃CONH—	—CONHCH₃ [c]	> 80 (Na); > 100 (M)	6,000	300	73	[174], [i]
CH₃CONH—	—CONHCH₂CH₂OH [d]	> 80 (Na); > 60 (M)	8,800	120	–	[11]
CH₃CONH—	—CONHCH₂CH₂OMe	>125	4,550	530	32	[i]
CH₃CONH—	—CONHC(CH₂OH)₃	65	14,000 [e]	705	150	[187]
CH₃CONH—	—CONHC(CH₃)(CH₂OH)₂	82	4,650	790	240	[187]
CH₃OCH₂CONH—	—CONHCH₃	65	6,000	480	40	[178]
			7,200 [f]	210	34 [f]	[178]
CH₃OCH₂CONH—	—CONHCH₂CH₂OH [g]	–	> 20 g/kg (salt)	–	–	[188]
CH₃OCH₂CONH—	—CONHC(CH₂OH)₃	64	6,000	150	< 20	[187]
CH₃OCH₂CONH—	—CONH—C(CH₃)₂—CH₂OH	–	20 g/kg (salt)	–	–	[189]
CH₃CONH—	—CH₂CONHCH₃	> 65 (M)	12.0 g/kg; 9.5 g/kg	< 30	< 25	[190]
CH₃CONH—	—CO₂CH₃	30	7,744	–	< 5	[i]

CH_3CONH-	$-C=N-C(CH_2OH)_2-CH_2O-$	95	5,522	485	55	[191]
CH_3CONH-	$-C=N-C(CH_3)(CH_2OH)CH_2-O-$	> 70	5,500	280	28	[191]
CH_3NHCO	$-N(COCH_3)CH_2CONHCH_3$[g]	—	—	480 (salt, pig)	—	[192]
CH_3OCH_3CONH-	$-CONHCH(CH_3)-CONHCH_3$[g]	—	> 20 g/kg (salt)	—	—	[193–195] [i]
CH_3CONH-	$-CONH(CH_2)_2-N(CH_2CH_2OH)COCH_3$ >100		4,100	138	< 10	[196]
$CH_3NHCONH-CO$	$-CONHCH_3$[g]	—	—	—	—	
$CH_2-CH_2-CO-N-$	$-CONHCH_3$[g]	—	—	—	—	[197]
$CH_3CO(CH_3)N-$	$-CONHCH_3$	—	—	350	—	[179]
$CH_3CO(CH_3)N-$	$-CONHCH_2CH_2OH$	—	—	350	—	[179]
$CH_3CO(HOCH_2CH_2-)N-$	$-CONHCH_3$[g]	—	—	400–260	—	[180]
$HOCH_2-(CHOH)_4-CONH-$	$-CONHCH_3$	100	5,040	620	355	[183]
$HO_2C(CH_2)_4-CONH-$	$-CONHCH_3$	80	8,700[e]	353[e]	198[e]	[i]
H_2N-	$-CONHCH_3$	—	—	—	37	[i]
H_2N-	$-CONH-C(CH_2OH)_3$	> 80	5,650	195	15	[i]
$NC-$	$-CO_2H$	—	~ 4,000[h]	—	—	[i]

[a] Na, sodium salt; M, meglumine salt

[b] In mice [intravenous (i. v.) or intracerebral (i. cereb.)] or rats [intracisternal (i. cis.)] as meglumine salt unless otherwise noted

[c] Iothalamic acid

[d] Ioxithalamic acid

[e] mg salt/kg

[f] Na salt

[g] Example of structural type. Data for analogous compounds in reference

[h] Rat

[i] Mallinckrodt, Research Department, St. Louis (unpublished data)

(β) *Carbamyl/Acyl Series* (Table 7). New Carbamyl functions include:

Carbamyl type	*Examples*
Hydroxyalkyl	$-CONHCH_2CH_2OH$
	$-CONHC(CH_2OH)_3$
Methylcarbamylmethyl	$-CONH-CH_2-CONH-CH_3$
Alkoxyalkyl	$-CONH-CH_2CH_2-OCH_3$
Oxazinyl	$\overset{\displaystyle\ \ \ \ \ \ \ \ CO\ \ \ \ \ \ \ \ }{-C=N-C(CH_2OH)_2-CH_2}$

Of these, CM containing THAM (trishydroxymethylaminomethane) had low toxicity but high viscosity:

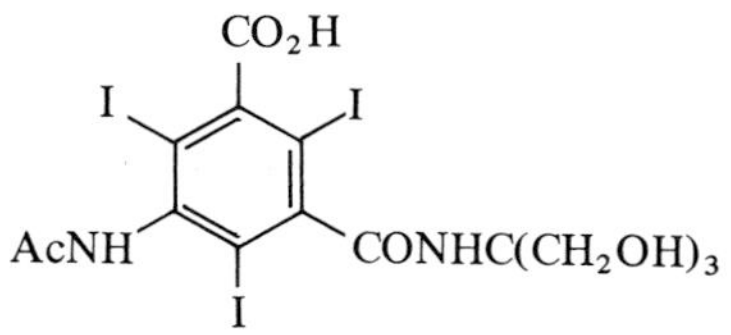

γ) Acylmethyl/Acyl Series (Table 8). Here improvements have been directed toward introducing more oxygen functions onto the side chain of the acylmethyl group, but without substantial improvement in acute systemic toxicity.

b) Bis Compounds (Table 9)

These compounds generally arise from the synthesis of novel side chains in the mononuclear series followed by conventional coupling through the amino function (Fig. 3). The Pharmacia and Bracco groups have used polyhydroxyalkoxy side chains to good advantage in preparing improved bis compounds [51–54]. These polyhydroxylated coupler chains do appear to offer advantages in safety and water solubility without appreciably affecting biliary clearance. It should be noted that having the "open" 5-position, (X=H), still provides useful compounds [55–58].

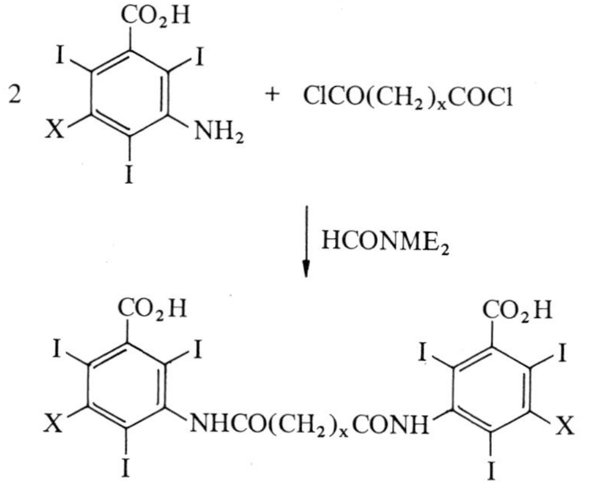

Fig. 3. Synthesis of ionic bis compounds

Table 8. Substituted triiodobenzoic acids: acylmethyl/acyl series

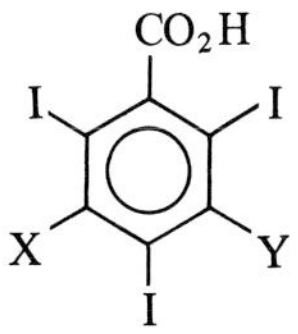

X	Y	Water solubility[a] (w/v)	Toxicity[b] i.v.	Toxicity[b] i.cereb.	Toxicity[b] i.cis.	Ref.
$CH_3CONHCH_2-$	$-NHCOCH_3$ [c]	>70 (M, Na)	6.6, 7.0	97	20[e]	[176, 198, 199]
$CH_3CONHCH_2-$	$-N(CH_2CHOHCH_2OH)COCH_3$		6.6	285	39	[176]
$CH_3CONHCH_2-$	$-N(CH_2CH_2OH)COCH_3$		5.7	120, 210	21	[176, 181]
$CH_3CHOHCONHCH_2-$	$-NHCOCH_2OH$ [d]	>65 (M, Na)	9.0	–	–	[199]
$CH_3CHOHCONHCH_2-$	$-NHCOCH_3$		9.6	–	–	[199]
$HOCH_2CONHCH_2-$	$-NHCOCH_2OH$		8.2	–	–	[199]
$CH_3CONHCH_2-$	$-NH-COCH_2OH$		6.2	–	–	[199]
$CH_3OCONHCH_2-$	$-NHCOCH_3$ [d]		7.8	–	–	[200]
$CH_3OCONHCH_2-$	$-NHCOCH_2OH$		7.7	–	–	[200]
$CH_3OCH_2CH_2OCONHCH_2-$	$-NHCOCH_2OCH_3$		7.0	–	–	[200]
$CH_3NHCOCH_2-$	$-NHOCH_3$	>64 (Na); >82 (M)	10.5 (rat, salt)	–	–	[201]
$CH_3CONHCH_2-$	$-NHCOCH_2OCH_3$ [e]	>75 (M)	–	–	–	[202]

[a] Na, sodium salt; M, meglumine salt

[b] In mice [intravenous (i.v.) or intracerebral (i.cereb.)] or rats [intracisternal (i.cis.)] as meglumine salt unless otherwise noted. Results, i.v. in mg I/kg; others mg I/kg

[c] Iodamide

[d] Example of structural type. Date for analogous compounds in reference

[e] Rabbit

Table 9. Bis compounds

X	Y	Z	Toxicity i.v. LD_{50} [a,b]	Ref.
$CH_3NHCOCH_3NHCO-$	$-NHCOCH_2-$	$-CH_2-O-(CH_2)_2-O-CH_2-$		[203, 204]
$CH_3CONHCH_2-$	$-N(COCH_3)CH_2-$	$-$		[205]
$CH_3NHCONH-$	$-CONHCH_2-$	$-(CH_2)_n-$		[206]
$CH_3NHCONH-$	$-NHCOCH_2-$	$-(CH_2)_n-$		[207]
CH_3CONH-	$-N(COCH_3)CH_2-$	$-(CH_2)_n-$		[208]
$CH_3CO(HOCH_2CH_2)N-$	$-N(COCH_3)CH_2-$	$-(CH_2)_n-$		[208]
CH_3CONH-	$-CH_2NHCO_2CH_2-$	$-CH_2^{c}-$	7.4 g/kg	[200]
CH_3CONH-	$-CH_2NHCO_2CH_2-$	$-CH_2-O-CH_2-$	10.5 g/kg	[200]
CH_3CONH-	$-N(COCH_3)CH_2-$	$-CHOHCH_2O-CH_2-CHOH-^{c}$		[209]
CH_3NHCO-	$-N(CH_3)COCH_2-$	$-(CH_2)_2-$	6.6 g I/kg	[210]
$CH_3CO(CH_3)N-$	$-N(COCH_3)CH_2-$	$-CHOH-CH_2-O-(CH_2)_4-O-CH_2-CHOH-$		[51–53]
CH_3NHCO-	$-NHCOCH_2-$	$-(CH_2)_6-^{c}$		[54]

CH₃CONHCH₂–	–NHCOCH₂–	–(CH₂)₂₋₆–		[54]
H–	–NHCOCH₂CH₂O–	–CH₂CH₂(OCH₂CH₂)₂– c,d	5.2 g/kg	[54]
CH₃NHCO–	–N(COCH₃)CH₂–	–CHOHCH₂OCH₂CHOH–		[211]
CH₂NHCOCH₂NHCO– c	–NHCO–	–CH₂–		[212]
CH₃NHCOCH₂NHCO– c	–NHCO–			[212]
CH₃CONH–	–N(CH₃)CO–			[213, 214]
CH₃NHCO–	–NHCO–	–CH₂OCH₂–		[189]
CH₃CONHCH₂– ⌐CO	–NHCO–	–CH₂SCH₂– (–CH₂OCH₂)ₓ– –(CH₂)₈–	10 g/kg	[215]
CH₂–CH₂–CH₂–N–CH₂–	–NH–CO–	–(CH₂)ₙ–		[226]
H	–NHCO–	–CH₂CH₂(OCH₂CH₂)₄–	5.1 g/kg	[55]
H	–NHCO–	–CH₂CH₂(OCH₂CH₂)₃–	4.4 g/kg	[56]
H	–NHCO–	–CHOHCH₂OCH₂CH₂CHOH–		[57]
H	–NHCO–	–(CH₂OCH₂)₃–		[58]
CH₃CON(C₂H₅)–	–NHCO–	–CH₂CH₂SO₂CH₂CH₂– e		[257]

[a] Na, sodium salt; M, meglumine salt

[b] In mice [intravenous (i. v.) or intracerebral (i. cereb.)] or rats [intra-cisternal (i. cis.)] as meglumine salt unless otherwise noted

[c] Example of structural type. Data for analogous compounds in reference

[d] Iodoxamic acid

[e] Iosulamide

Table 10. Structures of IVC agents [59]

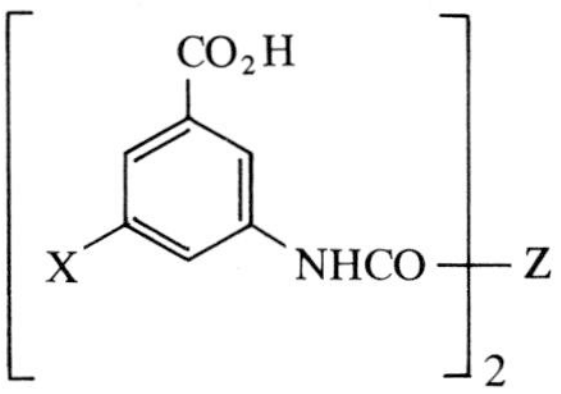

Compound			Protein binding	LD_{50} (g/kg)	Ref.
	X	Z			
Iodipamide	H–	$-(CH_2)_4-$	Strong	~2–3	[1]
Ioglycamate	H–	$-CH_2OCH_2-$	Strong	–	[1]
Iosefamate	CH_3NHCO-	$-(CH_2)_{10}-$	Moderate	~3	[46]
Iodoxamate	H–	$-(CH_2-CH_2O)_4-CH_2CH_2-$	Moderate	5.2	[52]
Iotroxate	H–	$-(CH_2OCH_2)_3-$	Moderate	~5–6	[56]
Iosulamide	$CH_3CON(C_2H_5)-$	$-(CH_2)_2-SO_2-(CH_2)_2-$	–	~6–8	[228]

With one exception (see discussion of iocarmate on p. 51) bis compounds have found their diagnostic utility as intravenous cholangiographic (IVC) agents (see Tables 9, 10). Iodipamide, an analog of acetrizoic acid, has been used clinically as a cholangiographic agent since 1954. It is strongly protein bound and relatively toxic. It is quite often administered by infusion with dextrose solution to minimize adverse reactions.

Synthesis efforts since the development of the first IVC agents have been directed toward the preparation of safer, better tolerated agents with comparable biliary uptake and excretion.

All the compounds in Table 10 have been evaluated as agents for enhancement of computed tomography scans, but as yet have not been found to be adequate, either providing little enhancement at usual clinical doses or requiring excessively large doses for only moderate enhancement.

Synthesis of ionic bis compounds is shown in Fig. 3.

c) Tris Compounds (Table 11)

Two series of compounds have been reported. Intravenous toxicity and water solubilities were improved when compared with the monomeric analogs. The somewhat improved osmotic properties did not outweigh the difficulty of preparing these compounds [49, 50, 60].

d) Miscellaneous Structures

α) *Aroylaminoacylamidobenzoic Acids* (Table 12). In an attempt to reduce osmotic activity and the charge, Tilly, Lautrou, and co-workers synthesized a

Table 11. Tris compounds

X	Y	Water solubility % w/v	Toxicity i.v.	i.cereb.	i.cis.	Ref.
CH$_3$NHCO–	–NHCOCH$_2$–	>65 (Na salt) >80% (NMG)	16.5 g/kg	480 mg I/kg	69 mg I/kg	[49, 50]
CH$_3$CONH–	–NHCOCH$_2$–	Sol.	14.3 g/kg	–	–	[49, 50]
CH$_3$CONH–	–NHCOCH$_2$–	Sol.	10.5 g/kg	–	–	[49, 50]
CH$_3$NHCO– CH$_3$CON(CH$_3$)– $\Big\}$ a						
CH$_3$CONH–	–CONH(CH$_2$)$_n$– b	Sol.	–	–	–	[60]
CH$_3$NHCO–NH–	–CONH(CH$_2$)$_n$– b	Sol.	–	–	–	[60]

a One each of indicated X group   b n=2–4

Table 12. Miscellaneous structures

Type	Water solubility (% w/v)	Toxicity (mg I/kg)			Ref.
		i.v.	i.cereb.	i.cis.	
Iodoaroylacylbenzoates					
X = CH$_3$CON(CH$_3$)– Y = –CONHCH$_3$ Z = –CH$_2$–CO– A = –CONHCH$_2$CH$_2$OH					[220]

series of aroylaminoacylamidotriiodobenzoic acid derivatives (the "monoacid dimers"), the most promising compound proving to be ioxaglic acid (Fig. 4) [61, 62].

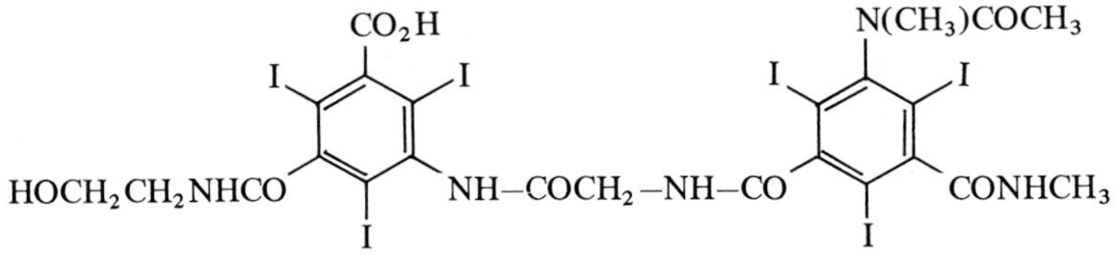

Ioxaglic acid

The molecular design provides six iodines per anion. In cardiovascular experiments in animals, ioxaglate's level of biological safety is similar to that of nonionic compounds. This CM is thus an improvement over classical ionic agents mainly because of lower osmolality. Due to its ionic nature ioxaglic acid is not suitable for intrathecal use. As would be expected, its viscosity is higher at a given

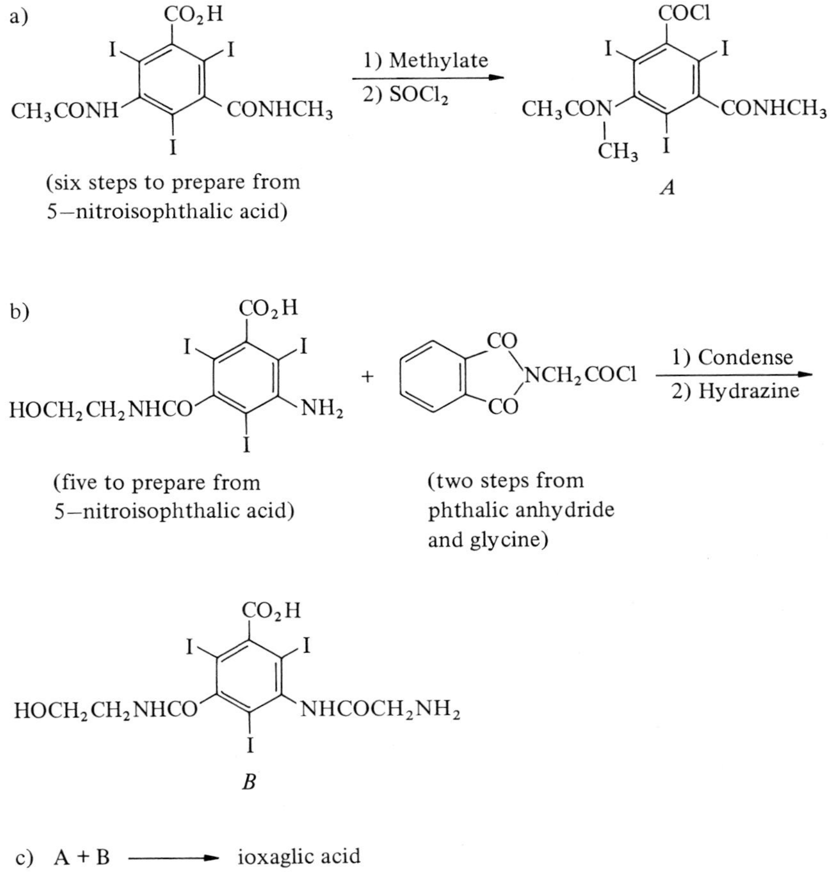

Fig. 4. Synthesis of ioxaglic acid

Table 13. Miscellaneous structures

Type			Water solubility (% w/v)	Toxicity (mg I/kg)			Ref.
X	Y	n		i. v.	i. cereb.	i. cis.	

C	Iodoaroylamino acids						
CH$_3$CO(CH$_3$)N−	−CONHCH$_3$	5		9,500 (M, 28)	−	−	[66]

Table 14. Miscellaneous structures

Type		Water solubility (% w/v)	Toxicity (mg I/kg)			Ref.
X	Y		i. v.	i. cereb.	i. cis.	

A	Triiodobenzoic acids					
H	H	9 (Na); 5 (M)	455	−	22.5	(Hoey et al., unpublished)
CH$_3$NH−	−H[a]					[217]
HOCH$_2$−	−NHCOC$_2$H$_5$[a]	6,450	92	−		[218]
CH$_3$CHOH−	−NHCOCH$_3$	5,910	47	−		[218]
CH$_3$−	−NHCOCH$_3$	2,800	−	−		[218]
CH$_3$O−	−CONHCH$_3$[a]					[219]
HO−	−NHCOCH$_3$[a]					[219]

[a] Example of structural type. Related compounds in reference

iodine concentration than those of comparable mononuclear triiodobenzoic acid compounds [12, 63–65].

Analogous to ioxaglate are the iodoarylamino acids (Table 13), likewise devised by Tilly and collaborators [66, 67].

Table 15. Miscellaneous structures

Type	CONHR$_1$			LD$_{50}$ rat, meg. (g/kg)	Urinary excretion rat, 3 h (% of dose)	Ref.

Structure:

$$\text{R}_2\text{CONH} \diagup \diagdown \text{COAOH}, \quad \text{I positions}$$

	A	R$_1$	R$_2$			
D	Aroylamino acids					
	DL-ala	CH$_3$–	CH$_3$–	18.5	78	
	gly	CH$_3$–	CH$_3$–	17.5	82	[221]
	gly	CH$_3$–	CH$_3$OCH$_2$–	20.0	74	
	DL-ser	CH$_3$–	CH$_3$–	7.5	77	

These compounds exhibit similar toxicity profiles to ioxaglate but as yet have not been clinically evaluated.

The "monoacid dimers" are compounds with potentially increased safety but are lengthy and tedious to synthesize. Thus ioxaglic acid is prepared in 18 steps from iothalamic acid, employing the amino precursor of ioxithalamic acid as the key intermediate.

β) Triiodobenzoic Acid Derivatives. Table 14 summarizes work reported with various substituted triiodobenzoic acid compounds. In general, these compounds contain either an acetamido or methylcarbamyl function, in addition to the novel side chain.

γ) Aroylamino Acids. KLIEGER and SCHROEDER [80] prepared and screened a series of substituted hippuric acids. These compounds, although structurally similar to the phenylalkanoates used as oral cholecystopaques, are highly water soluble in aqueous solution as salts, and on intravenous administration are excreted via the kidneys rather than via the biliary system. Excretion by this route is probably not only a function of the high water solubility but also the absence of protein binding resulting from the bis-acetamido function.

Table 15 summarizes the toxicity and excretion data for some of the compounds reported.

δ) Triiodobenzylamines. In 1970, HEBKY et al. published a series of triiodo-benzylamine derivatives (Table 16) [68–71]. This work culminated in the prepara-

Table 16. Miscellaneous structures

Type		Ref.
E	Benzyl amines	

1.

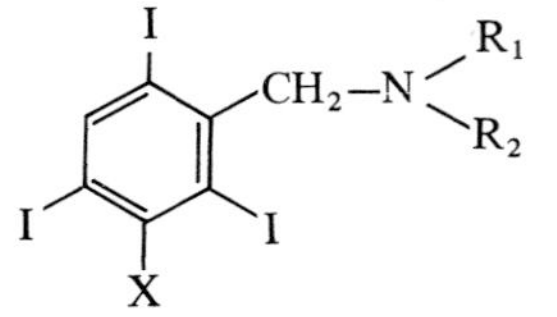

[68–71]

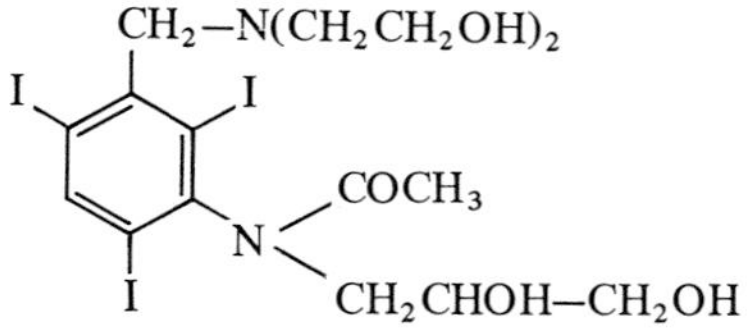

[68–71]

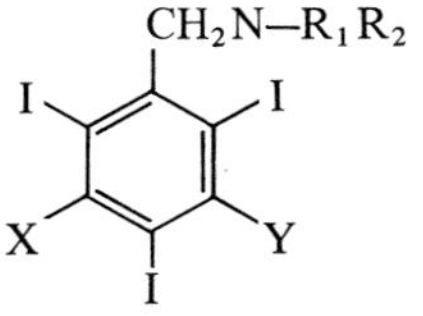

[68–71]

2. $Me_2-N^+-(CH_2)_n-N^+-Me_2 \cdot 2X^-$

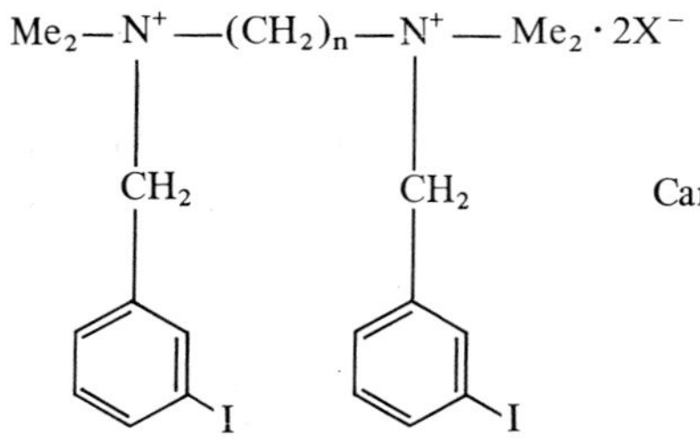

[72]

Cartilage binding

3.

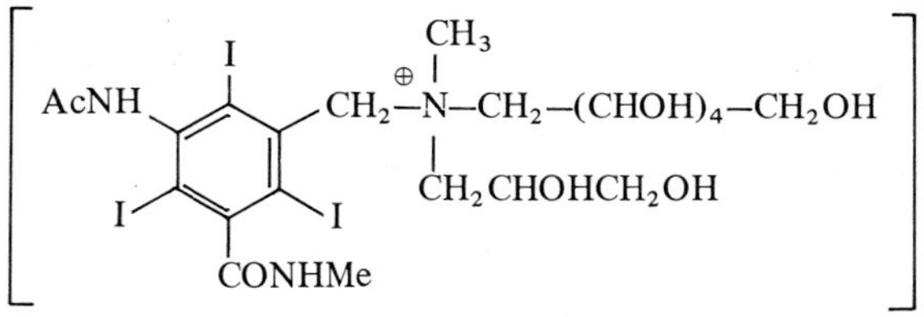

Cl^-

Iothalamate$^{\ominus}$

[73]

tion of the compound given below, which was clinically tested as a cholecystographic agent. These compounds are noteworthy in that they represent early examples of cationic media. Some of the compounds showed high water solubility.

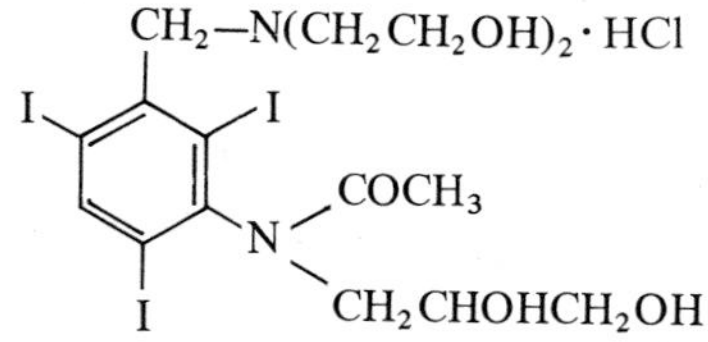

Oral LD$_{50}$(rat) 14 g/kg

VAN OOTEGHAM et al. [72] have reported the synthesis and evaluation of a series of bis iodophenylbenzylquaternary ammonium compounds postulated as cartilage-imaging agents. These compounds did not have significant cartilage affinity and were relatively toxic. SOVAK et al. [73] prepared several cationic CM in an attempt to improve both toxicity and osmotic properties of the molecules.

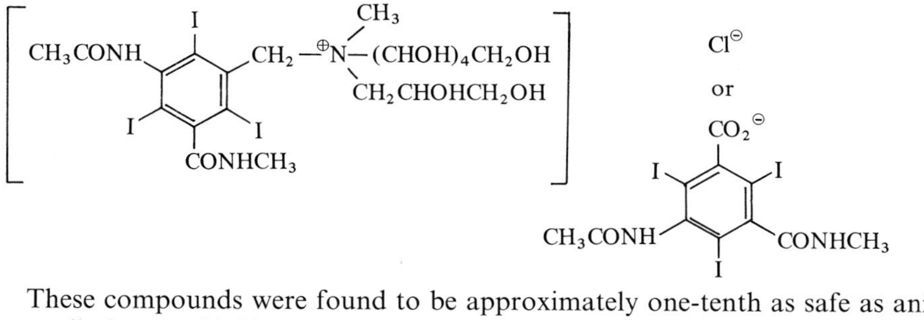

$$
\left[\begin{array}{c} CH_3CONH \quad CH_2 - \overset{\oplus}{N} \overset{CH_3}{\underset{CH_2CHOHCH_2OH}{-(CHOH)_4CH_2OH}} \\ \\ CONHCH_3 \end{array} \right]
$$

$$Cl^{\ominus}$$

or

$$CO_2^{\ominus}$$

$$CH_3CONH \quad CONHCH_3$$

LD$_{50}$

1,9 g/kg

2,4 g/kg

These compounds were found to be approximately one-tenth as safe as anionic media but are highly water soluble. Likewise, P. E. WIEGERT (unpublished data, Mallinckrodt, Inc., St. Louis) prepared the following compound and obtained comparable toxicity results:

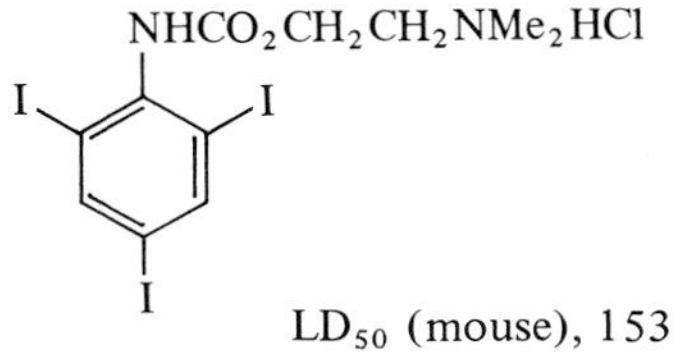

$$NHCO_2CH_2CH_2NMe_2HCl$$

LD$_{50}$ (mouse), 153 mg I/kg

More recently, however, SPECK et al. [74] disclosed a series of salts of X-ray CM wherein both the cationic and anionic portion of the molecule contain a 2,4,6-triiodobenzene moiety, for example:

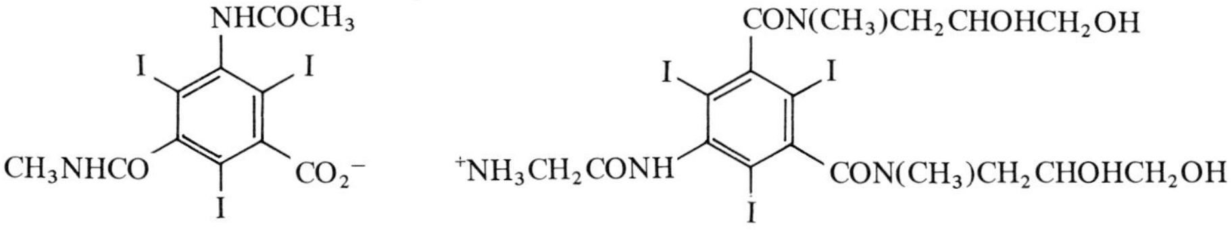

$$NHCOCH_3$$

$$CH_3NHCO \quad CO_2^-$$

$$CON(CH_3)CH_2CHOHCH_2OH$$

$$^+NH_3CH_2CONH \quad CON(CH_3)CH_2CHOHCH_2OH$$

Viscosity, 30% iodine solution, 37 °C = 2.4 cps
Molarity, 30% iodine solution   = 0.394 mol/liter
i.v. LD$_{50}$ mouse $\geq$ 10.5 g I/kg   i.v. LD$_{50}$ rat $\geq$ 10   g I/kg

Compounds of this series are reported to be highly water soluble with low toxicity. The osmolality is one-half that of conventional sodium or meglumine salts, which should provide greater tolerance in vivo.

ε) Miscellaneous. Through the years, a number of investigators have synthesized prototype compounds were stable carbon iodine bonds could be expected. The trisiodomethylacetamide compounds have been found to be relatively unstable. Iodomethanesulfonamides are known to be stable but of inadequate safety. Diiodofumaric acid proved to be too toxic for further consideration. Tetraiodoterephthalic acid derivatives appear to offer no advantage in terms of either water solubility or safety.

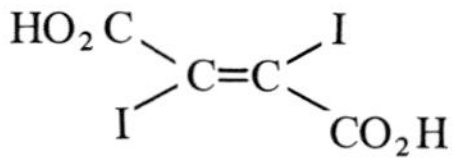

$$HO_2C \diagdown \atop I \diagup C=C \diagup ^I \diagdown _{CO_2H}$$

Diiodofumaric acids[75]

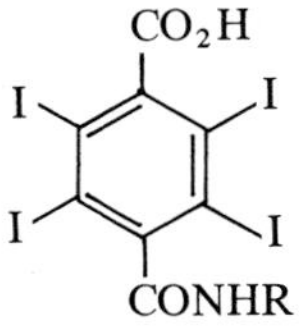

Tetraiodoterephthalic acids[77]

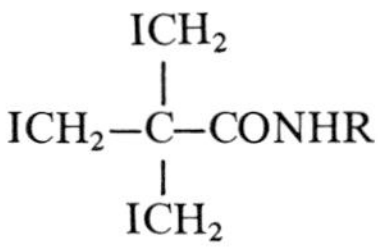

$$\begin{array}{c} ICH_2 \\ | \\ ICH_2-C-CONHR \\ | \\ ICH_2 \end{array}$$

Tris(iodomethylacetamides)[76]

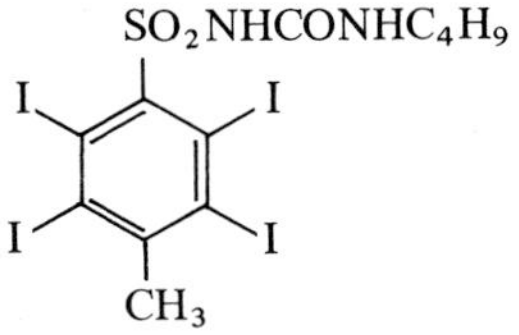

Iodosulfonylureas[78]

Table 17. Osmolality values for solutions of selected 2,4,6-triiodo-N-methylisophthalamic acid derivatives

Parent acid	Salt concentration[a] % (w/v)	Osmolality (mOsm/kg)
A	59.93	1,784
B	60.89	1,419
C	60.20	1,165

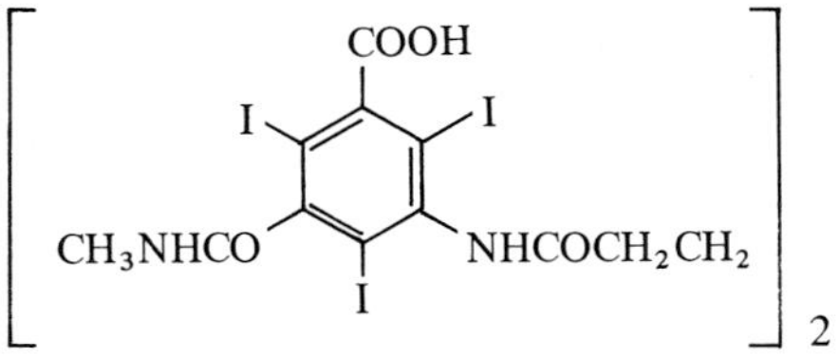

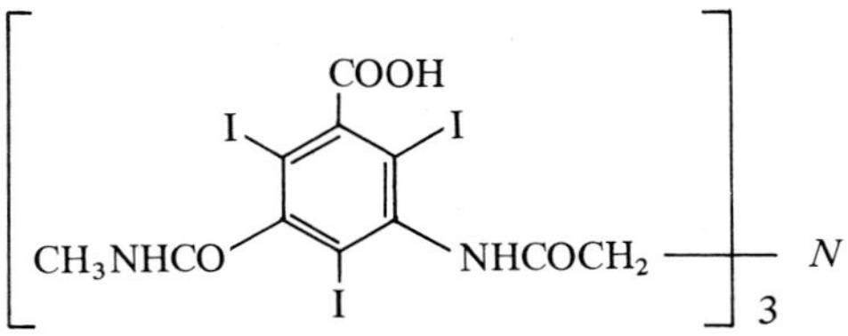

[a] As meglumine salt

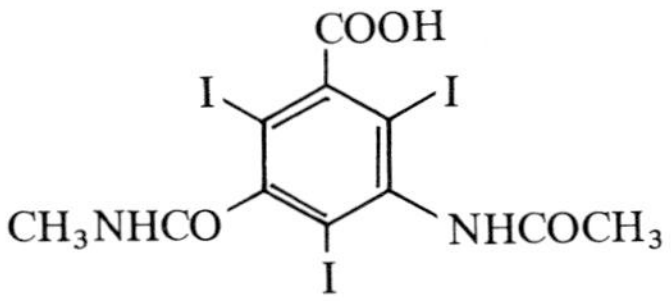

2. Reduction of Hypertonicity

a) Bis and Tris Compounds

Significant results have been achieved with this approach. Thus, the iothalamate molecule was converted to its bis analog by coupling with adipic acid to give the compound iocarmic acid. This compound has in the past been widely used clinically as an intrathecal (myelographic) agent. Most CM, as Tables 5, 1, 7 show, are too toxic for this application.

The "monovalent dimers" such as meglumine/sodium ioxaglate have resulted in significant improvements in osmotic properties and acute toxicity. This compound, while not suitable for myelography, as the nonionics are, is useful in angiography due to its low osmolality [30]. Compounds such as iocarmate and ioxaglate are more difficult to manufacture than the ionic monomers, but they are safer. The tris compounds described above are even more difficult to synthesize (Tables 17, 18), but their toxicity is not significantly improved.

b) Polymers

The ultimate extension of an ionic benzoic acid to minimum osmolality would be to form a polymer. Such polymers have been proposed and several synthesized [81–83]. A rational design of such a polymer would require that its molecular weight range be below the limits of permeability of the renal glomeruli, so that

Table 18. Bis compounds [79]

Compound	X	n	LD$_{50}$ (i. v. mice)	Protein binding Conc. $g \cdot 10^{-6}$	In albumin	In plasma
Iocarmate	$-CONHCH_3$	4	17.4 g/kg			
Iosefamate	$-CONHCH_3$	8	13.1 g/kg	700	–	93.97
				1,000	92.70	–
				10,000	81.69	80.87
MP-117	$-CONHCH_3$	10	4.8 g/kg	1,000	95.26	94.64
Intravenous cholecystopaques						
Iodipamide	$-H$	4	3.4 g/kg (rats)	1,000	98.44	98.70
				10,000	93.62	92.66
Ioglycamate	$-H$	5	~ 7.0 g/kg (rats)	1,000	95.27+	92.66
				10,000	85.60	–

Table 19. Polymeric X-ray CM

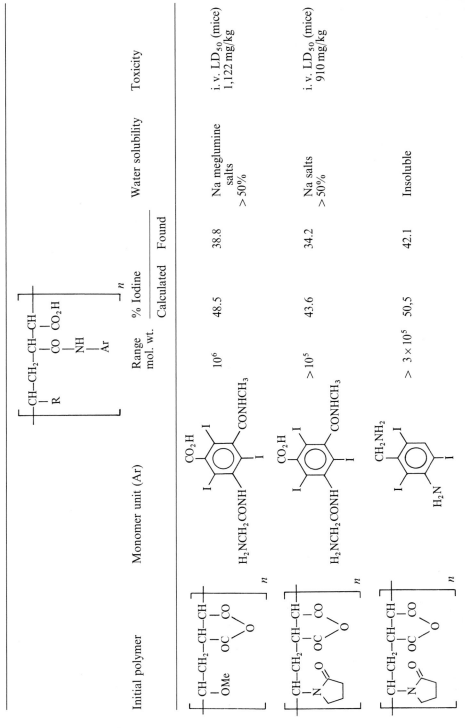

Initial polymer	Monomer unit (Ar)	Range mol. wt.	% Iodine Calculated	% Iodine Found	Water solubility	Toxicity
		10^6	48.5	38.8	Na meglumine salts > 50%	i. v. LD$_{50}$ (mice) 1,122 mg/kg
		>10^5	43.6	34.2	Na salts > 50%	i. v. LD$_{50}$ (mice) 910 mg/kg
		> 3×10^5	50,5	42.1	Insoluble	

(a) –A–B–A–B–A–B–A–B–A–B–A

(b)

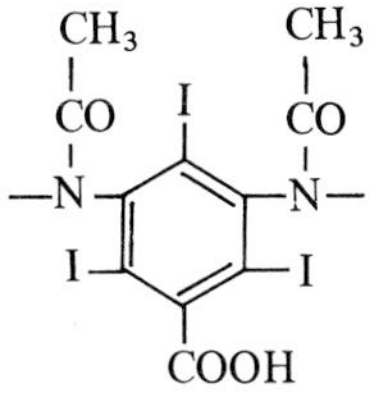

$$\text{(benzene ring with substituents: } CH_3\text{-}CO\text{-}N\text{-}, \; CH_3\text{-}CO\text{-}N\text{-}, \; COOH, \text{ and iodines)}$$

(c)

$$\text{(benzene ring with substituents: } CH_3\text{-}CO\text{-}N\text{-}, \; CH_3\text{-}CO\text{-}N\text{-}, \; COOH, \text{ and iodines)}$$

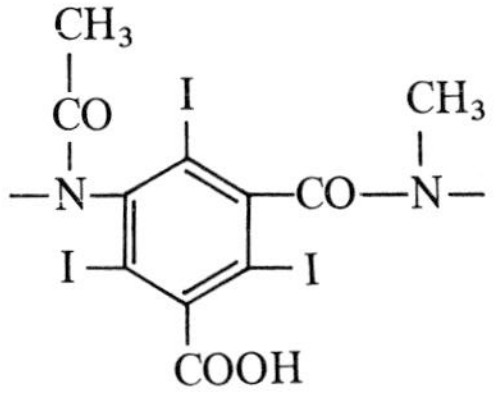

(d) $-CH_2CH(OH)CH_2OCH_2CH(OH)CH_2O(CH_2)_4OCH_2CH(OH)CH_2OCH_2CH(OH)CH_2-$

(e) $-CH_2CH(OH)CH_2O(CH_2)_4OCH_2CH(OH)CH_2-$

Type of iodine-containing unit A	Type of bridge B	Iodine content of dry polymer (1) as polyacid (2) as sodium salt	Mean mol. wt.	Type of salt in test solution[a]
c	e	46.1 (1)	–	M
c	e	45.5 (1)	4,000	M
c	e	46.1 (1)	5,000	M
c	e	44.7 (1)	14,000	M
c	e	44.7 (1)	41,000	Na
c	e	45.5 (1)	7,000	M
b	e	41.6 (2)	38,000	Na

[a] M, meglumine; Na, sodium

the compounds ultimately would be excreted. One would expect water solutions of polymer molecules to have a higher viscosity but lower osmotic activity and, therefore, greater safety, at least in some applications. Björk and Erikson synthesized a series of polymers based on both iothalamic acid and metrizoic acid (see Table 19 for structures). These compounds were found to be quite as water soluble as meglumine and, in some cases, as sodium salts and to have reasonably acceptable viscosities. They were evaluated as oral agents for gastrointestinal studies as well as in renal, thoracic, and cerebral angiography in several animal species. The results, while encouraging, did not justify pharmacological development.

In another approach, a suitably substituted triiodobenzoic acid was reacted with a commercially available polymer (see Table 19 for structure). These polymers had a high molecular weight and were too viscous and toxic (Mallinckrodt, Research Department, St. Louis, unpublished data).

D. Nonionic Contrast Media

Almen concluded that an ideal water-soluble CM should have low osmolality and low viscosity [84]. To achieve these objectives, he suggested that polymeric CM or nonionic CM containing no carboxyl or other solubilizing ionic functions be synthesized, as in principle they sould have one-half the osmotic effects of an analogous ionic compound. By 1970 it was well known that the water-solubilizing cations of ionic media, usually sodium and meglumine, are not biologically inert. Besides, many of the side reactions of the ionic media could be attributed to the hypertonicity and to the electrical imbalance of the solutions [85].

Polymeric ionic CM provided solutions which were substantially less hypertonic but viscous. Toxic manifestations resulted from low rate of excretion.

Prior to Almen's conclusions, two nonionic CM (1 and 2) [86, 87] were reported in 1966. However, compound 1 is insoluble in water; compound 2 is reportedly useful in an oral form for investigation of the biliary tract.

The first series of useful water-soluble, nonionic compounds was developed by ALMEN et al. [88, 89]. Some of these compounds were approximately twice as safe as conventional ionic CM when administered intravenously in animals and were one to two orders of magnitude safer than ionic media when injected intracisternally. Five compounds were selected for further evaluation and ultimately one of these – given the generic name metrizamide – has been made available clinically.

Metrizamide represents a pioneering development in water-soluble X-ray CM, since it has reached a new plateau in compound safety – particularly in the central nervous system. This compensates for its instability in aqueous solution under normal storage conditions. Metrizamide is available as a sterile, lyophilized powder which must be reconstituted prior to administration. The synthesis of metrizamide is more difficult than the synthesis of a conventional ionic CM. Its viscosity at 28%–35% iodine concentration is higher than for ionic monomers, but clinically acceptable. Unexpectedly the osmolality of solutions of metrizamide proved to be substantially below theoretical values (see Table 39).

The advent of nonionic CM has altered somewhat the requirements for improved water-soluble CM:

1. The compound must be stable in water solution when administered. Lyophilized dosage forms are acceptable where the dose is small and reconstitution of a powder is not impractical.
2. Viscosity of polyhydroxy compounds is generally acceptable. The low viscosity requirement prevails for some clinical applications.
3. In view of metrizamides certain clinical side effects, biological safety of new CM should be improved.
4. Polyhydroxy nonionic compounds should not be laborious and difficult to synthesize to avoid high manufacturing costs.

Since the first report of metrizamide, a number of laboratories have engaged in the synthesis and evaluation of a wide variety of nonionic CM, which meet the above criteria. The basic approach used in the design of new compounds is to couple a triiodinated aromatic moiety to one or more polyhydroxylated alkyl side chains:

Iodinated aromatic moiety	Coupler group	Polyhydroxylic group

The coupler groups which have been used are:

1. Amide
$$-\overset{\overset{\text{O}}{\|}}{\text{C}}-\underset{\underset{\text{R}}{|}}{\text{N}}-$$

2. Reversed amide
$$-\underset{\underset{\text{R}}{|}}{\text{N}}-\overset{\overset{\text{C}}{\|}}{\text{C}}-$$

3. Peptide $\quad -\overset{\overset{\displaystyle O}{\|}}{C}-\underset{\underset{\displaystyle R}{|}}{N}CH_2\overset{\overset{\displaystyle O}{\|}}{C}-\underset{\underset{\displaystyle R}{|}}{N}-$

4. Glycoside (ether, $-O-$)

5. Ureide $\quad -NH\overset{\overset{\displaystyle O}{\|}}{C}-\underset{\underset{\displaystyle R}{|}}{N}-$

6. Carbamate $\quad -NH\overset{\overset{\displaystyle O}{\|}}{C}-O$

7. Ester $\quad -\overset{\overset{\displaystyle O}{\|}}{C}-O-$

Several nonionic, iodinated methanesulfonamides have been discussed [88–90], but apparently these compounds did not offer advantages over available ionic media.

In the design of nonionic CM, three factors should be considered:

1. The coupler group
2. The X, Y groups on the aromatic nucleus
3. The stereochemistry of the polyhydroxyalkyl group

As is well known to those who concern themselves with the design and synthesis of new therapeutic or diagnostic compounds, water solubility, biological safety, and other physical and chemical parameters of a compound must await its synthesis and evaluation. In general, conclusions can be reached on a given homologous series after the chemical synthesis and animal testing, but it is impossible to predict either water solubility or biological safety, particularly in the field of CM, where there is a need for both high water solubility and very low toxicity for most clinical applications.

In general, based on the available data (see Tables 20–37), the order of safety for coupler groups appears to be as follows (the least toxic coupler group is given first):

Amide $\simeq$ reversed amide > peptide > glycoside (ether) > ureide > carbamate > ester

Interestingly, this order of toxicity appears to follow the relative hydrophilicity of the coupler groups given. It should be noted, of course, that these relationships could and probably would change with the synthesis and evaluation of additional compounds.

Many of the X, Y groups used for ionic CM have also been used for nonionic CM, and, in general, those groups which provide safe ionic CM also are safe for nonionic CM. However, the relative degree of safety may or may not correlate in a given series of ionic or nonionic compounds. The best X, Y groups, in terms of acute toxicity, are those which are hydrophilic. In the amide series of X, Y groups, mono-substituted amides are generally safer than are disubstituted amides, but exceptions can be noted.

Table 20. Nonionic X-ray CM: gluconanilides

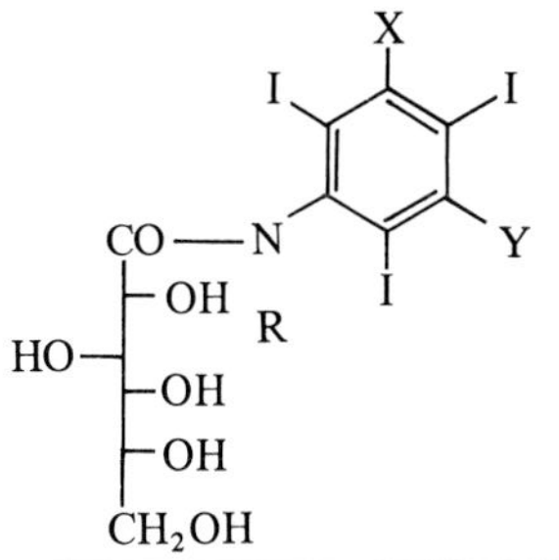

Compound No.	R	X	Y	Water solubility (% w/v)	% I	LD$_{50}$ (mg I/kg) i.v.	i.cis.	c.cereb.	Ref.
1	Me	-CONHMe	-CONHMe		48.99				[104]
2	H[a]	-CONHCH$_2$CH$_2$OH	-N(Me)Ac		48.00	9,000	> 58		[104]
3	Me	-CONHCH$_2$CH$_2$OH	-CONHMe		48.00		> 28		[104]
4	H[b]	-CONHMe	-CONHMe	1.2	49.89	>10,000	>150	> 750	[105]
5	H[c]	-CONHMe	-CONMe$_2$	28.4	48.99	8,085	100	2,350	[105]
6	H[d]	-CONHMe	-N(Me)Ac	> 100	48.99	6,400	75	1,175	[105]
7	H[e]	-CONHMe	-NHAc	8.6	49.90	11,000	180	~2,000	[105]
8	H	-CONHMe	-CH$_2$OH	1.86	51.73				[105]
9	H[f]	-CONHMe	-N(Ac)CH$_2$CH$_2$OH	14[k]	47.17	14,500	590	2,200	[105]
10	H[g]	-CONHMe	D-Gluconamido	3[k]	42.34	17,200	365	1,425	[105]
11	H[h]	-CONHMe	-CONHCH$_2$CH$_2$OH	40	48.87	~15,000	>400	>1,435	[105]
12	H[i]	-CONHMe	-CON(Me)CH$_2$CH$_2$OH	20	48.00	7,500	270	~1,800	[222]
13	H[j]	-CONHMe	-CON(Me)CH$_2$CHOHCH$_2$OH	22	46.25	~ 6,400	>270	~1,050	[222]

a P-297
b MP-5005
c MP-5007
d MP-5020
e MP-6012
f MP-6026
g MP-8000
h MP-7018
i MP-7017
j MP-7013
k Initially this compound was ~100% soluble in water for months

Table 21. Nonionic X-ray CM: 2-ketogulonamides

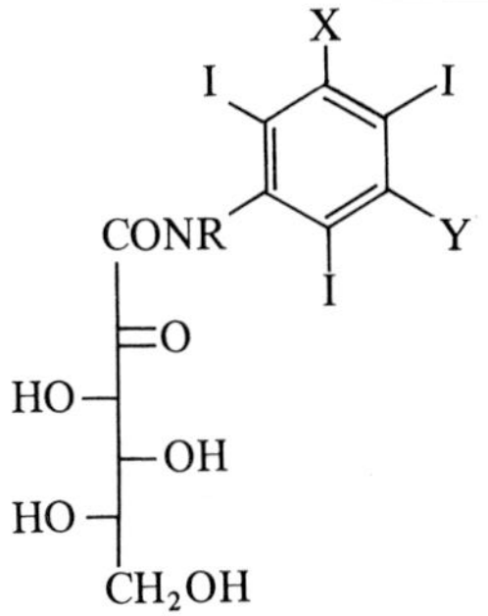

Compound No.	R	X	Y	Water Solubility (% w/v)	% I	LD₅₀ (mg I/kg) i.v.	i.cis.	i. cereb.	Ref.
1	H[a]	—CONHMe	—CONHMe$_2$	3.75	49.12				[105]
2	H[b]	—CONHMe	—N(Ac)CH$_2$CH$_2$OH	13	47.29	10,500	405	2,500	[105]
3	H[c]	—CONHMe	2-Ketogulonamido	100	42.60	~ 7,500	~740	–	[106]
4	H[d]	—CONHCH$_2$CH$_2$OH	2-Ketogulonamido	100	41.21	18,200	550	1,640	[107]
5	H[e]	—CONHCH$_2$CHOHCH$_2$OH	—CONHCH$_2$CHOHCH$_2$OH	93	43.21	19,300	744	1,470	[108]

[a] MP-5024
[b] MP-7014
[c] MP-10018
[d] MP-10007
[e] MP-10013

Table 22. Nonionic X-ray CM: miscellaneous reversed amides

Compound No.	Z	X	Y	Water solubility (% w/v)	%	LD$_{50}$ (mg I/kg) i.v.	i. cis.	i. cereb.	Ref.
1	CON(Me)– HO–OH HO–OH CHO	–CONHMe	–CONMe$_2$	>100	48.25	1,700	28	1,700	[105]
2	CONH– HO–OH HO–OH CHO	–CONHMe	–CONMe$_2$	13	49.11				[222]
3	CONH– HO–OH HO–OH CH$_2$OH	–CONHMe	–NHAc	1	48.87				[222]

Table 23. Nonionic X-ray CM: peptides

A—NR¹R²

Com-pound No.	X	Y	A	R¹	—NR²	% I	Water solubility (% w/v)	LD₅₀ (mg i/kg)			Ref.
								i. v.	i. cis.	i. cereb.	
1	—NHAc	—N(Me)Ac	—CONHCH₂CO—	H	2-Amino-2-deoxy-D-glucitol	44.89	100	~ 8,000	400	~1,100	[109]
2	—NHAc	—N(Me)Ac	—CONHCH₂CO—	Me	1-Amino-1-deoxy-D-glucitol	44.16	100	~ 9,600	438	1,030	[109]
3	—NHAc	—A—NR¹R²	—CONHCH₂CO—	Me	1-Amino-2.3-propanediol	42.81	100	>15,000	100	~1,425	[109]
4	—NHAc	—CONHMe	—CONHCH₂CO—	H	2-Amino-3-deoxy-D-glucitol	45.64	5	> 7,500	<200	> 543	[109]

Table 24. Nonionic X-ray CM: ureides

Compound No.	X	Y	R^1	$-NR^2$	% I	Water solubility (% w/v)	LD_{50} (mg I/kg) i.v.	i.cis.	i.cereb.	Ref.
1	H	–OMe	Me	1-Amino-1-deoxy-D-glucitol	52.72	< 1				[110]
2	–CONHMe	–N(Me)Ac	H	2-Amino-2-deoxy-D-glucose	57.35	100	6,800	~ 30	1,460	[110]
3	–CONHMe	–CONHMe₂	H	2-Amino-2-deoxy-D-glucose	47.35	100	4,800	16.9	1,720	[110]
4	–CONHMe	–N(Ac)CH₂CH₂OH	H	2-Amino-2-deoxy-D-glucitol	44.57	78	3,800	~ 35	~2,300	[110]
5	–CONHMe	–CONHMe₂	Me	1-Amino-1-deoxy-D-glucitol	46.42	100	1,900	21	1,500	[110]
6	–CONHMe	–CONHMe	H	2-Amino-2-deoxy-D-glucose	48.19	3		>266	> 900	[110]
7	–CONHMe	–NHAc	H	2-Amino-2-deoxy-D-glucose	48.19	18		62	> 350	[110]

Table 25. Nonionic X-ray CM: carbamates

Compound No.	X	R	% I	Water solubility (% w/v)	LD_{50} (mg I/kg) i.v.	i.cis.	i.cereb.	Ref.
1	CONHMe	1-L-Sorbose	47.29	20	3,000	13.0	1,450	[111]
2	N(Me)Ac	6-D-Galactose	47.29	100	~2,200	<20	222	[111]
3	N(Me)Ac	6-D-Glucose	47.29	100	~1,700	<50	1,670	[111]

Table 26. Nonionic X-ray CM: esters

Compound No.	X	Y	R	% I	Water solubility (% w/v)	LD_{50} (mg I/kg)			Ref.
						i.v.	i. cis.	i. cereb.	
1	−COOCH$_2$CHOHCH$_2$OH	−NHAc	−CH$_2$CHOHCH$_2$OH	50.83	5	~1,800	< 58		[a]
2	−COOCH$_2$CHOHCH$_2$OH	−N(Ac)CH$_2$CHOHCH$_2$OH	−CH$_2$CHOHCH$_2$OH	46.25	100	~2,300	<100		[a]
3	−CONHMe	−NHAc	6-Glucose	49.05 ~ 50	50	~ 450		<25	[a]

[a] Mallinckrodt, Reseach Department, St. Louis (unpublished results)

Table 27. Nonionic X-ray CM: glycosides and glucose derivatives

Compound No.	A	B	X	Y	R¹	Water-solubility (% w/v)	% I	LD$_{50}$ (mg I/kg) i.v.	i.cis.	i.cereb.	Remarks	Ref.
1	H	I	OR¹	OR¹	β-D-Glucosyl	∞	29.4	9,000			Code name: DTB Viscosity: 56.8 cps (66.6% w/v, 20°) 33.3 cps (66.6% w/v, 40°) Log P(BuOH/H$_2$O) = −1.24, (OcOH/H$_2$O) = −2.23	[94, 223, 225]
2	I	I	NHAc	−CONHMe	β-D-Glucosyl	∞	50.9	13,000			Log P(BuOH/H$_2$O) = −0.26 Log P(OcOH/H$_2$O) = −1.26	[94, 95, 225]
3	I	I	OR¹	−CONHMe	β-D-Glucosyl	∞	43.80				Log P(BuOH/H$_2$O) = −0.54	[95]
4	I	I	H–	H–	β-D-Glucosyl	0.4	46.08				Log P(BuOH/H$_2$O) = 0.30	[95]
5	H	I	OR¹	H–	β-D-Glucosyl	0.8	36.24				Log P(BuOH/H$_2$O) = −0.29	[95]
6	I	H	OR¹	H–	β-D-Glucosyl	0.2	36.24				Log P(BuOH/H$_2$O) = 0.53	[95]
7	I	I	OR¹	HOCH$_2$CONH–	3-Glucose		43.01	[a]		[a]	Code name: DL 2-98	[224]

[a] Similar to iopamidol and metrizamide

Table 28. Nonionic X-ray CM: benzamides/-2-glucose derivatives

Compound No.	X	Y	Z	Water solubility (% w/v)	% I	LD$_{50}$ (mg I/kg) i.v.	i.cereb.	Ref.
1	-N(Ac)CH$_2$CH$_2$OH	-N(Me)Ac	-CHO	>50	45.69	8,250	>1,500	[88, 89]
2	-NHAc	-N(Me)Ac	-CHO	>50 (80)^a	48.25	15,000 (10,200)^a	>1,500 (1,400)^a	[88, 89]
3	-N(Ac)CH$_2$CH$_2$OH	-N(Ac)ch$_2$CH$_2$OH	-CHO	>50	44.11	>12,000	>1,500	[88, 89]
4	-NHAc	-NHAc	-CHO	>50	49.12	>15,000		[88, 89]
5	-NHAc	-N(Me)Ac	-CH$_2$OH	>50	48.12		>1,500	[88, 89]
6	-NHAc	-NHAc	-CH$_2$OH		48.98			[88, 89]
7	-NHAc	-CONHMe	-CHO		49.11			[88, 89]
8	-NHAc	-CONHMe	-CH$_2$OH		48.99			[88, 89]
9	-N(Ac)CH$_2$CH$_2$OH	-CONHMe	-CHO		46.47			[88, 89]
10	-N(Ac)CH$_2$CH$_2$OH	-CONHMe	-CH$_2$OH		46.36			[88, 89]
11	-N(Me)Ac	-H	-CHO	>50	52.10			[88, 89]
12	-NHAc	-N(Me)Ac	-CHO^b		48.25			[88, 89]

^{a} See Ref. [97, 98]

^{b} Mannose isomer rather than glucose

Table 29. Nonionic X-ray CM: benzamides/1-glucamine derivatives

Compound No.	X	Y	R	Water solubility (% w/v)	% I	LD$_{50}$ (mg I/kg) i.v.	i. cereb.	Ref.
1	−N(Me)Ac	−H	H	>50	51.87			[88, 89]
2	−N(Ac)$_2$	−N(Me)Ac	ME		44.93			[88, 89]
3	−NHAc	−N(Me)Ac	Me	>50	47.29	6,000	>750	[88, 89]
4	−NHAc	−CONHMe	Me	>50	48.11	10,000	>1,500	[88, 89]
5	−NHAc	−CH$_2$NHAc	Me	>50	47.29			[88, 89]
6	−N(Me)COCH$_2$CH$_2$CH$_3$	−H	Me		48.18			[88, 89]
7	−NHCOCH$_2$CH$_2$CH$_3$	−H	Me		49.05			[88, 89]
8	−NHAc	−NHAc	H		48.98			[88, 89]
9	−NHAc	−CONHMe	H		48.99			[88, 89]
10	−N(Ac)CH$_2$CH$_2$OH	−CONHMe	H		46.36			[88, 89]
11	−NHAc	−NHAc	Me	7.9	48.11			[88, 89]
12	−H	−H	Me		56.28			[88, 89]
13	−NHAc	−H	Me	>50	51.87			[88, 89]
14	−N(Me)Ac	−H	Me	>50	51.0			[88, 89]
15	−N(Me)Ac	−NHAc	H		48.12	14,250	>750	[88, 89]
16	−N(Me)Ac	−N(Ac)CH$_2$CH$_2$OH	Me		44.83		>2,000	[88, 89]
17	−N(Me)Ac	−N(Ac)CH$_2$CH$_2$OAc	Me	20–50	42.72			[88, 89]
18	−N(Me)Ac	−N(Ac)CH$_2$CHOHCH$_2$OH	Me		43.20			[88, 89]
19	−N(Ac)CH$_2$CH$_2$OH	−N(Me)Ac	Me	>50	43.20	7,500	>2,000	[88, 89]
20	−NHAc	−CONHMe	−CH$_2$CH$_2$OH		46.36	15,000	>1,500	[88, 89]

Table 30. Nonionic X-ray CM: benzamides/heptitol derivatives

Compound No.	X	Y	Polyhydroxylamine (—NHR)	% I	Water solubility (% w/v)	LD_{50} (mg I/kg)			Ref.
						i. v.	i. cis.	i. cereb.	
1	—NHAc	—N(Me)Ac	1-Amino-1-deoxy-D-glycero-1-mannoheptitol	46.37	25	~12,500	100	>2,736	[222]
2	—NHAc[a]	—N(Me)Ac	1-Amino-1-deoxy-D-glycero-D-idoheptitol	46.37	~100	13,000	370	1,300	[222]
3	—NHAc	—N(Me)Ac	1-Amino-1-deoxy-D-glycero-D-guloheptitol	46.37	~100	~11,300	>525		[222]
4	—NHAc	—CONHMe	1-Amino-1-deoxy-D-glycero-D-idoheptitol	47.17	7	>2,600	>66	>233	[222]

[a] MP-7011

Table 31. Nonionic X-ray CM: benzamides/alkanol derivatives

Compound No.	$CONR_1R_2$				Water solubility (%, w/v)	% I	Ref.
	R_2	R_1	X	Y			
1	$-CH_2CHOHCH_2OH$	H	$N(Ac)CH_2CH_2OH$	$-N(Me)Ac$	>50	50.20	[88, 89]
2	$-CH_2CH_2OH$	$-CH_2CH_2OH$	$N(Ac)CH_2CH_2OH$	$-N(Ac)CH_2CH_2OH$	>50	45.47	[88, 89]
3	$-CH_2CH_2OH$	$-CH_2CH_2OH$	$-N(Me)Ac$	$-NHAc$	21.3	53.23	[88, 89]
4	$-CH_2CH_2OH$	$-H$	$-N(Me)Ac$	$-N(Ac)CH_2CH_2OH$	0.4	53.23	[88, 89]
5	$-CH_2CH_2OH$	$-Me$	$-N(Me)Ac$	$-N(Ac)CH_2CH_2OH$	25.5	52.52	[88, 89]
6	$-CH_2CH_2OH$	$-CH_2CH_2OH$	$-N(Me)Ac$	$-N(Ac)CH_2CH_2OH$	>50	50.20	[88, 89]
7	$-CH_2CHOHCH_2OH$	$-H$	$-N(Me)Ac$	$-N(Ac)CH_2CH_2OH$	0.26	51.10	[88, 89]
8	$-C(CH_2OH)_3$	$-H$	$-N(Me)Ac$	$-N(Ac)CH_2CH_2OH$	0.86	49.10	[88, 89]
9	$-CH_2CHOHCH_2OH$	$-Me$	$-N(Ac)CH_2CH_2OH$	$-N(Ac)CH_2CH_2OH$	>50	48.23	[88, 89]
10	$-CH_2CH_2OH$	$-H$	$-N(Ac)CH_2CH_2OH$	$-N(Ac)CH_2CH_2OH$	21.4	51.10	[88, 89]
	$-CH_2CHOHCH_2OH$	$-H$	$-N(Ac)CH_2CHOHCH_2OH$	$-N(Ac)CH_2CHOHCH_2OH$	∞		[259]

Table 32. Nonionic X-ray CM: isophthalamides

Compound No.	X	R₁	R₂	Water solubility (% w/v)	% I	LD₅₀ (mg I/kg) i.v.	i.cis.	i.cereb.	Ref.
1	$-NHAc$	$-CH_2CHOHCH_2OH$	Me	$>50^a$	49.11	$13,500^a$		ca. $1,500^a$	[88, 89, 97, 98]
2	$-N(Ac)CH_2CH_2OH$	$-CH_2CHOHCH_2OH$	Me		46.47				[88, 89]
3	$-NHAv$	$-CH_2CH_2OH$	$-CH_2CH_2OH$		49.11				[88, 89]
4	$-NHAc$	$-CH_2CHOHCH_2OH$	H	0.5	50.95				[88, 89, 97, 98, 222]
5	L-$CH_3CHOHCONH-$	$-CH_2(CH_2OH)_2$	H	89	48.99	21,800	250 (rabbits)	1,500	[97, 98]
6	D,L-$CH_3CHOHCONH-$	$-CH(CH_2OH)_2$	H	30	48.99				[97, 98]
7	L-$CH_3CHOHCONH-$	$-CH_2CHOHCH_2OH^b$	H	15.7	48.99				[87, 98]
8	D,L-$CH_3CHOHCONH-$	$-CH_2CHOHCH_2OH$	H	14	48.99				[97, 98]
9	$-NHAc$	$-CH_2(CH_2OH)_2$	H	0.2	50.95				[97, 98]
10	D,L-$HOCH_2CHOHCONH-$	$-CH_2(CH_2OH)_2$	H	"Good"	48.00				[97, 98]
11	D,L-$HOCH_2CHOHCONH-$	$-CH_2CHOHCH_2OH$	H		48.00				[97, 98]
12	$-NHAc$	$(+)-CH_2CHOHCH_2OH$	H		50.95				[226]
13	$-NHAc$	$(-)-CH_2CHOHCH_2OH$	H		50.95				[226]
14	$-N(Ac)CH_2CH_2OH$	$(+)-CH_2CHOHCH_2OH$	H	$83-104^c$	48.12				[226]
15	$-N(Ac)CH_2CH_2OH$	$(-)-CH_2CHOHCH_2OH$	H	$83-104^c$	48.12				[226]
16	$-N(Ac)CH_2CHOHCH_2OH$	$(\pm)-CH_2CHOHCH_2OH$	H	$83-104^c$	48.12				[226]
17	$-N(Ac)CH_2CHOHCH_2OH$	$(\pm)-CH_2CHOHCH_2OH$	H	$86-108^c$	46.36				[226]
18	$-NHCOCH_2OCH_3$	$(\pm)-CH_2CHOHCH_2OH$	CH_3, H^d		48.1				[228]
19	$(\pm)-HOCH_2CHOHCH_2N(CH_3)CO-$	$(\pm)-CH_2CHOHCH_2OH$	CH_3		46.8				[229]

a Ref. [91] reports a water solubility of 55%, an i.v. LD₅₀ of 15,700 and an i.cereb. LD₅₀ of 820

b Substitution of the pure D or L form of the amine provides compounds which are practically infinitely soluble in water

c These solutions may be supersaturated

d $R_1=CH_2-$ at C_1 carbamyl group; $R_2=H-$ at C_3 carbamyl group

Table 33. Nonionic X-ray CM: bis compounds (amide coupler)

Compound No.	R¹	R²	X	Water solubility (% w/v)	% I	Osmotic pressure (atm.) 300 mg I; 37°C	LD$_{50}$ (mg I/kg) i.v.	i.cereb.	Osmolality (300 mg I/ml) mOsm/kg H$_2$O	Protein binding 1.2 mg I/ml	Erythrocite damage 43 mg I/ml	Ref.
1	$-CH_2CHOHCH_2OH$	Me		>60	50.1	4.5	>10,000	Good	175	1.4[a]	0.33[a]	[100]
2	$-CH_2CH_2OH$	H			56.66							[100]
3	$-CH_2CH_2OH$	Me			55.50							[100]
4	$-CH_2CH_2OH$	$-CH_2CH_2OH$			50.1							[100]
5	$-C(CH_2OH)_3$	H			50.1							[100]
6	$-CH_2CH_2CH_2OH$	H			55.5							[100]
7	$-CH_2CHOHCH_3$	H			55.5							[100]
	$-CHCHOH(CH_2OH)_2$[b]		CH_2	∞	46.7		>24,000		300		0.2	[100, 101]
	$-CHCHOH(CH_2OH)_2$[b]		CH_2-CH_2	∞			>24,000		300			

[a] For comparison, the authors state that metrizamide has a protein-binding value of 6.2 and an erythrocyte index of 3.86 (scale 0–5)

[b] D,L threitol

Table 34. Nonionic X-ray CM: bis compounds (amide coupler)

Compound No.	X	R	Y	Water solubility (% w/v)	% I	Osmotic pressure (atm.) 37°C 400 mg I	LD$_{50}$ (mg I/kg) i.v.	i.cis	i.cereb.	Ref.
1	$-NHCH(CHOH)_2$	H	$-(CH_2CH_2O)_2CH_2CH_2-$	~ 50 (20 °C) 100 (boiling)	50.09	8.15			1,100	[102, 103]
2	$-NHCH(CHOH)_2$	H	$-CH_2-(CH_2CH_2O)_4(CH_2)_3-$	~100	46.53				990	[102, 103]
3	$-N(H)CH(CH_2OH)_2$	CH$_3$	$-(CH_2CH_2O)_3CH_2CH_2-$	Dissolves readily	47.28	10.59	14,000	233 (rabbit)		[102, 103]
4	$-N(H)CH(CH_2OH)_2$	CH$_3$	$-CH_2-(CH_2CH_2O)_4-(CH_2)_3-$	Dissolves readily	45.74	9.42			1,420	[102, 103]
5	$-NHCH(CH_2OH)_2$	H	$-(CH_2CH_2O)_3CH_2CH_2-$		48.29					[102, 103]
6	$-NHCH_2CHOHCH_2OH$	Me	$-CH_2-(CH_2CH_2O)_4-(CH_2)_3-$	Dissolves readily	45.74					[102, 103]
7	$-NHC(Me)(CH_2OH)_2$	H	$-CH_2-(CH_2CH_2O)_4-(CH_2)_3-$	Dissolves readily	45.74					[102, 103]
8	$-NHC(Me)(CH_2OH)_2$	H	$-(CH_2CH_2O)_4-CH_2CH_2-$	Dissolves readily	46.53					[102, 103]
9	$-NHC(Me)(CH_2OH)_2$	H	$-CH_2CH_2OCH_2CH_2-$	100	50.62					[102, 103]
10	$-NHCH(CH_2OH)_2$	H	$-(CH_2CH_2O)_4-CH_2CH_2CH_2-$		47.34					[102, 103]
11	$-NHCH(CH_2OH)_2$	H	$-(CH_2CH_2O)_5CH_2CH_2-$		46.07					[102, 103]

Table 35. Nonionic X-ray CM: bis compounds (amide coupler)

Compound No.	R	X	% I	i.v. LD_{50}	Ref.
1	(±)-NHCH(CH$_2$OH)CHOHCH$_2$OH (D,L-threitol)	$-CH_2-$	46.8	> 26 g I/kg	[101]
2	(±)-NHCH(CH$_2$OH)CHOHCH$_2$OH (D,L-threitol)	$-CH_2O-CH_2-$	46.0	> 26 g I/kg	[101]

Table 36. Nonionic X-ray CM: bis-polyhydroxylated acylamides (hexaiodinated)

Compound No.	X	Y	Z	Water solubility (% w/v)	% I	Osmolality (mOsm/kg) (28% I)	Viscosity	LD$_{50}$ (mg I/kg) i.v.	i.cis	i.cereb.	Ref.
1	−N(Me)Ac	−N(Me)Ac	−NHCH$_2$CH$_2$NH−	~ 51	49.06	200	7.4 cps (25% I, 37 °C)	15,000			[108]
2	−N(Me)Ac	−N(Me)Ac	−NHNH−		49.96	204		6,000			[108]
3	−N(Me)Ac	−N(Me)Ac	−N(Me)N(Me)−		49.06	140		9,000			[108]
4	−CONHCH$_2$CH$_2$OH	−CONHCH$_2$CH$_2$OH	−NHNH−		48.93						[108]
5	−CONHCH$_2$CH$_2$OH	−CONHCH$_2$CH$_2$OH	−NHCH$_2$CH$_2$NH−		48.06						[108]
6	−CONHCH$_2$CH$_2$OH	−CONHMe	−NHCH$_2$CH$_2$NH−		48.99						[108]
7	−CONHMe	−CONHMe	−NH(CH$_2$)$_4$NH−	3	49.06			> 10,000	> 177	~1,188	a
8	−N(Ac)CH$_2$CH$_2$OH	−N(Ac)CH$_2$CH$_2$OH	−NH(CH$_2$)$_4$NH	100	46.42			~ 7,500	≦ 70		a

a Mallinckrodt, Research Department, St. Louis (unpublished results)

Table 37. Nonionic X-ray CM: iodomethane sulfonamides

$$I-CH_2-SO_2N\overset{R_1}{\underset{R_2}{|}}$$

Compound No.	R_1	R_2	Water solubility (% w/v)	% I	LD$_{50}$ i.v. mg/kg	i. cis mg I/kg	i. cereb. mg I/kg	Ref.
1	$-CH_2CH_2OH$	H	50	47.87	4,150	58.9	214	[90]
2	$-CH_2(CH_2OH)_2$	H	153	43.01	10,900	89	385	[90]
3	$-CH_2CHOHCH_2OH$	H	45 (55)	43.01	9,500	99	370	[90]
4	$-CH_2CHOHCH_2OH$	Me		41.06	6,900		310	[90]
5	$-CH_2CH_2OCH_2CH_2OH$	H	50	41.06	6,100	96	262	[90]
6	$-H$	H	0.2	57.42				[90]
7	D-Gluco- $-CH_2(CHOH)_4CH_2OH$	Me	~10	31.8	> 1,000			[88–90]
8	$-CH_2CH_2OH$	$-CH_2CH_2OH$	6	40.9				[88–90]

A review of the tables reveals the following trends:

1. (Poly)hydroxyalkylacylamides (e.g., $CH_3CHOHCONH-$) > acylamides (e.g., $AcNH-$) > N-(hydroxyalkyl)acylamides [e.g., $AcN(CH_2CH_2OH)-$] > N-alkyl amides [e.g., $AcN(Me)-$]
2. N-(Poly)hydroxyalkylcarbamoyl (e.g., $CONHCH_2CHOHCH_2OH$) > N-alkylcarbamoyl (e.g., $-CONHMe$) > N,N-dialkylcarbamoyl (e.g., $-CONMe_2$)

Although there are fewer examples (Tables 20–22, 25), the stereochemistry of the polyhydroxyalkyl group can influence the properties of the candidate CM as can be seen in the reversed amide series of compounds wherein: 2-ketogulonamido ≧ gluconamido > galacturonamido, and in the carbamate series wherein the order of toxicity (LD_{50} value) is: L-sorbose > D-galactose > D-glucose.

Nonionic compounds which have been evaluated for both intravascular and intrathecal administration are shown in Fig. 5.

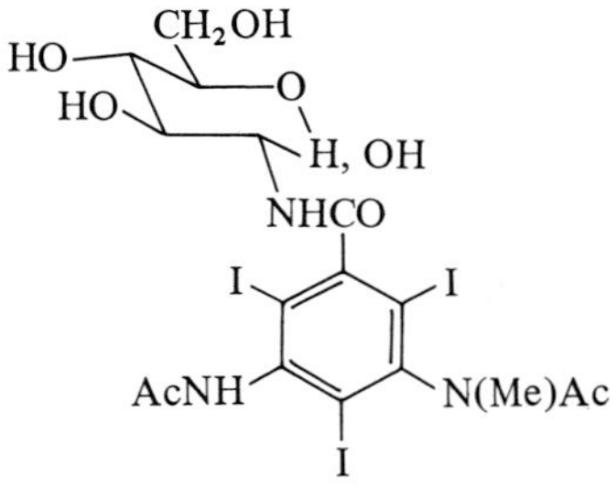

Metrizamide
(amide coupler, Table 28)

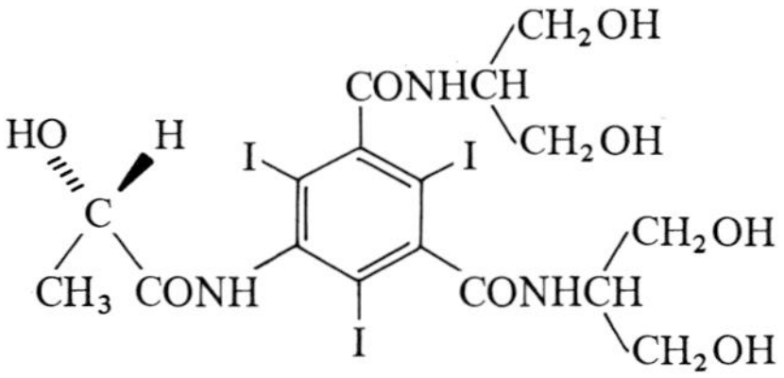

Iopamidol
(amide and reversed amide coupler,
Table 32)

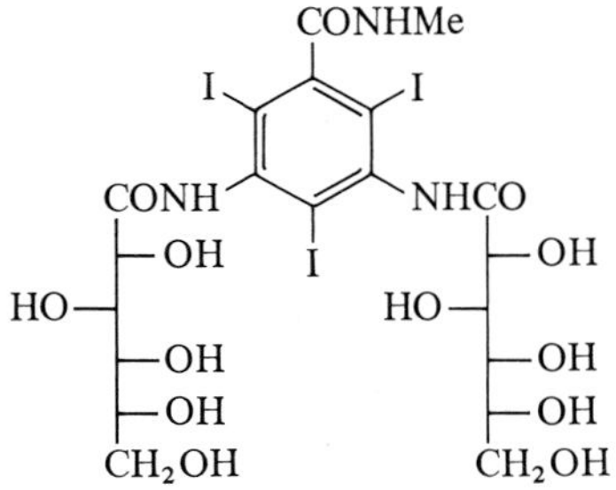

Ioglucomide (MP–8000)
(reversed amide coupler, Table 20)

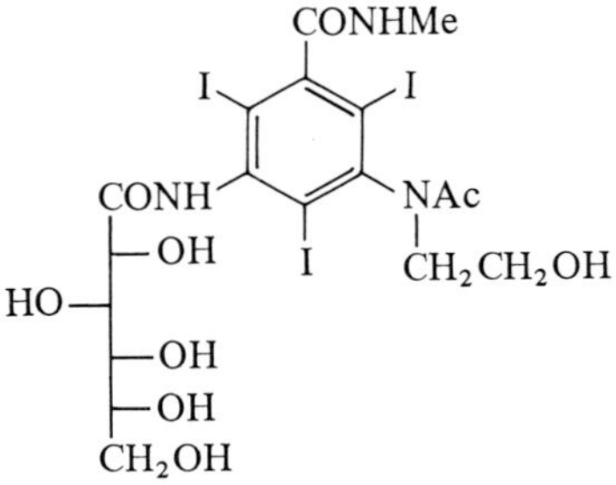

Ioglucol (MP–6026)
(reversed amide coupler, Table 20)

Fig. 5. Nonionic compounds

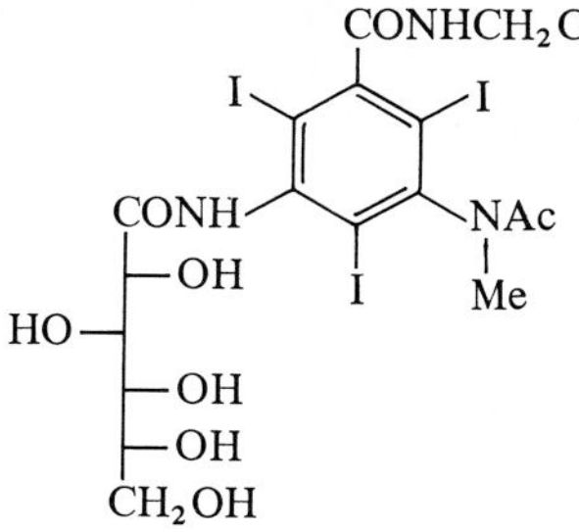

P–297
(reversed amide coupler, Table 20)

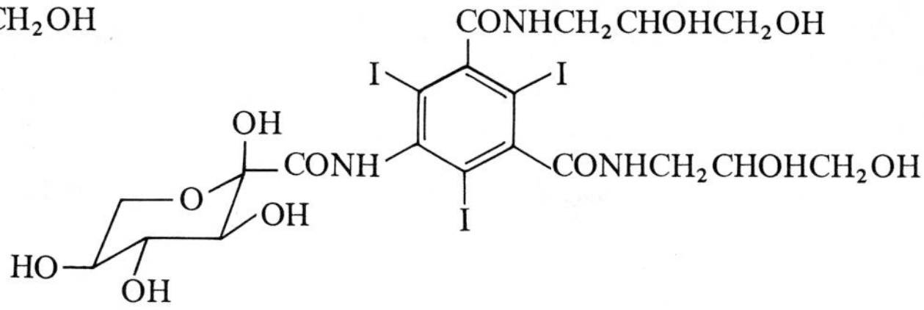

Iogulamide (MP–10013)
(reversed amide coupler, Table 21)

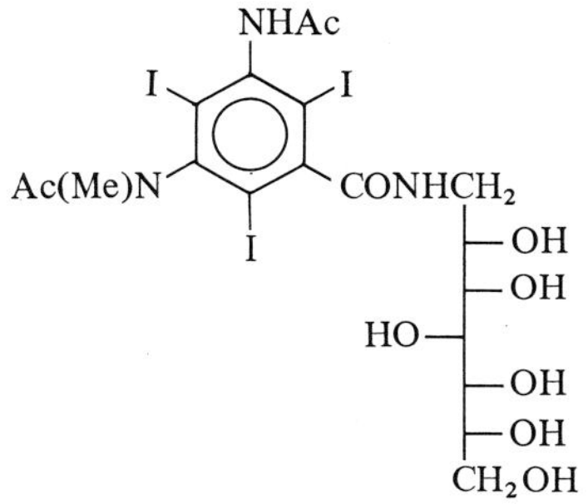

MP–7011
(amide coupler, Table 30)

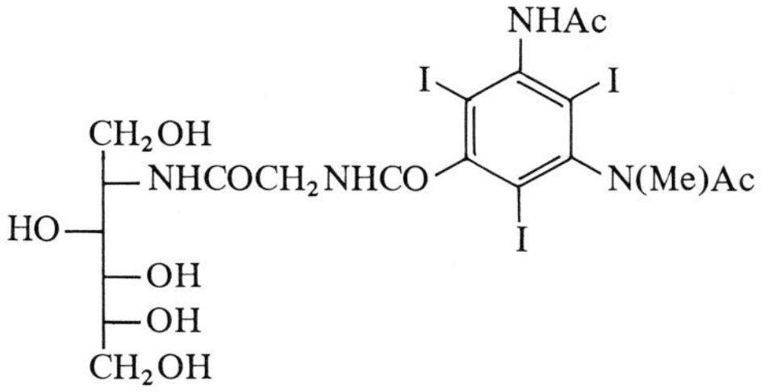

MP–7012
(peptide coupler, Table 23)

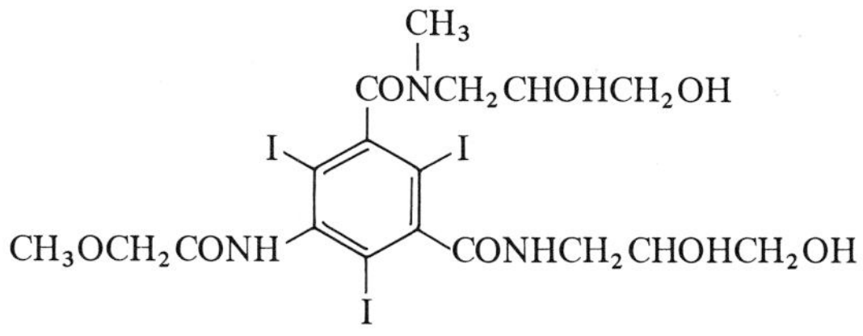

Iopromide
(amide coupler, Table 32)

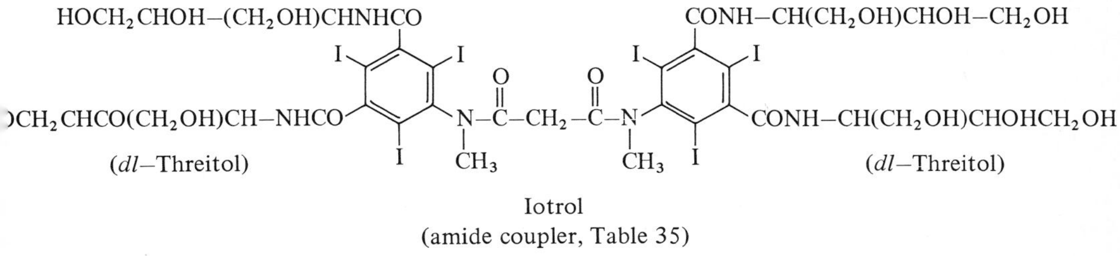

Iotrol
(amide coupler, Table 35)

Fig. 5 (Legend see p. 74)

I. Solubility Aspects of Nonionic Media

The concentration requirements for CM are largely dependent on their intended clinical use. To obtain maximum opacity for myelography, the clinically useful myelographic iodine concentrations are in the range of 170–280 mg iodine/ml. To achieve these iodine concentrations, a molecule which contains 50% iodine (molecular weight: 761 g mol^{-1}) must be soluble to the extent of 34%–56% w/v, and correspondingly a compound which contains only 40% iodine (molecular weight: 952 g mol^{-1}) must be 42.5%–70% water soluble. In angiography (such as coronary arteriography), the clinically useful dose lies in the range of 320–400 mg iodine/ml. Accordingly, the compound which contains 50% iodine must be 64%–80% w/v water soluble, and the compound with 40% iodine should be 80%–100% water soluble. In either case, little water is used for these formulations as can be seen from Table 38.

Few organic compounds with molecular weights in the range of 761–956 g mol^{-1} show high solubility in water irrespective of their structures. It is thus indeed surprising that the high molecular weight CM essentially nonpolar molecules, exhibit such a high degree of water solubility.

In the design of such agents, the basic chemical approach is to attempt to solubilize a triiodobenzene moiety with appropriate hydrophilic functions coupled to the ring with suitable organic functional groups. For most applications stability is also a consideration (see p. 26). Many polyhydroxy nonionic compounds exhibit the phenomenon of supersaturation, i.e., they form metastable solutions at 100% w/v and higher. These solutions may remain clear for months or even years, but ultimately a crystalline compound may precipitate. Sometimes it may have water solubility substantially lower than that initially observed. For this reason, the researcher must always be careful to crystallize the candidate compound, preferably from water and/or at the least from an organic solvent and thus confirm its water solubility in the thermodynamically most stable crystalline form.

Table 38. Compound and water requirements, for the formulation of nonionic CM

1. For a compound containing 40% iodine with a bulk density of 2 g ml^{-1}

Desired iodine concentration (mg I/ml)	Weight of compound (g)	Volume of water (ml)
170	425	787
280	700	650
320	800	600
400	1,000	500

2. For a compound containing 50% iodine with a bulk density of 2 g ml^{-1}

Desired iodine concentration (mg I/ml)	Weight of compound (g)	Volume of water (ml)
170	340	830
280	560	720
320	640	680
400	800	600

It is important to recognize that many organic compounds may exist in several hydrate or polymorphic forms and that one hydrate or polymorph may be substantially more water soluble than another. The authors have experienced and heard a sufficient number of "horror stories" from their colleagues in other laboratories to appreciate the importance of experimental crystallization. Indeed compounds have remained in highly concentrated water solutions for months only to crystallize just prior to or after a decision to formulate them pharmaceutically. Nonionic CM are rendered soluble by an unpredictable effect from the combination of hydrophilic, hydrogen-bonding groups such as alcohols and amides. Therefore, only the most general rules can be observed in the design of CM and even these are speculative.

1. The number of the hydroxyl groups in the aliphatic chain(s) affects water solubility. The minimum number of hydroxyl groups to confer water solubility appears to be four to six; the addition of more hydroxyl groups does not necessarily provide higher water solubility (compare MP-6026 with MP-8000 in Table 20) and may increase viscosity.
2. Many useful compounds possess some element of dissymmetry as a result of isomers due to restricted rotation (see below) or to the use of optically active hydroxylic side chains derived, for example, from glucose.
3. The coupler group does not necessarily affect the water solubility of the various classes of compounds.
4. The better X, Y groups in terms of systemic and especially neural safety (myelography, angiography) are those which have a higher degree of hydrophilic character. More specifically, X, Y groups which are –H or –NH$_2$ typically provide less water solubility than hydroxylated ethers, or acetamido or carbamyl groups (see tables for examples).

II. Viscosity Considerations

In contrast to the monomeric ionic CM, there are pronounced differences in the viscosities of the nonionic agents particularly as the concentration increases. At a 37% iodine concentration, most nonionic compounds have a viscosity of 20 cps or higher, except iopamidol as is illustrated in Fig. 6 [85]. Accordingly, most nonionic agents are not well suited for procedures such as arteriography at a 37% iodine concentration; however, provided sufficient contrast may be seen, they may be suitable at lower concentrations.

At the present time, there exist no data correlating the effects of minor structural variations in a series of CM to the viscosity of their solutions. ALMEN [84] suggested that in analogy with a study carried out by EINSTEIN in 1906 of gold sols a more globular particle would be less viscous. However, Einstein's equation [Eq. (1)] is only applicable to spherical particles at infinite dilution and subsequently for higher solute concentrations. Equation (2) was developed wherein the coefficient C' represents the contribution of solute-solute interactions.

$$\eta = \eta_0 (1 + 2.5\,\Phi) \tag{1}$$

$$\eta\eta_0 = 1 + 2.5\,\Phi + C'\Phi^2 \tag{2}$$

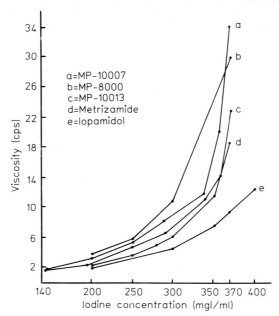

Fig. 6. Nonionic CM viscosities at 37 °C

where η = viscosity, η_0 = solvent viscosity, and Φ = volume fraction of the particles.

Subsequent work on aqueous solutions of alcohols, amides, and ureas has shown that these compounds do not obey either equation. Reasons for these deviations are complex, but some of them may be attributed to the size of the solute relative to the solvent, structure formation, structure breaking of the solvent by the solute, reduction of the spatial volume of water, and extensive hydration of the molecule [92].

III. Osmolality

As previously discussed, one of the prime reasons for development of nonionic CM was to provide solutions with a high iodine content which were not hypertonic and would not have any electrical effects. For comparison, the osmolalities of several ionic and nonionic CM are shown in Table 39. The osmolalities of several nonionic compounds as a function of concentration are plotted in Fig. 7 (MALLINCKRODT, Research Department, St. Louis, unpublished results). Interestingly iopamidol and metrizamide show a negative deviation from the theoretical values [85, 91], however, MP-10013 exhibits a negative deviation from the theoretical value at low concentrations and a positive deviation at high concentrations. FELDER et al. [91] have suggested that the negative deviation for iopamidol is a result of iopamidol forming molecular aggregates (by hydrogen bonding) and hydrates. The tendency to form molecular aggregates was confirmed by determining the critical micellar concentration [91].

Table 39. Osmolalities of several ionic and nonionic CM

Medium	Osmolality (30% I mOsm/kg)
Metrizoate[a]	1,460
Diatrizoate[a]	1,520
Iothalamate[a]	1,485
Iocarmate[a]	1,040
Iopamidol	616
Metrizamide	480
MP-8000	1,205
MP-10007	1,120
MP-10013	967
MP-6026	590
Iotrol	320
Human blood	300
CSF	300

[a] Meglumine salt

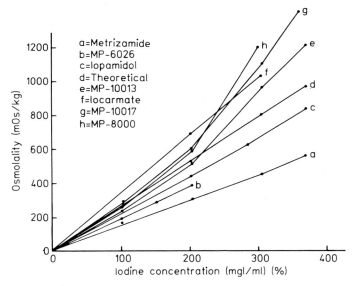

Fig. 7. Osmolality profiles for several nonionic CM

IV. Stability

Stability requirements for X-ray CM depend upon intended use. A compound intended for infusion urography must be stable in water solution and susceptible to either terminal sterilization or a sterile fill process. Compounds given in low dosages at relatively high concentrations such as in myelography must first of all be biologically safe. Stability to withstand the terminal sterilization process is desirable but not indispensable with these agents. Agents intended for oral administration are required to be autoclavable but must be stable in the gastrointestinal tract. Thus, in general terms, CM can fall into three stability classes: (a) stable in aqueous solution under conditions of autoclaving; (b) stable in lyophilized or powder form, yet suitable for reconstitution with an appropriate vehicle to provide a sterile pyrogen-free solution; and (c) oral compounds stable in the dry state and in the gastrointestinal tract.

Principally there are three modes of decomposition of nonionic CM, which can be detected as follows:

Mode of decomposition	*Parameter changed*
Deiodination	Iodide ion, pH, color
Instability of the polyhydroxyalkyl group	Assay, color, precipitation
Hydrolysis of the coupler group	Assay, pH, color (free amine)

In ionic media, these modes of decomposition can be monitored by the methods in Tables 40 and 41.

1. Deiodination

It has been reported that iopamidol does not deiodinate on autoclaving as readily as diatrizoic acid without chelating agents; this was explained by the carboxyl group of diatrizoic acid coordinating with trace levels of copper in solution, which in turn catalyzes deiodination. In contrast, it has been reported that the deiodination of the experimental compounds C-29 and C-545 (Nyegaard Co.) can be almost completely circumvented by weakly basic amine buffers such as tris-(hydroxymethyl) methylamine (Tris) or 1-deoxy-1-methylamino-D-glucitol [N-methylglucamine (NMG)]. The authors suggest that deiodination for these compounds might occur by intramolecular displacement of iodine as shown in Fig. 8, but the deiodinated product(s) was(were) not isolated [93]. It is entirely possible that other mechanisms are applicable [44].

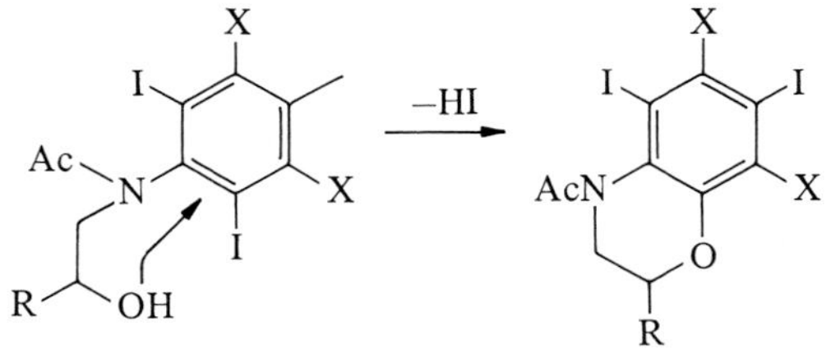

C–29:   R = H, X = CONHCH$_2$CHOHCH$_2$OH

C–545:   R = CH$_2$OH, X = CONHCH$_2$CHOHCH$_2$OH

Fig. 8. Proposed mode of deiodination for C-29, C-545, and analogous compounds

2. Instability of the Polyhydroxylalkyl Group

Metrizamide is unstable because the polyhydroxylic group, even under mild conditions, undergoes epimerization at C-2 (i.e., glucose→mannose epimerization, Fig. 9 [88, 94, 116]. Also, the glucosamine portion of metrizamide can undergo typical aldehydic reaction (e.g., multiple aldol condensations, furan formation,

Table 40. Stability of X-ray CM (meglumine iothalamate 30% w/v)

Tests and their specification limits

Storage temp.	Storage time (months)	Meglumine iothalamate 95.0%–105.0% of label	Meglumine 22.9%–25.3% of labeled amount (300 mg/ml)	pH 6.5–7.7	Calcium disodium edetate 0.085–0.135 (mg/ml)	Sodium biphosphate 0.10–0.15 (mg/ml)	Iodine and iodide (as I) 0.02% Max.	Free amine 0.05% Max.	Heavy metals 0.0020% Max.	Color @450 nm 0.200 Max.[a]	Color @500 nm 0.100 Max.[a]
25 °C	Initial	103.1%	25.0%	7.5	0.101	0.12	0.01%	0.03%	<0.0005%	0.042	0.028
	1	—	—	7.5	—	—	0.01	0.03	—	0.008	0.007
	3	—	—	7.4	—	—	0.01	0.03	—	0.032	0.015
	6	102.6	25.2	7.6	0.096	0.12	0.00	0.03	<0.0005	0.032	0.015
	12	101.1	25.1	7.4	0.109	0.12	0.00	0.03	<0.0010	0.042	0.021
	24	100.3	25.1	7.5	0.106	0.13	0.00	0.03	<0.0010	0.036	0.015
	36	100.2	25.3	7.3	0.101	0.13	0.00	0.03	0.0010	0.042	0.021
	48	100.6	25.0	7.3	0.106	0.13	0.01	0.04	<0.0005	0.042	0.021
37 °C	1	—	—	7.5	—	—	0.01	0.03	—	0.013	0.012
	3	—	—	7.4	—	—	0.01	0.03	—	0.037	0.015
	6	98.6	25.1	7.5	0.096	0.12	0.01	0.03	<0.0005	0.038	0.017
	12	98.5	25.1	7.4	0.110	0.12	0.01	0.04	<0.0010	0.053	0.024
	24	100.3	25.1	7.3	0.106	0.13	0.01	0.04	<0.0010	0.055	0.025
50 °C	½	—	—	7.4	—	—	0.01	0.03	—	0.032	0.015
	1	—	—	7.4	—	—	0.01	0.03	—	0.013	0.011
	3	—	—	7.3	—	—	0.01	0.04	—	0.051	0.022
	6	102.5	25.2	7.3	0.096	0.12	0.01	0.05	<0.0005	0.050	0.026
	12	102.7	25.1	7.0	0.109	0.12	0.01	0.07	<0.0010	0.075	0.038

Unpublished data from formal stability submitted to U.S. Food and Drug Administration in support of New Drug Application for indicated formulation. Container: 300-ml Type I USP glass bottle. Lot: S73107

[a] One-month color results were obtained using a 1-cm cell rather than a 5-cm cell

Table 41. Stability of X-ray CM (sodium iothalamate 54.3% w/v)

Tests and their specification limits

Storage temp.	Storage time (months)	Sodium iothalamate 95.0%–105.0% of label (543 mg/ml)	pH 7.0–7.6	Calcium disodium edetate 0.085–0.135 mg/ml	Sodium biphosphate 0.10–0,15 mg/ml	Iodine and iodides (as I) 0.02% Max.	Free amine 0.05% Max.	Heavy metals 0.0020% Max.	Color @ 450 nm 0.200 Max.	@ 500 nm 0.100 Max
25 °C	Initial	99.4%	7.2	0.115	0.13	0.00%	0.04%	<0.0010%	0.071	0.043
	1	99.4	7.2	0.112	0.12	0.00	0.04	<0.0005	0.067	0.041
	3	99.3	7.2	0.123	0.12	0.00	0.04	<0.0015	0.078	0,051
	6	99.0	7.1	0.121	0.12	0.00	0.05	<0.0010	0.068	0,050
	12	99.8	7.1	0.114	0.12	0.00	0.04	<0.0010	0.096	0.085
	24	100.0	7.1	0.124	0.13	0.00	0.04	<0.0010	0.110	0.083
	36	102.0	7.0	0.116	0.13	0.00	0.04	0.001	0.165	0.127
	48	100.2	7.0	0.117	0.13	0.00	0.05	0.001	0.180	0.140
	60	102.4	7.0	0.114	0.13	0.00	0.04	<0.0005	0.165	0.105
37 °C	1	98.8	7.1	0.115	0.12	0.00	0.04	<0.0005	0.061	0.041
	3	99.3	7.1	0.120	0.12	0.00	0.04	<0.0015	0.084	0,059
	6	99.1	7.0	0.120	0.13	0.00	0.05	<0.0010	0.100	0.071
	12	100.9	6.9	0.122	0.13	0.00	0.04	<0.0010	0.125	0.087
50 °C	1	99.8	7.0	0.117	0.12	0.00	0.04	<0.0005	0.067	0.045
	3	99.6	7.0	0.122	0.12	0.00	0.05	<0.0010	0.112	0.076
	6	100.4	6.8	0.127	0.12	0.00	0.06	<0.0010	0.160	0.120
	12	100.8	6.7	0.109	0.13	0.00	0.06	<0.0010	0.215	0.150

Unpublished data from formal stability submitted to U.S. Food and Drug Administration in support of New Drug Application for indicated formulation. Container: 300-ml Type I USP glass vial. Lot: S74101-1704

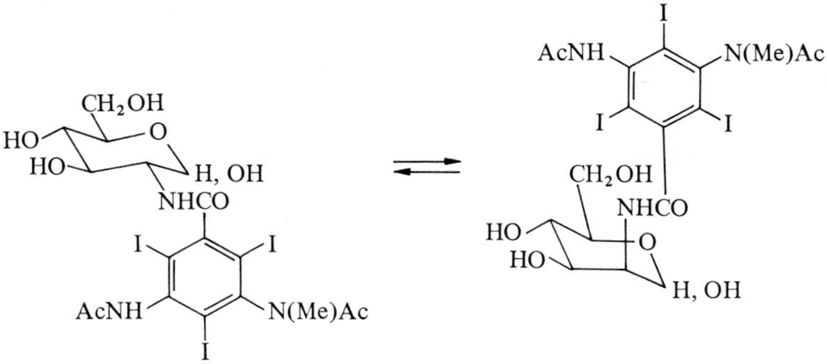

Metrizamide

Fig. 9. Epimerization of metrizamide

etc.) [225] leading to principitates and highly colored impurities. For these reasons, metrizamide must be dispensed as a sterile, lyophilized powder which is reconstituted with dilute aqueous bicarbonate solute just prior to administration.

3. Hydrolysis of the Coupler Group

Based on available data, the relative order of stability to conditions of terminal sterilization for the coupler groups is as follows (the most stable coupler is listed first) (MALLINCKRODT, Research Department, St. Louis, unpublished data; [94, 95]):

Amide $\simeq$ simple reversed amides without γ- or δ-hydroxyls (e.g., $HOCH_2-CONH-$, $CH_3CHOHCONH-$, $HOCH_2CHOHCONH$) $\simeq$ esters $>$ 2-ketogulonamides $>$ gluconamides $\geqq$ peptides $>$ ureides $\simeq$ carbamates $\simeq$ glycosides

The amide group is perhaps the most stable coupler linkage because the steric bulk of the two ortho iodines helps to prevent nucleophilic hydrolysis by water (or hydroxide ion) as is shown in Fig. 10 (unhindered amides generally will hydrolyze slightly under autoclave conditions).

In a similar vein, compounds with an ester coupler or simple reversed amide coupler (i.e., those that do not possess a γ- or δ-hydroxyl) are protected from hydrolysis by the two adjacent iodine atoms. Reversed amides which have a γ- or δ-hydroxyl (e.g., D-gluconamides) are more susceptible to vigorous hydrolysis because of the tendency for intramolecular lactonization (Fig. 11) to form five- or six-membered ring lactones [44].

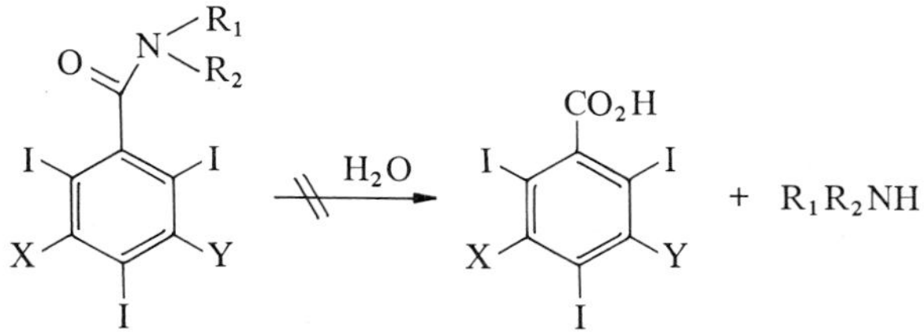

Fig. 10. Stability of the amide group

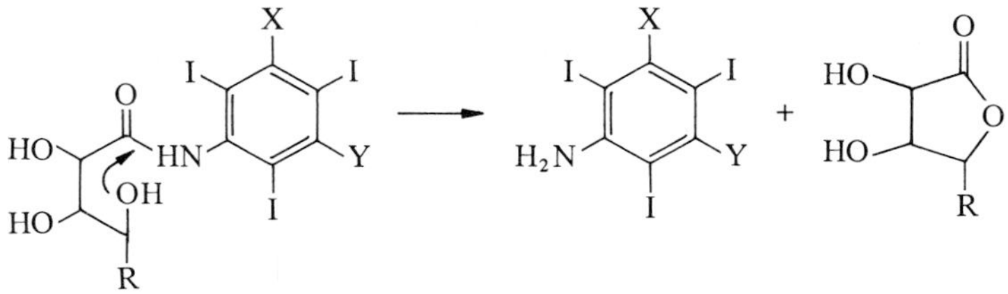

Fig. 11. Mechanism for the hydrolysis of reversed amides containing γ- or δ-hydroxylic groups [222]

In contrast, the reversed amides formed from the cyclic sugar acids (e.g., 2-keto-L-gulonic acid) appear in general more stable than reversed amides formed from the straight chain sugar acids (e.g., D-gluconic acid). This may be explained by the γ- or δ-hydroxyls not being close enough to allow intramolecular lactonization:

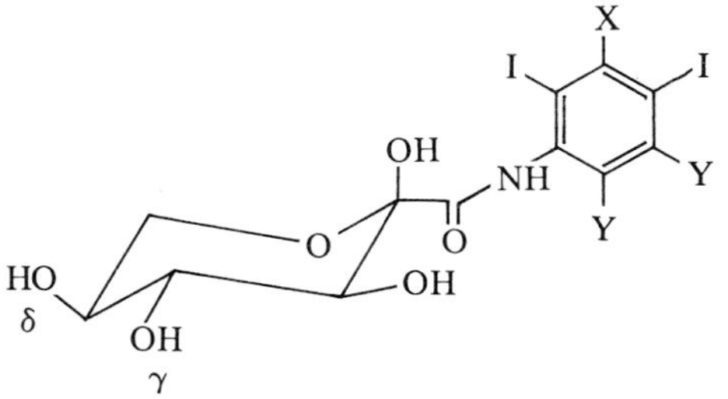

At 120 °C in aqueous solution, the peptide couplers slowly hydrolyze to their corresponding hippuric acids probably by direct hydrolysis and by intramolecular ester formation followed by hydrolysis (Fig. 12). Both the ureide and carbamate coupler groups probably hydrolyze by the same mechanisms as the reversed

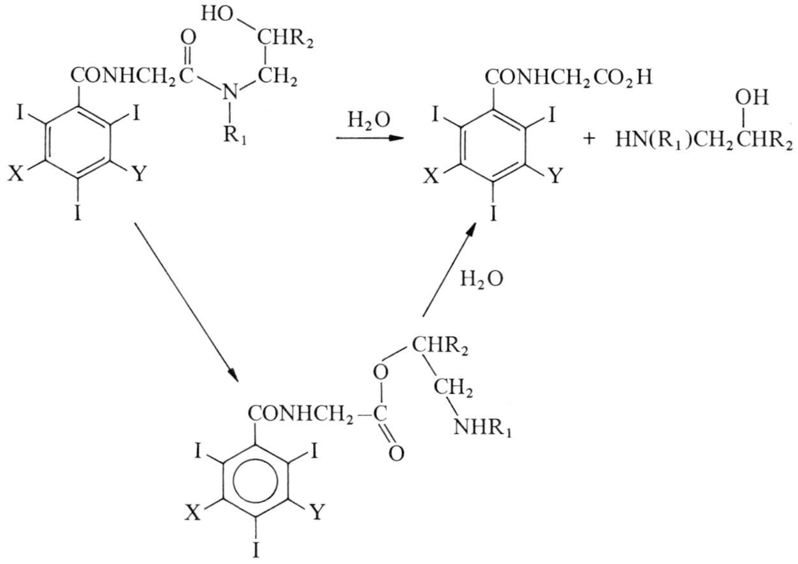

Fig. 12. Hydrolysis of the peptide coupler

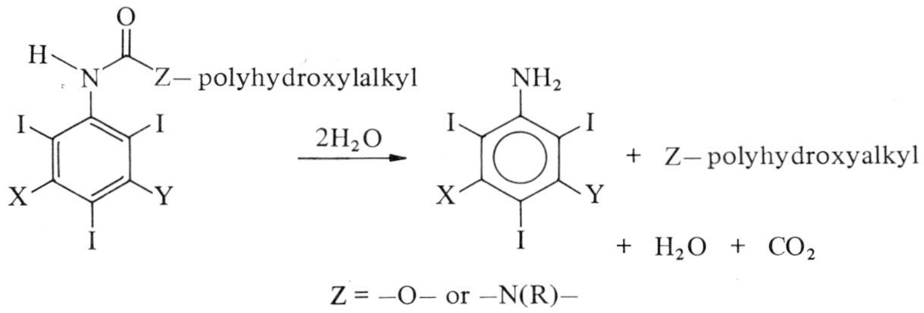

Fig. 13. Hydrolysis of the ureide and carbamate coupler groups

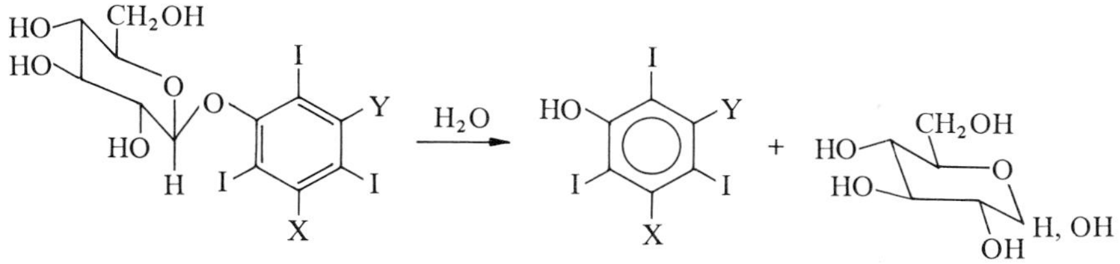

Fig. 14. Hydrolysis of glycosides

amide with a γ- or δ-hydroxyl group. In each case the aromatic amine is formed (Fig. 13). Similarly the glycosides [94, 95] readily hydrolyze to the free sugar and iodinated phenol (Fig. 14).

V. Synthesis of Nonionic Compounds

1. Synthetic Approaches

Currently nonionic CM are more expensive to manufacture than conventional ionic compounds since they require more costly raw materials and generally more manufacturing steps [96].

The synthesis of the various nonionic media will be classified by their respective coupler groups. More attention will be devoted to the amide and reverse amide groups since both types of compounds appear generally more useful and are presently being evaluated for clinical use.

a) Amide Couplers

α) *Synthesis of Metrizamide* [88]. Metrizamide is manufactured in three steps from the intermediate *1* used in the manufacture of metrizoic acid, with overall yields of 35%–40% (Fig. 15). Treatment of the acid with phosphorus pentachloride gives the acid chloride *2*, which is acetylated in toluene using acetic anhydride to produce compound *3*. The acid chloride *3* is condensed with 2-amino-2-deoxy-D-glucose in *N,N*-dimethylformamide using potassium carbonate as an acid scavenger to give metrizamide *4*, which is purified by treatment with ion exchange resins and crystallized from isopropyl alcohol. The purified metrizamide is dissolved in water and the water is removed by vacuum distillation to provide purified metrizamide *4* as an amorphous powder.

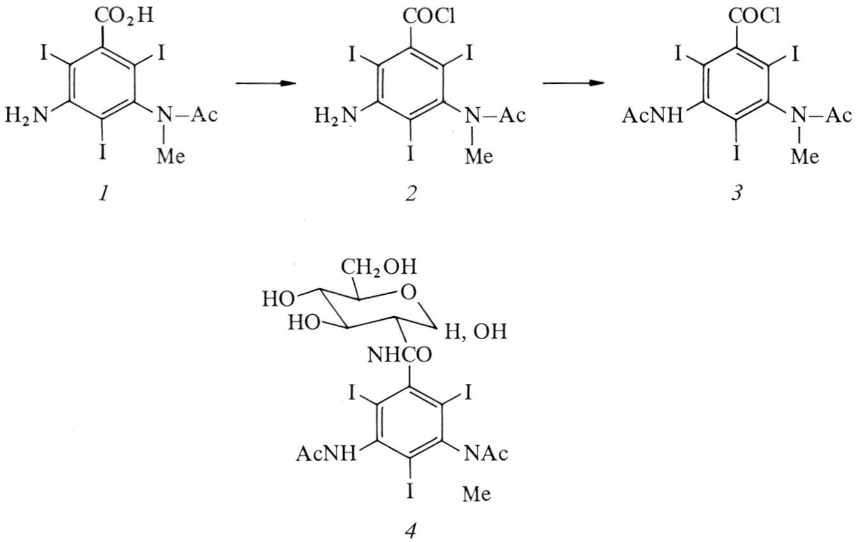

Fig. 15. Synthesis of metrizamide

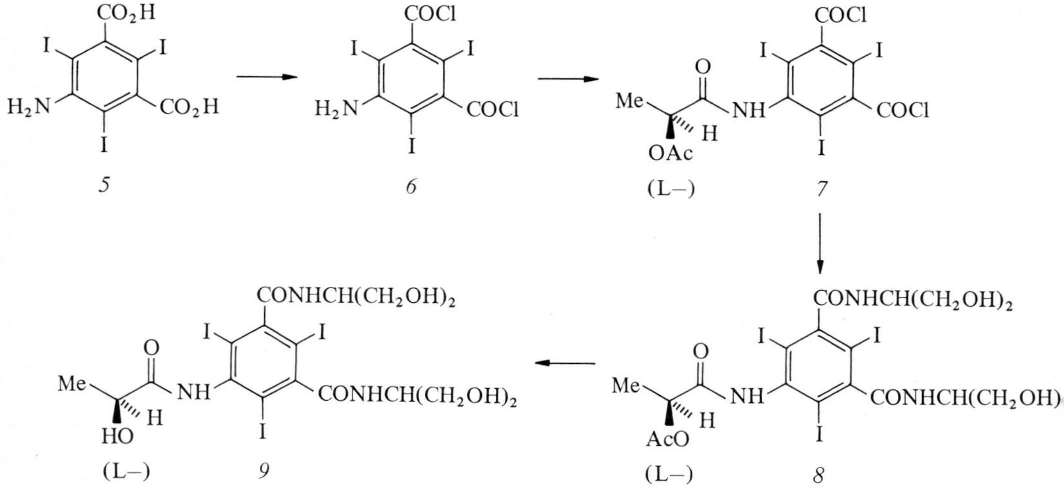

Fig. 16. Synthesis of iopamidol

β) Synthesis of Iopamidol and Iohexol. In contrast to the synthesis of metriza-mide, the manufacturing process for iopamidol has not been published. However, Felder et al. [97, 98] have described three different methods for preparing iopa-midol. Actual yields, ease of synthesis, and costs of raw materials will dictate which method is used.

The first method (Fig. 16) involves the preparation of diacid chloride 6 from 5-amino-2,4,5-triiodoisophthalic acid 5 (readily prepared by the catalytic reduc-

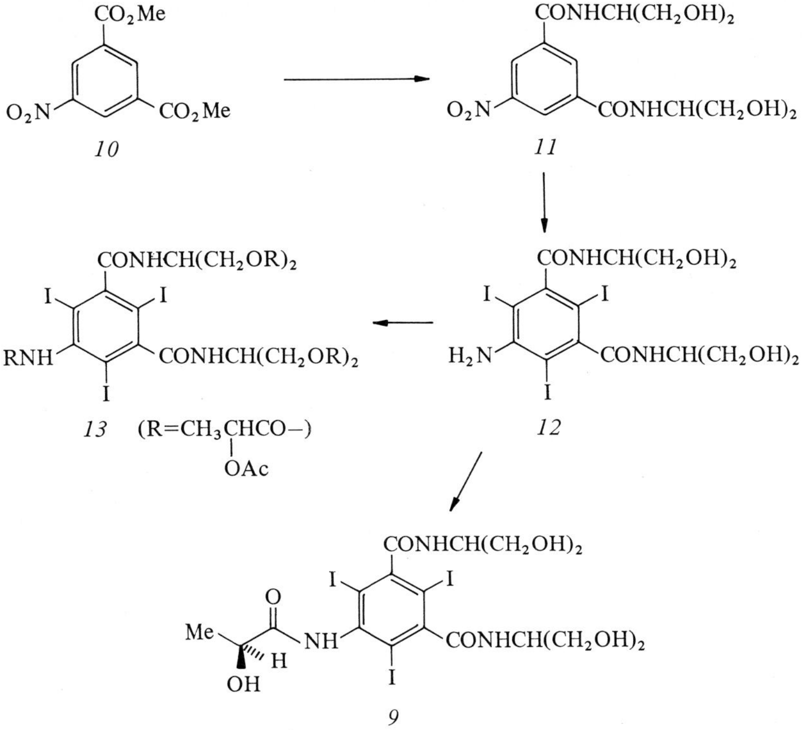

Fig. 17. Synthesis of iopamidol

tion of 5-nitroisophthalic acid followed by iodination) using thionyl chloride. The diacid chloride *6* is acylated in *N,N*-dimethylacetamide with L-2-acetoxypropionyl chloride prepared in two steps from L-lactic acid to provide the acylamido diacid chloride *7*. This diacid chloride *7* is treated with serinol (2-amino-1,3-propanediol) in *N,N*-dimethylacetamide with tri-*n*-butylamine as an acid scavenger to yield after purification the *O*-acetyl derivative *8*. Simple saponification of *8* with dilute sodium hydroxide, removal of the ionic by-products with cationic and anionic ion exchange resins, and recrystallization from ethanol yields 65% iopamidol *9*.

The amino alcohol, serinol, is prepared by several methods, with perhaps the best being that described by PFEIFFER, utilizing nitromethane and formaldehyde to give in situ the intermediate $[(HOCH_2)_2C=NO_2]^-$, which is reduced catalytically with hydrogen to yield $(HOCH_2)_2CHNH_2$ [99].

The alternative synthesis (Fig. 17), which appears to be more costly, involves the aminolysis of dimethyl 5-nitroisophthalate *10* with serinol to give the nitro-bis-amide *11*, which is catalytically reduced and subsequently iodinated with potassium iododichloride to give the iodinated bis-amide *12* (this intermediate can also be obtained by reacting the diacid chloride *6* with serinol). Treatment of the iodinated bis amide *12* with excess L-2-acetoxypropionyl chloride gives the

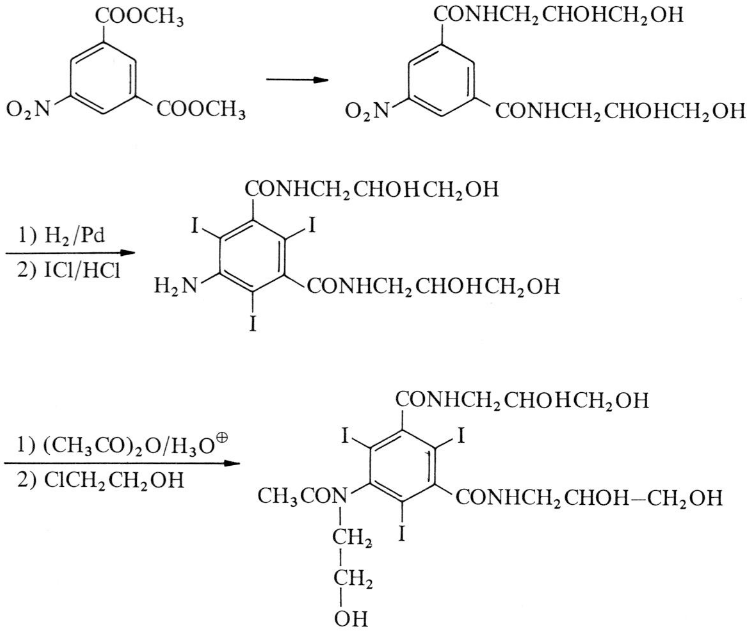

Fig. 18. Synthesis of iohexol

peracylated intermediate *13*, which is saponified with alkali and purified as above to yield iopamidol *9*.

The synthesis reported for iohexol [198] proceeds in a straightforward fashion (Fig. 17).

γ) Bis Compounds. To date two classes of bis compounds (Tables 41–44) have been prepared. The principal difference between these classes is the manner in which the two triiodoaromatic rings are coupled together. In the first class (Fig. 19) [88, 100] a triiodinated aniline derivative *14* is coupled using a diacid chloride (e.g., oxalyl chloride, adipyl chloride) to provide *15*, which is then treated with a polyhydroxylic amine to give the desired product *16*.

Recently SOVAK et al. [101] reported on the preparation and testing of a water-soluble bis compound ("dimer") derived from the polyhydroxyamine, *dl*-2-aminothreitol (DL-3-117, iotrol).

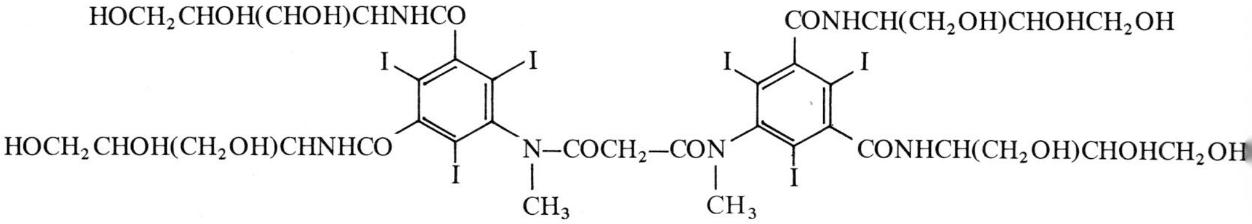

Iotrol

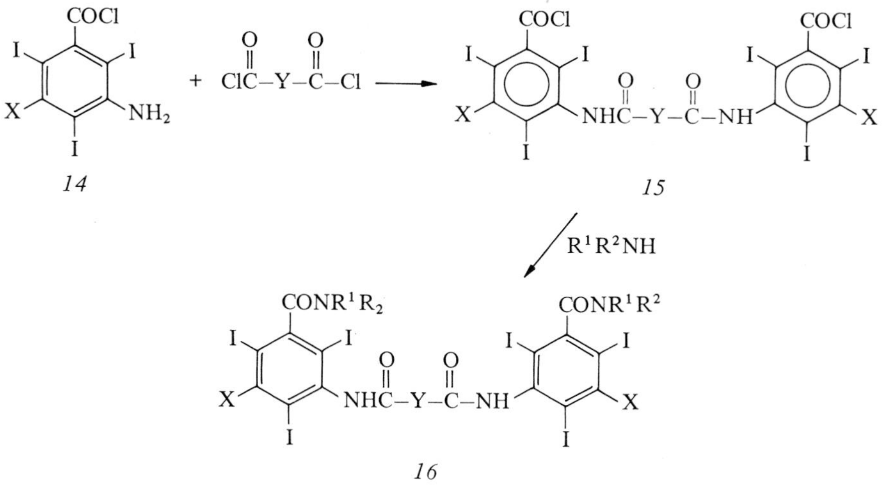

COCl
I ⟍⟍ I
X ⟋⟋ NH$_2$
I

14

$+$ ClC–Y–C–Cl (each C bears =O)

$\longrightarrow$

COCl
I ⟍⟍ I
X ⟋⟋ NHC–Y–C–NH ⟍⟍ X
I (each C bears =O) I

COCl
I ⟍⟍ I
I

15

R^{1}R^{2}NH

CONR^{1}R$_2$
I ⟍⟍ I
X ⟋⟋ NHC–Y–C–NH
I (each C bears =O)

CONR^{1}R^2
I ⟍⟍ I
X
I

16

R^1,R^2 = H, alkyl, hydroxyalkyl
X = H, –CONR^{1}R^2
Y = single bonds or alkylene

Fig. 19. Synthesis of the first class of bis compounds

The introduction of an additional asymmetrical center with a concomitant increase in the number of isomers resulted in high water solubility, whereas for the second class of bis compounds, the triiodinated aromatics are coupled using a diamine (Fig. 20) [102, 103].

b) Reversed Amide Couplers

α) *Monomeric Compounds.* Several reversed amides have been reported. These include the experimental compounds P-297 [104], MP-8000 and MP-6026 [105], MP-10007 [106], and MP-10013 [107]. Since none of these compounds has yet reached the stage of commercial development, the following discussion will be centered on the two basic methods for preparing reversed amides. The essential difference between the two methods lies in the protected sugar acid chloride which is used. In the one case (Fig. 21) a per-*O*-acetylated sugar acid chloride (e.g., 2,3,4,5,6-penta-*O*-acetyl-D-gluconyl *17* is used to acylate a 3,5-disubstituted-2,4,6-triiodoaniline *18*, giving an amide of structure *19* which is deprotected with either dilute acid or base (preferably base) to give the desired product *20*. In the other case (Fig. 22), acylation to provide the amide *22* is carried out using a di-*O*-isopropylidene-protected sugar acid chloride such as 2,3,4,6-di-*O*-isopropylidene-2-keto-L-gulonyl chloride *21*, and the protecting groups can only be removed by treatment with mild acid to give the final product *23*.

β) *Bis Compounds.* Relatively few bis reversed amides have been prepared; generally these compounds are synthesized according to Fig. 23 [108].

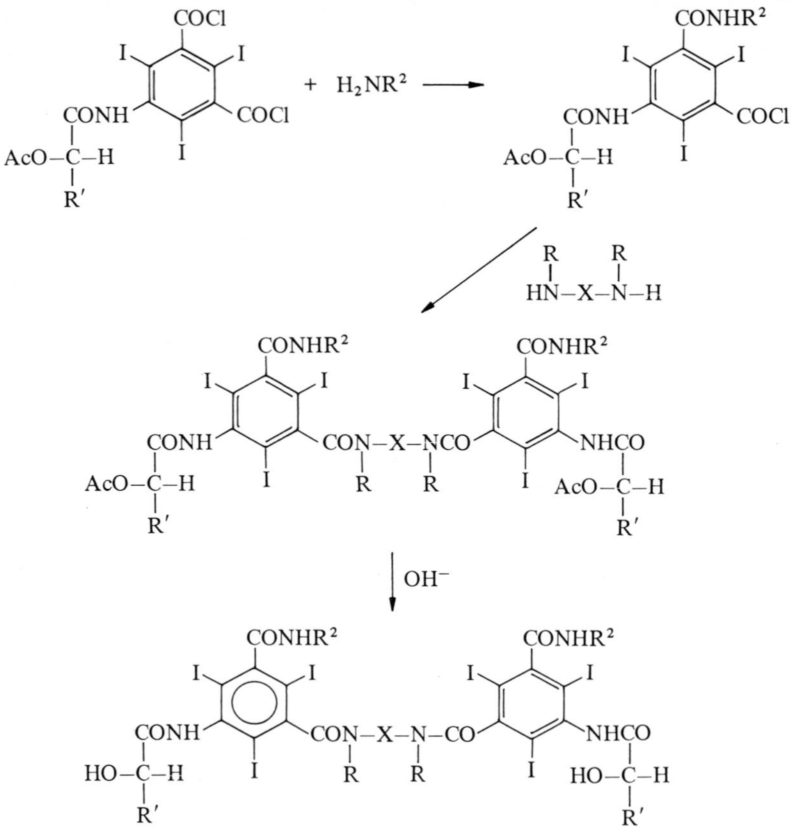

Fig. 20. Synthesis of the second class of bis compounds

R and R′ = H or Me

R² = dihydroxypropyl or dihydroxybutyl

X = $-C_nH_{2n}-(OC_nH_{2n})_m-$

$n = 2$ or 3

$m = 1-5$

c) Peptide Coupler

The peptides *26* were synthesized either by aminolysis of the 3,5-disubstituted-2,4,6-triiodohippuric acid ester *24* (Fig. 24, *top*) or by acylation of the glycylamino polyol with a 3,5-disubstituted-2,4,6-triiodobenzoyl chloride *25* (Fig. 24, *bottom*) [109].

d) Ureide Coupler

The ureide *29* was prepared by the condensation of an aminopolyol with a 3,5-disubstituted-2,4,6-triiodophenylisocyanate (or carbamoyl chloride) *28* in *N,N*-

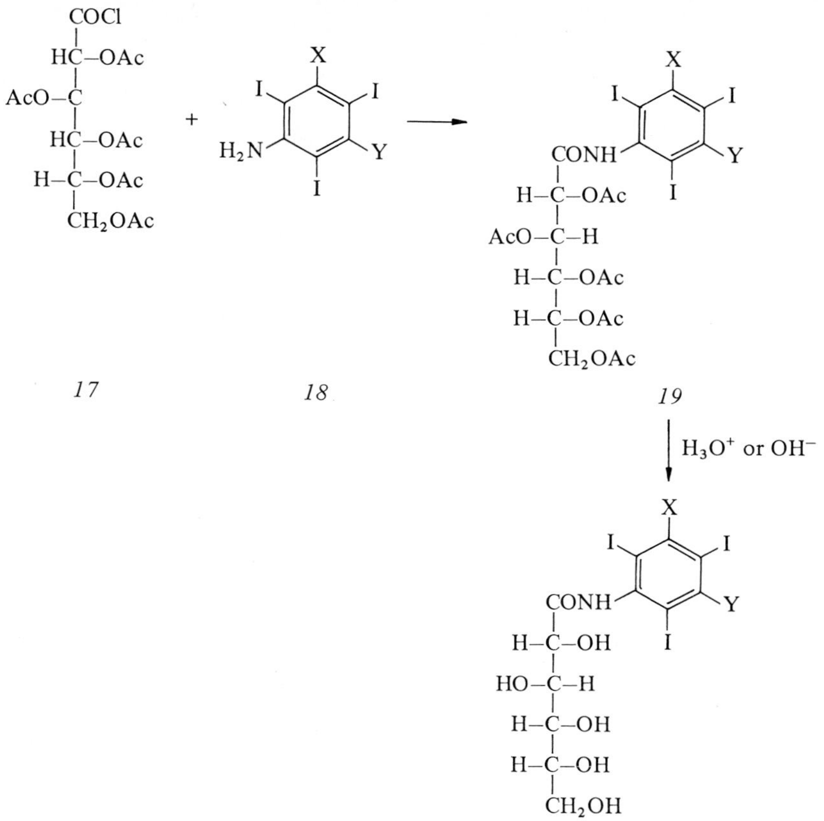

Fig. 21. First method for the synthesis of reversed amides. Partial synthesis of P-297, MP-6026, or MP-8000

dimethylformamide (Fig. 25) [110]. The isocyanate is prepared from the appropriately substituted aniline 27 and excess phosgene at room temperature.

e) Carbamate Coupler

The carbamate coupler 30 was prepared by reaction of the isocyanate 28 with a di-O-isopropylidene protected sugar [111]. The protecting groups 29 were easily removed by treatment with mild, aqueous acid (Fig. 26).

f) Ester Coupler

An ester-coupled nonionic compound was prepared by alkylation of a lithium salt of 3,5-disubstituted-2,4,6-triiodobenzoic acid with a protected sugar tosylate with subsequent deprotection (Fig. 27, top), or by reaction of a partially protected polyol with a 5-substituted-2,4,6-triiodoisophthaloyl dichloride 34 and removal

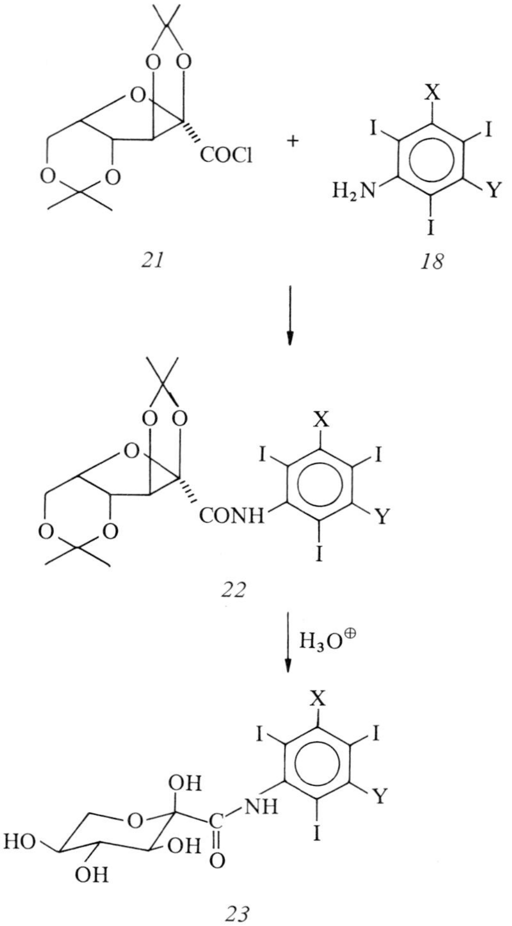

Fig. 22. Second method for the synthesis of reversed amides

of the protecting groups (Fig. 27, *bottom*) (Mallinckrodt, Research Department, St. Louis, unpublished results).

g) Glycoside Coupler

The glycosides are generally prepared by the alkylation of a phenol *37* with 2,3,4,6-tetra-*O*-acetyl-α-D-glucopyranosyl bromide *38* followed by deacetylation of *39* with methanolic ammonia (Fig. 28) [94, 95].

2. Manufacturing Costs

The cost of nonionic (as well as ionic) CM may be separated into the cost of the bulk chemical (iodinated compound) and the cost of pharmaceutical formulation.

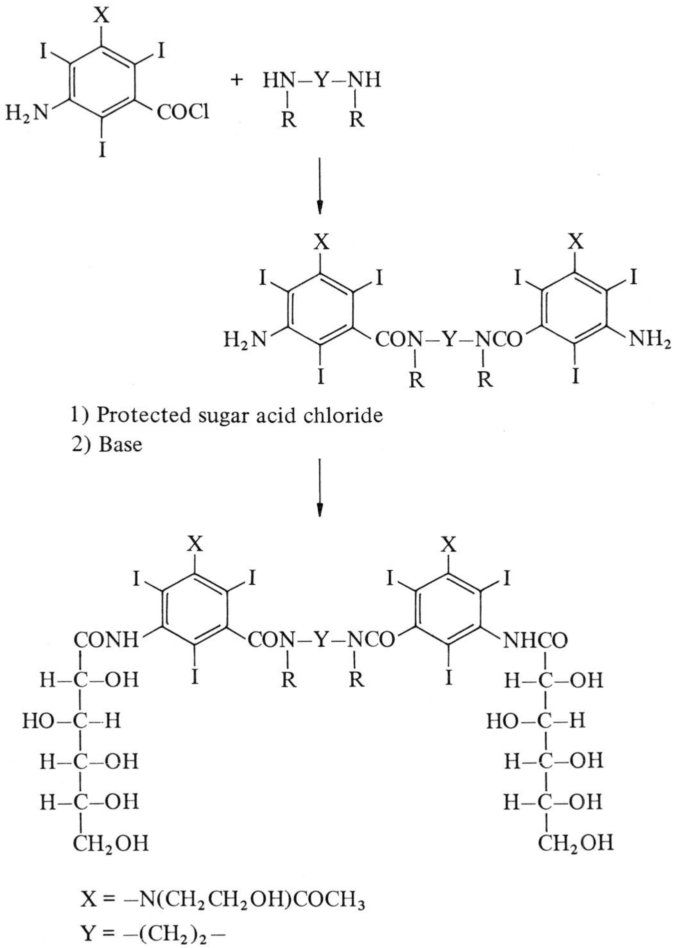

Fig. 23. Synthesis of bis reversed amides

a) Cost of Bulk Chemical

Manufacturing costs of a CM are influenced by several factors, which include:

1. The cost and availability of the basic raw materials.
2. The scale of manufacture. The amount of labor required to carry out a reaction and isolate a product for a 1,000- to 2,000-liter scale reaction is about the same as for a 10,000- to 15,000-liter scale reaction, if comparably sized equipment is used.
3. The number of manufacturing steps, which is best defined as the number of chemical isolations which are required rather than the number of chemical reactions which are carried out.
4. The yields in each synthesis step.

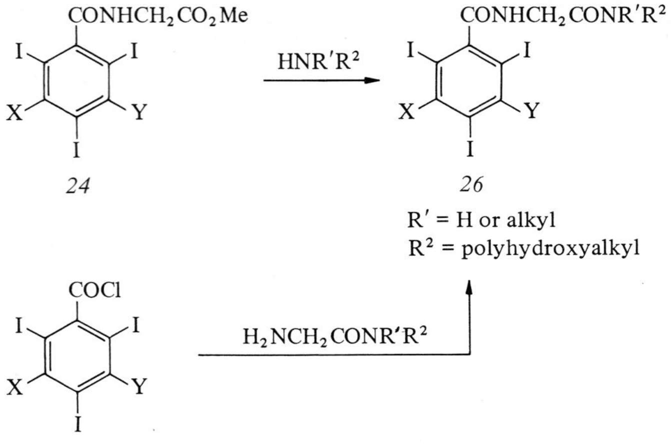

Fig. 24. Synthesis of peptides

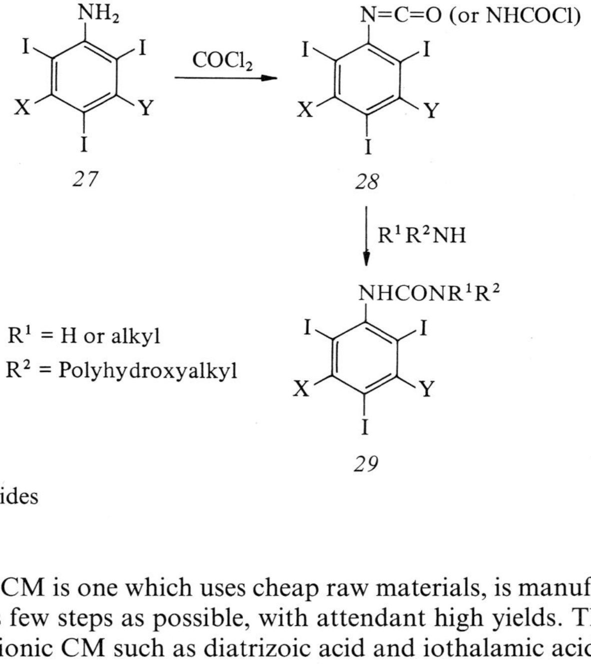

Fig. 25. Synthesis of ureides

Thus, a practical CM is one which uses cheap raw materials, is manufactured on a large scale in as few steps as possible, with attendant high yields. This generally is the case for ionic CM such as diatrizoic acid and iothalamic acid. However, the nonionic agents developed to date suffer in one or more of the above aspects. Therefore, they are generally more costly to synthesise.

b) Formulation of Contrast Media

Contrast media are formulated in water solution and rendered sterile by thermal sterilization. Compounds unstable under autoclaving conditions can be sterile

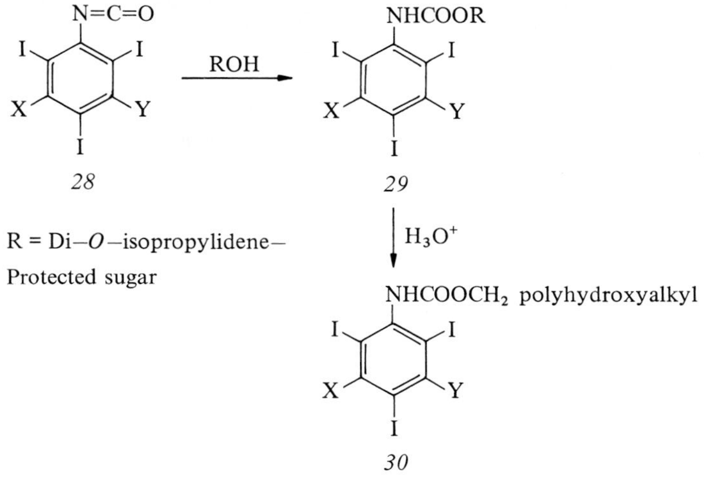

Fig. 26. Synthesis of carbamates

filled by an aseptic process to give either a solution or a lyophilized powder. The cost of formulating CM is not higher than that for other parenteral formulations.

In general, steam sterilization is used with aqueous CM, usually at 121 °C for 15–20 min [112]. The quality and type of container and closure (rubber stopper) are prescribed by each countries' pharmacopoeial group. Usually a high-quality borosilicate glass (Pyrex) and an essentially completely chemically inert rubber stopper (butyl) are employed.

VI. Stereochemical Aspects of Contrast Media

Depending upon its structure, a CM may exist in isomeric forms. The existence of isomeric forms may affect the physicochemical properties of the compound, e.g., water solubility and chemical stability. Isomers arise as a result from several characteristic structural features of CM such as (a) restricted rotation about the aromatic bonds adjacent to the iodine atoms and (b) restricted rotation about the carbonyl nitrogen bond in alkylamido substituents. If the compound contains a sugar moiety or other group with asymmetrical centers, additional isomers will be present.

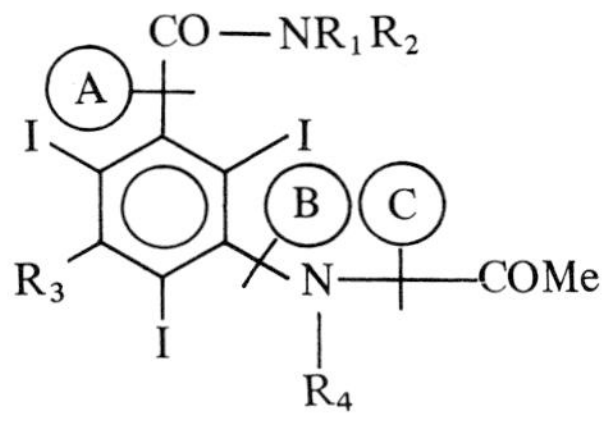

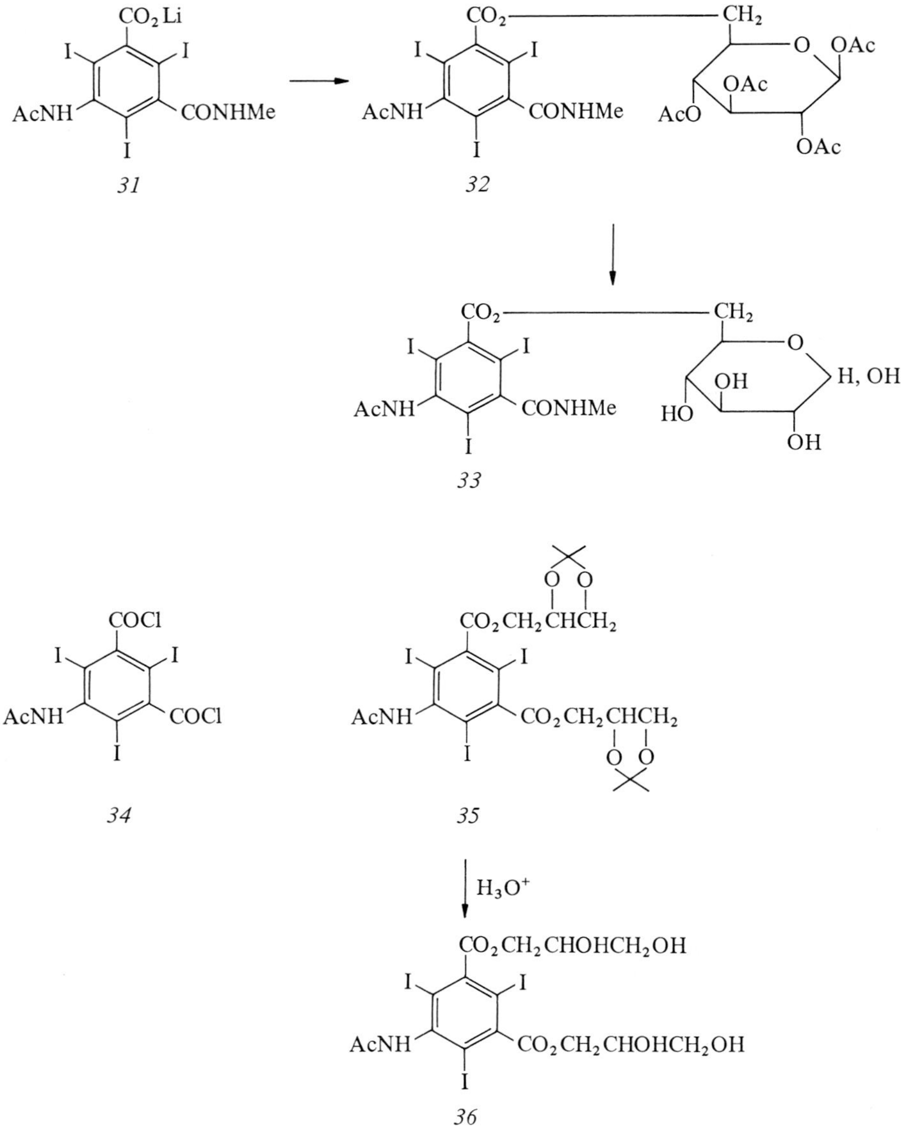

Fig. 27. Synthesis of ester-coupled nonionic compounds

1. Isomers Resulting from Restricted Rotation

ACKERMAN et al. [113–115] clearly demonstrated that optical and geometrical isomers could be isolated as a result of restricted rotation about bond "A" ($R_1 = R_2 = $ alkyl).

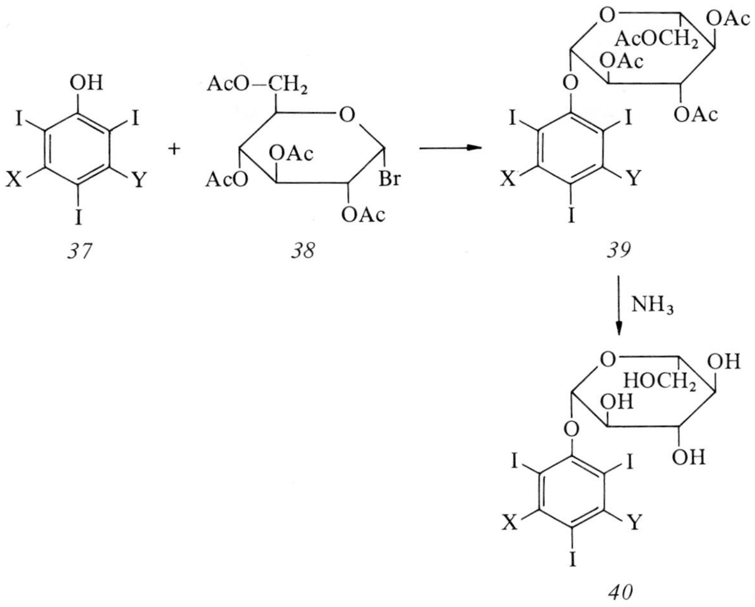

Fig. 28. Synthesis of glycosides

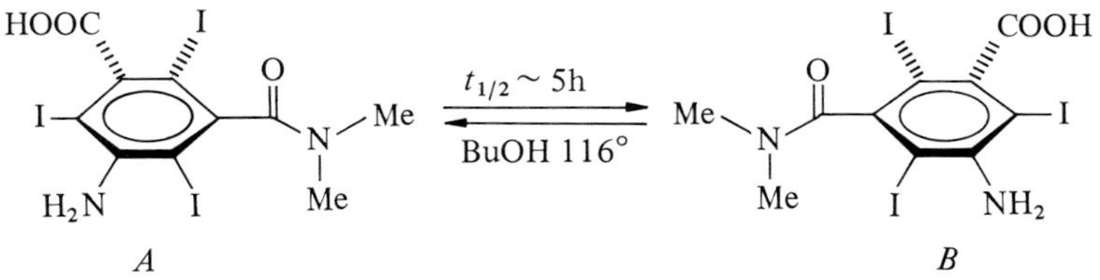

Fig. 29. Optical isomerism

a) Optical Isomerism

The authors isolated optically active A and found that A racemized at 116 °C (Fig. 29).

b) Geometrical Isomerism

Cis and trans isomers are formed due to restricted rotation. The same authors prepared cis isomer C and the optically active isomers (+) and (−) D. The cis isomer was a meso due to a plane of symmetry. The optically active trans isomer D was equilibrated and the half-life at 117 °C (nBuOH) was found to be about 9 h (Fig. 30).

In contrast to the information available for an N,N-disubstituted carbamyl group, there are no reports of restricted rotation at the aromatic-carbon, car-

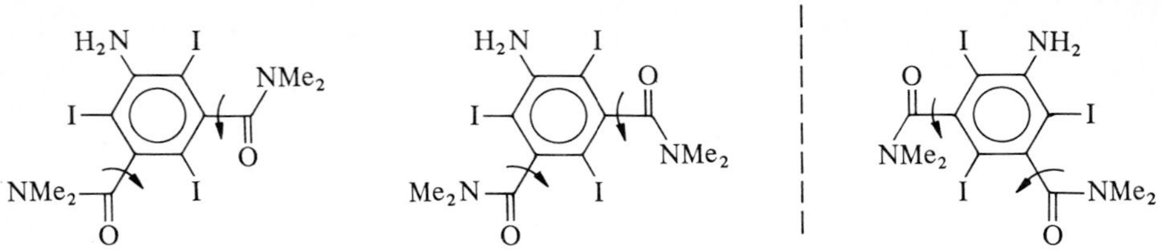

C "*cis*" — (+) *D* "*trans*" — Mirror plane — (–) *D* "*trans*"

Fig. 30. Geometrical isomerism

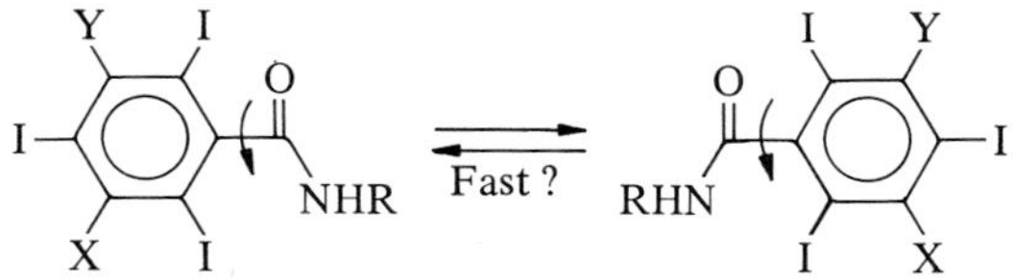

R = alkyl

Fig. 31. Equilibration at room temperature

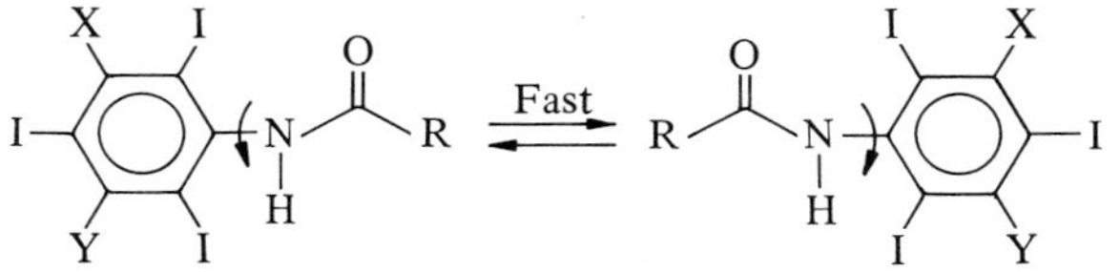

R = alkyl

Fig. 32. Rotation about bond "B"

bonyl-carbon bond in compounds with a monosubstituted carbamyl group (R_1 = H, R_2 = alkyl, hydroxyalkyl ... etc.). Possibly the barrier to rotation in the monosubstituted carbamyl group is lower than that of the disubstituted carbamyl group; therefore, equilibration is very fast at room temperature (Fig. 31).

Bond "B". There have been no reports of restricted rotation about bond "B" in iodinated aromatic compounds when R_4 = H (see Fig. 32). When R_4 = alkyl, such isomers were proposed for iocetamic acid [96]. The two diastereoisomers were isolated in a crystalline form (Fig. 33). In another communication, the occurrence of these isomers was reported [116] but the isomers were not isolated (Fig. 34).

Bond "C". When R_4 = alkyl, restricted rotation of the acyl group (bond "C") results in two thermodynamically preferred orientations of the acyl group [198]. In one form, the carbonyl of the acyl group is directed inward toward the aromatic nucleus (endo form). In the second, it points outward (away) from the aromatic nucleus (exo form). These isomers are in equilibrium in solution and are separable by thin-layer chromatography or liquid chromatography (Fig. 35).

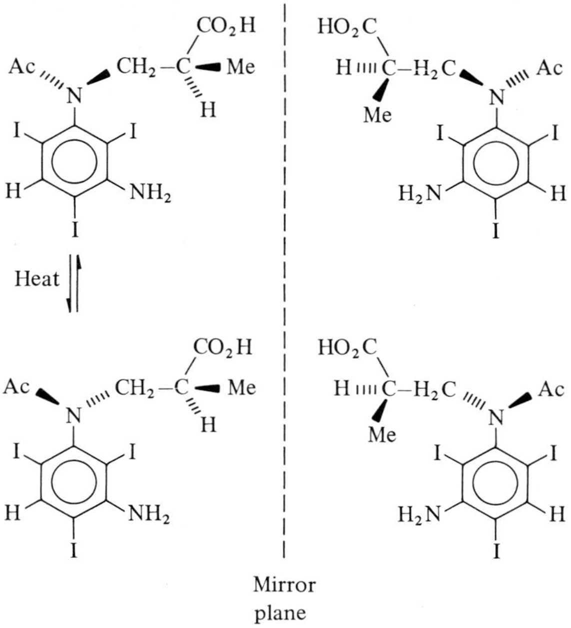

Fig. 33. Isolation of two diastereoisomers

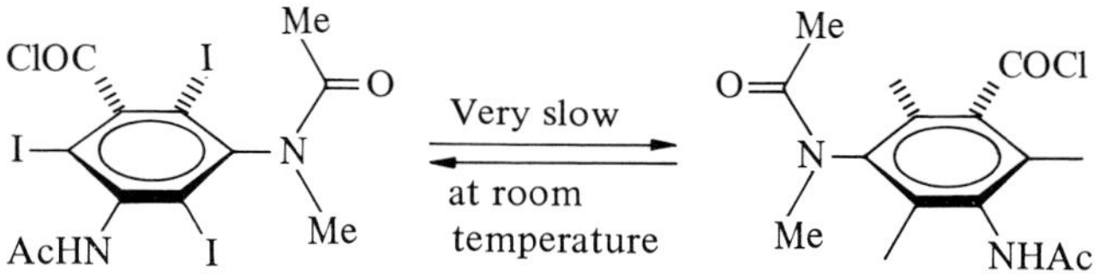

Fig. 34. Occurrence of two diastereoisomers [116]

VII. High-Pressure Liquid Chromatography

The classical method for determining oil/water partition coefficients is to partition the compound between an organic solvent (e.g., CHCl$_3$, butanol, octanol) and water and to measure the conentration of the compound in each solvent by a sensitive analytical technique. The partition coefficient (P) is then calculated and the logarithm (log P) is related to the hydrophobicity of the compound (i.e., a negative log P indicates that the compound is not very hydrophobic; rather it is highly hydrophilic). Many of the nonionic CM are too hydrophilic for an accurate measurement of log P (in other words, the compound does not partition well into an organic solvent) [95].

A rapid and dynamic method for measuring the oil/water partition coefficients involves the use of high-pressure liquid chromatography (HPLC) [117]. By this method, a compound is injected onto a reverse-phase column of absorbant

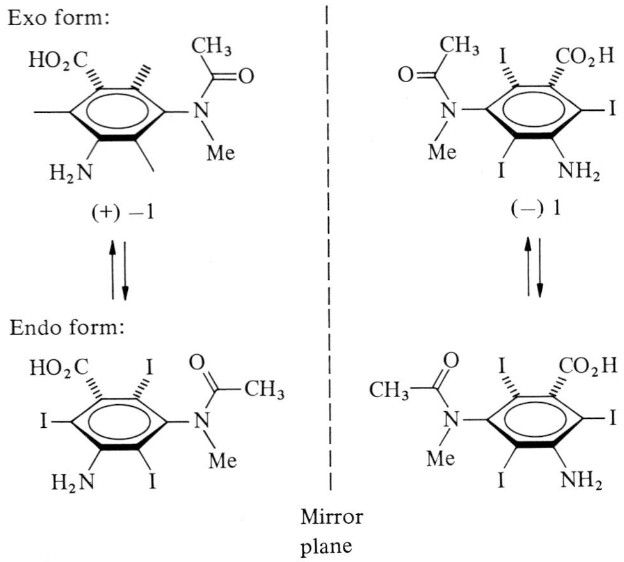

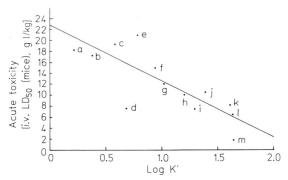

Exo form:

$(+) -1$

Endo form:

Mirror
plane

Fig. 35. Isomers from restricted rotation about bond "C"

Fig. 36. Correlation of the retention factor ($\log K'$) with acute toxicity (i.v. LD_{50}) of several nonionic reversed amide compounds. *a*, MP-10007 (Table 29); *b*, MP-8000 (Table 28); *c*, MP-10013 (Table 29); *d*, MP-10018 (Table 29); *e*, Iopamidol (Table 40); *f*, MP-7018 (Table 28); *g*, MP-6012 (Table 28); *h*, MP-5005 (Table 28); *i*, MP-7017 (Table 28); *j*, MP-7014 (Table 29); *k*, MP-5007 (Table 28); *l*, MP-5020 (Table 28); *m*, MP-6004 (Table 30) (compound 1)

consisting of a silica gel which is bonded with octadecylsilyl groups. It is thus non-polar and for the purpose of this discussion can be considered "an oil". The compound tested is eluted from the column with water. The retention (or capacity) factor K' is determined by Eq. (3); K' is related to the oil/water partition coefficient (a large K' is indicative of a highly hydrophobic compound).

$$K' = \frac{V - V_o}{V}, \tag{3}$$

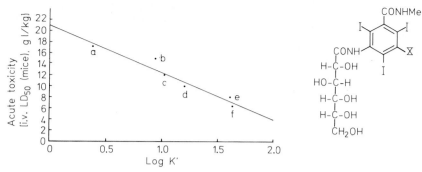

Fig. 37. Correlation of the retention factor (log K') with acute toxicity (i.v. LD$_{50}$) within a series of nonionic gluconanilides (reversed amides). Effects of varying the X group. *a*, Gluconamido; *b*, *N*-Hydroxyethylcarbamyl; *c*, Acetamido; *d*, *N*-Methylcarbamyl; *e*, *N,N*-Dimethylcarbamyl; *f*, *N*-Methylacetamido

where V is the volume of eluant required to elute the compound and V_o is the void volume of the column.

This method has been used for several series of nonionic CM [118]. Within a series of compounds with analogous structure, there appears to be a good correlation of acute toxicity (LD$_{50}$ i.v.) with log K'. For example, it was found that the acute toxicities for the reversed amides (Fig. 36) when treated by regression analysis could be described by Eq. (3). Within a series of gluconanilides (Fig. 37) there was even better correlation. However, acute toxicity values correlated poorly for compounds with different X, Y and coupler groups, which suggests that the determination of hydrophobicity by physical means (i.e., partition) cannot determine the biological toxicity of CM accurately.

Correlation of acute toxicity values of a series of nonionic reversed amides with log K':

$$LD_{50}(i.v.) = 10.2 \log K' + 22.8 \quad n = 13, \quad r = 0.7761, \quad s = 3.71 . \tag{4}$$

Correlation of acute toxicity values of a series of 3-*N*-methylcarbamyl gluconanilides with log K':

$$LD_{50}(i.v.) = 8.47 \log K' + 21.0 \quad n = 6, \quad r = 0.9628, \quad s = 1.02 . \tag{5}$$

VIII. Water-Insoluble Nonionic Contrast Media

Nonionic contrast media in water-insoluble forms have been used since the early days of radiography. These include both ester and amide derivatives, primarily ester derivatives of iodinated poppyseed oil, safflower oil, and rapeseed oil. For reviews on the use of these oil compounds in bronchography and lymphography, see the appropriate chapters in the work edited by KNOEFEL [1]. The second category in this class includes insoluble esters of iodinated organic compounds, such as the propyl ester of 3,5-diiodo-4-pyridone-*N*-acetic acid and the esters of triiodobenzoic acids designed to be hydrolyzed relatively quickly and completely in vivo.

The perfluorocarbons are nonionic but display entirely different chemical, physical, and biological characteristics [145].

1. Oily Contrast Media

The uses of these compounds have been previously reviewed [1]. Within the past several years a new application of these oils has developed. They have been used in an emulsified form in computed tomography (CT) [119–122]. Thus these materials given in doses of 0.2–0.3 ml/kg of a 3% iodine emulsion have been shown to enhance the contrast of the liver in patients, making diagnoses of metastases possible. The oils are trapped in the liver by the reticuloendothelial system (RES). A 10%–15% enhancement required for good visualization has been achieved with emulsion EOE-13, which is trapped primarily in the liver due to a particular particle size; the emulsion is relatively rapidly excreted (Mallinckrodt, Research Department, St. Louis, unpublished results).

Lipiodol Ultrafluid has been reported to represent an improvement over previous agents such as Ethiodol in that a stable, more reproducible formulation is provided (an emulsion of triglycerides of iodinated poppyseed oil) [123, 124].

Several formulations for emulsified oils have been tested [108, 110]. An iodinated poppyseed or sesame seed oil was formulated with glycerine and ethanol-soluble lecithin. The anhydrous mixture was emulsified with sterile water and mixed with isotonic sodium chloride or glucose solution prior to intravenous administration [125].

An iodinated fatty acid ester of glycerol emulsified with a polyoxyethylene-sorbitan-fatty acid emulsifier and water gave a formulation with an average droplet diameter of less than 1 ψm. The formulation was stable to sterilization by gamma irradiation [126].

An emulsion for lymphography of iodinated poppyseed oil combined with an emulsifier made from ethylene oxide and castor oil mixed with glycerol and 5% glucose solution contained a wide spectrum of particle sies (0.85–19 ψm). The viscosity was 48 cp at 20 °C. The formulation was reportedly unstable [127].

Another widely used oil is the ethyl ester of iodiophenylundecenoic acid (iophendylate). This material has been used for many years in myelography but has recently almost been replaced by the water-soluble CM. In an attempt to improve the safety and excretion characteristics of iophendylate, Newton and co-workers have synthesized a series of oily carbonate ester and thiocarbonate ester compounds [128–131]. Little difference was noticed between the approximate lethal dose (ALD_{50}) of p-iodo, m-iodo, and 3,5-diiodobenzylalcohols, while 3-amino-2,4,6-triiodobenzyl alcohol and 3-acetamido-2,4,6-triiodobenzyl alcohol had higher ALD_{50} values (Tables 42, 43).

The results suggest a definite relationship between toxicity and the aromatic substituent.

An advantage of the carbonates over iophendylate is lower viscosity and more rapid excretion. The thiocarbonate compounds appeared to be comparable to the carbonates [128–131].

Table 42. Approximate lethal doses of iodinated aromatic alcohols

Structure	Approximate lethal dose (g/kg)
I—⟨◯⟩—CH₂OH	1
(I, ◯)—CH₂OH	0.75
(I, ◯, I)—CH₂OH	<0.5
I—⟨◯⟩—CH₂OH (I, H₂N, I)	7.5
I—⟨◯⟩—CH₂OH (I, H₃COCHN, I)	7.5

2. Benzoate Esters

The esters of triiodobenzoic acid were investigated in applications wherein insolubility might offer certain advantages in terms of delayed excretion, e.g., in bronchography or lymphography. It would be expected that such esters would be hydrolyzed in vivo to give relatively nontoxic products, namely an acid and the alcohol analog. The ester compounds are readily synthesized by standard organic chemistry techniques, such as by Fischer esterification or by alkylation of the sodium salt of the acid with an alkyl halide. The ester compounds were formulated into aqueous suspensions intended for entrapment by the RES, depending on the particle size. In one of the earlier reports, esters of diatrizoic acid such as the hydroxyethyl or 2-3-dihydroxypropyl compounds gave LD_{50} values substantially greater than those of acetrizoate esters [133].

FELDER and co-workers have prepared and tested derivatives of both triiodo and tetriiodo-benzoic acid compounds [134–136].

$$CO_2CH_2CH_2OH$$

$$CO_2CH_2CH_2OH$$

Table 43. Approximate lethal doses of iodinated aromatic alcohols

Structure	Approximate lethal dose
I—⟨O⟩—OH	0.7 g/kg
I—⟨O⟩—CH$_2$OH	1.0 g/kg
I—⟨O⟩—CH$_2$CH$_2$OH	1.0 ml/kg
I—⟨O⟩—CHMeCH$_2$CH$_2$OH	0.5 ml/kg
I—⟨O⟩—CH$_2$CHEtCH$_2$OH	0.5 ml/kg
I—⟨O⟩—CHMe(CH$_2$)$_2$CH$_2$OH	2.2 ml/kg

These hydroxyalkyltetraiodoterephthalates were formulated in isotonic saline suspension with additives such as carboxymethylcellulose (CMC) and used in experimental lymphangiography; localized inflammatory reaction resulted [137].

In contrast to esters of tetraiodophthalic acid, esters of tetraiodoterephthalic acid are hydrolyzed to the well-tolerated tetraiodoterephthalic acid. Acute i.v. (LD$_{50}$) values obtained for 50% suspensions are 5,600 mg/kg and 380 mg/kg for the two acids. Their corresponding esters gave values generally higher than 10,000 mg/kg. Metabolism and excretion or the esters were evaluated in rats. A suspension of bis-2-hydroxyethyltetraiodoterephthalate in normal saline containing 200 mg I/ml was injected either intravenously or intraperitoneally at dosages of 1 g I/kg. Within 7 days after i.v. administration, 18% of the injected iodine was excreted in the urine and 23% in the feces. Later chromatographic studies indicated the excretion of unchanged ester, half acid ester, and the free acid. Within 8 days after intraperitoneal administration, 8.5% of the iodine had appeared in the urine [134–136].

ZUTTER and BRUNNER reported on a series of 22 amides of terephthalic acid [138]. Esters of 3,5-diiodo-4-pyridone-N-acetic acid have also been reported [139–141].

More recently, VIOLANTE and FISCHER have evaluated esters of iothalamic acid and of other CM as potential enhancing agents for liver and CT (see Chap. 13, this volume).

A novel type of ester has been reported by SOULAL and UTTING [142, 143]. They designed an ester of benzoic acid containing either an ester or acetal linkage, thus providing not only a stable crystalline solid but one which could be readily hydrolyzed in vivo. HOEY et al. [unpublished, 144] adopted a similar approach using ether (ketal) derivatives rather than ester linkages. Tables 44 summarize the results obtained with both types of molecules. Limited excretion data indicated that

Table 44. Hydrolytic esters

X	Y	R	Stability[a]	Toxicity (mice, i.p.)
CH_3CONH-	H	$-CH_2OC_2H_5$[b]	Unstable in H_2O suspension	3,100 mg/kg
CH_3CONH-	CH_3NHCO-	$-CH_2OC_2H_5$[b]	Unstable in H_2O suspension	16,000 mg/kg
CH_3CONH-	CH_3NHCO-	$-C_2H_5$[b]	Stable	1,900 mg/kg
CH_3CONH-	CH_3NHCO-	1-Glucopyranosyl-[b]	—	>10,000 mg/kg (i.p., oral)
Iobenzamic acid		$-CH_2OC_2H_5$[b]	—	>10 g/kg (i.p., oral)
CH_3CONH-	CH_3NHCO-	6-Glucose[b]	Soluble 50% w/v	Mouse i.v. $LD_{50} \sim 800$ mg/kg Mouse i.cereb. < 50 mg/kg Mouse oral < 10 g/kg
CH_3CONH-	$-CONHCH_3$	$-CH_2-O-COCH_3$[c]	—	—
CH_3CONH-	$-N(CH_3)COCH_3$	$-CH_2-O-COCH_3$[c]	—	—
CH_3CONH-	$-CONHCH_3$	(see structure)	—	—

[a] All H_2O insoluble. Tested in H_2O suspension in 0.5% methocel and 0.1% Na lauryl sulfate
[b] Hoey GB, Weigert PE, Kneller MT, VanDeripe DR (unpublished data, research Dept., Mallinckrodt, Inc.)
[c] Ref. [142]

these compounds are more rapidly hydrolyzed than the corresponding alkyl ester analogs and are also somewhat less toxic.

3. Perfluoroalkyl Halides

Perfluorohydrocarbon compounds have been studied as vehicles for oxygen transport, as synthetic blood substances, and as potential CM because of their high oxygen solubility and lack of chemical reactivity. Perfluorohexylbromide and perfluorooctylbromide have been studied extensively in animals and humans, suggesting application in gastrointestinal radiology, myelography, bronchography, lymphography, and CT enhancement of the liver [145–147]. Perfluorooctylbromide is a neutral, colorless, odorless, and tasteless liquid with a low surface tension (16–18 dynes/cm), which enables it to wet any surface and to flow freely

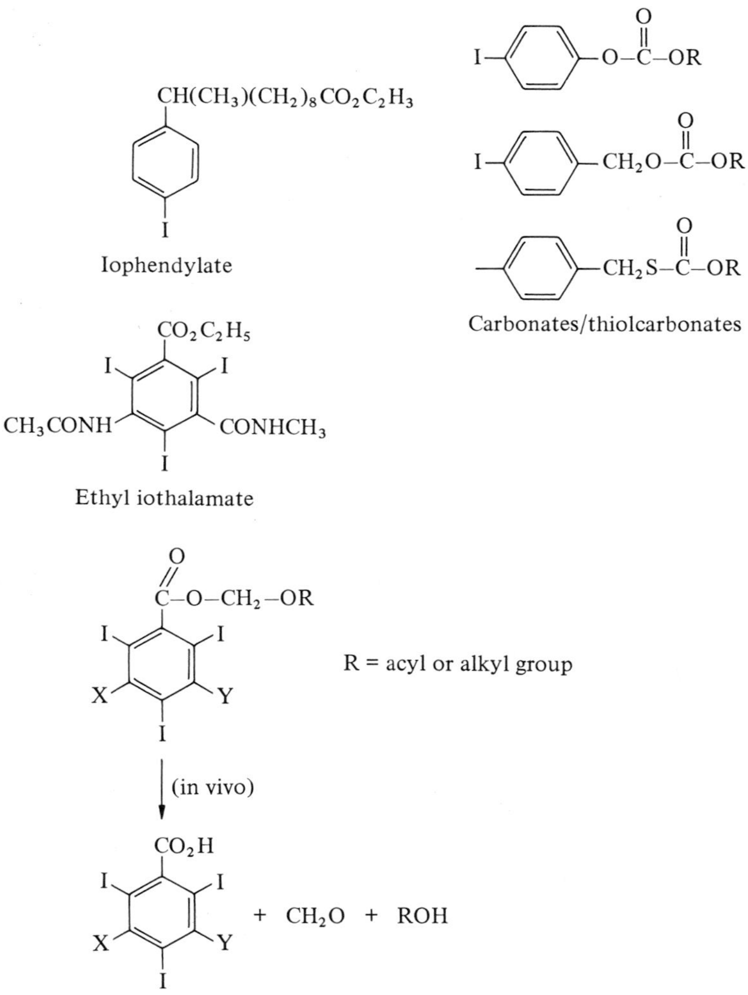

Fig. 38. Benzoate esters

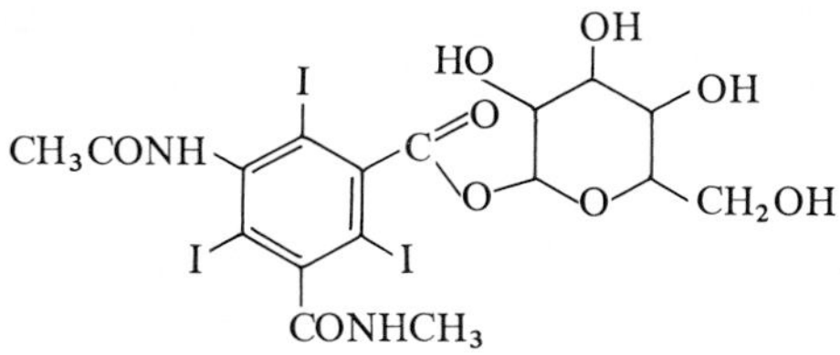

HOEY et al. [unpublished, 144]

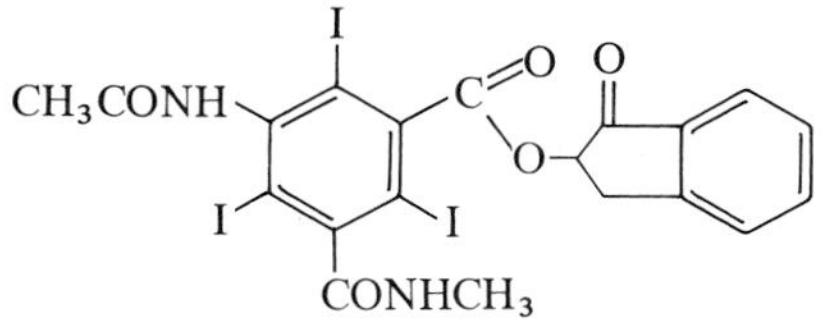

SOULAL and UTTING [142, 143]

into small folds and orifices. It is chemically stable and has a low boiling point. Perfluorohexylbromide has a boiling point of 98 °C and a vapor pressure of 90 mm.

E. Oral Cholecystographic Agents

The requirements for an oral cholecystopaque have been defined as follows [1, 148]

1. The compound must be orally absorbed.
2. The compound should be excreted from the liver and bile ducts in sufficient concentration to provide opacity to X-rays.
3. The compound should be nontoxic and exhibit minimal side effects.

The compounds are usually formulated as the free acid or as sodium or calcium salts in the form of tablets, suspensions, or liquids. it has been shown that the solid state of iopanoic acid greatly affects its dissolution rate; thus the amorphous form has a tenfold greater rate of dissolution than the crystalline form which is commercially available [149].

Generally useful agents are described by the general structure:

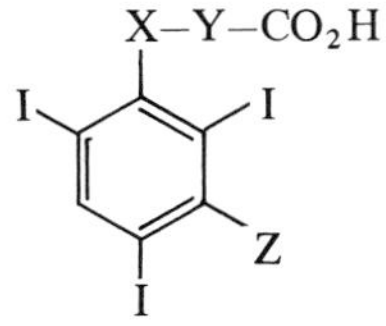

In this structure, X is an oxygen, a methylene group, a carbamoyl group, or an acylamino radical which connects a hydrophilic/lipophilic group Y to the triiodinated aromatic ring (Tables 45–48). The group Z (–NH$_2$ or –OH group) allows

Table 45. Oral cholecystopaques with X as an oxygen atom

Benzene ring substituted with $X-Y-CO_2H$, Z, and H and three iodine (I) atoms.

X	Y	Z	Toxicity data	Biliary visualization	Comments	Ref.
$-O-$	$-(CH_2)_3-$	$CON{\bigcirc}$ (morpholine)	0.62 (i. v.) 5.9 g/kg (Os)	Yes	Formulated with sucrose, Na carrageenin; $p\text{-}PrO_2CC_6H_4OH$, $pMeO_2CC_6H_4Me$	[227]
$-O-$	$-(CH_2)_n-O-CH_2CH-$ $\mid$ R' ($n=2$–4 $R'=Me, Et$)	$-NHC-R^2$ $\overset{O}{\parallel}$ ($R^2=Me, Et$)	Yes	Yes	Contains formulations – tablets, capsules, syrups. Iopronic acid $n=2$, $R'=Et$, $R^2=Me$	[90, 94, 95, 108–111, 223–225], [a]
$-O-$	$-CH_2CH_2OCH_2CH-$ $\mid$ R ($R=Me, Et$)	$-C-NR^1R^2$ $\overset{O}{\parallel}$ ($R^1=H$ $R^2=Me, Et$ $R^1R^2=CH_2CH_2OCH_2CH_2-$)				[230]
$-O-$	$-CH_2CH-$ $\mid$ NH_2 (attached to benzene ring)	$-OH$	?			[231]

[a] Mallinckrodt, Research Department, St. Louis (unpublished results)

Table 46. Oral cholecystopaques with X as a methylene or methine group

$X-Y-CO_2H$

Structure: benzene ring bearing I (×3), Z, and H substituents, with $X-Y-CO_2H$ attached.

X	Y	Z	Toxicity data	Biliary visualization	Comments	Ref.
$-CH_2-$	Et $-CH-$ $\mid$ R (R = Me, Et)	$-H-Ac$				[232]
$-CH_2-$	$-CH-$ $\mid$ R^1 (R^1 = H or A^a)	$-N=C-N$ with R^3, R^2, R^4 R_2 = H, alkyl R_3, R_4 = H or A^a R_3, R_4 = $-(CH_2)_4-$, $-CH_2CH_2OCH_2CH_2-$ $-CH_2CH_2NHCH_2CH_2-$	No	Claimed	Formulations are claimed. Suspensions, dragees, tablets, capsules (may use Ca salt)	[233]
$-CH_2-$	$-CH-$ $\mid$ R^1 [R^1 = H, A^a(Et), Ph]	ring structure with O, Y, N, O [Y = $-(CH_2)_{2,3}-$, $-(CH_2)_y O(CH_2)_3-$, $-(CH_2)_y-S-(CH_2)_3-$]	R^1 = Et Y = $-CH_2CH_2-$ LD_{50} = 595 mg/kg	Yes		[234]
$-CH_2-$	$-CH-$ $\mid$ R^1 R^1 = H, alkyl	$-N-C-Y-CO_2R^3$ with O, R^2 (R^2 = H, A^a, HO$-A^a$; R^3 = H, A^a)				[234]

Table 46. (continued)

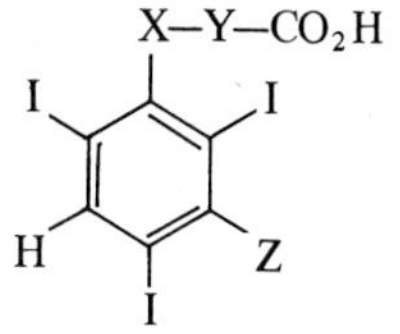

Structure: $X-Y-CO_2H$ on a benzene ring bearing three I substituents, one H, and substituent Z.

X	Y	Z	Toxicity data	Biliary visualization	Comments	Ref.
$-CH_2-$	$-CH-$ R (R = H, alkyl)	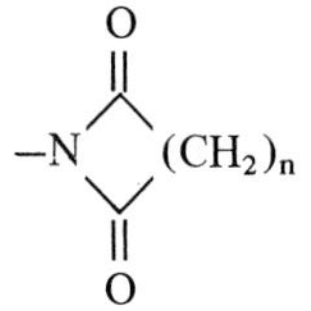 cyclic imide $-N(CH_2)_n$ with two $C{=}O$ (R^1 = H, Me, Et, n = 2, 3)				[235]
$-CH_2-$	$-CH-$ R (R = Et)	$O{=}\ \ {=}O$ $-NC{-}(CH_2)_n{-}CO_2H$, R^1				[236]
$-CH-$ R (R = H, Me, Et, Pr)	Single bond	$-NR^1R^2$ (R^1 = H, Ac, $-COEt$, $-COPr$; R^2 = H, Me, Et, Pr, Bu, CH_2Ph)	Yes	Yes		[237]
$-O-$ or $-CH_2-$	$-CH-$ R (R = H, Me, Et, Ph)	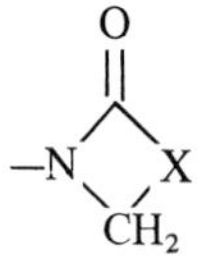 azetidinone $-N{\Big(}^{X}_{CH_2}$ with $O{=}$ (X = $-CH_2CH_2-$, $-CH_2OCH_2-$, $-CH_2CH_2CH_2-$)	Yes	Yes	B 8560 (X = CH_2, R = Et) was selected for pre-clinical studies	[238]
$-CH_2-$	$-CH-$ Et	$-NHCOPr$			Sustained release formulation of the sodium of tyropanoate	[239, 240]

[a] Lower alkyl

Table 47. Oral cholecystopaques with X as an acyl amino group

Structure: X–Y–CO$_2$H on a benzene ring bearing I, I, I, Z and B substituents.

B	X	Y	Z	Toxicity data	Biliary vizualization	Comments	Ref.
H	O=C–, –N–R, R=CH$_2$CH$_2$OH, CH$_2$CHOHCH$_2$OH	–CH$_2$CH$_2$–	–H		Yes		[241]
H	O=C–, –N–R^1, R=A[a]	–(CH$_2$)$_{1-2}$–CH–R^2, R^2=H, A[a]	–NH$_2$	Yes – LD$_{50}$ 750–1,175 (mg/kg) (Os)	Yes		[242, 243]
H	O=C–, –NC–, Me	–CH$_2$CH$_2$–	–CONEt$_2$				[244]
H	O=C–, –NC–, Et	–CH$_2$CH$_2$–	–NHMe		Yes	Tablet formulation Iosumetic acid	[245]
–NR$_2$R$_3$	–N–, Ac	–CH$_2$CH–R^1, (R^1=H or Me)	–NR^{2}R^3 (R^2=H, A, R^3=C–Me, –C–Et, =O)	Less toxic than iodipamide in mice	Yes		[246]
H	–N–, Ac	–CH$_2$CH–R, (R=H, Me)	–N=CHNMe$_2$	Yes	Yes		[247]

[a] Lower alkyl

Table 48. Oral cholecystopaques with X as a carbamyl group

$$X-Y-CO_2H$$

(benzene ring substituted with I, I, I, B, and Z; X–Y–CO₂H group attached)

B	X	Y	Z	Toxicity data	Visualization	Comments	Ref.
H	$O=C-NH$ (carbamyl)	phenyl, $X-(CH_2)_n-$, $X = -O-$ or single bond	$-NH_2$	Yes "Better tolerance in humans"	Yes	High bile/urine ratio 4.1–19.5. Formulated as pills, granules, capsules, dragees, globules, suspensions. Formulations given	[248]
H	$\overset{O}{\overset{\|}{C}}-\overset{R^2}{\underset{}{N}}$ (R = Me, Et)	phenyl, $X-(CH_2)_n CO_2H$, $X = -O-$ or single bond, $n = 2, 3$	$-NRR^1$ (R = H, Et) (R^1 = H, Ac)				[243, 249]
H	$-\overset{O}{\overset{\|}{C}}-N-$ / $-CH_2$	$-CH_2CH_2-$ / $-CH_2-$	$-N=$ (pyrrolidine ring with N–R^1) [R^1 = H, Me, Et, CH$_2$CH$_2$OH, Ph, -cyclo-C$_6$H$_{12}$, or (CH$_2$)$_n$OMe] ($n = 0, 2,$ or 3)	Yes			[250]

R^5				References
H, CO_2H, CONHMe	$\begin{array}{c}O\\\parallel\\-C-N\\\quad\mid\\\quad R\end{array}$ R = H, A^a, Ph, CH_2Ph, A^aOMe	$-CH_2CH-$ or $\quad\mid$ $\quad$ Me $-(CH_2)_n-$ $n = 1, 2,$ or 5	$-N=C-NR^3R^4$ $\quad\mid$ $\quad R^2$ $R^2 =$ H, Me, Et, or $CH_2CH_2CO_2H$ $R^3 =$ H, Me, Et $R^4 =$ Me, Et, or Ph $R^3R^4 = (-CH_2)_5-$ or $-CH_2CH_2OCH_2CH_2-$ Yes	[251]
H	$\begin{array}{c}O\\\parallel\\-C-N\\\quad\mid\\\quad R^1\end{array}$ $R^1 =$ H, A^a, HO–A^a, MeO–A, cyclo-A^a, Ph, Ph–A^a, allyl	$-(CH_2)_2$ (straight or branched chain) $-CH_2CH-$ $\quad\mid$ $\quad R^2$ $R^2 =$ H, Me, Et	(pyrrolidine imine structures with N–R^1) Tablet formulation	[252–254]
H	$\begin{array}{c}O\\\parallel\\-C-N-\\\quad\mid\\\quad R\end{array}$ R = H, A^a, AO^aA^a, AOAOA	$-(CH_2)_n-$ $n = 1-5$	$-N=CH-NMe_2$ $\begin{array}{c}O\\\parallel\\-NHC-(CH_2)_n-\end{array}$ $O(CH_2)_m-OR^1$ $n = 1-5,\ m = 2-3$ $R^1 =$ H, A^a	[255, 256]

^{a} Lower alkyl

Table 49. Cholecystopaques in use

Compound	X	Y	Z	Ref.
Iopanoic acid	$-CH_2-$	$-CH-$ Et	$-NH_2$	[170]
Ipodic acid (ipodate)	$-CH_2-$	$-CH_2-$	$-N=CHNMe_2$	[171]
Iobenzamic acid	$-CON-$ Ph	$-CH_2CH_2-$	$-NH_2$	[172]
Iocetamic acid	$-N-$ Ac	$-CH_2CH-$ Me	$-NH_2$	[173]
Tyropanoic acid	$-CH_2-$	$-CH-$ Et	$-NHCOPr$	[174]
Iopronic acid	$-O-$	$-(CH_2)_2OCH_2CH-$ Et	$-NHAc$	[163]

introduction of three iodine atoms into the aromatic ring. Subsequently it is usually modified to provide chemical stability and/or to reduce chemical toxicity and/or to provide greater biliary excretion. In the past 10 years, several workers have patented compounds in which the 5-position is not hydrogen, but none of these compounds has found clinical utility.

Numerous compounds have been evaluated clinically; however, the only compounds which are in current use are iopanoic acid, ipodic acid (ipodate), iobenzamic acid, iocetamic acid, and tyropanoic acid (Table 49). Iopronic acid has been extensively evaluated in animals and man and reportedly is much safer than iopanoic acid [158–169].

References

1. Hoey GB, Wiegert PE, Rands RD Jr (1971) Organic iodine compounds as X-ray contrast media. In: Knoefel PK (ed) Radiocontrast agents, sect 76, vol 1. Pergamon, New York, pp 23–131
2. Ackerman JH (1970) Diagnostic Agents. In: Burger AA (ed) Medicinal chemistry, 3rd edn. Wiley, New York, pp 1686–1699
3. Doerge RF, Wilson CO (1977) Diagnostic agents. In: Wilson CO, Gisvold O, Doerge RF (eds) Textbook of organic medicinal and pharmaceutical chemistry. Lippincott, Philadelphia, p 939
4. Lasser C (1967) Dynamic factors in roentgen diagnosis. Williams and Wilkins, Baltimore
5. Miller RE, Skucas J (1977) Radiographic contrast agents. University Park Press, Baltimore, pp 329–418, 451–494
6. Contrast Material Symposium (1980) Invest Radiol [Suppl] 15/6
7. Wallingford VH (1953) The development of organic iodine compounds as X-ray contrast media. J Am Pharmacol Assoc 42:721–728
   See also: Wallingford VH, Becker HH, Kruty M (1952) X-ray contrast media. I. Iodinated acylaminobenzoic acids. J Am Chem Soc 74:4365

8. Knoefel PA (1971) Binding of iodinated radiocontrast agents to plasma proteins. In: Knoefel PA (ed) Radiocontrast agents, sect 76, vol 1. Pergamon, New York, pp 133–145

9. Baker CE (1979/1980) Physicians desk reference for radiology and nuclear medicine. Medical Economics, Oradell, p 75

10. Aspelin P (1979) Effect of ionic and nonionic contrast media on red cell deformability in vitro. Acta Radiol [Diagn] (Stockh) 20:1–12

11. Guerbet M, Tilly G (1969) 2,4,6-Triiodo-3-(N-hydroxyethyl)carbamoyl)-5-(acetylamino) benzoic acid as an opaquing agent for radiography. French patent 6777, 21 April 1969

12. Grainger RD (1979) A clinical trial of a new low osmolality contrast medium. Sodium and meglumine ioxaglate (Hexabrix) compared with meglumine iothalamate (Conray) for carotid arteriography. Br J Radiol 52:781–786

13. Lehninger AL (1975) The molecular basis of cell structure and function. In: Biochemistry, 2nd ed. Worth, New York, p 174

14. Harrington C, Michie C, Lynch PR, Russel MA, Oppenheimer MJ (1966) Blood brain barrier changes associated with unilateral cerebral angiography. Invest Radiol 1:431–440

15. Sorensen SE (1971) Changes in vascular permeability after local application of roentgen contrast media in the hamster cheek pouch. Acta Radiol [Diagn] (Stockh) 11:274–288

16. Waldron RL, Bridgenbraugh RB, Dempsey EW (1974) Effect of angiographic contrast media at the cellular level in the brain: hypertonic vs. chemical action. AJR 122:469–476

17. Rapoport SI, Hori M, Klatzo I (1972) Testing of hypothesis for osmotic opening of the blood brain barrier. Am J Physiol 223:323–331

18. Sterrett PR, Bradley IM, Kitten TG, Janssen FH, Holloway SL (1976) Cerebrovasculature permeability changes following experimental cerebral angiography. A light and electron microscopic study. J Neurol Sci 30:385–403

19. Chaplin H, Carlsson E (1961) Change in human red blood cells during in vitro exposure to several roentgenologic contrast media. AJR 86:1127–1137

20. Giammona ST, Lurie PR, Segar WE (1963) Hypertonicity following selective angiocardiography. Circulation 28:1096–1101

21. Meyer MW, Read RC (1964) Red cell aggregation from concentrated saline and angiographic media. Radiology 82:630–635

22. Friesinger GC, Schaffer J, Criley JM, Gartner RA, Ross RJ (1965) Hemodynamic consequences of the injection of radiopaque material. Circulation 31:730–740

23. Cohen LS, Kokko JP, Williams WH (1969) Hemolysis and hemoglobinuria following angiography. Radiology 92:329–332

24. Von Bubnoff M, Riecker G (1961) Zellosmolaritat und Zellwassergehalt. Klinische und experimentelle Untersuchungen an Erythrozyten. Klin Wochenschr 39:724–733

25. Raininko R (1979) Role of hypertonicity in the endothelial injury caused by angiographic contrast media. Acta Radiol [Diagn] (Stockh) 20:410–416

26. Almen T (1971) Toxicity of radiocontrast agents. In: Knoefel PK (ed) Radiocontrast agents, vol 2. Pergamon, New York, pp 443–550

27. Fischer HW (1968) Hemodynamic reaction to angiographic media. A survey and commentary. Radiology 91:66–73

28. Rapoport SI, Thompson HK, Bidinger JM (1974) Equi-osmolal opening of the blood brain barrier in the rabbit by different contrast media. Acta Radiol [Diagn] (Stockh) 15:21–32

29. Oldendorf WH (1971/1972) Blood brain barrier permeability to lactate. Eur Neurol 6:49–55

30. Hilal SK, Dauth GW, Hess KH, Gilman S (1978) Development and evaluation of a new water-soluble iodinated myelographic contrast medium with markedly reduced convulsive effects. Radiology 126:417–422

31. Haughton V, Ho K-C, Unger GF (1977) Arachnoiditis following myelography with water-soluble agents. Radiology 125:731–733

32. Rapoport SI, Levitan H (1974) Neurotoxicity of X-ray contrast media. AJR 122:186–193

33. Binz A (1937) History of the uroselectans. Z Urol 31:73–84

34. Long L Jr, Burger A (1941) Synthesis of some iodinated aromatic compounds. J Am Chem Soc 63:1586–1589

35. Wang JY-C (1980) Deiodination kinetics of water-soluble radiopaques. J Pharm Sci 69/6:671–675

36. Fischer H (1978) Contrast media in coronary arteriography: a review. Invest Radiol 13:450–457

37. Mohl MH, Rizzolo RR, Hoey GB, Gorman AD (1979) Determination of diatrizoic acid in X-ray contrast media by high performance liquid chromatography. 15th Midwest regional meeting, American Chemical Society, St. Louis, 8 November 1979

38. Hoey GB, Wiegert PE, Rands RD Jr (1971) Organic iodine compounds as X-ray contrast media. In: Knoefel PK (ed) Radiocontrast agents, sect 76, vol 1. Pergamon, New York, p 23

39. Lasser C (1967) Dynamic factors in roentgen diagnosis. Williams and Wilkins, Baltimore, pp 77–79

40. Kodama JK, Butler WM, Tusing TW, Hallett FP (1963) Iothalamate: a new intravascular radiopaque medium with unusual pharmacotoxic inertness. Exp Mol Pathol [Suppl] 2:65–80

41. Melartin E, Tuohimaa PJ, Dabb R (1970) Neurotoxicity of iothalamates and diatrizoates. I. Significance of concentration and cation. Invest Radiol 5:13–21

42. Haley TJ, McCormick WG (1957) Pharmacological effects produced by intracerebral injection of drugs in the conscious mouse. Br J Pharmacol 12:12–15

43. Valzelli L (1964) A simple method to inject drugs intracerebrally. Med Exp 11:23–26

44. Sovak M, Ranganathan R (1980) Stability of nonionic water-soluble contrast media: implications for their design. Invest Radiol 15:S323–S328

45. Hopkins RM, Tusing TW (1979) Preclinical pharmacology and toxicology evaluation for diagnostic X-ray contrast media. R&D Division, Mallinckrodt, St Louis

46. Gries H, Pfeiffer H, Speck U, Mützel W (1981) Ionic 5-C-substituted-2,4,6-triiodoisophthalic acid derivatives. German Offen 3,001,293, 16 July 1981

46a. Gries H (1981) 3,5-Dicyano-2,4,6-triiodobenzoic acids. German Offen 3,001,294, 16 July 1981

47. Priewe H, Rutkowski R, Pirner K, Junkman K (1954) Derivatives of 2,4,6-triiodo-3-aminobenzoic acid. Chem Ber 87:651–658

48. Hoey GB, Rands RD, Wiegert PE, Chapman DW, Zey RL, DeLaMater GB (1966) X-ray media. II. Synthesis of alkanoylbis(isophthalamic acids) and X-ray contrast agents. J Med Chem 9:964–966

49. Wiegert PE (1972) 5,5′,5′-(Nitrilotriacetamido)tris-(2,4,6-triiodobenzoic acids). German Offen 2,132,614, 17 Aug 1972

50. Wiegert PE (1974) (Nitrilotriacyltriimino)tris-(2,4,6-triiodobenzoic acid) compounds for X-ray contrast media. British patent 1,346,795, 13 Feb 1974

51. Bjork L, Erickson U, Ingelman B (1972) New type of contrast medium in selective coronary arteriography. Ups J Med Sci 77/1:19–21

52. Bjork L, Erickson UE, Ingelman BGA (1970) New type of contrast medium in arthrography. AJR 109/3:505–510

53. Bjork L (1959) X-ray contrast agent. French patent M 7251, 8 Sept 1969

54. Felder E, Pitre D, Fumagalli L, Lorenzotti E (1973) Radiopaque contrast media. XXIV. Synthesis and structure-activity relations of new hexaiodinated radiopaque compounds. Farmaco [Sci] 28/11:912–924

55. Felder E, Pitre D (1971) 3′,3″-Dicarboxy-2′,2″,4′,4″,6′,6″ hexaiodo-4,7,10,13-tetra-oxohexadecane-1,16-dianilide as X-ray contrast agent. German Offen 1,937,211, 4 Feb 1971

56. Felder E, Pitre D (1969) Nontoxic 4,7,10-trioxatridecanebis(3-carboxy-2,4,6-triiodo-anilide) for cholecystography. German Offen 1,922,578, 13 Nov 1969

57. Pharmacia AB (1970) Hydroxyalkylene bis(acylamino-2,4,6-triiodobenzoic acid) derivatives for use as X-ray visualization agents. British patent 1,207,974, 7 Oct 1970

58. Pfeiffer H, Speck U, Kolb H (1975) 3,5,9-Trioxaundecane-1, 11-dioxyl-bis(3-carboxyl-2,4,6-triiodoanilide) and its salts. German Offen 2,405,652, 21 Aug 1975

59. Weinmann HJ, Mützel W, Souchon R, Wegener OH (1981) Experimental water soluble contrast media for computed tomography of the liver. Excerpta Med Int Congr Ser 561:95–100

60. Bernstein J, Losee KA (1971) Tris(2-(2,4,6-triiodo-3-carboxy-5-acetamido-benzamido) ethyl)amine. German Offen 2,039,214, 25 Feb 1971

61. Tilly G, Hardouin MJC, Lautrou J (1977) X-ray contrast media. US patent 4,014,986, 29 March 1977

62. Tilly G, Hardouin MJC, Lautrou J (1977) X-ray contrast media. US patent 4,065,554, 27 Dec 1977

63. Thomson KR, Evill CA, Fritzche J, Benness GT (1980) Comparison of iopamidol, ioxaglate and diatrizoate during coronary arteriography in dogs. Invest Radiol 15:234–241

64. Owman T, Hoevels J (1979) Comparison of monomer, dimer and non-ionized medium at urography with simulated compression. ROEFO 131/3:309–317

65. Higgins CB, Sovak M, Schmidt WS, Kelley MJ, Newell JD (1980) Direct myocardial effects of intracoronary administration of new contrast material with low osmolality. Invest Radiol 15:39–46

66. Tilly G, Hardouin JC, Lautrou J (1974) Improvements in or relating to new X-ray contrast media. British patent 1,488,904, 31 May 1974

67. Tilly G, Hardouin MJG, Lautrou J (1979) New ionic polyiodo benzene derivatives useful as X-ray contrast media. British patent 2,002,583A, 19 Dec 1979

68. Hebky J, Polacek J (1970) Preparation of 3,5-diaminobenzyl alcohol and its iodinated derivatives. Coll Czech Chem Commun 35/2:667–674

69. Hebky J, First B, Polacek J, Karasek M (1970) Synthesis of iodinated benzylamine X-ray diagnosis. Coll Czech Chem Commun 35/3:867–881

70. Hebky J (1970) X-ray contrast agents. Pharm Ind 32/10A:938–940

71. Hebky J, Polacek J, Tikal I, Lupinek V, Sova M (1976) Synthesis of iodinated derivatives of 3-aminobenzylamine and 3,5-diaminobenzylamine for X-ray diagnosis. Coll Czech Chem Commun 41/10:3094–3105

72. Van Ootegham SP, Smith RG, Daves G Jr, Chang EM, El-Mazati A, Olsen GD, Riker WK (1976) Iodo-bis(quaternary ammonium) salts. Potential cartilage-selective X-ray contrast agents. J Med Chem 19/11:1349–1352

73. Sovak M, Weitl FL, Lang JH, Higgins CB (1979) Development of a radiopaque cation: toxicity of the benzylammonium group. Eur J Med Chem Chim Ther 14/3:257–260

74. Speck U, Klieger E, Mützel W (1981) Triiodinated aminoacetamido isophthalamide X-ray contrast agents. US patent 4,283,381, 11 Aug 1981

75. Suter H, Zutter H (1975) Diiodofumaric acid derivatives as possible new X-ray contrast agents. Pharm Acta Helv 50/5:151–152

76. Carnmalm B, Gyllander J, Jonsson HA, Mikiver L (1974) Potential X-ray contrast agents. III. Synthesis of some derivatives of iodomethanesulfonic acid and tris (iodomethyl) acetic acid. Acta Pharm Suec 11/2:161–166

77. Suter H, Zutter H, Brunner J (1971) Tetraiodoterephthalic acid derivatives as X-ray contrast agents. Helv Chim Acta 54/7:2097–2107

78. Bedford AJM (1973) Radiographic contrast medium. German Offen 2,136,255, 22 March 1973

79. Hoey GB (1970) The symposium on contrast media toxicity of the Association of University Radiologists. Invest Radiol 5/6:453

80. Kleiger E, Schroeder E (1975) Synthesis of N-(3-acylamino-5-alkylcarbamoyl-2,4,6-triiodobenzoyl) amino acids as X-ray contrast agents. Eur J Med Chem Chim Ther 10/1:84–88

81. Bjork L, Erickson U, Ingelman B (1970) Polymeric contrast media for roentgenologic examination of gastrointestinal tract. Invest Radiol 3:142–148 (and references therein)

82. Bjork L, Erickson U, Ingelman B, Zaar B (1974) Improved polymeric contrast agents for roentgenologic examination of the gastrointestinal tract. Upsala J Med Sci 79:103–105 (and references therein)

83. Bjork L, Erickson U, Ingelman B (1976) Preliminary report on angiography with polymeric contrast agents in rabbits and dogs. Ups J Med Sci 81:183–187 (and references therein)

84. Almen T (1969) Contrast agent design. Some aspects of the synthesis of water soluble contrast agents of low osmolarity. J Theor Biol 24:216–226

85. Holtermann H (1973) Metrizamide, a nonionic, water soluble contrast medium. Acta Radiol [Suppl] (Stockh) 335:1–4

86. Kejha J, Radek O, Jelinek V, Nemecek O (1966) X-ray opaque agents. Czech patent 118,444, 15 May 1966 (cf Chem Abstr 66:55207r, 1967)

87. Kocourek J (1966) A method for the manufacture of 6-O-(2,4,6-triiodophenyl)-D-glucose. Czech patent 120,380, 15 Oct 1966

88. Almen TO, Haavaldsen J, Nordal N (1971) Nonionic iodinated X-ray contrast media. German Offen 2,031,724, 7 Jan 1971 (cf Chem Abstr 74:99662e, 1971)

89. Torsten HO, Almen TO, Haavaldsen J, Vegard T (1972) N-(2,4,6-triiodobenzoyl)-sugar amines. US patents 3,701,771, 31 Oct 1972 (and 4,021,481, 3 May 1977)

90. Suter H, Zutter H, Mueller HR (1971) Iodomethansulfonamides. German Offen 2,201,578, 23 March 1971 (cf Chem Abstr 78:3694a, 1973; see also British patent 1,359,908, 17 July 1974)

91. Felder E, Pitre D, Tirone P (1977) Radiopaque contrast media. XCIV. Preclinical studies with a new nonionic contrast agent. Farmaco [Sci] 32:835–844

92. Herskovits TT, Kelly TM (1973) Viscosity studies of aqueous solutions of alcohols, ureas, and amides. J Phys Chem 77:381–388 (and references cited therein)

93. Rakli FB, Keely MJ (1980) A process for the preparation of a sterile injectable physiologically acceptable solution of an X-ray contrast agent and solutions of the contrast agent and a buffer. British patent 2,031,405, 23 April 1980

94. Weitl FL, Sovak M, Ohno M (1976) Synthesis of a potential water soluble radiographic contrast medium, 2,4,6-triiodo-3-acetamido-5-N-methylcarboxamidophenyl β-D-glucopyranoside. J Med Chem 10:353–356

95. Weitl FL, Sovak M, Williams TM, Lang JH (1976) Studies in the design of X-ray contrast agents. Synthesis, hydrophobicity, and solubility of some iodoresorcyl bis β-glucosides. J Med Chem 10:1359–1362

96. Sovak M (this volume) Introduction

97. Felder E, Vitale RS, Pitre DF (1977) Water soluble, non-ionizing hydroxy-containing amide derivates of 2,4,6-triiodo-isophthalic acid. US patent 4,001,323, 4 Jan 1977

98. Felder E, Pitre DE (1976) Easily water-soluble nonionic X-ray contrast agents. German Offen 2,547,789, 24 Jan 1976 (cf Chem Abstr 8s:94103r, 1976)

99. Pfeiffer H (1979) Method for the preparation of serinol (1,3-dihydroxy-2-aminopropane). German Auslegeschrift 2,742,981, 22 March 1979)

100. Pfeiffer H, Speck U (1978) New dicarboxylic acid-bis-(3,5-dicarbamoyl-2,4,6-triiodoanilides). German Offen 2,628,517, 5 Jan 1978

101. Sovak M, Ranganathan R, Speck U (1982) Nonionic dimer: Development and initial testing of intrathecal contrast agents. Radiology 142:115–118

102. Felder E, Pitre D (1978) Water soluble, nonionic X-ray contrast agent. German Offen 2,805,928, 5 Oct 1978 (cf Chem Abstr 90:127532p, 1979)

103. Felder E, Vitale RS, Pitre D (1979) Water-soluble, nonionizing, radiopaque compounds and contrast compositions containing the same. US patent 4,139,605, 13 Feb 1979

104. Tilly G, Hardouin M, Michel JC, Lautrou J (1975) X-ray contrast medium. German Offen 2,456,685, 12 June 1975 (cf Chem Abstr 83:114021b, 1975; see also British patent 1,436,357, 19 May 1976)

105. Hoey GB, Murphy GP, Wiegert PE, Woods JW (1977) 3,5-Disubstituted-2,4,6-triio-doanilides of monobasic polyhydroxy acids. German Offen 2,643,841, 7 April 1977 (cf Abstr 87:136300, 1977)

106. Lin Y, Smith KR (1979) N-(2-Hydroxyethyl)-2,4,6-triiodo-3,5-bis-(2-keto-L-gulona-mido) benzamide and radiological compositions containing same. 15th American Chemical Society Midwest Meeting, St Louis, 8 Nov 1979

107. Lin Y (1981) N,N′-Bis(2,3-dihydroxypropyl)-2,4,6-triiodo-5-(2-keto-L-gulonamido) isophthalamide and radiological compositions. US patent 4,256,729, 17 March 1981

108. Tilly G, Hardouin MJC, Lautrou J (1976) X-ray contrast material. German Offen 2,624,153, 23 Dec 1976 (cf Chem Abstr 87:157183, 1977; see also US patent 4,062,934, 13 Dec 1977)

109. Smith KR (1977) N-Triiodobenzoylaminoacyl derivates of polyhydroxyamines. German Offen 2,710,730, 22 Sept 1977 (cf Chem Abstr 88:2337w, 1978)

110. Smith KR (1976) L-(3,5-Disubstituted-2,4,6-triiodophenyl)-3-(polyhydroxy-alkyl) urea compounds. German Offen 2,610,500, 25 Nov 1976 (cf Chem Abstr 86:190410e, 1977; see also US patent 4,109,081, 22 Aug 1978)

111. Smith KR (1976) Polyhydroxyalkyl 3,5-disubstituted-2,4,6-triiodocarbanilate. German Offen 2,541,491, 15 April 1976 (cf Chem Abstr 85:63296, 1976; see also US patent 4,125,706, 14 Nov 1978)

112. United States Pharmacopoeia, 20th revision. US Pharmacopoeial Convention, Rockville, p 1037 (and references therein)

113. Ackerman JH, Laidlaw GM, Snyder CA (1969) Restricted rotational isomers I. Hindered triiodoisophthalic acid derivatives. Tetrahedron Lett 44:3879

114. Ackerman JH, Laidlaw GM (1969) Restricted rotational isomers II. Maleimido derivatives of the cis and trans isomers of 5-amino, 2,4,6-triiodo-N,N,N′,N′-tetra-methylisophthalimides. Tetrahedron Lett 51:4487

115. Ackerman JH, Laidlaw GM (1970) Restricted rotational isomers III. Cis and trans 3′,5′-(dimethylcarbamoyl)-2′,4′,6′-triiodooxalanilic acid and their N-methyl derivatives. Tetrahedron Lett 27:2381

116. Hol L, Kelly M, Salvesen S (1977) Metrizamide. In: Goldberg ME (ed) Pharmacological and biochemical properties of drug substances. American Pharmacological Association, Washington (Academy pharmaceutical sciences, vol 1, pp 387–412)

117. McCall JM (1975) Liquid-liquid partition coefficients by high pressure liquid chromatography. J Med Chem 18:549–552

118. Rizzolo RR, Smith KR, Hoey GB, Reed RD, Ehrhard EJ (1979) Relationship between toxicity and HPLC retention times of nonionic iodinated X-ray contrast media. 15th American Chemical Society Midwest Meeting, St Louis, 8 Nov 1979

119. Larmaque JL, Bruel JM, Dondelinger B, Vendrell B, Pelissier O, Rouanet JP, Michel JL, Boulet P (1979) The use of iodolipids in hepatosplenic computed tomography. J Comput Assist Tomogr 3/1:21–24

120. Vermess M, Chatterji BC, Doppman JL, Grimes G, Adamson RH (1979) Development and experimental evaluation of a contrast medium for computed tomographic examination of liver and spleen. J Comput Assist Tomogr 3:25–31

121. Vermess M, Adamson RH, Doppman JL, Rapson AS, Herdt JR (1976) Intravenous hepatospleenography. Experimental evaluation of a new contrast material. Radiology 119/1:31–37

122. Grimes G, Vermess M, Galielli JF, Girton M, Chatterji BD (1979) Formulation and evaluation of ethiodized oily emulsion for intravenous hepatography. J Pharm Sci 68/1:52–56

123. Roth SL, Dumbrowski H, Heiort U, Kalbfleisch H, Ludwig J, Siefart F, Saeher A, Vielhauer E (1979) A new contrast medium emulsion for lymphography. ROFO 131/3:317–321

124. Villemein T, Morre J, Laval-Jeantet AM, Laval Jeantet M (1973) Experimental hepatography in the rat by selective intraarterial injection of an iodolipid emulsion. Ann Radiol (Paris) 16/7–8:527–532

125. Arbadus BT, Ferno OB, Linderot TO (1971) X-ray contrast agent. German patent 1,617,275, 13 May 1971

126. Roth S (1977) X-ray contrast agent based on an emulsion of iodinated oils. German patent 2,602,907, 28 July 1977
127. Fritsch G, Voigt R, Lleuning M (1970) Preparation of a contrasting emulsion agent for lymphography. Pharmazie 25/4:248–252
128. Newton BN (1976) Iodine containing organic carbonates as investigative radiopaque compounds. J Med Chem 19/12:1362–1366
129. Newton BN (1977) Iodine containing organic carbonates for use as radiographic agents. US patent 4,022,814, 10 May 1977
130. Newton BN (1978) Structure-toxicity relationships of iodinated organic carbonates and related compounds. J Pharm Sci 67/8:1154–1157
131. Newton BN (1978) Iodinated thiolcarbonates for use as radiographic contrast agents. US patent 4,125,554, 14 Nov 1978
132. Deleted in production
133. Larsen AA (1964) Iodinated esters of substituted benzoic acids and preparations thereof. US patent 3,119,858, 20 Aug 1964
134. Felder E, Pitre D, Tirone P, Zingales AH (1978) Radiopaque contrast media. XLV. Experimental lymphography with crystal suspensions. Farmaco [Sci] 33/4:302–314
135. Felder E, Pitre E (1976) New X-ray media and methods for their preparation. German Offen 2,625,826, 23 Dec 1976
136. Felder E, Vitale RS, Pitre D (1977) Radiopaque esters of tetriiodoteraphthalic acid. US patent 4,044,048, 23 Aug 1977
137. Kaude JE, Abrams RM, Daly JW (1978) Percutaneous indirect lymphography with a new experimental contrast medium – a preliminary report. Angiology 29/2:162–168
138. Zutter H, Brunner J (1970) New X-ray contrast media, their use and methods for their preparation. German Offen 1,958,333, 27 Aug 1970
139. Schic M, Povse T, Zupet T (1971) Bronchography using an iodine contrast agent substituted at the ester of 3,5-diiodo-4-pyridone in N-carboxylic acid ester. Tekhnika 26/4:158–159
140. Povse T, Zupet T, Japelj N (1971) Tekhnika 26/4:333–336
141. French Patent 2,180,568 (1974) Contrast material for radiologic examinations, 4 Jan 1974
142. Soulal MJ, Utting K (1974) Acetoxymethyl and peivaloyloxymethyl 5-acetamido-2,4,6-triiodo-N-methylisophthalamates. US patent 3,795,698, 3 May 1974
143. Soulal MJ, Utting K (1975) Derivatives of 3-acetamido-2,4,6-triiodobenzoic acid. German Offen 2,428,140, 23 Jan 1975
144. Hoey GB (1980) Lower alkoxymethyl esters of 2,4,6-triiodobenzoic acid derivatives. US patent 4,225,725, 30 Sept 1980
145. Long EM, Liu MS, Dobben GB, Scanto PF, Aranbulo AS (1976) Radiopaque applications of brominated fluorocarbon compounds in experimental animals and human subjects. Am Chem Soc Ser 28:171–189
146. Enzmann D, Young SY (1979) Applications of perfluorinated compounds as contrast agents in computed tomography. J Comput Assist Tomogr 3/5:622–626
147. Brahme F, Sovak M, Powell H, Long DM (1975) Perfluorocarbon bromides as contrast media in radiography of the central nervous system. Acta Radiol [Suppl] (Stockh) 347
148. Felder E, Tanara CB (1976) Radiopaque contrast media. XXXIII. Oral cholecystography, a review. Farmaco [Sci] 31:283–294
149. Stagner WC, Guillory JK (1979) Physical characterization of solid iopanoic acid forms. J Pharm Sci 68:1005–1009
150. Deleted in production
151. Deleted in production
152. Deleted in production
153. Deleted in production
154. Deleted in production
155. Deleted in production
156. Deleted in production
157. Deleted in production

158. Pitre D, Felder E (1976) Radiopaque contrast media. XLII. Metabolism of iopronic acid in human. Farmaco [Sci] 31:540–546

159. Pitre D (1976) Radiopaque contrast media. XL. Isolation and identification of the metabolites of iopronic acid in the urine and bile of the dog. Farmaco [Sci] 31:516–528

160. Pitre D, Fumagalli L (1976) Radiopaque contrast media. XLI. Isolation and identification of the metabolites of iopronic acid in the rat. Farmaco [Sci] 31:529–539

161. Raffaeli E, Facino RM, Salmona M, Pitre D (1977) In vitro binding and metabolism of iopronic acid by rat liver microsomes. Pharmacol Res Commun 9:833–846

162. Pitre D, Facino RF (1976) Radiopaque contrast media. XXXIX. Metabolism of iopronic acid by rat liver microsomes: characterization and identification of the metabolites. Farmaco [Sci] 31:755–762

163. Felder E, Pitre D (1972) 3[ω[3-(Acylamino)-2,4,6-triiodophenoxy]alkoxy]-2-alkyl-propinoic acids. German Offen 2,128,902. 22 June 1972

164. Felder E, Pitre D, Fumagalli L, Lorenzotti E (1976) Radiopaque contrast media. XXXIV. Derivatives of ω-(3-amino-2,4,6-triiodophenoxy)alkoxyalkanoic acids. Farmaco [Sci] 31:349–363

165. Felder E, Pitre D, Frandi M (1976) Radiopaque contrast media. XXXV. Physical properties of iopronic acid, a new oral cholecystographic agent. Farmaco [Sci] 31:426–437

166. Felder E, Zingales MF, Tiepolo U (1976) Radiopaque contrast media. XXXVI. Iopronic acid: proposed analytical monograph. Farmaco [Prat] 31:383–396

167. Pitre D, Frigerio A, Maffei-Facino R (1976) Identification of some urinary metabolites of iopronic acid in human, rat and dog. Mass spectrum drug metab, Proc int symp, pp 13–30

168. Tirone P, Rosati G (1976) Radiopaque contrast media. XXXVII. Iopronic acid, a new contrast medium for oral chelecystography: pharmacologic investigation. Farmaco [Prat] 31:397–412

169. Tirone P, Rosati G (1976) Radiopaque contrast media. XXXVIII. Iopronic acid, a new contrast medium for oral cholecystography: toxicologic investigation. Farmaco [Prat] 31:437–446

170. Lewis TR, Archer S (1949) Preparation of some iodinated aminophenylalkanoic acids. J Am Chem Soc 71:3753–3755

171. Priewe H, Poljak A (1960) Foramidino derivatives of β-(2,4,6-triiodo-3-aminophenyl) alkanoic acids. Chem Ber 93:2347–2352

172. Obendorf W (1962) 3-Amino-2,4,6-triiodoaminobenzoyl compounds for use as X-ray contrast agents. German patent 1,085,048. Appl 6 Aug 1958 (ch Chem Abstr 56:5884h, 1962). US patent 3,051,745, 28 Aug 1962

173. Archer S, Hoppe JO (1959) Acylated triiodoaminophenylalkanoic acids. US patent 2,895,988, 21 July 1959

174. Almen T (1971) 2,4,6-Triiodobenzoic acid derivaties: methods for their preparation and properties as X-ray contrast media. In: Knoefel P (ed) Radiocontrast agents, vol 2. Pergamon, New York, p 688

175. Salvesen S, Haugen LG, Haavaldsen J, Nordal V (1971) Triiodobenzoic acid derivatives as X-ray contrast agents. Norwegian patent 122430, 28 June 1971
See also: Haugen LG, Salvesen S, Haavaldsen J, Nordal V (1969) Substituted 2,4,6-triiodobenzoic acids, X-ray contrast media. German Offen 1,928,838, 11 Dec 1969

176. Felder E, Pitre D, Grandi M (1977) Radiopaque contrast media. XLIII. Physico-chemical properties of iodamide. Farmaco [Sci] 32/10:755–766

177. Bernstein J, Losee KA (1972) 2,4,6-Triiodobenzoic acid derivatives. Methods for their preparation and properties as X-ray contrast media. German Offen 2,129,936, 27 Jan 1972

178. Wiegert PE (1976) 2,4,6-Triiodo-5-methoxyacetamido-N-methylisophthalamic acid compounds and their use in X-ray contrast media. German Offen 2,528,795, 12 Feb 1976

179. Tilly G (1971) Opaquing agents for radiography. French demande 2,074,734, 12 Nov 1971

180. Tilly G (1971) Iodinated radiocontrast agents. German Offen 211,750, 28 Oct 1971 (and French demande 2,085,636, 4 Feb 1972: Iodinated radiocontrast agents; also Norwegian patent 122430, 28 June 1971)

181. Haugen LG, Salvesen S, Haavaldsen J, Nordal V (1969) Substituted 2,4,6-triiodobenzoic acids, X-ray contrast media. German Offen 1,928,838, 11 Dec 1969

182. Pfeiffer H, Zoellner G, Beich W (1972) 3-Acetamido-5-(hydroxyacetamido)-2,4,6-triiodobenzoic acid-containing contrast media. German Offen 211,829, 26 Oct 1972 (and references therein)

183. Wiegert PE (1978) 2,4,6-Triiodobenzoic acid derivatives. Methods of preparation and use as X-ray contrast media. German Offen 2,732,825, 23 Feb 1978

184. Sterling Drug Co. (1970) Iodonated imido-benzoic acids. British patent 1,191,015, 5 May 1970

185. Ackerman JH (1969) Triiodoaniline derivatives. German Offen 1,915,196, 20 Nov 1969

186. Zupet P, Povse T, Japelj M, Sehic M, Obrez I, Bulic D (KRKA Inst. Raziskave Razvo) (1975) Novo Mesto, Yugoslavia. Kem Ind 24/7:379–381

187. Wiegert PE (1976) Substituted 2,4,6-triiodoisophthalamic acids for use in X-ray contrast media. German Offen 2,526,848, 2 Jan 1976

188. Kleiger E, Speck U (1978) Iodinated isophthalamic acid derivatives. German Offen 2,629,228, 5 Jan 1978 (see also Belgian patent 856,095, 27 Dec 1977)

189. Schering AG (1977) Iodinated isophthalamic acid derivatives. Belgian patent 856,095, 27 Dec 1977

190. Dagra NV (1971) X-Ray contrast medium containing a shielding component. Netherlands Appl 6,912,102, 10 Feb 1971 (CA 75:35436 (19), 1971)

191. Kneller MT (1978) Oxazolinylacetamidotriiodobenzoic acid X-ray contrast agents., US patent 4,066,743, 3 Jan 1978

192. Tilly G (1972) Triiodobenzene derivatives as X-ray contrast media. German Offen 2,216,627, 19 Oct 1972

193. Kleiger E, Schroeder E (1973) Synthesis of N-(carbamoylalkyl)triiodoisophthalamic acids and their use as X-ray contrast media. Arch Pharm (Weinheim) 306/11:834–845

194. Kleiger E, Beich W, Schroeder E (1976) Triiodoisophthalamic acid monoamino acid amides. US patent 3,953,501, 27 April 1976

195. Kleiger E, Beich W, Schroeder E (1973) N-3-Carbamoyl(or carboxy)-5-acetamido-2,4,6-triiodobenzoyl amino acids (or amides) for X-ray contrast media. German Offen 2,207,950, 23 Aug 1973

196. Bernstein J, Losee KA (1972) Substituted triiodoisophthalamic acids. US patent 3,666,800, 30 May 1972

197. Ackerman JH (1970) Iodinated imido-benzoic acids. British patent 1,191,015, 6 May 1970

198. Felder E, Pitre D, Zutter H (1974) 5-(Acetamidomethyl)-3-acetyl(2,3-dihydroxypropyl) amino-2,4,6-triiodobenzoic acid. German Offen 2,229,360, 7 Nov 1974 (see also French demande 2,150,805, 26 Aug 1971; US patent 3,360,436, 26 Dec 1967)

199. Felder E, Pitre D (1975) 3-Hydroxyacylaminomethyl-5-acylamino-2,4,6-triiodobenzoic acids and their use as X-ray contrast materials. German Offen 2,425,912, 20 March 1975

200. Felder E, Pitre D (1975) X-ray contrast medium. German Offen 2,422,718, 13 Feb 1975

201. Kleiger E (1972) Synthesis of triiodo-phenylacetic acid derivatives and their use as X-ray contrast agents. Chim Ther 7/6:475–478

202. Pfeiffer H, Zoellner G, Geich W (1972) Circulation-compatible 5-hydroxy (and alkoxy) acetamido-3-(acetamidomethyl)-2,4,6-triiodobenzoic acids for X-ray contrast media. German Offen 2,124,904, 7 Dec 1972

203. Kleiger E, Schroeder E (1976) Preparation of new hexaiodated X-ray contrast materials. Eur J Med Chem Chim Ther 11/3:283–286

204. Kleiger E, Speck U, Schroeder E (1976) Dicarboxylic acid derivatives of triiodoisophthalic acid monoamino acid amides and their use as X-ray contrast media. German Offen 2,505,320, 5 Aug 1976

205. Ekstrand TKIV, Ronlan A, Wickberg BV, Munksgaard AH (1973) X-ray contrast agent. German Offen 2,038,263, 22 Feb 1973
206. Bernstein J, Loese KA (1971) *N,N'*-Trimethylenebis(5-(3-methylureido)-2,4,6-triiodoisophthalamic acid as X-ray contrast medium. German Offen 2,038,263, 18 Feb 1971
207. Bernstein J, Losee KA (1971) *N,N'*-Bis 5-(3-methylureido)-3-carboxy-2,4,6-triiodophenyl adipamide. German Offen 2,130,369, 23 Dec 1971
208. Ekstrand TKI, Munksgaard A, Ronlan A, Wickberg BV (1971) *N,N'*-Bis(triiodophenyl) alkylenediamines as X-ray contrast media. German Offen 2,111,127, 21 Oct 1971
209. Bjork L, Erickson UE, Ingelman BGA (1973) Derivative of 3,5-dialkanoylamino-2,4,6-triiodobenzoic acid and its use as X-ray contrast medium. Swedish patent 354,853, 26 March 1973
210. Tilly G (1975) *N,N'*-Dimethyliocarmic acid derivatives useful as radiography opacifiers. British patent 1,385,684, 26 Feb 1975
211. Ingelman BGA (1969) Radiopaque iodocompounds. German Offen 1,816,844, 24 July 1969
212. Klieger E, Speck U, Schroeder E (1977) Triiodoisophthalamic acids, useful as X-ray contrast agents. German Offen 2,554,148, 6 Aug 1977 (see also Belgian patent 856,095, 23 Dec 1977)
213. Gries H, Pfeiffer H (1977) Triiodized *N*-methyldicarboxylic acid anilides. US patent 4,001,298, 4 Jan 1977
214. Gries H, Pfeiffer H (1977) Dicarbopylic acid derivatives of triiodoisophthalic acid mono-amides. Methods for their preparation and their use as X-ray contrast media. German Offen 2,554,148, 6 Aug 1977
215. Felder E, Pitre D (1969) Alkanedioylbis(3-acylaminomethyl-5-carboxy-2,4,6-triiodoanilides). German Offen 1,922,606, 13 Nov 1969
216. Felder E, Pitre D (1969) New X-ray contrast media. German Offen 1,922,613, 2 May 1969
217. Gries H (1972) 3-(Methylamino)-2,4,6-triiodophenyl derivatives. German Offen 2,050,217, 6 April 1972
218. Felder E, Pitre D (1974) 3-(Acylamino)-5-(alpha-hydroxyalkyl)-2,4,6-triiodobenzoic acids as X-ray contrast media. German Offen 2,317,535, 30 May 1974
219. Bernstein J, Sowinski FA (1975) 3,5-Disubstituted-2,4,6-triiodobenzoic acids. US patent 3,914,294, 21 Oct 1975
220. Tilly G, Hardouin MJC, Lautrou J (1975) X-ray contrast media. German Offen 2,523,567, 11 Dec 1975
221. Klieger E, Schroeder E (1975) Synthesis of *N*-(3-acylamino-5-alkylcarbamoyl-2,4,6-triiodobenzoyl)amino acids as X-ray contrast agents. Eur J Med Chem Chim Ther 10/1:84–88
222. Murphy GP, Hoey GB, Wiegert PE, Smith KR, Lin Y, El-Antably SM, Friedman MD, Kneller MT, Reed RD, Hopkins RM, VanDeripe DR, Adams MD, Lau DHM, Valenti A (1979) Synthesis and toxicological evaluation of nonionic iodinated X-ray contrast media. 15th Midwest American Chemical Society Meeting, St Louis, 8 Nov 1979
223. Sovak M, Nahlovsky B, Lang J, Lasser ES (1975) Preliminary evaluation of di-iodotriglucosyl benzene. An approach to the design of nonionic water-soluble radiographic contrast media. Radiology 117:717–719
224. Sovak M, Johnson M, Ranganathan R (1979) Improved screening of acute toxicity of novel contrast media. Invest Radiol 14:378
225. Sovak M, Ranganathan R (1980) Stability of nonionic water-soluble contrast media. Invest Radiol [Suppl], p 3327
226. Nordal V, Holterman H (1977) Iodine-containing isophthalamide derivates. German Offen 2,727,196, 22 Dec 1977 (cf Chem Abstr 88:152269z, 1978; see also US patent 4,250,113, 10 Feb 1981)
227. Tilly G (1968) 4-[2,4,6-Triiodo-3-morpholino carbonyl)phenoxy]-butyric acid. French CAM 202, 24 June 1968 (cf Chem Abstr 72:43699p, 1970)

228. Speck U, Blasskiewicz P, Seidelmann D, Kleiger E (1980) New nonionic X-ray contrast media. German Offen 2,909,439, 19 Sept 1980
229. Gries H, Pfeiffer H, Speck U, Mützel W (1981) Nonionic 5-C-substituted 2,4,6-triiodoisophthalic acid derivates. German Offen 3,001,292, 16 July 1981
230. Felder E, Pitre D (1972) 2-Alkyl-3-[2-(3-carbamoyl-2,4,6-triiodophenoxylethoxy] propionic acids as X-ray contrast media. German Offen 2,212,741, 28 Dec 1972 (cf Chem Abst 78:71710c, 1973)
231. Bernstein J, Sowinski FA (1972) 3-[4-(3-Hydroxy-2,4,6-triiodophenoxy)phennyl-alanine. French demande 2,182,161, 27 April 1972 (cf Chem Abstr 80:133827y, 1974)
232. Felder E, Pitre D (1969) Aminotriiodophenylpropionic acids as contrast agents. Swiss patent 480,071, 15 Dec 1969 (cf Chem Abstr 72:100292b, 1970)
233. Pfeiffer H, Kolb KH, Harwart A, Schulze PE (1971) 3-(2,4,6-Triiodo-3-amidinophenyl) propionic acids as X-ray contrast media. German Offen 1,956,844, 19 May 1971 (cf Chem Abstr 75:35474b, 1971)
234. Ackerman JH (1972) 3-(Carboxyalkanoylamino)-2,4,6-triiodohydrocinnamic acids. US patent 3,637,825, 25 Jan 1972
235. Ackerman JH (1968) 3-Cyclic imides of 3-amino-2,4,6-triiodohydrocinnamic acids. US patent 3,655,669, 25 March 1968
236. Ackerman JH (1977) 3-Acylamino-2,4,6-triiodobenzoic acids. US patent 4,031,088, 21 June 1977
237. Felder E, Pitre D, Fumagalli L, Lorenzotte E (1970) Radiopaque contrast media. XVIII. Derivatives of 2-(3-amino-2,4,6-triiodophenyl)alkanoic acids. J Med Chem 13:559–561
238. Pitre D, Fumagalli L, Lorenzotti E (1972) Radiological contrast media. XXI. Iodo derivatives of aryl [3-(N-alkylacylamino)phenoxy]acetic acid. Formaco [Sci] 27:408–418
239. Skulan TW (1977) Diagnostic process using sodium tyropanoate. US patent 4,002,711, 11 Jan 1977
240. Hoppe JO, Ackerman JH, Larsen AA (1970) Sodium tyropanoate, a new oral cholecystographic agent. J Med Chem 13:997–999
241. Holtermann H (1969) N-(Hydroxyalkyl)-2′,4′,6′-triiodosuccinanilic acids, cholecystographic contrast media. German Offen 1,927,557, 18 Dec 1969 (cf Chem Abstr 72:66587q, 1970)
242. Cassebaum H, Dierbach K (1969) Alkyl substituted-N-(2,4,6-triiodo-3-aminophenyl)-glutaramidic acids. German (East) patent 67,209, 5 June 1969 (cf Chem Abstr 72:66654j, 1970)
243. Cassebaum H, Dierback K, Bekker H (1972) Iodinated N-aryldicarboxylic acid monoamides as orally applied bile contrast media. Pharmazie 27:391–395
244. Obendorf W, Lindner I (1969) 3-Amino-2,4,6-triiodobenzamide derivatives as X-ray contrast agents. Austrain patent 275,025, 10 Oct 1969 (cf Chem Abstr 72:78726x, 1970)
245. Clauss W, Speck U, Jentsch D (1976) Oral X-ray contrast medium. German Offen 2,505,218, 19 Aug 1976 (cf Chem Abstr 85:166652u, 1976)
246. Korver JA (1977) Radiographic contrast agents containing N-acetyl-N-(3,5-diamino-2,4,6-triiodophenyl)aminopropionic acid derivatives. French demande 2,313,917, 7 Jan 1977 (cf Chem Abstr 88:16159m, 1978)
247. Dagra NV (1979) Triiodophenylaminopropionic acids and their use in X-ray contrast media. Belgian patent 874,988, 16 July 1979 (cf Chem Abstr 91:175027v, 1979)
248. Suter H, Pitre D, Fumagalli L (1969) Amino-triiodobenzamidophenylalkanoic acids as contrast media. Swiss patent 480,070, 15 Dec 1969 (cf Chem Abstr 72:100300c, 1970)
249. Suter H, Pitre D, Fumagalli L (1970) Roentgen contrast media containing [(3-amino-2,4,6-triiodobenzoyl)aminophenyl]alkanoic acid as shadow imaging component. Swiss patent 490,090, 30 June 1970 (cf Chem Abstr 73:112947c, 1970)
250. Obendorf W, Lindner I, Schwarzinger E, Krieger J (1974) Cyclic amidines for X-ray contrast medium. German Offen 2,235,915, 7 Feb 1974 (cf Chem Abstr 80:108538p, 1974)

251. Obendorf W, Lindner I, Schwarzinger E, Krieger J (1974) [(Aminoalkylidene)-amino]triiodobenzamide derivatives for X-ray contrast media. German Offen 2,235,935, 7 Feb 1974 (cf Chem Abstr 80:108545x, 1974)

252. Obendorf W, Schwarzinger E, Krieger J, Lindner I (1974) X-ray contrast medium. Austrian patent 319,463, 27 Dec 1974 (cf Chem Abstr 82:160245e, 1975)

253. Obendorf W, Schwarzinger E, Krieger J, Lindner I (1974) Iodine-substituted cyclic amidines as X-ray contrast agents. Austrian patent 319,226, 10 Dec 1974 (cf Chem Abstr 83:9777e, 1975)

254. Obendorf W, Schwarzinger E, Krieger J, Lindner I (1975) X-ray contrast material. Austrian patent 320,139, 27 Jan 1975 (cf Chem Abstr 83:654998b, 1975)

255. Obendorf W, Lindner I, Schwarzinger E (1978) N-Acyl derivatives of 3-amino-2,4,6-triiodobenzoic acid. German Offen 2,732,599, 20 April 1978 (cf Chem Abstr 89:42838x, 1978)

256. Obendorf W, Schwarzinger E (1979) N-Acyl derivatives of 3-amino-2,4,6-triiodobenzoic acid. US patent 4,152,526, 1 May 1979

257. Ackerman JH (Sterling Drug Inc.) (1969) 3,3'-[Alkylenebis(carbonylimino)]bis[2,4,6-triiodobenzoic acids]. British patent 1,164,526, 17 Sept 1969 (cf Chem Abstr 71:123989c, 1969; see also US patent 3,542,861 and/or German Offen 1,618,001)

258. Rosenberg FJ, Ackerman JH, Nickel AR (1980) Iosulamide: A new intravenous cholangiocholecystographic medium. Invest Radiol [Suppl] S142

259. Sovak M, Ranganathan R, Douglass I, Gallagher I, Nagavajan G (1983) New concepts in CM synthesis: development of a new nonionic contrast medium. Invest Rad (Suppl) 19

CHAPTER 2

Urographic Contrast Media and Methods of Investigative Uroradiology

K. GOLMAN and T. ALMÉN

A. Introduction

Clinical diagnostic radiology is based on the differences of X-ray attenuation in the body. Urographic contrast media (CM) are used to enhance the differences between the urinary tract structures and the surrounding tissues. In this way morphological details of diagnostic importance are revealed on the roentgenograms. Examples include:

1. Visualization of details of the renal surface (for instance, a localized atrophy or a tumor) as a result of the difference between the *concentration* of CM in the renal cortex and the tissue outside the cortex.
2. Detection of a cyst inside the renal parenchyma if there is sufficient difference between the CM *concentration* in the fluid of the cyst and the surrounding renal parenchyma.
3. Visualization of the entire lumen of the renal pelvis or the ureter. Accurate visualization of ureteral patency depends again on a sufficient difference between the ureter volume and the CM *concentration* inside the ureter.
4. Detection of the presence of an irregular tumor surface in a small sector of the wall surrounding the ureter or pelvis lumen, which is also dependent on the difference in attenuation between the tumoral tissue surrounding the clefts in the tumor and the urine penetrating these clefts, i.e., tumor detection depends more on CM *concentration* in the urine penetrating the clefts than on the size or volume of the renal pelvis or ureter.

Besides visualizing urinary tract structures, a urographic CM must be low in toxicity. Therefore, research has concentrated on developing a CM that increases X-ray attenuation in the urinary tract and is at the same time of low toxicity.

This chapter discusses X-ray attenuation of urographic CM within the urinary tract, the pharmacodynamics of urographic CM, and methods applicable to investigative urography.

The *urinary tract* can be taken to include the renal parenchyma with its cortex and medulla, renal pelvis, ureter, bladder, and urethra. A *nephrogram* is the X-ray image of the CM-containing parenchyma and may be either a *cortical nephrogram* or a *medullary nephrogram,* images of the CM-filled renal cortex and renal medulla, respectively. A *pyelogram* is the image of the renal pelvis with its calyces and the ureter opacified by CM.

Increased attenuation of radiation by the renal parenchyma increases the diagnostic quality of the nephrogram. The expressions "quality of cortical nephrogram" and "quality of medullary nephrogram" refer to the diagnostically meaningful information. Increased X-ray attenutation of the renal pelvis and ureter increases the diagnostic value of the pyelogram and the expression "quality of pyelogram" refers to such value.

B. Historical Remarks

In 1918, CAMERON introduction sodium iodide as a radiographic contrast medium [1]. This medium was used in the first study of excretory urography in 1923 by OSBORNE et al. [2].

Urography was introduced into clinical use in 1929, as a result of the collaboration of researchers in different countries [3–6]. Later, different iodine compounds were synthesized by BINZ [3, 4] and RATH and tested in human urography, first by SWICK [5] and later by HRYNTHSCHAK [7]. The sodium salt of 5-iodo-2-pyridone-N-acetic acid (Fig. 1a), under the commercial name Uroselektan, was

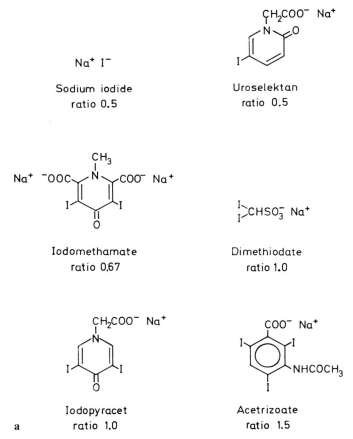

Sodium iodide
ratio 0.5

Uroselektan
ratio 0.5

Iodomethamate
ratio 0,67

Dimethiodate
ratio 1.0

Iodopyracet
ratio 1.0

Acetrizoate
ratio 1.5

a

Fig. 1. a Structures of previously used CM. b Structures of recently used urographic CM

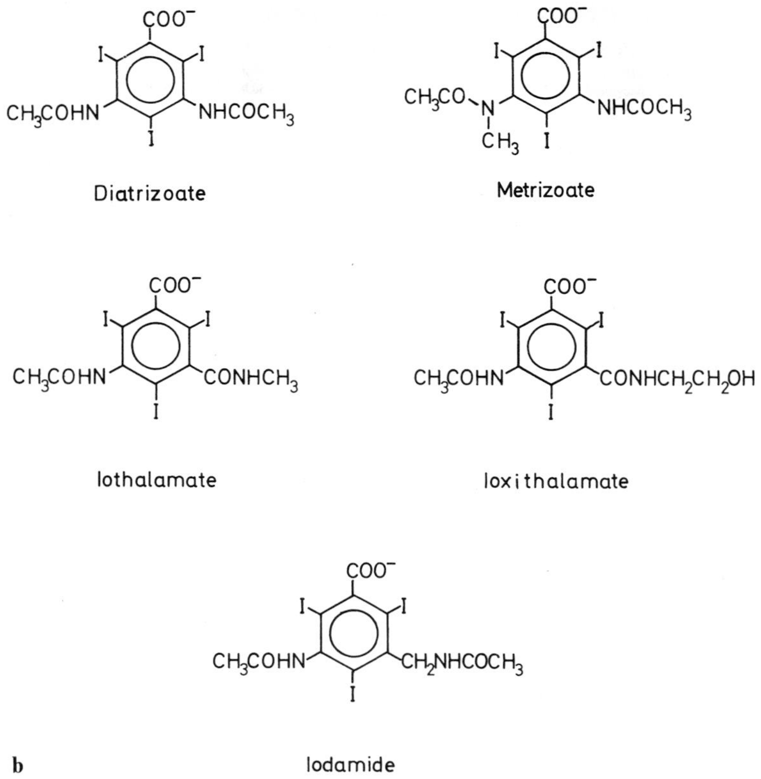

Diatrizoate

Metrizoate

Iothalamate

Ioxithalamate

b   Iodamide

introduced for clinical urography. Uroselektan contained one iodine atom per molecule; thus, a solution of this ionic medium contained for every iodine atom two ions (one cation and one anion); the ratio between the number of iodine atoms and the number of the particles in solution was $1/2 = 0.5$. The compound was found acceptable, but was actually used only on a limited basis.

Uroselektan was replaced by the ionic media iodomethamate, dimethiodal sodium and iodopyracet (Fig. 1 a), all of which contained two iodine atoms per molecule; thus, for every two iodine atoms there were two ions (one cation and one anion), giving a ratio of $2/2 = 1$. During the 1930s and 1940s, these compounds dominated the urographic field.

A major improvement was achieved by WALLINGFORD, who synthesized acetrizoate, which contained three iodine atoms per molecule (Fig. 1 a) [8]. The ratio between the number of iodine atoms and the number of particles in the solution was $3/2 = 1.5$.

In the mid-1950s, another CM with a ratio of 1.5 (diatrizoate) (Fig. 1 b) was introduced by LANGECKER et al. [9] in Germany and by LARSEN in the United States [10, 11]. These new CM were mixtures of sodium salts and methylglucamine salts, or of pure methylglucamine salts. These compounds were developed because sodium diatrizoate had insufficient water solubility to form highly con-

Table 1. Product names of the presently used ratio-1.5 urographic CM

Nonproprietary name	Product name
Diatrizoate – Na and/or meglumine	Renografin, Renovist, Hypaque, Urografin, Angiografin, Urovison, Pielografin, Urotrast, Radioselectan, Triombrin, Visotrast
Iothalamate – Na and/or meglumine	Conray, Angio-Conray, Conray, Meglumine, Contrix, Angio-Contrix, Cardio-Conray
Metrizoate – Na, Ca, Mg, and/or meglumine	Isopaque, Ronpacon, Triosil
Iodamide – Na and/or meglumine	Uromiro, Uromiron, Iodamide, Iodoradiopaque, Iodomiron
Ioxihalamate – Na and/or meglumine	Telebrix, Vasobrix

centrated solutions. Methylglucamine salts had a higher solubility but also the disadvantage of a higher viscosity than the sodium salts.

In 1962, two more ratio-1.5 CM were introduced which, as sodium salts, had higher water solubilities than diatrizoate, and consequently lower viscosities at high concentrations; these media were metrizoate [12] and iothalamate [13]. Later, two similar media, iodamide [14] and ioxithalamate [15] (Fig. 1 b), were also introduced for urography.

Today, the most commonly used CM for clinical urography are salts of diatrizoate, iodamide, iothalamate, ioxihalamate, and metrizoate. All these media are derivatives of 2,4,6-triiodobenzoic acid (Figs. 1 b, 3). Their intravenous toxicity surpasses the media used in the 1930s and the 1940s. They are available in iodine concentrations ranging from 111 to 480 mg/ml, as sodium or meglumine salts or mixtures. Metrizoate mixtures containing Mg^{2+} and Ca^{2+} have been shown to decrease intravenous toxicity [16, 17]. Some nonproprietory names and product names of presently used urography CM are listed in Table 1.

Urography with these CM has been extensively reviewed by several authors [18–26]. Though mainly diatrizoate, both metrizoate and iothalamate were the substances reviewed most extensively; the conclusions drawn from these studies are in principle valid also for iodamide and ioxihalamate. These CM have similar osmolality in iodine equivalent concentrations [27] and are, under normal conditions, excreted mainly by the kidney by the same excretion mechanisms [28–42]. The extrarenal excretion is negligible [43–45].

Contrast media of this type have several adverse effects, however. In angiography, high iodine concentrations (280 mg/ml or more) are needed. Such solutions have an osmolality of more than 1,500 mOsm/kg water, thus being highly hypertonic in relation to human serum, which has an osmolality of approximately 300 mOsm/kg. Hypertonicity of the injected CM solutions results in withdrawal of water from the red blood cells and the tissues. Other osmotic effects include damage to the vessel wall and pain during angiography.

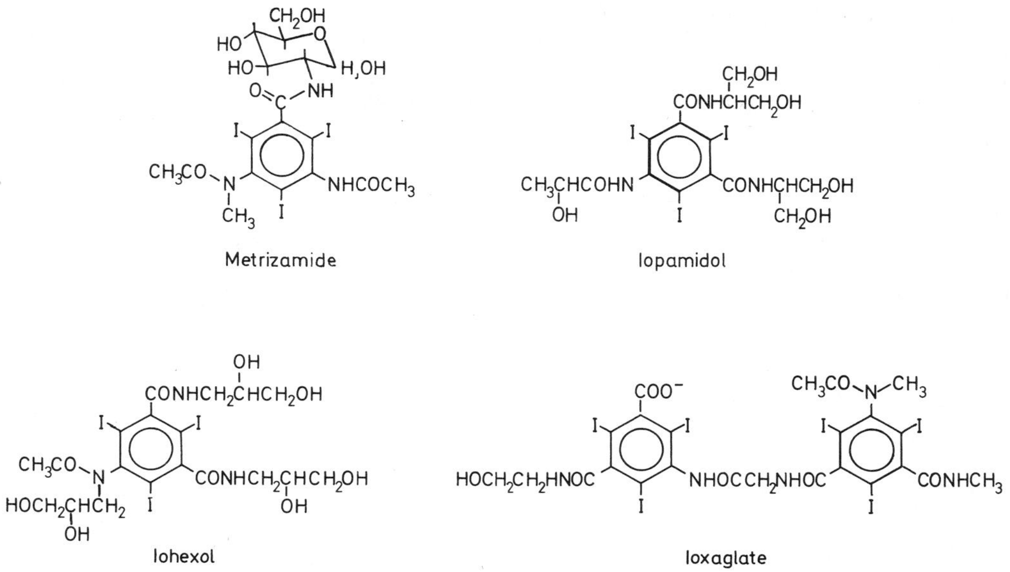

Fig. 2. Structures of the recently developed CM, which may all be used for urography

Table 2. Product names of the ratio-3 CM

Nonproprietary name	Product name
Metrizamide	Amipaque
Iopamidol	Iopamiro
Iohexol	Omnipaque
Ioxaglate – Na and/or meglumine	Hexabrix

In the kidney, the ratio-1.5 media are excreted with the glomerular filtrate and are not reabsorbed in the tubuli. They therefore induce osmotic diuresis.

In order to decrease osmolality for the same iodine content, a nonionic medium, metrizamide, was developed [46, 47]. It contains three iodine atoms per molecule and dissolves in water as a complete nondissociated molecule, thereby forming an aqueous solution with a ratio of 3 iodine atoms to one particle. Other nonionic CM with a ratio of 3 have since been developed (iopamidol [48] and iohexol [49]) (Fig. 2, Table 2).

Another approach to the design of a CM with a ratio of 3 is based on an ionic concept. Ioxaglate (Table 2, Fig. 2) contains six iodine atoms per molecule; thus, for every six iodine atoms there are two particles in solution (one anion and one cation) $(6/2 = 3)$ [50].

Experimental nonionic dimers containing six iodine atoms for every dissolved molecule achieve a ratio of $6/1 = 6$ (Fig. 3) [51, 51 a]. Unfortunately, these com-

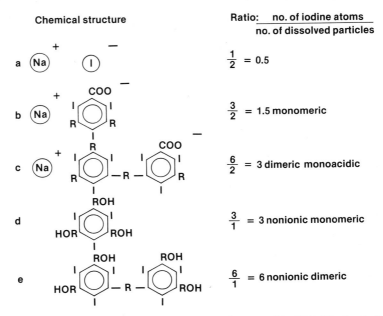

Fig. 3. Development in the fundamental structure of urographic CM. The "ratio" concept is demonstrated. **a–b**, previous and present media; **c–e**, future media?

pounds, although essentially isotonic with blood at 300 mg I/ml, have a viscosity which so far makes them unsuitable for clinical urography.

For fifty years in the development of iodine-containing CM researchers have thus been striving for a decrease in the chemotoxicity of the CM and an increase in the ratio of number of iodine atoms to number of dissolved particles in solutions in order to decrease hyperosmolality (Fig. 3).

C. Attenuation of X-Rays

The attenuation of X-rays by urographic CM within the urinary tract structures (such as the renal cortex, medulla, pelvis, or ureter) is dependent on the following factors: heavy elements in the CM; concentration of CM in the urinary tract; and structure thickness in the path of the primary radiation ("depth of attenuating layer"). The dose and injection rate of CM influence these factors and in this way affect the diagnostic yield of a urograph.

Atomic Number of Heavy Elements of the Contrast Medium. All current CM molecules for urography contain iodine, an element with an atomic number of 53, which, because of its physical characteristics, availability, chemical suitability, and compatibility with X-ray equipment, is the source of attenuation of choice at the present time. The rest of the CM molecule contains hydrogen, carbon, nitrogen, and oxygen and does not contribute essentially to the attenuation of radiation, but seems to be only an iodine carrier conferring water solubility and low toxicity on the entire molecule. Therefore, when comparing the effects or toxicities of different urographic CM, iodine equivalence rather than moles or weights should be employed.

I. Contrast Medium Concentration in Different Regions of the Urinary Tract; Factors Influencing the Nephrogram and Pyelogram

Importance of the CM concentration in different regions of the urinary tract for visualization is illustrated in a simplified way by two examples (Figs. 4, 5): Figure

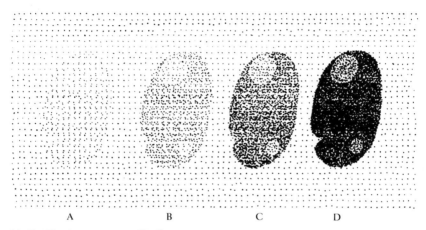

Fig. 4A–D. The importance of iodine concentration in the renal parenchyma. See text for explanation

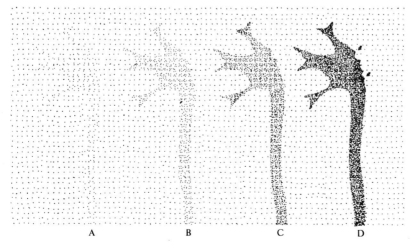

Fig. 5A–D. The importance of iodine concentration in the renal pelvis and ureter. See text for explanation

4 shows a schematic roentgenogram of the renal parenchyma (nephrogram). Each black point represent the presence of CM. In *A, B, C*, and *D* the number of black points in the renal parenchyma is respectively 2, 4, 8, and 16 times higher than in the background. In *A* only the size of the kidney silhouette can be seen. In *B* renal size can be evaluated and the presence of two cysts suspected. In *C* and *D* it is possible to see the cysts and in *D* it is also possible to appreciate a defect in the renal parenchyma at the lower pole of the kidney.

Similarly, Fig. 5 shows a schematic roentgenogram of the renal pelvis and ureter (pyelogram). In *A, B, C*, and *D* the number of black points is respectively 2, 4, 8, and 16 times higher in the renal pelvis than in the background. In *A*, the size of the pelvis and ureter cannot be estimated, in contrast to *B* and *C*. In *D*, the highest CM concentration, an irregular surface (a tumor?) in the renal pelvis, between the *arrows*, can be discerned.

Obviously, with higher CM concentrations in an organ, the diagnostic information increases. Urographic CM should therefore be chosen and used to yield a high concentration in the urinary tract.

The question is what CM should be chosen for a urograph and how should it be used to obtain an "optimal urograph" from the diagnostic point of view?

It must be realized that an "optimal urograph" in one diagnostic situation requires "an optimal nephrogram"; in another diagnostic situation an "optimal pyelogram" is desirable; sometimes both "nephrogram" and "pyelogram" would be optimal; furthermore, the toxic effects of CM must be minimized for patients in poor condition.

Factors which influence urography are as follows:

1. For a cortical nephrogram quality is dependent mainly on iodine (CM) concentration in the plasma because:
   a) The renal cortical parenchyma has a very high blood volume
   b) The CM concentrations are equal in blood plasma, in the primary urine inside Bowman's space, and in the most proximal portion of the tubuli
   c) Intracellular CM concentration is almost zero
2. For a pyelogram quality is dependent mainly on the iodine concentration in the final urine in the renal pelvis and ureter and on the depth of the attenating layer because:
   a) There are no blood vessels in the lumen of the renal pelvis or ureter
   b) The volume of the renal pelvis and ureter changes depending on the degree of diuresis produced by the different CM
3. For a medullary nephrogram quality is dependent mainly on iodine concentrations in tubular urine and tubular volume because:
   a) Iodine concentration in the tubular urine is between that of plasma and the final urine in the renal pelvis
   b) The volume of the medullary tubule is affected by the degree of osmotic diuresis produced by the different media.

Thus, the quality of the cortical nephrogram, medullary nephrogram, and pyelogram is related to plasma iodine concentration, urine iodine concentration, renal volume, and urine volume.

1. Effects of Plasma Iodine Concentration

The plasma iodine concentration following intravenous injection of a urographic CM depends on (a) dose and injection rate and (b) distribution in the body.

a) Dose and Injection Rate

The plasma level of iodine *during the first minutes after injection* is strongly influenced by the dose and injection rate. The larger the dose and the faster the injection rate, the higher the plasma level. Since the amount of CM excreted into the glomerular filtrate is directly related to CM plasma level, a rapid CM injection produces a higher attenuation of X-rays in Bowman's space, in the early proximal tubules, and in the renal vessels. Based on this aspect, several authors [52–54] have suggested injection of the entire dose (1 ml/kg) within 2–15 s. Such rapid injection gives, within the 1st min, first a cortical, then a corticomedullary, and finally a medullary nephrogram. The mean concentration of CM in the cortical tubular lumen, immediately after a rapid injection, is nevertheless only a few times higher than that of plasma. This is a consequence of a high osmotic diuresis produced by a suddenly injected solute load.

The high quality of a cortical nephrogram following rapid injection is attributable to the high plasma iodine concentration. The poor quality of cortical nephrograms resulting from slow injection is caused by the low plasma CM concentration, and the nephrogram obtained is attributable to the accumulation of iodine within the tubular lumen [55–57]. Intracellular ingress of current CM is unlikely.

The "ratio-3 media" all have a higher *viscosity* than the ratio-1.5 media sodium salts (Tables 3, 4). This may be of importance when a very rapid injection is needed for a cortical nephrogram. The advantage of the high plasma iodine concentration resulting from low-volume distribution of ratio-3 media does not necessarily have to compensate for the effects of a slow delivery.

Table 3. Physical properties of urographic CM in solutions of 280 mg I/ml

Type	Compound	Osmolality (mOsm/kg) (approx.)	Viscosity at 37 °C (mPa·s⁻¹)	
			Meglumine salt	Sodium salt
Ratio 1.5	Diatrizoate salts Metrizoate salts Iothalamate salts Iodamide salts Ioxithalamate salts	1,500	4	2
Ratio 3	Ioxaglate salts	500	6	4
	Metrizamide	500	5	
	Iopamidol	600	4	
	Iohexol	700	5	

The data have been extrapolated from published results

Table 4. Relationship between concentration and viscosity

Compound	Concentration (mg I/ml)	Viscosity (mPa·s^{-1} at 37 °C)	Δ Viscosity
Diatrizoate, meglumine	370	8 ⎫	
Iohexol	370	13 ⎭	5
Diatrizoate, meglumine	280	4 ⎫	
Iohexol	280	5 ⎭	1
Metrizoate, meglumine	370	8 ⎫	
Metrizamide	370	16 ⎭	8
Metrizoate meglumine	280	4 ⎫	
Metrizamide	280	5 ⎭	1

b) Volume of Distribution

Immediately after intravenous injection, a CM is diluted in the circulating plasma and begins to diffuse into the extravascular space. The diffusion is rapid; about 70% of the dose disappears from plasma within 2 min after the injection. Reverse diffusion of extracellular water also takes place (Fig. 6), diluting the plasma and reestablishing the equilibrium between the tonicity of intra- and extravascular fluids. The rate of CM diffusion from plasma declines exponentially with time (Fig. 7a) [58, 59], and although the final volume of distribution is not reached until about 2 h after the injection (Fig. 7b), 10 min later only 10%–15% of the CM dose remains in the vascular space [28, 29, 60].

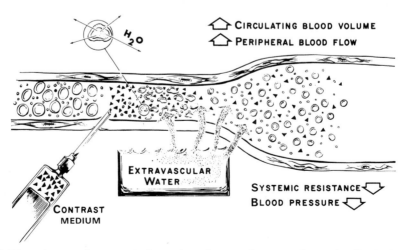

Fig. 6. The extravascular water is drawn into the vascular space due to the CM-induced increase in plasma osmolality

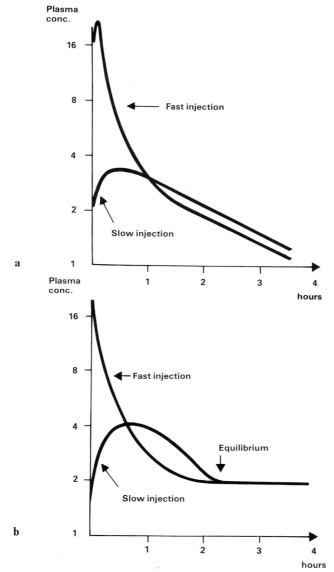

Fig. 7 a, b. Plasma iodine level after CM injection into a subject with **a** normal renal function. **b** No renal function has been assumed to demonstrate that distribution in the body takes about 2 h

The smaller the distribution volume of a CM, the higher the iodine concentration in the blood for a given dose. A higher iodine concentration in the blood increases the absolute difference in X-ray attenuation between the kidney and the surrounding tissue because of the higher blood volume in the kidney. Theoretically, due to the difference in blood volume, attenuation would increase without limits with an increasing dose of a CM.

The CM concentration in the plasma also determines the amount of CM excreted across the glomerular membrane into the urine; therefore, it is advantageous to use a CM with a low distribution volume and a slow reverse diffusion of extracellular water into the vascular space. Among the ratio-1.5 CM, measurements of distribution volume have been determined for diatrizoate [29, 59, 61, 62], metrizoate [43, 62], and ioxithalamate [63]. As expected from the similarity of their molecular structures, all these CM have a similar distribution volume, i.e., about 25% of body weight. Comparison of experimental data on the nonionic ratio-3 CM indicate that the distribution volume of these CM is about 10% less than that of the ratio-1.5 media [63–65]. This is probably due to less movement of intracellular water into the extracellular space during the first minutes after injection. This can be expected, since a smaller osmotic load has been introduced into the body with a ratio-3 CM.

Other factors which could conceivable influence the distribution phase of CM are metabolism and protein-binding. No important differences in these parameters are expected between the ratio-3 and ratio-1.5 CM. No significant CM metabolism has been found [65–70] and binding of urographic CM to proteins at relevant plasma concentrations is less than 5% of the injected dose [31, 71–73].

2. Effects of Urine Iodine Concentration

a) Dose and Injection Rate

As stated above, the quality of the nephrogram is dependent on the iodine content in both the renal vascular space and the tubules. Therefore, high plasma iodine levels obtained shortly after CM injection are important for the nephrogram. The pyelogram is not related to the plasma iodine level, i.e., volume of distribution and injection rate, in the same way as the nephrogram. Although no direct study on the relationship between the injection rate and a maximum urine concentration has been performed, it has been shown that an injection of a urographic dose (0.2–0.5 g I/kg) in less than 1 min does not achieve maximum urinary iodine concentration for 5–20 min [74, 75]. Some of this delay is due to the mixing of the CM with urine present in the urinary tract before the injection. The delay is attributable to the kidney's concentrating a certain solute load. If the solute load exceeds the limit of maximal negative free water clearance, the iodine concentration in the final urine decreases below the maximally attainable level. For this reason, rapid CM injection previously suggested for "dense cortical nephrograms" [52, 53] produces osmotic diuresis [76, 77] which results in very diluted urine during the first minutes after the injection. Consequently, the X-ray absorption within the urinary tract distal to the proximal tubuli is low and a low-density medullary nephrogram and pyelogram result.

On the other hand, infusion urography [78, 79] with infusion periods of about 15 min tends to decrease the osmotic load below the limit of the maximal concentrating capacity, and the "loss" of CM into the extravascular space makes it necessary to increase the dose in order to obtain the same urinary iodine concentration which otherwise could have been obtained with a lower dose and a faster injection.

Data on the urinary CM concentration after injection of different doses suggest that a maximum CM concentration is obtained if a urographic dose (200–500 mg I/kg) is injected in 5–10 min [23, 65].

To summarize, slow injection rates give the best quality pyelograms and low frequency of adverse effects; fast injections give the best quality cortical nephrograms but the incidence of adverse effects is higher.

A ratio-3 CM would permit a doubling of the plasma iodine concentration compared with a ratio-1.5 CM, either by increasing the injection rate or the dose, without increasing the kidney "work" by a high solute load in the glomerular filtrate.

b) Excretion Mechanisms

The way that the kidney handles different substances varies greatly. Figure 8b, demonstrates how albumin with a molecular weight of 60,000 and proteins larger than albumin do not pass the glomerular filter and thus do not normally appear in the final urine.

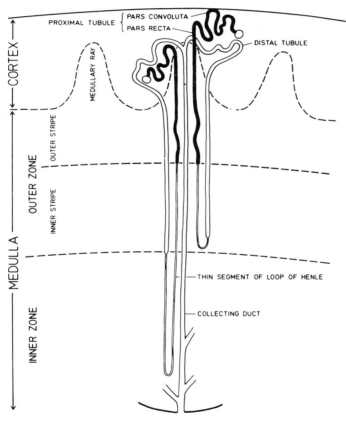

Fig. 8. a diagram of the nephrons, showing the relations of segments of the nephrons to the zones of the kidney. The diagram has been further simplified in **b** and **c** [244]. **b** Albumin is not excreted. **c** Water passes the glomerular filter and is heavily reabsorbed

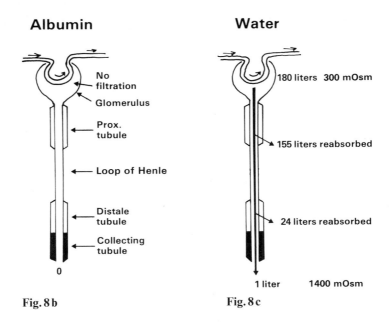

Albumin   **Water**

No
filtration

Glomerulus   180 liters 300 mOsm

Prox.
tubule

                                    155 liters reabsorbed

Loop of Henle

Distale
tubule   24 liters reabsorbed

Collecting
tubule

0

                                    1 liter   1400 mOsm

Fig. 8 b   Fig. 8 c

The glomerular filtrate is formed as long as there is adequate blood pressure in the glomerular capillaries. The filtrate volume in adult humans is 180 liters/day. The filtrate osmolality is 300 mOsm, similar to that of serum (Fig. 8 c).

Because of the water reabsorption by the tubular cells, the final urine is concentrated to about 1 liter/day; the osmolality can be as high as 1,400 mOsm. The work of the tubular cells requires considerable metabolic energy.

Most textbooks of physiology consider the polysaccharide inulin as the substance of choice for determination of glomerular filtration rate based on its solubility in serum with no protein binding, its ability to pass freely through the glomerular filter, and a similar concentration in serum and ultrafiltrate, as well as its inertness toward the tubular cells, which neither absorb nor secrete this substance (Fig. 9 a).

Both the ratio-1.5 and ratio-3 CM do not bind appreciably to the plasma proteins; they dissolve easily in the serum and freely pass the glomerular filter (Fig. 9 b). They will therefore attain the same concentration in both the plasma and the glomerular filtrate.

It is generally agreed that glomerular filtration is the main excretory pathway for all the urographic CM (Table 1). Diatrizoate and iothalamate, labeled with ^{125}I or ^{131}I, have been used instead of inulin as tracers of glomerular filtration [28–30, 34].

For iodamide, some tubular secretion has been shown nevertheless [33, 80] and some reabsorption of metrizamide has been reported [81]. The capacity of the tubular secretion and reabsorption of these CM is, at the urographic dose level (0.2–0.5 g I/kg), about 10% of the amount excreted by glomerular filtration [33, 81]. Even for these media, glomerular filtration can therefore be considered by far the most prevalent excretory pathway.

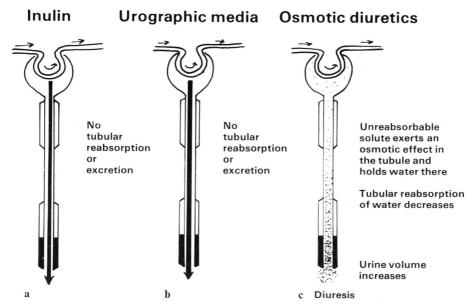

Inulin   Urographic media   Osmotic diuretics

No tubular reabsorption or excretion

No tubular reabsorption or excretion

Unreabsorbable solute exerts an osmotic effect in the tubule and holds water there

Tubular reabsorption of water decreases

Urine volume increases

a   b   c   Diuresis

Fig. 9. a Diagram of the nephron. Inulin passes the glomerular filter and is not reabsorbed. **b** Urographic CM are treated mainly the same way as inulin. **c** Osmotic diuretics increase in concentration along the nephron and "withhold" water

c) Osmotic Diuresis

When large quantities of unreabsorbed solutes appear in the renal tubules, the volume of water in the tubules increases, causing an increase in urine volume. Osmotic diuresis is produced by the administration of compounds which are filtered but not reabsorbed, such as inulin or CM. Diuresis caused by CM in urography is attributed to the high osmotic load (Fig. 10).

The ratio-1.5 CM are strong osmotic diuretics. Following intravenous injection of clinical doses, a 20-fold or even higher increase in urine volume can ensue. It follows that in order to achieve high urine iodine concentration during urography it is desirable to decrease the osmotic diuretic effects of the CM.

As a ratio-3 and a ratio-1.5 CM move along the renal tubule important differences emerge. Both the ratio-3 and the ratio-1.5 media are freely filtered through the basement membrane of glomeruli. This means that inside the initial part of the proximal tubules the iodine concentration is almost the same as the iodine concentration in plasma. As the ultrafiltration moves along the proximal tubules, water is continuously reabsorped, as a consequence partly of the active Na^+-K^+ transport, and partly of the passive Na^+ or HCO^- transport [82–85]. In the terminal portion of the proximal tubules the ionic composition is changed [82], but the filtrate is still isotonic with blood. About 85% (six-sevenths) of the water in the ultrafiltrate is reabsorbed in the proximal tubules under normal conditions, but if foreign molecules, e.g., CM, are present, this is no longer possible. The osmotic gradient necessary for the water reabsorption is counteracted by the

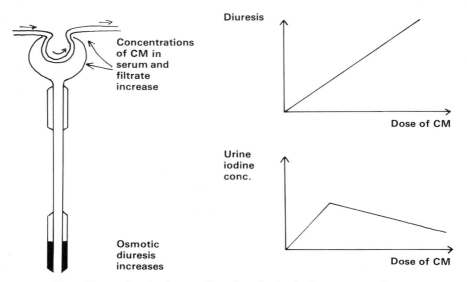

Fig. 10. Effect of increasing the dose on diuresis and urine iodine concentration

foreign molecules in the tubular fluid. Instead of the expected increase in concentration about seven times that of plasma (six-sevenths of the water should have been reabsorbed), the concentration of 1.5-ratio CM at the end of the proximal tubules is probably only about twice that of plasma during the first minutes after injection of 500 mg I/kg.

As mentioned above, the osmotic pressure of the alien unreabsorbable molecules in the tubular fluid determines the amount of intratubular water. It can therefore be concluded that in the proximal tubules a *sodium* rather than a *methylglucamine* salt of a ratio-1.5 CM produces a higher attenuation of X-rays in the cortex of the kidney, because methylglucamine is a foreign unreabsorbable cation while sodium is not. Visualization of the kidney cortex is also enhanced by compounds of low osmotic pressure, i.e., the ratio-3 media (metrizamide, iopamidol, iohexol, the sodium salt of ioxaglate, etc.). The concentration of these ratio-3 media in the proximal tubules is high because they withhold less water per molecule than the ratio-1.5 media.

Active transport takes place also in the ascending limb of Henle loop, to the end of the collecting duct, although it is chloride rather than sodium which is transported actively in this case [86]. Akin to the proximal tubules, reabsorption of water is inversely related to the osmotic pressure of the alien unreabsorbable molecules in the tubular fluid. This has been experimentally confirmed in studies in which the relationship between the maximum iodine concentration in the final urine obtained after injection of ratio-3 and ratio-1.5 CM was found [87–89] to be close to the theoretically expected ratio of 2:1 (Fig. 11).

In order to obtain the same iodine concentration after injection of a ratio-1.5 medium as after injection of a ratio-3 medium, the kidney tubular cells must "work" twice as hard. The concentrating "work" also increases with increasing

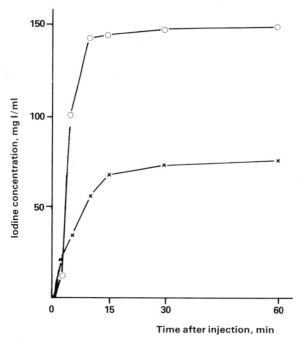

Fig. 11. Urinary iodine concentration after injection of CM (500 mg I/kg) into rabbit. ○, ratio-3 medium (metrizamide); **x**, ratio-1.5 medium (diatrizoate)

dose. The "work" the kidney can perform when concentrating the CM has a certain limit.

Figure 12 a, b illustrates the effects of an increasing CM dose on diuresis and urine CM concentration. Assuming a steady blood pressure, glomerular filtration of an increasing CM dose parallels increasing CM concentration in serum and, consequently, a higher CM concentration in the glomerular filtrate and the proximal tubular urine. This results in increased osmotic diuresis. Increasing diuresis means that the fluid in the tubules passes by the tubular cells faster and the effects of tubular cells on the composition of the final urine decrease. The efforts of the tubular cells to concentrate urine become less effective. The combined effects of the glomerular filtration and the work of tubular cells on CM concentration in urine can be summarized as follows: With an increasing dose, the CM concentration in urine increases up to a maximum. Beyond this point, further increase in CM dose decreases CM concentration in urine, mainly because of an increase in the volume of urine. Even when sodium salts of the conventional monomeric benzoates are used, a level is reached when further dosage increases will cease to produce an improved concentration [19]. This also applies to the new CM (ratio-3 media), due mainly to the limit for maximum concentrating work which the kidney can perform.

Figure 12 a, b also compares the effects on diuresis and urine iodine concentration of increasing doses of ratio-3 and ratio-1.5 media at equal levels. It can

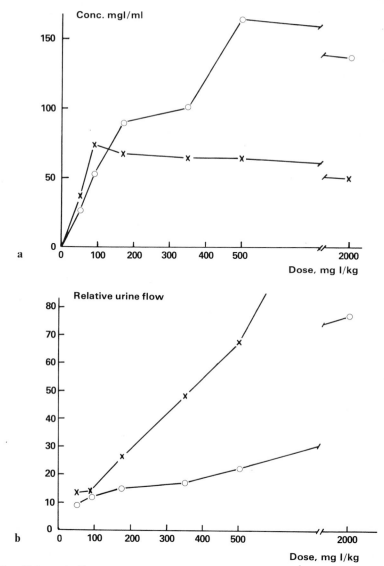

Fig. 12. a Urinary iodine concentration and **b** urinary flow as a function of dose during the first 30 min after injection of CM (500 mg I/kg) into rabbits. ○, ratio-3 medium; **x**, ratio-1.5 medium

be seen that the medium with a higher ratio (lower osmotic effects) produces the smallest diuresis and reaches a higher concentration in urine.

Experimental data suggest that the maximum iodine concentration in urine could be obtained with a dose of about 300 mg I/kg of ratio-1.5 media [90,91] while the dose has to be increased to 500–600 mg I/kg for ratio-3 media [65,75]. Such doses increased the urine flow about ten times during the first 10 min after the injection [87], producing a nearly maximal dilatation in tubular diameter [92]. It follows that any dose increase beyond a dose level which produces maximum urinary iodine concentration can only increase X-ray absorption in the kidney by higher levels of iodine in the vascular bed and only to a small extent by additional dilatation of the tubules. Although such high doses prolong the period of maximum urinary iodine concentration, it should be remembered that the toxicity (adverse reactions) to contrast agents significantly increases with increasing dose.

It should be noted that at doses below that where maximum iodine concentration is obtained with ratio-1.5 media, the advantage of using the ratio-3 media over the ratio-1.5 media lies more in the reduction of the concentrating work of the kidney than in the improvement of the diagnostic yield. At usual clinical dose levels, the differences in iodine concentration are relatively small. Using a ratio-3 medium rather than a ratio-1.5 medium, an improvement of visualization can be expected with dose levels where the kidney is close to performing maximum "concentrating work." It should, however, be stressed that such levels may be relatively low in patients with impaired renal functions (see Sect. C.I.2.e).

d) Antidiuretic Hormone

The ratio-3 CM can give twice as high maximal iodine concentration in the urine as the ratio-1.5 CM. This fact should be considered in connection with the concentrating ability of the kidney. Normal man can excrete in 24 h as little as 500 ml urine with an osmolality of up to 1,400 mOsm/liter or as much as 20 liters urine with an osmolality as low as 40 mOsm/liter. Up to 60% of total urine osmolality can be attributed to exogeneous substances. The solute concentration in final urine is mainly determined by the plasma levels of antidiuretic hormone (ADH). Apparently plasma levels of ADH, and hence the state of hydration, are of utmost importance for the quality of the pyelogram. The ADH level in blood influences the concentration of urinary solutes by its effect on the terminal portion of the distal tubules. Higher plasma levels of ADH result in higher concentration of urinary solutes. An increase in iodine concentration in final urine is obtained by factors which influence the release of ADH secretion from the posterior lobe of the pituitary gland, i.e., for the urographic patient mostly (a) emotional stress (anger, fear of the procedure) and (b) the effect of preliminary dehydration [93].

The value of dehydrating the patient has been studied by measuring the effect of fluid deprivation on urinary iodine concentration during urographic examination. It was found that the urinary iodine concentration was increased by about 50% after 18 h of fluid deprivation [94].

At least 30 h of fluid deprivation are needed to achieve maximum CM urinary concentration. Thirty hours of fluid restriction are certainly undesirable to the patient and other ways have therefore been tried to increase urinary solute concentration. It has been reported that the urinary iodine concentration during urography nearly doubles after 12 h of dehydration forced by diuretics [74].

An improvement of the X-ray attenuation in parts of the urinary tract is thus to be expected during this relatively short dehydration procedure. Further, overnight fluid restriction prevents the patient from coming to the urogram overhydrated and with his stomach full.

Dehydration, however, may be dangerous in the presence of some diseases of the kidney (myeloma) and of the heart. Dehydration or artifically increased plasma levels of ADH are without value in azotemic patients.

e) Renal Failure

In patients with normal renal function, the volume of the urinary tract increases during osmotic diuresis [95]. Therefore, both the increase in urine flow and the iodine concentration affect the attenuation of X-rays in the urinary tract.

In polyuria, the urinary tract may be chronically fully distended by diuresis. In this case, the CM cannot further increase the diameter of the tubules, and the depth of the X-ray absorbing layer remains unchanged. The urinary iodine concentration in patients becomes the only parameter of importance for the attenuation of X-rays within the urinary tract, and use of ratio-3 media instead of ratio-1.5 media might therefore be warranted to obtain diagnostically useful results.

Another potentially useful area of ratio-3 CM is in children with renal failure. The dehydration produced by the ratio-1.5 media diuresis can negatively affect the fluid balance of such patients.

II. Urinary Tract Volume Changes

1. Urine Flow

The relationship in man between urine formation (V_u) and osmotic load excreted (L) was found experimentally to be [96]:

$$V_u = \frac{L}{0.847e^{-0.21L} + 0.33}.\qquad(1)$$

From this equation it can be seen that increase in osmotic load increases urine volume exponentially with consequent dilution of the substance used for increasing the load. Injection of a ratio-1.5 CM would be expected to increase the urine formation more than injection of iodine-equivalent amounts of a ratio-3 medium. This would have no effect on the depth of X-ray attenuating layer in the kidney if the renal tubuli and renal pelvis were completely rigid. However, increase in kidney size has often been noted during urographic examinations [97–100], and a dilatation of the tubuli must be expected during osmotic iduresis.

As mentioned above a ratio-3 CM (with lower osmolality per iodine equivalent) compared with a ratio-1.5 medium (with higher osmolality per iodine equivalent) would produce a higher iodine concentration in the urinary tract, while the ratio-1.5 medium caused the largest volume and thereby the greatest depth of the attenuating layer of the urinary tract.

The relative influence of these two parameters determining the attenuation of X-rays in the urinary tract has been considered theoretically [65] and experimentally [101].

2. Theoretical Effects of Changes

The theoretical consideration may be exemplified as follows:

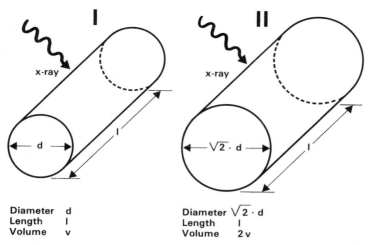

Fig. 13. Two cylinders (nephrons). *l*, length of cylinder; *d*, diameter. Cylinder *II* is twice the volume of cylinder *I*. For calculation of the X-ray absorption see Table 5

Table 5. X-ray absorption in an elastic cylinder containing equal amounts of either a ratio-1.5 CM or a ratio-3 CM (see also Fig. 13)

Contrast medium	Concentration (arbitrary unit)	Diuresis (arbitrary unit)	X-ray absorption: conc × $\sqrt[3]{\text{diuresis}}$
Ratio 1.5	1	2	$\sqrt[3]{2}$
Ratio 3	2	1	$\dfrac{\sqrt[3]{2}}{2}$

Let us compare the X-ray attenuation by two different kinds of CM (one ratio-1.5 medium and one ratio-3 medium) in the urinary tract. The media are compared at a dose level at which the ratio-3 medium reaches twice as high an iodine concentration in the urine as the ratio-1.5 medium while the diuretic effect of the ratio-1.5 medium is twice that of the ratio-3 medium. If we assumed that the renal tubuli were elastic cylinders always within the elastic limit, they would then be able to contain twice the volume of urine, while the depth of the attenuating layer, the diameter of the cylinders (Fig. 13), would be increased by a factor $\sqrt[3]{2}$ ($= 1.41$, Table 5). Similarly, considering the renal pelvis as a cone, a doubling of urine volume would, under stasis conditions, also increase the thickness of the attenuating layer in the renal pelvis by a factor $\sqrt[3]{2}$.

Under free flow conditions, the flow through the nephron may, however, be considered as a laminar flow through cylinders [102]. If this is so, a doubling of the flow without changes in the glomerular filtration pressure would, according to Poiseuille's rules, only increase the diameter of the cylinder, i.e., the depth of the X-ray attenuating layer, by a factor $\sqrt[4]{2}$ ($= 1.19$). Assuming this to be the case, it should be possible, after injection of ratio-3 CM to increase the attenuation of X-rays in the urinary tract by a factor in the range of $\frac{2}{1.41}$ to $\frac{2}{1.19}$ times that obtained after injection of ratio-1.5 CM.

3. Experimental Effects of Changes

The relationship between diuresis and volume of the whole urinary tract and the renal pelvis has been examined in the rabbit. It was suggested that if the *third root* of the renal pelvis volume is multiplied by the urine iodine concentration a reasonable value of pelvic X-ray absorption capacity ("estimated density") corresponding to radiographic opacification at urography (density of pyelogram) can be obtained. This approach was recently used by others, who compared a series of ratio-3 media with a ratio-1.5 medium during experimental urography [103, 104]. As can be seen from Fig. 14 a, b the curves of "estimated density" are very similar to those obtained using ordinary iodine concentration [103, 104].

Increase in ureter hydrostatic pressure under conditions simulating abdominal compression during urography was measured. The ratio-3 medium was found to produce a lower increase in pressure inside the ureter than the ratio-1.5 medium examined (Fig. 15) [104]. The difference obtained in rabbits between the two media was in the order of 15 cm H_2O after 25 min of complete ureter stasis. Direct measurement [105] demonstrated that increase of the proximal intratubular pressure of 15 cm H_2O increased the diameter of the proximal tubules by less than 20%, and the above-mentioned theoretically calculated factor ($\frac{2}{1.41} - \frac{2}{1.19}$) may therefore be valid during urography carried out either during free urinary flow or by using abdominal compression.

Use of experimental roentgenograms to estimate CM attenuation in kidneys has been reported [106]. Metrizamide (ratio 3) reached the highest score when compared with metrizoate (ratio 1.5). In this study, X-rays of both kidneys were obtained simultaneously, exluding possible errors due to differences in film processing and development. Visual determination will, however, always be subjec-

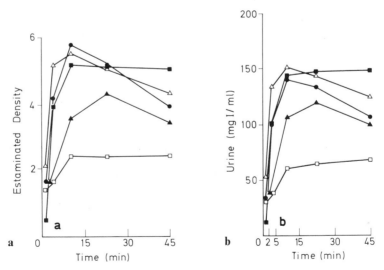

Fig. 14. a "Estimated density" and **b** urinary iodine concentration following injections of ratio-3 media and a ratio-1.5 medium into rabbits (500 mg I/kg). □–□, ratio-1.5 medium (diatrizoate); ▲–▲, iohexol; ●–●, iopamidol; ■–■, metrizamide; △–△, sodium ioxaglate

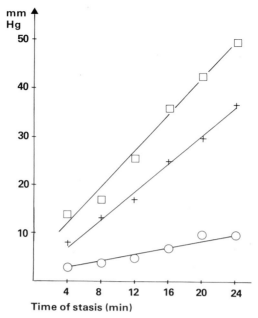

Fig. 15. Pressure increase in the ureter of rabbit during a period of ureter stasis after injection of: □–□, ratio-1.5 medium (diatrizoate); +–+, ratio-3 medium (iohexol): and ○–○, control solution (0.9% NaCl)

tive, which, together with the problem of patient standardization, is probably the main reason why no final conclusions on the technique and CM choice for improved nephrograms and pyelograms have been drawn [107–111].

D. Pharmacodynamics

I. Intravenous Lethal Dose

Compared with most drugs, urographic contrast media have a very low toxicity. They do, however, as do all other drugs, show a dose-response relationship. Animal experiments have shown that increasing the dose or injection rate of CM (which means higher plasma concentration of CM) increased mortality, vasodilatation, previous renal damage, effects on red blood cells, effects on myocardial contractility, and effects on vascular endothelium [112].

Increasing dose or injection rate of CM increases their toxic effects in both animal and man. This does not mean that a patient receiving a large rapid intravenous dose of urographic must be damaged by the CM to the extent that clinical symptoms occur. It does mean, however, that *the statistical chance that a patient may be damaged by CM increases with increasing dose and injection rate of the CM*.

The relationship between CM toxicity and injection rate and dose is shown in Fig. 16; with a constant injection rate, an increased CM dose increases the mor-

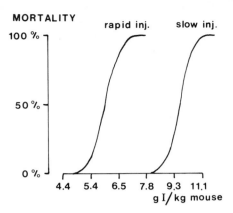

Fig. 16. Typical dose-response curves after 370 mg I/ml (metrizoate) intravenous CM injection. The effects of rapid (2 ml/10 s) and slow (0.1 ml/10 s) injections CM-induced osmolality are shown

Table 6. Intravenous LD_{50} of urographic CM in mice

Ratio	Contrast medium	LD_{50} (g I/kg)
1.5	Diatrizoate, Na	9
	Methylglucamine	9
	Iothalamate, Na	9
	Iothalamate, meglumine	10
	Metrizoate, Na	9
	Metrizoate, Na, Ca, Mg	10
	Metrizoate, Na, Ca, Mg, meglumine	10
	Iodamide, meglumine	6
	Ioxithalamate	8
3.0	Ioxaglate, Na, meglumine	12
	Metrizamide	18
	Iopamidol	22
	Iohexol	23

tality rate in animals. Conversely, increasing the injection rate increases the mortality rate even though the CM dose is low. The dependency of CM toxicity on the delivery rates has been amply demonstrated [113, 114]. It should be noted that these factors also greatly influence determination of the systemic CM toxicity by intravenous lethal dose (LD_{50}). Furthermore, LD_{50} data from different laboratories are not always suitable for direct comparison, presumably because of such factors as minute species differences, diet, and weather. Table 6 gives the dose of intravenously injected CM killing 50% of the mice in a group. For the commonly used ratio-1.5 media (diatrizoate, iothalamate, metrizoate, iodamide, ioxithalamate), the intravenous LD_{50} ranges from 5 to 10 g I/kg, varying with the nature of the cation, CM concentration, and injection rate.

The ratio-3 media are less toxic. The intravenous LD_{50} of ioxaglate varies from 10 to 15 g I/kg, that of metrizamide from 15 to 20 g I/kg [110], and those of iopamidol and iohexol from 20 to 25 g I/kg. The systemic toxicity of CM as reflected by LD_{50} in animals does not, however, correlate directly with the death frequency in clinical situations. Yet, the new media are safer, affording a clinical dose in the range of one-fifth to one-tenth of the LD_{50} for the ratio-1.5 media and $1/15$–$1/30$ of the LD_{50} of the ratio-3 media.

II. Causes of Death

The causes of death by intravenous LD_{50} are: (a) edema and hemorrhages of the lungs and dilatation of the right side of the heart; (b) renal failure after some days in animals who survive the first few hours: (c) other not yet investigated mechanisms in some animals.

1. Lung Edema and Red Blood Cell Changes

Edema in the lungs and dilation of the heart result from effects of CM on pulmonary vessels, on red blood cells, and on the pulmonary blood flow. Following rapid intravenous injection, CM or other hypertonic solutions increase the pulmonary arterial pressure in both animals and man [117]. This is to some extent due to the effect of CM on erythrocytes [115, 116].

The hypertonic CM withdraw water from the red blood cells. Further, they exert a direct effect on the membrane. This deforms the erythrocytes into echinocytes and desiccocytes (Fig. 17 a–c) [115], which become rigid. The rigid red blood cells then occlude pulmonary capillaries or pass through them with increased resistance. The consequence is increased pulmonary arterial resistance, increased

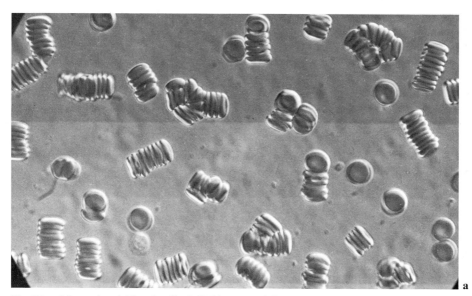

Fig. 17. a Normal red blood cells. **b** Echinocyte deformation of red blood cells after exposure to CM. **c** Desiccocyte deformation of red blood cells after exposure to CM

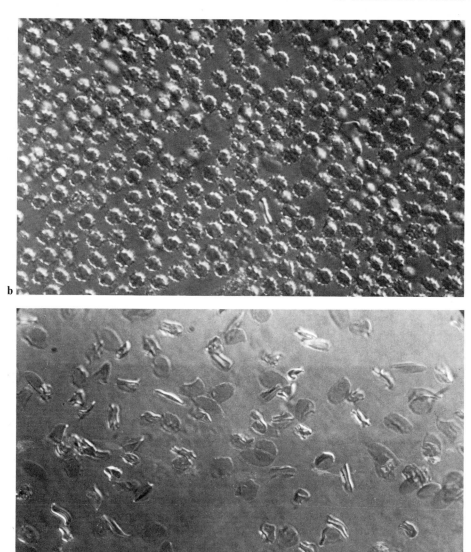

Fig. 17 b, c

pressure, reduced blood flow through the lungs, and prolonged contact time between CM and lung vessels. As a result, the potential for CM damage to vessel walls increases.

In animal experiments, ratio-1.5 media produced a three times higher increase in pulmonary arterial pressure than the ratio-3 media metrizamide and iohexol [117, 118]. All ratio-3 media can be expected to produce less rigidity of red blood cells than presently used ratio-1.5 media.

The adverse effects of CM on red blood cells increase with increasing CM concentration and injection rate. It is therefore advisable in patients with pulmonary or cardiac probleme undergoing urography to employ low concentrations and injection rates as well as to consider using the new ratio-3 media.

2. Nephrotoxicity

More than 90% of the i.v. dose of the ratio-1.5 or ratio-3 CM is normally excreted through the kidneys. For this reason, the kidney is a target organ for the CM toxic action.

Nephrotoxicity of the ratio-1.5 CM (diatrizoate, iodamide, iothalamate, metrizoate, ioxithalamate) is generally considered very low. Renal angiography is performed in patients with severely impaired renal functions [119, 120], and high-dose urography is considered admissible in oliguric patients [121]. Recent data, however, suggest revision of these indications.

Contrast-media-induced renal damage is being reported with increasing frequency: during the past 5 years more than 100 cases have appeared in the literature [122–136]. Some studies suggest that the incidence of renal failure following angiography may be as high as 10%–12% in high-risk groups of patients [137, 138]. High-risk diseases were identified as diabetes mellitus, arteriosclerosis, myeloma, arterial hypertension, and renal diseases. The clinical course of CM-induced renal failure may vary. Often there is only a transient increase in serum creatinine or urea, with a return to normal values within 1 or 2 weeks. Occasionally, oliguria or anuria starts within 24 h, necessitating temporary dialysis.

A few patients have been described who developed chronic renal failure. These patients required chronic dialysis or even renal transplantation [139, 140].

Why do CM induce renal failure? The exact pathogenic mechanisms are unknown. Probably individual differences are involved. There are three main pathways by which CM could produce renal failure (Fig. 18): (a) vascular damage, (b) glomerular damage, and (c) tubular damage.

a) Vascular Damage

Most vascular beds respond to CM with a decrease in peripheral resistance and an increase in blood flow. In the kidneys, however, CM produce a decrease in renal blood flow following an initial increase (Fig. 19) [95, 141–145]. These changes in renal blood flow were attributed to release of vasoactive substances such as renin, prostaglandins, and kallikreins; deformation and rigidification of red blood cells; or platelet accumulation in the areas of denuded vessels, with endothelium damaged by CM [146]. The relative contribution of these factors to changes in renal blood flow is not known. Both chemotoxicity and hypertonicity of CM solutions seem to be the etiological factors. Thus, hypertonic solutions of control substances (i.e., saline, dextrose, urea) elicit hemodynamic responses qualitatively similar to CM, whereas isotonic solutions do not produce significant hemodynamic changes. Changes in renal blood flow after renal angiography with ratio-3 media are smaller than with ratio-1.5 media [145].

Factors other than CM can influence the renal blood flow. Practically all commercial CM vials, rinsing solutions, and angiographic equipment are contami-

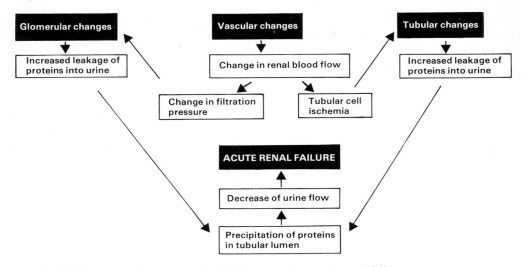

Fig. 18. The main pathways by which CM may produce acute renal failure

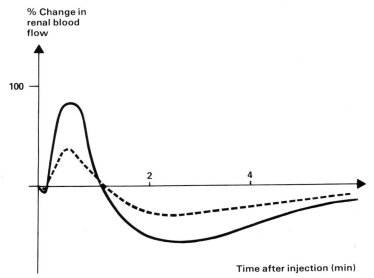

Fig. 19. Change in renal blood flow measured after nephroangiography with the equivalent dose of: ——— ratio-1.5 CM and ––– ratio-3 CM

nated with foreign bodies (Fig. 20) [147]. The significance of such foreign body contamination is currently under evaluation [148].

b) Glomerular Damage

Nephroangiography and urography increase glomerular permeability, thus causing leakage of the proteins into the urine [149]. In both man and dog the urinary

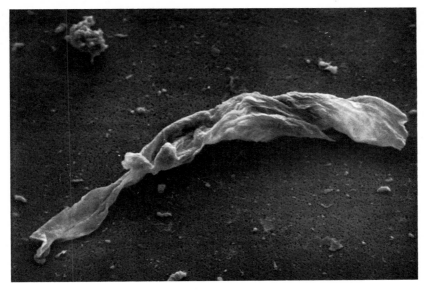

Fig. 20. Foreign body contamination. Scanning electron micrograph of a foreign body (particle) found in a CM for urography. The particle consists of organic material (possibly plastic), longest dimension approximately 105 cm. Courtesy of O. Winding × 1,000

Table 7. The excretion pattern of proteins after nephroangiography. Concentrations of prealbumin, albumin, and IgG in urine before and after unilateral selective nephroangiography with diatrizoate [150]

Dog No.	Protein concentration in urine					
	Prealbumin		Albumin		IgG	
	Before	After	Before	After	Before	After
1	ND	150	0.074	260	ND	73
2	ND	100	0.096	160	0.043	26
3	ND	70	ND	69	ND	20
4	ND	34	ND	49	ND	14
5	ND	32	ND	23	0.11	9.2
6	ND	6.3	ND	6.1	ND	2.3
7	0.63	3.0	0.13	3.4	0.19	1.9
8	ND	1.8	ND	1.2	ND	0.87

Clearance ratios: Albumin/prealbumin: median 0.78, range 0.51–1.3; IgG/prealbumin: median 0.39, range 0.26–0.63. Correlations: prealbumin after – albumin after: $r = 0.98$; prealbumin after – IgG after: $r = 0.94$; albumin after – IgG after: $r = 0.96$

excretion of albumin may increase several thousand times after renal angiography. Proteins larger than albumin have also been found, and their excretion pattern (Table 7) suggests damage of the glomerular membrane [150, 151]. The method is more sensitive than electron microscopy, which failed to demonstrate the morphological changes in the glomerular membrane [150]. The effects on the glomerular membrane of ratio-1.5 media (diatrizoate and metrizoate) seem to be equal to those of the ratio-3 medium (metrizamide), producing a similar degree of proteinuria in dog, rat, and man [152–154]. This finding rules out hyperosmolality of the CM solutions as the causative mechanism. It has been shown that ioxaglate and iohexol elicit a lesser degree of albuminuria than ratio-1.5 media during nephroangiography in dog and rat [154, 155]. The glomerular damage is not necessarily proportional to the degree of exposure to CM.

Renal failure has been produced by intravenous injection of CM, which would not be expected to expose the glomerular endothelium to high CM concentration. On the other hand, albuminuria found in dogs after intravenous injection of twice the dose used in nephroangiographic procedures was only in the order of 1/300 of what was found after the selective renal artery injection. This indicates that different causative mechanisms of renal failure may be present following urography or nephroangiography.

Massive proteinuria produced by the glomerular damage might in some cases lead to a tubular precipitation of proteins, which can obstruct the urine flow, causing oliguria and/or anuria. Tubules can also be obstructed by proteins released from CM-damaged tubular cells.

c) Tubular Damage

Tubular-cell toxicity of CM has been demonstrated in man [156]. Review of 211 renal biopsies performed within 10 days after excretory urography or renal arteriography employing diatrizoate, iothalamate, or ioxithalamate revealed vacuolization of proximal-tubular-cell cytoplasma (Fig. 21) [157] on about one-fourth of the cases. Later work has shown that such vacuolization, reminiscent of osmotic nephrosis, was also produced by metrizamide [158, 159]. Quantitative differences among the CM were not established, and the vacuolization was attributed to chemotoxicity of CM rather than to their osmotic effects.

Enzymuria is another indicator of tubular-cell damage. Enzymes highly specific for different locations within the nephron have been described [160]. High-dose urography in rabbits has shown that iothalamate and metrizamide lead to an increased excretion of enzymes normally localized in all tubular cells and at the brush border of cells of proximal tubules [146]. Apparently, damage produced by ratio-3 media is not different from that produced by ratio-1.5 media. The urinary concentration of the intracellular enzyme, leueinearylpeptidase, has been found to increase after injection of diatrizoate [161, 162] or iothalamate [163, 164] in man.

Renal arteriography also produces increased urinary excretion of the enzymes lactate dehydrogenase, glutamic oxaloacetic transaminase, creatine phosphokinase, catalase [165], and reduced glutathione (GSH) [166], and it is thought that this increase, which mainly occurs during the first minutes after the injection, represents tubular-cell damage. Further to this has been furnished by finding an increased mitotic rate among the tubular cells in animals following renal angiography [167, 168]. Such an increased rate was attributed to the healing, i.e., regeneration, of tubular cells damaged by angiography.

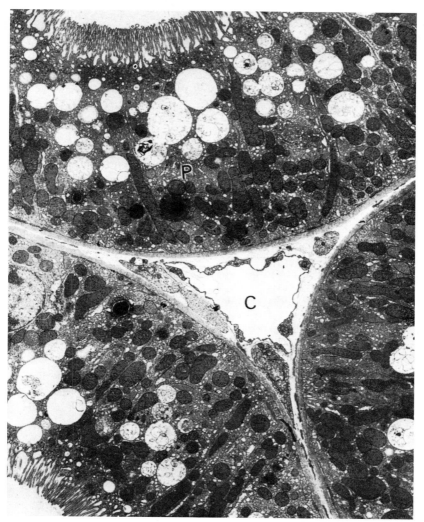

Fig. 21. Osmotic nephrosis vacuolization of proximal tubular cell, *P,* cytoplasma; *C,* capillary [157]

It is possible that CM damage the tubular cells by affecting the cell membrane. CM were shown to interfere with the potential difference across the cell membrane [169–171].

Both ratio-1.5 media and ratio-3 media can induce tubular damage; in fact, there seems to be no significant difference between these CM groups.

d) Conclusions

Urographic contrast media can produce acute renal failure. Because of the increasingly aggressive use of urographic and angiographic diagnosis in older patients with multiple medical problems, acute renal failure after CM may increase. The ratio-3 media with limited glomerular and vascular effects, and thus lower renal toxicity, may find application in high-risk patients.

III. Other Adverse Reactions

The systemic adverse reactions elicited by urography with a ratio-1.5 medium include cough, metallic taste, sensation of heat, nausea, vomiting, headache, pain, hypotension, angioedema, urticaria, laryngeal edema, bronchospasm, seizures, systemic anaphylaxis, and even death. The metallic taste and warmth sensation are by far the most frequent. The rate with which the adverse reactions occur varies considerably (3%–63%) [172–185]. It has not been possible to show any difference between the anions within the ratio-1.5 media group with regard to the frequency of the adverse reactions [175, 176, 181, 182]. The basic mechanisms underlying the adverse reactions to CM can be considered under two major categories: idiosyncratic and pseudoallergic, and chemotoxic [183, 186, 187]. Most of the chemotoxic adverse reactions can be explained by a general damaging effect of the CM on the cells of the organism. In contradistinction, the "allergic" type of reactions are mediated through the immunological system and include release of vasoactive substances from the basophils or the mast cells.

The frequency of idiosyncratic reactions of animals to CM has not been established, mainly due to the difficulties in producing a suitable animal model. Adverse reactions involving immunological mechanisms may constitute a clinical problem at least as severe as kidney toxicity. Mortality rate has been reported as 1 : 20,000 and 1 : 50,000 [184–186], but "clinically important" reactions, such as hypotension, laryngeal edema, and anaphylaxis, have been shown to occur in 0.1% [172] of procedures [174, 177, 178, 188]. Possible mechanisms of these types of reactions are discussed elsewhere in this book (Chap. 11).

IV. Advantages of Ratio-3 Media

In comparison with the ionic monomers, ratio-3 media have a lower toxicity and can therefore be tolerated at high plasma concentrations. A higher plasma concentration results in a better cortical nephrogram and thus, despite a higher viscosity, the ratio-3 media offer the best nephrogram at the least risk to the patient.

Ratio-3 media can produce a high iodine concentration in the urine. A higher urinary iodine concentration results in a better pyelogram, and despite a lower diuresis, the ratio-3 media produce the best pyelograms at a reduced risk to the patient.

E. Methods of Investigative Uroradiology

I. Introduction

When designing an experiment, it is essential to consider carefully: (a) choice of species; (b) choice of anesthetic; (c) choice of surgical procedure; and (d) how will these choice affect the response to the question being investigated?

1. Choice of Species

The rat, rabbit, and dog are predominantly employed for research on the effects of CM on the kidney. Some advantages and disadvantages of these species are summarized in Table 8. Other species which have been used for CM research are mouse, cat, and monkey.

Table 8. Advantages and disadvantages of the three species most commonly used for renal CM research

Species	Advantage	Disadvantage
Rat	Cheap. The species which has been most extensively used in the world literature both for morphological and functional studies. Small amounts of CM are necessary. Barbiturate anesthesia. Easy to control	Surgical procedures difficult without stereomicroscope. Small urine and blood samples make clinical chemical analysis difficult. Difficult to simulate CM kidney toxicity. Higher urine osmolality and protein concentration
Rabbit	Easy to handle. Much reference literature. Used for micropuncture technique. Possible to produce CM kidney toxicity. Reabsorption of some ratio-3 media as in man	Barbiturate anesthesia difficult to control. Urine often filled with insoluble crystals. Higher urine protein concentration than in man
Dog	Abundant reference literature. Used for kidney perfusion studies. Surgical procedure easy. Large urine and blood samples	Tubular transport of creatinine and ratio-3 media not present as in man. Expensive. Higher urine osmolality than in man

2. Anesthesia

In experimental procedures involving anesthesia it is important to consider the effects of anesthetics on the animal's physiology. Since PRINGLE observed in 1905 that ether anesthesia produced oliguria [190], a number of studies on the effects of anesthesia on kidney function have been performed [191–193]. Table 9 shows the effect of some commonly used anesthetics on renal blood flow and glomerular filtration. It can be seen that renal blood flow may decrease to about one-third and glomerular filtration rate to about one-half the control values with some anesthetic agents. These effects must be carefully controlled when the renal pharmacodynamics of CM are investigated.

Sodium pentobarbital has been by far the most commonly used drug in studies on the effects of CM on the kidney. Sodium pentobarbital or other barbiturates have also been generally used in clearance studies of diuretics and other drugs, and the minimal effects of this type of anesthesia are therefore relatively well known.

Table 9. Renal effects of some anesthetics

Compound	Anesthetic depth	Change (% of control)	
		RBF	GFR
Ether [192]	Light	65	78
	Deep	42	57
Cyclopropane [192]	Light	72	74
	Deep	34	45
Halothane [192]	0.5%–1.0%	39	52
	1.2%–3.0%	31	42

Nevertheless, a certain effect on tubular transport and renal blood flow and on intrarenal distribution away from the outer cortex must be expected from barbiturates [193–195].

A review of the renal effects of anesthesia is available [196]. In one study, the effect of anesthesia was investigated by renal angiography [197].

3. Surgical Procedures

Surgical procedures may severely affect kidney function. Renal blood flow, renal vascular resistance, and glomerular filtration rate can be changed by more than 10% by retroperitoneal dissection; and profound changes can be produced even by slight manipulation of the renal artery [198]. Renal circulation is soon affected by any surgical trauma [199]. In general, it should always be the aim to measure as few parameters as possible in a single experiment, as the surgical procedure introduced to measure one parameter may affect the result of another.

Comprehensive reviews of the effects of the surgical trauma on renal function are available [198, 200, 201].

II. Assays for Contrast Media

a) Radiographic Densitometry

The attenuation of X-rays in the kidney during urography can be determined from the radiographic contrast on the X-ray film.

Contrast as used in photography and X-ray film can be defined as:

$$C = D_1 - D_2 ,$$

where C is the radiographic contrast and D_1 and D_2 are the optical densities of the regions of interest on the radiogram. Optical density (D) of the radiogram is defined as:

$$D = \log \frac{I_o}{I} ,$$

where I_o/I is the reciprocal of the fractional light transmission through the radiogram. Optical density of films can be measured with high accuracy using densitometers.

The problem with this method is not the reading of the optical density but the presence of many factors affecting the optical density of the films [202]. The main factor is the sensitivity of the film (film speed), which can be affected by the quality and quantity of radiation, temperature of the films and screen during exposure, film-processing conditions, and reciprocity failure [202].

The in vivo measurements of contrast of the kidney by radiodensitometry may also be influenced by movement of the intestinal contents or by the surrounding tissue.

Scientific work has therefore mainly dealt with separate methods for determination of the actual concentration of CM within the kidney and calculations about the depth of the attenuating layer (the latter, for instance, directly determined through the diuresis).

b) UV Spectrophotometry

When CM is present in the urine at a concentration higher than 10 mg I/ml, the analytical procedure is simple [203]. The urine is diluted about 10,000 times with water. By doing this, the endogenous UV light absorption of the urine becomes insignificant compared with the CM absorption, which can be read directly from the spectrophotometer. All urographic CM have a maximum absorption in the range of 230–245 nm.

When the concentration drops below 10 mg I/ml, it is necessary to use other and more laborious methods.

c) Combustion

The oxygen flask combustion method determines total iodine content by titration. It is an old, well-established but laborious method which requires but simple analytical equipment to determine iodine concentrations down to about 0.1 mg/ml [204]. The method may be applied to urine, serum, and tissue.

d) Alkaline Ashing

Alkaline ashing, originally developed by Foss et al. [205] for the determination of endogenous iodide and serum protein-bound iodine (PBI), is sufficiently sensitive to assay iodine concentrations in the order of 1 ng/ml. The method is, however, applicable to serum only.

e) Neutron Activation

This method has the advantage of being applicable to any samples; its sensitivity is in the order of 10 ng I/g. Samples of urine, serum, or tissue are activated by neutrons until a certain level of radioactivity has been reached. Following separation procedures, the amount of ^{128}I is read on a gamma-spectrophotometer [206, 207]. Due to the requirement of neutron activation equipment (a reactor), the method has seldom been used for CM analysis.

f) Radioactive Labeling

Use of radioactive labeling of CM has been common. Either ^{125}I or ^{131}I has been chemically built into the CM molecules. Both ^{125}I and ^{131}I isotopes emit gamma rays, with half-lives of 60 and 8 days, respectively. The energy of gamma rays emitted from ^{131}I-labeled material is sufficient for in vivo measurements of the CM concentration in the kidney when external detectors are employed. High sensitivity requires high specific activity, i.e.

$$\left(\text{high ratio of: } \frac{\text{labeled molecules}}{\text{total number of molecules}} \right)$$

of the CM solution. The higher specific activity of the solution, the more unstable it is. It is thus advisable always to check the I$^-$ content of the solution when working with the radio-labeled CM.

Radioactive labeling is a suitable method for simultaneous examination of the fate of two or more different CM in the kidney. To this end, detection of the different energies of gamma rays emitted from, e.g., ^{125}I and ^{131}I isotopes can be used for separation of the sources.

g) X-Ray Fluorescence

A method for both in vivo and in vitro measurement of unlabeled iodine concentration has been developed. This method, X-ray fluorescence analysis, is based on the characteristic X-rays of elements heavier than $Z = 25$, measured by semiconductor detectors. When iodine is irradiated with gamma-rays from, e.g., a ^{241}Am source, electrons are ejected from the iodine K shell, and the resulting characteristic radiation with an energy of 33.8 keV is emitted. The number of photons emitted with this energy is directly related to the amount of iodine irradiated. The method is, in practice, sensitive to 1 µg I/g when applied in vitro [208, 209] or in vivo [209–211] on urine, serum, and kidney tissue.

h) High-Pressure Liquid Chromatography

All the above-mentioned methods use the amount of iodine in the sample as an indication of CM content. This is a valid assumption since iodine in urographic CM is firmly bound to the benzene ring. The I$^-$ content of commercial CM solutions varies but in general is less than 100 µg I$^-$/g (0.01%).

A sensitive method for direct assay of CM should be preferred when available. High-pressure liquid chromatography (HPLC) has proved capable of separating the different urographic CM, thus making it possible specifically to determine mixtures of CM in blood and urine with the sensitivity of 1 µg/ml. The detector unit in this equipment is a UV spectrophotometer. The other advantage of HPLC is that very small sample volumes (about 1 µl) can be analyzed.

i) Computed Tomography

The development of computed tomography scanners and computerized fluoroscopy techniques seems to offer a new approach to determining X-ray attenuation within the kidney. Recent reports show that total kidney iodine content in vivo at different times after injection can be estimated [212–214]. Until further prog-

Table 10. Available methods of measuring urographic CM concentration in blood, urine, and kidney fluids

Method	Advantage	Disadvantage
UV spectrophotometry	Simple equipment. Easy to perform	Low sensitivity. Urine only. (Unreliable at low serum concentrations)
UV spectrophotometry after chromatography (HPLC)	Very specific. Sensitive	Expensive equipment. Technically difficult
Combustion	Simple equipment	Low sensitivity. Laborious
Alkaline ashing	Very sensitive	Technically difficult. Serum only
Neutron activation	Very sensitive. Urine, serum, and tissue	Advanced expensive equipment. Technically difficult
Radioactive labeling ^{125}I or ^{131}I (^{14}C and ^{3}H) radiation	Very sensitive. In vivo and in vitro	Does not separate CM and iodide.
X-ray fluorescence	Easy to perform. In vivo and in vitro	Advanced equipment
Radiographic contrast	Radiologically relevant. Easy to interpret	Difficult to control. Low sensitvity
Computed tomography, computed fluoroscopy	Radiologically relevant. Easy to interpret. Applicable in vivo and in vitro	Advanced expensive equipment. Low specificity, low sensitivity. Unsuited for small laboratory animals

ress has been made, the sensitivity of the methods (in the order of 0.1 mg I/g) and the resolution (size of pixel) may, however, limit the use of CT scanners for scientific work with small laboratory animals. Subtraction techniques in connection with "digital angiography" might become useful for iodine determination in vivo.

j) Other Methods

In addition to the above-mentioned methods of CM analysis, other chemical methods have been described in the literature [216–220] but none have gained general acceptance. The advantages and disadvantages of the presented methods are summarized in Table 10.

III. Methods for the Measurement of the Depth of the X-Ray Attenuating Layer

1. Planimetry

The increase in kidney size during urography in vivo can be examined by planimetry of the kidney image on the X-ray film (Fig. 22) or on the fluoroscopic screen [95, 221–224].

Using a rapid-freezing technique, it has been possible to evaluate the volume changes of the different compartments within the renal cortex influencing the ma-

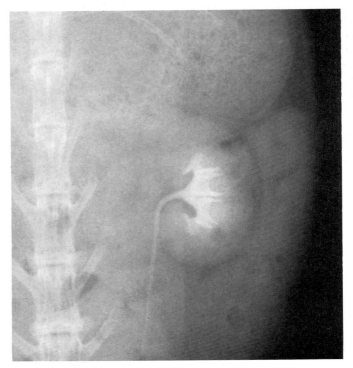

Fig. 22. Experimental urography in rabbit 7 min after injection of 500 mg I/kg of a ratio-3 medium

croscopic volume changes of the kidney during urography [225]. Using this technique, however, it has not been possible to obtain information about volume variation of the deeper (noncortical) part of the kidney, and the depth of the X-ray absorbing layer has in most studies been estimated indirectly by measuring urine flow.

2. Urine Flow

Urine flow may be determined by placing a catheter in the bladder through the urethra. This method is applicable in the rat, rabbit, and dog and has the advantage of not inflicting a surgical trauma. The disadvantage of the method is that the bladder often empties incompletely even if the catheter has side holes and the bladder is compressed externally. In addition, the "dead space," i.e., the urine volume from the glomerular membrane to the end of the catheter often becomes unacceptably large relative to urine flow in the sampling period.

For this reason, it may be preferable to introduce the catheter into the ureters. Ureteral catheterization is possible in rat, rabbit, and dog at any point of the ureter. In rabbits, the most favorable point is 1.2 cm above the entry of the ureters into the bladder (Fig. 23). It can be exposed with a minimal surgical trauma; the area is relatively poorly vascularized.

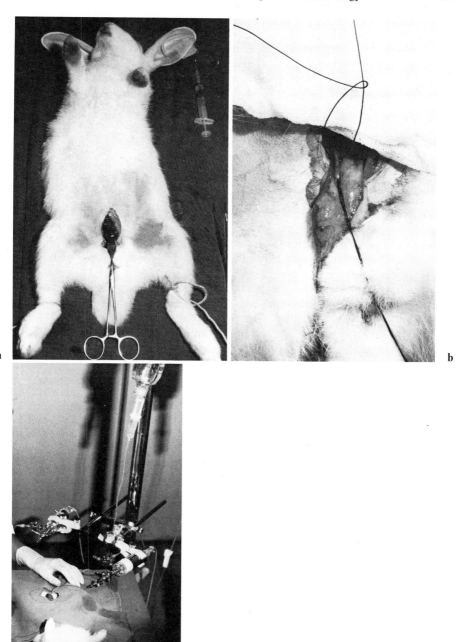

a

b

c

Fig. 23a–c. Method for collection of ureter urine. **a** The bladder is exposed through a small incision. **b** The ureter is ligated. **c** A catheter is introduced into the ureter

IV. Methods for Studying Excretion Mechanisms

Secretion and reabsorption of CM in the renal tubules have been reported of both some ratio-3 and some ratio-1.5 media. The fraction transported across the tubular cells may be relevant both for the X-ray absorption in the kidney and for the evaluation of possible kidney toxicity. Several methods are available for the examination of the excretion mechanisms.

1. Clearance of Contrast Media

a) Infusion of Contrast Media

The basic method for determining CM clearance is based on collection of urine and plasma samples at regular 20-min intervals after a continuous infusion has brought the plasma concentration to a stable level. The equation $U_x V/P_x$ gives the CM clearance rate (where U_x and P_x are the urine and plasma concentrations of the substance and V is the rate of urine flow).

Since clearance of inulin is equivalent to the glomerular filtration rate (GFR) in most species, a comparison of the CM clearance with that of inulin indicates whether the CM is either secreted or reabsorbed in the renal tubules. When CM and inulin are infused as a mixture, the relation between the clearance of the two substances is:

$$\frac{\dfrac{U_{contrast}V}{P_{contrast}}}{\dfrac{U_{inulin}V}{P_{inulin}}} = \frac{U_{contrast}P_{inulin}}{U_{inulin}P_{contrast}}$$

Therefore, it is sufficient to determine the concentration of the substance in the blood and urine alone to determine the rate of CM excretion compared with inulin.

Inulin, unfortunately, is difficult to analyze and obtain in a defined molecular size. Other substances such as [^{169}Yb]-EDTA, [^{99}Tc^m]-DPTA, and [^{51}Cr]-EDTA have been used [226–229] as markers for glomerular filtration, and in fact the ^{125}I- and ^{131}I-labeled, as well as the unlabeled, CM iothalamate, diatrizoate, and metrizoate have also been advocated for this purpose.

b) Single-Injection Technique

Estimation of clearance can be made from plasma samples taken more than 2 h after a single injection of the CM [228]. This is because 2 h after the injection, the body distribution of the CM is complete and the decrease in plasma concentration reflects exclusively the kidney activity (Fig. 7 a, b). Extrarenal excretion of urographic media is insignificant, especially when high doses (> 0.1 g I/kg) are given [43, 45].

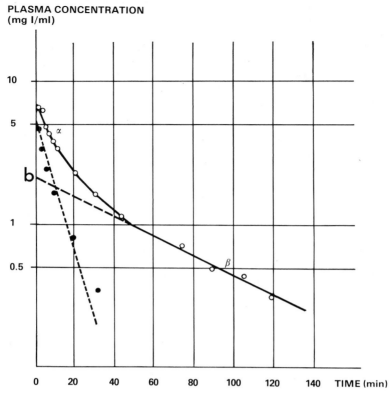

Fig. 24. Typical semilog plot of plasma iodine concentration after intravenous injection of a urographic CM in dog

From plasma samples obtained in the late period (3–4 h after a single CM injection), it is possible to get an estimation of the clearance using the equation:

$$Cl = V_d \times k = \frac{\text{dose} \times ln2}{b \times T_{1/2}},\tag{3}$$

where

V_d is the distribution volume of the CM,

k is the elimination constant $= \dfrac{1}{T_{1/2}} = \dfrac{1}{\text{'biological half-life'}}$, and

b is the intercept with the ordinate in a semilog plot of the plasma concentration versus time (Fig. 24).

For CM, the "single-injection technique" can be further refined as a noninvasive method. Using X-ray fluoroscence equipment for in vivo measurement of the iodine concentration in a well-perfused organ, it has been shown that more than 2 h after the injection the organ's iodine concentration decreases proportionally to the serum level [62]. Rabbit nose or patient's fingertip [229 a] has been used for this (Figs. 25, 26); the CM clearance can then be estimated from the organ iodine disappearance curve using Eq. (3) and a correction factor.

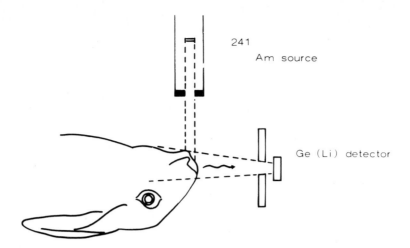

Fig. 25. Experimental "set up" for in vivo measurements of iodine in a well-perfused organ using the X-ray fluorescence technique

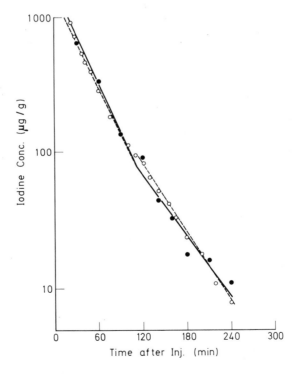

Fig. 26. Semilog plot of: ●─●, serum iodine and +─+, tissue iodine concentration (multiplied by a correction factor) after intravenous injection of a urographic CM in rabbit using the technique shown in Fig. 25

c) Stop-Flow Technique

There is no noninvasive technique available for precise localization of the tubular transport. The "stop-flow technique," however, is a relatively nontraumatic procedure. It has considerable value in localizing the transport processes along the length of the nephron [230–232].

The ureter of an animal is clamped for several minutes allowing a relatively static column of urine to remain in contact with the various tubular segments for longer than usual periods. Thus, the operation of each segment on the tubular fluid is exaggerated. After release of the ureteral occlusion, small serial samples are collected rapidly, the earliest sample representing fluid which had been in contact with the most distal nephron segments. Since the column of urine is not completely static and since nephrons vary appreciably in length and behavior, there is some slurring of the "stop-flow" patterns and only fairly gross differences in localization can be appreciated. Users of this technique must also appreciate that tubular segments downstream from the proximal segments may modify the tubular fluid during its egress. Despite these limitations, a fairly large body of useful information on basic renal physiology has emerged from the application of this method. Thus, comparative clearance of CM have been established using creatinine as a marker of glomerular filtration [232]. Figure 27 shows a typical result of a "stop-flow" analysis. The "stop-flow" method has been extensively applied to CM [233].

A useful variant of the "stop-flow" technique is based on injecting intravenously the test substance along with a glomerular marker after several minutes of ureteral occlusion [234]. If, in the subsequently collected samples, the glomerular marker is preceded by the test substance, it is evidence for the latter's transtubular permeability. The technique has been of value in demonstrating the secretory component of bidirectionally tubularly transported compounds by separating the effect of reabsorption [235, 236].

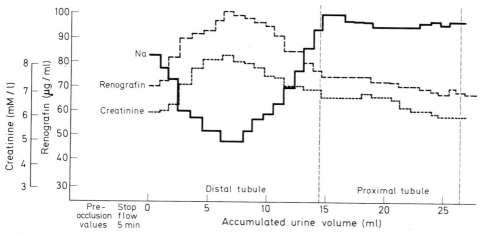

Fig. 27. Stop-flow analysis curve for Renografin [233]. Note that the slope is the same as that for creatinine, indicating that it is excreted by glomerular filtration alone

2. Tubular Micropuncture and Microperfusion

This technique was designed to study the localization of a transport process at the level of a single nephron [237–239]. The technique's major potential is precise localization of tubular functions. Since the majority of tubules visible on the kidney surface are convolutions of the proximal tubule, other nephron components have to be made accessible by direct dissection (Fig. 28) [240] and mounting between two pipettes, one for perfusion and one for collection (Fig. 29) [241–244]. The test compound can be introduced with the perfusion fluid, or dissolved into the bath surrounding the tubule, or both. This technique was successfully applied to iothalamate [244]. Since the composition of both perfusate and the bath must be rigorously defined, the technique is eminently suited for study of the effects of various ions and other constituents on transport of the CM, and for the study of

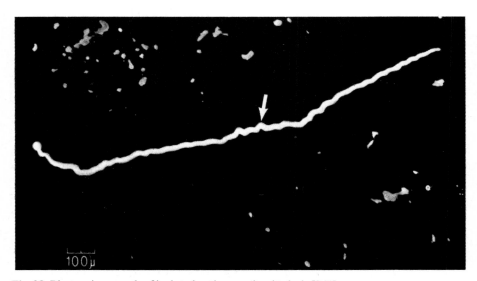

Fig. 28. Photomicrograph of isolated entire proximal tubule [241]

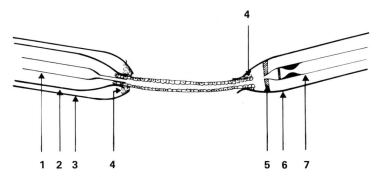

Fig. 29. Isolated tubule perfusion arrangement of concentric perfusion and collecting pipettes [245]. *1,* perfusion pipette; *2,* holding pipette; *3,* Sylgard pipette; *4,* Sylgard; *5,* oil; *6,* collecting pipette; *7,* volumetric collecting pipette

transport kinetics. In addition, it is possible to determine the concentration of transported materials in intracellular water.

Microtechnique is considerably difficult. To be successful it requires experience and patience. An excellent textbook is available [240].

3. Cell Culture

Cell culture is the basic approach for studies of CM cellular transport [245]. Different kinds of kidney cells from different species (monkey, rabbit, rat) are now commercially available. The cells are delivered growing in nutritious solutions, suitable for addition of CM. After incubation, intracellular accumulation of the CM suggests that active transport has taken place. The cell cultures are also well suited for studies of CM cell toxicity [246, 247].

V. Methods for Studying Renal Pharmacodynamics

1. Urine Osmolality

Some of the reduced toxic effects of the ratio-3 media compared with the ratio-1.5 media are related to the lower osmotic pressure exerted by ratio-3 media. As discussed above, the osmotic properties of a CM determine the urinary iodine concentration and flow during urography.

To assay the osmolality of a CM solution, two methods are available: (a) freezing point depression or (b) vapor pressure.

For determination of the body fluids and CM osmolality contained in body fluids [248], the freezing point depression method is by far the simplest. Modern equipment requires only very small samples (less than 50 µl). Freezing point depression, however, is not applicable when CM concentration is high (>200 mg I/ml), because of CM crystallization [249]. In such a situation, the vapor pressure method should be used [27].

Urine osmolality is greatly affected by the state of hydration. Therefore, when comparing urinary iodine concentration after CM injections, it is important to control the state of hydration of the animal. The state of hydration can be determined by measuring the plasma level of antidiuretic hormone or, more conveniently, by measuring the preinjection urine osmolality.

2. Ability to Concentrate Urine

Decrease of the renal capacity to concentrate urinary solutes is a useful sign of kidney damage [250, 251]. In unanesthetized rats, monkeys, or dogs a maximally concentrated urine should be produced after 2 days of water deprivation [252]. A number of factors can influence the concentrating ability of the kidney. To determine whether production of endogenous vasopressin has been impaired, lysine vasopressin (about 0.5 IU/kg body wt.) or other peptides with antidiuretic activity are injected subcutaneously [253]. The concentrating ability may be depressed by a variety of nephrotoxic agents that damage the corticomedullary osmotic gradient [250, 254, 255]. Primary changes which interfere with the establishment of the normal corticomedullary sodium gradient (major depression of glomerular filtration rate, disturbances of proximal tubule fluid reabsorption, disturbance of chloride transport out of the ascending limb of Henle's loop, blood flow changes in the renal medulla) impair the maximal urine concentration. Any extensive functional renal damage depresses urinary-concentrating ability [256].

3. Urine Flow

Oliguria is often the first sign of renal failure after CM injection. Experimentally it is easily measured by some of the previously mentioned urine collection methods. It is important that initially the fluid equilibrium of animals is maintained, insomuch as urine flow may change dramatically within a 15-min period.

4. Vascular Changes

The response of the renal vascular bed to CM is biphasic (Fig. 19). To investigate the nature of the response, blood flow must be measured accurately. Electromagnetic flowmeters, p-aminohippurate (PAH) clearance, and the dye dilation technique are applicable methods.

a) Electromagnetic Flowmeters

The renal blood flow is most commonly measured directly by electromagnetic flowmeters. The principle is outlined in Fig. 30. The disadvantage of this technique lies in the necessity for a traumatic dissection and need for a strictly perpendicular placement of the flow probe around the renal artery. Poor placement or manipulation of the probe will result in erroneous measurement.

b) p-Aminohippurate Clearance

In small animals, the renal plasma flow can be measured by the urinary clearance of PAH, diodrast, or the dye-dilution technique.

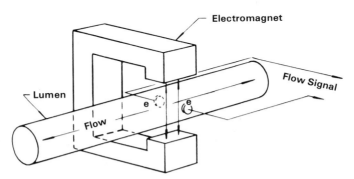

Fig. 30. Diagram of the arrangement of the electromagnetic cuff around the renal artery. The electromagnetic cuff produces a magnetic field through the renal artery. The flowing blood disturbs this field, and the disturbances, which are related to blood flow, are detected by the electrodes (*e*)

PAH or diodrast clearance does not actually measure total plasma flow through the kidneys since 15%–20% of PAH or diodrast entering the kidney by the renal artery escapes excretion and returns to the circulation. Plasma flow is obtained by dividing the marker clearance by the extraction rate:

Plasma flow

$$= \frac{\text{conc. of marker in renal artery} - \text{conc. of marker in renal vein}}{\text{conc. of marker in renal artery}}.$$

Marker extraction can be measured in anesthetized animals by repeated blood sampling from the renal vein through a fine cannula. A decrease of marker clearance after administration of a nephrotoxic agent signifies either fall of renal plasma flow or an impaired tubular secretion of the marker in the proximal tubule. PAH extraction should be determined before making conclusions about changes in renal blood flow, since a decrease in PAH secretion may or may not be accompanied by a decrease in renal plasma flow.

c) Dye Dilution

The dye-dilution techniques consist of injections of a known amount of dye (which may also be a CM) into the renal artery concomitant with the withdrawal of renal venous blood at a constant flow rate. The renal venous blood is drawn into a cuvette and a dye-dilution curve is obtained. An experimental model is shown in Fig. 31.

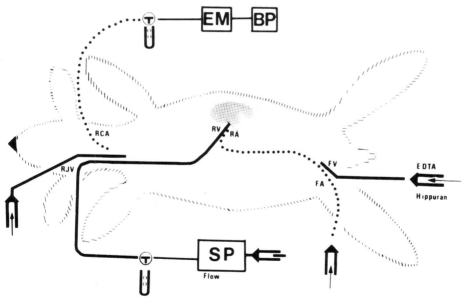

Fig. 31. Schematic drawing of experimental arrangement for using the dye-dilution technique [199]. *EM*, electromanometer; *BP*, registration of arterial blood pressure; *RCA*, right carotid artery; *RJV*, right jugular vein; *RV*, renal vein; *RA*, renal artery; *SP*, spectrophotometer cuvette; *FV*, femoral vein; *FA*, femoral artery

From the dye-dilution curve, renal blood flow (RBF) can be calculated from the equation:

$$RBF = D \int_o^t c\, dt \simeq D/A$$

where D is the amount of dye injected, c is the dye concentration, and A is the area of the recorded dye concentration-time curve.

The methodological problems of the dye-dilution technique in RBF measurements have been discussed thoroughly [257]. RBF changes in nephroangiography, measured with dye dilution, have been reported [258].

The dye-dilution technique is superior to other blood flow measurements in that it affords calculation of "mean transit time" and "intrarenal blood volume," parameters useful in studying CM renal hemodynamics [95].

In addition to techniques measuring total renal blood flow, methods have been developed for studying the regional blood distribution within the kidney. Osmotic diuresis redistributes blood from the outer cortex to the medulla; since CM are osmotic diuretics, such RBF redistribution is to be expected.

Measurements of regional renal blood flow are performed using either the inert gas washout method [259–262] or the radioactive microsphere method [263–265].

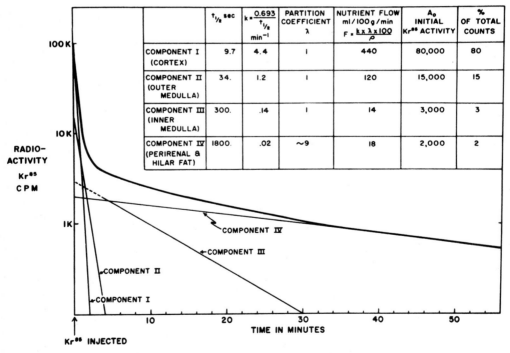

Fig. 32. A typical ^{85}Kr washout curve in a normal conscious dog. The figure also shows the compartmental analysis dividing the washout curve into four components: *I,* cortex; *II,* outer medulla; *III,* inner medulla; and *IV,* perirenal and hilar fat [267]

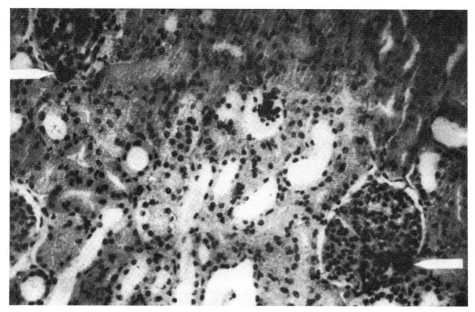

Fig. 33. Localization of 15-μm microspheres in a peripheral glomerular capillary loop [268]

d) Inert Gas

The inert gas technique is preferably carried out with either ^{133}Xe or ^{85}Kr. The gas is dissolved in saline and injected within seconds into the renal artery. The disappearance of gas from the kidneys can then be followed with a scintillation detector of radioactivity located over the kidney. An example of the gas washout is shown in Fig. 32. The data allow separation of blood flow contribution to the cortex, outer and inner medulla, as well as perirenal fat [266].

e) Microspheres

The microsphere technique has been developed to measure the total body blood distribution, but it is readily adaptable to intrarenal blood distribution studies. Radiolabeled microspheres (with a diameter of 15–50 μm) have been developed, which, after injection into the left ventricle, embolize arterioles of the glomeruli (Fig. 33) [267]. The spheres, being stable, remain at the site of embolization. The radioactivity of a given area of the kidney is considered representative of the blood flow through that area at the time of injection. A detailed description of the handling and use of microspheres is available [267].

5. Glomerular Damage

a) Clearance

Decrease of the glomerular filtration rate by a CM can be evaluated indirectly by measuring the plasma level of the endogenous waste products, urea or creatinine. Interpretation of the plasma urea levels is difficult since in most species this compound, in addition to being filtered through the glomeruli, is also transported across the membrane of the nephron at several sites. For this reason, creatinine is considered a far better marker of glomerular filtration than urea [268], although creatinine lacks the sensitivity to detect functional renal damage. Thus, even when 50% of the kidney function is missing, there may be no measurable increase in the creatinine plasma levels.

When detailed information on the glomerular function is needed, clearance studies should employ the other previously mentioned glomerular markers [226–234]. The effects of CM on the single nephron glomerular filtration rate can be studied using micropuncture and microperfusion technique [237–244].

b) Proteinuria

The proteinuria after nephroangiography is taken as evidence of glomerular membrane changes. Since conventional chemical determination of proteins is neither sensitive nor specific enough, specific immunological methods are applicable. The sensitive "radial immunodiffusion" and the "rocket" techniques have been described in detail [269, 270].

6. Tubular Damage

Damage inflicted on the tubuli can be studied by measuring the enzymes excreted into the urine. Increased enzyme excretion appears to be the more sensitive and earlier indicator of renal damage compared with most other tests (Table 11) [252].

Table 11. Comparison between different renal function tests with regard to sensitivity and/or early occurrence of changes after administration of various nephrotoxic agents

Test indicating renal damage earlier than other tests or at the lowest dose levels of nephrotoxic agent	Other tests performed	Species	Agent investigated	Ref.
Enzymuria (GOT)	Increase of blood urea nitrogen (BUN)	Rat	Various nephrotoxic agents	[272]
Enzymuria (AP, GOT, GPT)	Routine urinalysis, GFR, Tm_{PAH}	Rabbit	Uranyl ions	[273]
Enzymuria (AP, Ac), loss of body weight	Routine urinalysis, GFR, Tm_{PAH}	Rabbit	Cadmium ions	[274]
Enzymuria (AP, Ac)	Routine urinalysis, GFR, Tm_{PAH}	Dog	Mercuric chloride	[275]
Enzymuria (lysosomal hydrolases)	Creatinine clearance, increase of BUN	Rat	Gentamicin	[276]
Enzymuria (AP, maltase)	Increase of BUN	Rat	Mercuric chloride, neomycin	[278]
Enzymuria (LAP, arylsulphatase A)	Creatinine		Diatrizoate, iothalamate	[161–163]
Enzymuria (LAP, AP)	BUN, creatinine	Rabbit	Iothalamate, metrizamide	[146]

AP, alkaline phosphatase; Ac, acid phosphatase; GOT, glutamic oxalacetic transaminase; GPT, glutamic pyruvic transaminase; LAP, leucine-alanine peptidase

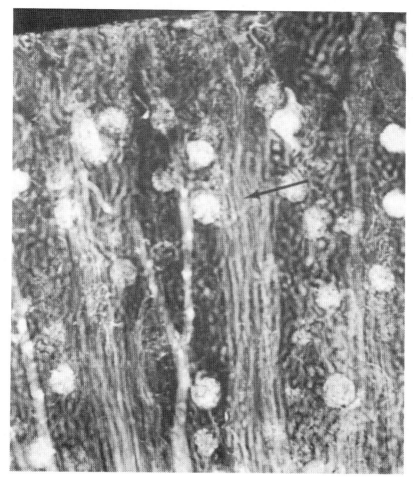

Fig. 34. An antegrade injection of BaSO$_4$-gelatine suspension using the microradiographic technique demonstrating a cluster of collecting ducts, pars recta of the proximal convoluted tubules as well as ascending loops of Henle (*arrow*). This represents the medullary ray [283]

a) Urinary Enzymes

The mechanisms of a rise in urinary enzyme activity may, as previously discussed, represent: (a) a glomerular leakage of serum enzymes; (b) a decreased reabsorption by damaged tubules of filtered enzymes; or (c) a release of enzymes from the renal tubular cells. The latter mechanism is thought to be involved in the types of enzymuria most commonly observed in renal diseases or toxic damage to the kidney. Experimentally, the type and localization of damage can be determined. Maps of the enzyme location in the nephron are available (Tables 12, 13) [155, 271–278].

Determination of the enzyme concentration in the urine is relatively simple using commercial kits. It is important to realize that many urinary enzymes are unstable and that their activity may decrease rapidly.

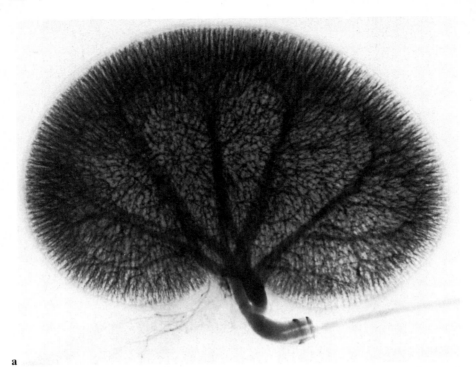

a

Fig. 35 a–b. An arterial injection of BaSO$_4$-gelatine suspension using the microangiographic technique allowing a detailed study of the microvascular bed. **a** Whole kidney placed on X-ray film. **b** Slice (1 mm) placed on X-ray film. (Courtesy of Hegedüs)

b) Histology

One aspect of the tubular damage by CM is that it resembles the "osmotic nephrosis" [156, 157]. Vacuoles inside the tubular cells are demonstrated by conventional fixation technique and light microscopy. Techniques for morphological studies of

Table 12. Main localization sites of some enzymes within the kidney [160]

Enzyme	Localization
Alkaline phosphatase	Proximal tubule basement membrane
Acid phosphatase	Proximal tubule cytoplasma, lysosomes
Arylesterase	Microsomes
β-Glucuronidase	Lysosomes
Glucose-6-phosphatase	Smooth endoplasmatic reticulum
Arylsulfatase	Lysosomes
Arylaminopeptidase	Tubular basement membrane
α-Glycerophosphate dehydrogenase	Mitochondria and cytoplasm
Succinic dehydrogenase	Mitochondria
Malate dehydrogenase	Mitochondria and cytoplasm
Phospholipase A$_2$	Subcellular membranes

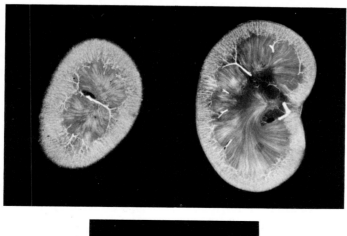

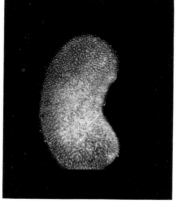

b

the kidney have been described in detail [279]. Renal microradiography allows examination of both the urinary (Fig. 34) and the vascular side (Fig. 35) of the kidney [280–282]. This technique is useful both for examination of CM toxicity and for the anatomical basis for the radiographic appearance of the renal structure.

While both microangiography and conventional light microscopy have frequently been used to investigate the effects of CM on the kidney, only a few stud-

Table 13. Enzyme activities measured in different membrane fractions [278]

Membrane fraction	Alkaline phosphatase (mU/mg protein)	Na-K-ATPase (mU/mg protein)	Succinic dehydrogenase (µg/mg protein)
Plasma membrane fraction	1.1 ± 0.2	0.16 ± 0.02	4.0 ± 0.2
Brush-border membranes	1.8 ± 0.2	0.05 ± 0.02	2.1 ± 0.1
Lateral-basal plasma membranes	0.3 ± 0.1	0.42 ± 0.02	3.6 ± 0.2

ies have taken advantage of electron and scanning electron microscopy. The fixation procedures often involve use of fixatives which are osmotically active [283, 284], and thus introduce artifacts.

The continuing advancements in electron microscopy technology and sample fixation techniques (especially within the freezing preparation) make it likely that both transmission and scanning electron microscopy will be increasingly used in future evaluation of the many effects of contrast media in the kidney.

Acknowledgment. This work was supported in part by Research Grant 3483, Swedish Medical Research Council.

References

1. Cameron DF (1918) Aqueous solution of potassium and sodium iodide as opaque medium in roentgenography. JAMA 70:754–759
2. Osborne ED, Sutherland CG, Scholl AJ, Rowntree LG (1923) Roentgenography of urinary tract during excretion of sodium iodide. JAMA 80:368–375
3. Binz A (1931) The chemistry of Uroselectan. J Urol 25:297–301
4. Binz A (1937) Geschichte des Uroselectans. Z Urol 31:73–84
5. Swick M (1929) Darstellung der Niere und Harnwege im Röntgenbild durch intravenöse Einbringung eines neuen Kontraststoffes, des Uroselectans. Klin Wochenschr 8:2087–2089
6. Tondreau R (1964) Roentgenography of the urinary tract. In: Lasser E (ed) Classic descriptions in diagnostic radiology, vol 2. Thomas, New York, pp 1605–1728
7. Hryntschak T (1929) Studien zur röntgenologischen Darstellung von Nierenparenchym und Nierenbecken auf intravenösem Wege. Z Urol 23:893–904
8. Wallingford V (1953) The development of organic iodine compounds as X-ray contrast media. J Am Pharm Assoc Sci Ed 42:721–728
9. Langecker H, Harwart A, Junkmann K (1954) 3,5-Diacetylamino-2,4,6-trijodbenzoesäure als Röntgenkontrastmittel. Naunyn Schmiedebergs Arch Pharmakol Exp Pathol 222:584–590
10. Larsen A, Moore C, Sprague J, Cloke B, Moss J, Hoppe J (1956) Iodinated 3,5-diaminobenzoic acid derivatives. J Am Chem Soc 78:3210–3216
11. Hoppe J, Larsen A, Coulston F (1956) Observations on the toxicity of a new urographic contrast medium, sodium 3,5-diacetamido-2,4,6-triiodobenzoate (Hypaque Sodium) and related compounds. J Pharmacol Exp Ther 116:394–403
12. Holtermann H (1962) Symposium on metrizoate sodium (Isopaque), a new contrast medium for angiography and urography. Farmakoterapi 18:1–29
13. Hoey G, Ronds RD, Delamater J, Chapman DW, Wiegert PE (1963) Synthesis of derivatives of isophthalamic acid as X-ray contrast agents. J Med Chem 6:24–26
14. Felder E, Pitre D, Fumagalli L (1965) Röntgenkontrastmittel. 6. Mitteilung. Iodierte derivat der Triaminomethylbenzosäure. Helv Chim Acta 48:259–274
15. Guerbet M, Tilly G (1967) 2,4,6-Triiod-3-(N-oxäthyl)-carbamyl-5-acetaminobenzosäure, deren Salze und Ester sowie Verfahren zu deren Herstellung. Offenlegungsschrift P 1643440, 1967
16. Salvesen S, Nilsen PL, Holtermann H (1967) Ameliorating effects of calcium and magnesium ions on the toxicity of isopaque sodium. I. Acute toxicities and toxicities in the brain. Acta Radiol [Suppl] (Stockh) 270:17–29
17. Salvesen S, Nilsen PL, Holtermann H (1967) Effects of calcium and magnesium ions on the systemic and local toxicities of the N-methylglucamine (meglumine) salt of metrizoic acid (Isopaque). Acta Radiol [Suppl] (Stockh) 270:180–193
18. Meschan I (1965) Background physiology of the urinary tract for the radiologist. Radiol Clin North Am 3:13–28
19. Saxton HM (1969) Review article. Urography. Br J Radiol 42:321–346

20. Sherwood T (1971) The physiology of intravenous urography. Sci Basis Med XX:336–348
21. Knoefel PK, Carrasquer G (1971) Radiocontrast agents for the urinary system. In: Knoefel PK (ed) Radiocontrast agents, sect 76/1. Pergamon, Oxford, pp 261–298
22. Fischer HW, Rothfield NJH (1972) Whither urography? J Urol 107:120–125
23. Mudge GH (1974) Renal function during intravenous urography. In: Knoefel PK (ed) Recent advances in renal physiology and pharmacology. University Park Press, Baltimore, pp 349–359
24. Elkin M (1975) Radiology of the urinary tract: Some physiological considerations. Radiology 116:259–270
25. Talner LB (1972) Urographic contrast media in uremia. Physiology and pharmacology. Radiol Clin North Am 10:421–432
26. Dure-Smith P (1977) Urographic agents. In: Knoefel PK (ed) Radiographic contrast agents. University Park Press, Baltimore, pp 273–306
27. Børdalen BE, Wang H, Holtermann H (1970) Osmotic properties of some contrast media. Invest Radiol 5:559–565
28. Stokes JM, Ter-Pogossian MM (1964) Double isotope technique to measure renal functions. JAMA 187:120–123
29. Denneberg T (1965) Clinical studies on kidney function with radioactive sodium diatrizoate. Acta Med Scand [Suppl] 442:1–49
30. Elwood CM, Sigman EM (1967) The measurement of glomerular filtration rate and effective renal plasma flow in man by iothalamate ^{125}I and iodopyracet ^{131}I. Circulation 36:441–448
31. Engelen AJM (1968) Renal contrast media. Thesis, University of Nijmegen
32. Israelit AH (1973) Measurement of glomerular filtration rate utilizing a singel subcutaneous injection of ^{125}I-iothalamate. Kidney Int 4:346–349
33. Bollerup AC, Hesse B, Steiness E (1975) Renal handling of iodamide and diatrizoate. Evidence of active tubular secretion of iodamide. Eur J Clin Pharmacol 9:63–67
34. Bianchi G, Toni CP (1963) La determinazione delle clearances renali mediante traccianti radioactivi. Minerva Nefrol 10:110–115
35. Blaufox MD, Sanderson DR, Tauxe WN (1963) Plasmatic diatrizoate I^{131} disappearance and glomerular filtration in the dog. Am J Physiol 204:536–540
36. Burbank MK, Tauxe WN, Maher FT (1963) Utilisation des substances marquées dans les épreuves classiques de clearance rénale. J Physiol (Paris) 55:433–437
37. Farmer CD, Tauxe WN, Maher FT (1967) Measurement of renal function with radioiodinated diatrizoate and o-iodohuppurate. Am J Clin Pathol 47:9–13
38. Meschan J, Deyton WE, Schmid HF (1963) The utilization of I^{131}-labelled renografin as an inulin substitute for renal clearance rate determination. Radiology 81:974–979
39. Meschan J, Watts FC, Lathem E (1966) Simultaneous PAH, inulin and renografin-I^{131} renal clearance determinations and a method for calculating renografin clearance from renograms in patients. AJR 97:909–913
40. Morris AM, Elwood C, Sigman EM (1965) The renal clearance of ^{131}I-labelled meglumine diatrizoate (Renografin) in man. J Nucl Med 6:183–188
41. Tauxe WN, Burbank MK, Maher FT (1964) Renal clearance of radioactive ortho-iodohippurate and diatrizoate. Mayo Clin Proc 39:761–764
42. Woodruff MW, Malvin RL (1960) Localization of renal contrast media excretion by stop flow analysis. J Urol 84:677–681
43. Dawson JB, McChesney EW, Teller FF (1968) Excretion of metrizoate in man. Acta Radiol (Stockh) 7:502–508
44. Van Waes PFGM (1972) High-dose urography in oliguric and anuric patients. Thesis. Excerpta Medica, Amsterdam, pp 7–15
45. Golman K (1973) Excretion of metrizamide. I. Comparison with diatrizoate and iothalamate after intravenous administration in rabbits. Acta Radiol [Suppl] (Stockh) 335:253–258
46. Almen T (1969) Contrast agent design. Some aspects on the synthesis of water-soluble contrast agents of low osmolality. J Theor Biol 24:216–222
47. Almen T, Nordal V, Haavaldsen J (1968) British patent no 1,321,591

48. Felder E, Pitre D (1974) Swiss patent no 16588/74
49. Nordal V, Holtermann H (1976) Triiodoisophthalic acid amides. British patent no 1,548,594
50. Tilly G, Hardoin MJ-C, Lautrou J (1975) Kontrastmittel für Röntgenaufnahmen. Offenlegungsschrift 2523567, 1975
51. Pfeiffer H, Speck U (1976) Neue Dicarboxysäure-bis-(3,5-dicarbamoyl-2,4,6-triiodoaniliden). Offenlegungsschrift P 2628517, 1976
51a. Sovak M, Ranganathan R, Speck U (1982) Nonionic dimer: development and initial testing of an intrathecal contrast agent. Radiology 142:115–118
52. Delahaye RP, Metges PJ, Lomazzi R, Flageat JR, Mathiot JL (1976) Les accidents et les incidents aux produits de contraste iodés au cours de l'urographie intraveineuse. Fréquence, clinique, physiopathologie. Med Arm 4:153–157
53. Sablayrolles J-L, Joffre F, Ecoiffier J, Suc JM, Putots J (1975) Etude systématique des temps néphrographiques de l'urographie intraveineuse. 1re partie: Problèmes techniques et aspects normaux. Ann Radiol (Paris) 18:543–558
54. Wells S, Dixon D, Rabinowitz J (1976) Renal cortical outline evaluation in excretory urography. J Urol 116:402–408
55. Kelsey Fry I, Catel WR (1972) The nephrographic pattern during excretion urography. Br Med Bull 28:227–232
56. Golman K (1973) Distribution and retention of ^{125}I-labelled metrizamide after intravenous and suboccipital injection in rabbit, rat, and cat. Acta Radiol [Suppl] (Stockh) 335:300–311
57. McChesney EW, Hoppe JO (1957) Studies of the tissue distribution and excretion of sodium diatrizoate in laboratory animals. AJR 78:137–144
58. Kormano M, Dean PB (1976) Extravascular contrast material: the major component of contrast enhancement. Radiology 121:379–382
59. Dean PB (1977) Early pharmacokinetics of an intravascular contrast medium. Thesis, University of Turku
60. Pihl B (1974) The single injection technique for determination of renal clearance. Scand J Urol Nephrol 8:147–154
61. Knoefel PK, Kraft RP, Knight RD (1974) Sodium versus meglumine diatrizoate in excretory urography. Invest Radiol 9:117–125
62. Sjöberg S, Almen T, Golman K, Grönberg T, Mattsson S (to be published) Noninvasive estimation of kidney function by X-ray fluorescence analysis. Invest Radiol
63. Gardeur D, Lautrou J, Millard JC, Berger N, Metzger J (1980) Pharmacokinetics of contrast media: Experimental results in dog and man which CT implications. J Comput Assist Tomogr 4:178–185
64. Benness GT, Glazer M (1973) Urographic contrast agents. Comparison of sodium and methylglucamine salts of iothalamate monomer and dimer. Clin Radiol 24:445–448
65. Golman K (1979) Experimental urography. Thesis, University of Oslo
66. Frey K (1973) Thin-layer chromatography of ^{125}I-labelled metrizamide in urine from laboratory animals. Acta Radiol [Suppl] (Stockh) 335:286–292
67. Talner LB, Coel MN, Lang JH (1973) Salivary secretion of iodine after urography. Radiology 106:263–268
68. McChesney EW (1971) The biotransformation of iodinated radiocontrast agents. In: Knoefel PK (ed) Radiocontrast agent, 1st edn. Pergamon, Oxford, pp 147–163
69. Kelly M, Golman K (1981) Metabolism of urographic contrast media. Invest Radiol 16:159–164
70. Felder E, Pitre D, Tirone P (1977) Radiopaque contrast media. XLIV. Preclinical studies with a new nonionic contrast agent. Farmaco [Sci] 32:835–844
71. Lasser EC, Farr RS, Fujimagari T, Tripp WN (1962) The significance of protein binding of contrast media in roentgen diagnosis. AJR 87:338–360
72. Salvesen S, Frey K (1973) Protein binding of metrizamide and the effect on various enzymes. Acta Radiol [Suppl] (Stockh) 335:247–252
73. Mützel W, Siefert H-M, Speck U (1980) Biochemical-pharmacological studies with iotexol. Acta Radiol 73 [Suppl] (Stockh) 362:111–117

74. Cattell WR, Fry IK, Spencer AG, Purkiss P (1967) Excretion urography. I. Factors determining the excretion of hypaque. Br J Radiol 40:561–580
75. Golman K, Almen T (1976) Metrizamide in experimental urography. VI. Effect of renal contrast media on urinary solutes. Acta Pharmacol Toxicol (Copenh) 38:120–136
76. Cunningham JJ, Friedland GW, Thurber B (1974) Immediate diuretic effects of intravenous sodium diatrizoate injections. Radiology 111:85–89
77. Mudge GH, Cooke WJ, Berndt WO (1975) Electrolyte excretion and free-water production during onset of acute diuresis. Am J Physiol 228:1304–1312
78. Jørgensen J (1967) Infusion urography. Acta Radiol [Suppl] 270:171–179
79. Schenker B (1964) Drip infusion pyelography. Radiology 83:12–21
80. Bonati F, Rosati GF, Poletto MG (1965) Röntgenkontrastmittel. 7. Mitteilung: Jodamid, ein neues Kontrastmittel, biologische Daten. Arzneimittelforsch 15:222–229
81. Golman K, Almen T, Denneberg T, Nosslin B (1977) Metrizamide in urography II. Invest Radiol 12:353–356
82. Burg MB (1976) Mechanism of fluid absorption by proximal convoluted renal tubules. In: Berlyne GM (ed) Proceedings of the 6th international congress on nephrology, Florence, 1975. Karger, Basel, pp 102–107
83. Hierholzer K (1976) Recent advances in renal physiology. In: Berlyne GM (ed) Proceedings of the 6th international congress on nephrology, Florence 1975. Karger, Basel, pp 19–37
84. Kill F (1976) Editorial mechanism of isotonic fluid transport in the intestinal tract and kidney tubules. Scand J Clin Lab Invest 36:609–615
85. Windhager EE (1976) Proximal sodium and fluid transport. Kidney Int 9:121–133
86. Burg MB (1976) Tubular chloride transport and the mode of action of some diuretics. Kidney Int 9:189–187
87. Evill CA, Benness GT (1975) Solute excretion during intravenous urography. A comparison of sodium iothalamate and sodium iocarmate (iothalamate dimer). Invest Radiol 10:552–556
88. Evill CA, Benness GT (1977) Urographic excretion studies with metrizamide and "dimer": A high dose comparison in dogs. Invest Radiol 12:169–174
89. Sjöberg S, Almen T, Golman K (1979) Excretion of contrast media for urography. Urine volume and iodine concentration during free urine flow in rabbits. J Belge Radiol 62:451–457
90. Doyle FH, Sherwood T, Steiner RE, Breckenridge A, Dollery CT (1967) Large dose urography. Is there an optimum dose? Lancet I:964–966
91. Fischer HW, Rothfield JH, Carr JD (1971) Optimum dose in excretory urography. AJR 113:423–426
92. Omvik P, Raeder M, Kill F (1971) Determinants of renal cortical volume. Am J Physiol 221:1560–1567
93. Wright S (1965) Applied physiology. Oxford University Press, London, pp 449–452
94. Keates PG (1953) Improving the intravenous pyelogram: an experimental study. Br J Urol 25:366
95. Dorph S, Sovak M, Talner LB, Rosen L (1977) Why does kidney size change during i.v. urography? Invest Radiol 12:246–250
96. Rapoport S, Brodsky WA, West CD, Mackler B (1949) Urinary flow and excretion of solutes during osmotic diuresis in hydropenic man. Am J Physiol 156:433–439
97. Wolpert SM (1965) Variation in kidney length during the intravenous pyelogram. Br J Radiol 38:100–103
98. Wolf GL, Wilson WJ (1972) Vasodilated excretory urography: An improved screening test for renal arterial stenosis. AJR 114:684–691
99. Dorph S, Øigaard A (1973) Variations in renal size in the diagnosis of renovascular hypertension. Br J Radiol 46:187–194
100. Wolf GL (1973) Rationale and use of vasodilated excretory urography in screening for renovascular hypertension. AJR 119:692–697
101. Owman T (1978) Excretion of urographic contrast media. Experimental studies in the rabbit. Thesis, University of Lund

102. Omvik P, Raeder M, Kiil F (1980) Relationship between tubular driving force and urine flow. Am J Physiol 226:982–987
103. Sjöberg S, Almén T, Golman K (1980) Excretion of contrast media for urography. Urine volume and iodine concentration during free urine flow in rabbits. Acta Radiol [Suppl] (Stockh) 362:93–98
104. Sjöberg S, Almén T, Golman K (1980) Excretion of contrast media for urography. Iohexol and sodium diatrizoate during ureteric stasis in rabbits. Acta Radiol [Suppl] (Stockh) 362:99–104
105. Jensen PK, Steven K (1979) Influence of intratubular pressure on proximal tubular compliance and capillary diameter in the rat kidney. Pfluegers Arch 382:179–187
106. Golman K (1973) Metrizamide in experimental urography. II. Iodine concentration following intravenous injection of an ionic and a non-ionic contrast medium in rats. Acta Radiol [Suppl] (Stockh) 335:323–329
107. Pinet A, Lyonnet O, Guillot M, Bret P (1977) Nouveau produit de contraste en urographie intraveineuse. XII. International congress of radiology, Rio de Janeiro
108. Hayek HW, Fleischhauer G (1978) Metrizamid (Amipaque®) in der Ausscheidungsurographie von Neugeborenen und Säuglingen. Untersuchungen zur Verträglichkeit und Bildqualität. Amipaque Workshop, Berlin, Excerpta Media: 182–190
109. Brun B, Egeblad M (1979) Metrizamide in pediatric urography. Ann Radiol (Paris) 22:198–201
110. Kolbenstvedt A, Andrew E, Christophersen B, Golman K, Kvarstein B, Lien HH (1979) Metrizamide in high-dose urography. Acta Radiol [Diagn] (Stockh) 20:39–45
111. Stake G, Borgnes J, Monn E (1979) Urography in children. A double blind study of metrizamide and metrizoate. Ann Radiol (Paris) 22:202–207
112. Almén T (1971) Toxicity of radiocontrast agents. In: Knoefel PK (ed) Radiocontrast agents, vol 2. Pergamon, Oxford II:443–550
113. Aspelin P, Almén T (1976) Studies of the acute toxicity of ionic and nonionic contrast media following rapid intravenous injection. Invest Radiol 11:309–313
114. Salvesen S (1977) Toxicity of metrizamide. Radiology 123:241–242
115. Aspelin P (1976) Effect of ionic and non-ionic contrast media on red blood cell morphology and rheology. Thesis, University of Lund
116. Bollman G, Jäger B, Freitag G (1979) In vitro effects of contrast media on the water content of human erythrocytes. Acta Radiol [Diagn] (Stockh) 20:681–687
117. Almén T, Aspelin P, Lewin B (1975) Effect of ionic and nonionic contrast medium on aortic and pulmonary arterial pressure. An angiocardiographic study in rabbits. Invest Radiol 10:519–525
118. Almén T, Aspelin P, Nilsson P (1980) Effect of ionic and nonionic contrast medium on aortic and pulmonary arterial pressure. Acta Radiol [Suppl] (Stockh) 362:37–43
119. Abrams H (1971) Angiography, 2nd edn. Little, Brown, Boston, p 22
120. Kong T, Meany T, Dustan H, Sones F (1963) Safety of selective renal arteriography. Am J Med Sci 246:527–532
121. Ansari Z, Baldwin S (1976) Acute renal failure due to radiocontrast agents. Nephron 17:28–40
122. Alexander R, Berkes S, Abuelo J (1978) Contrast media induced oliguric renal failure. Arch Intern Med 138:381–384
123. Borra S, Hawkins D, Duguid W, Kaye M (1971) Acute renal failure and nephrotic syndrome after angiocardiography with meglumine diatrizoate. N Engl J Med 284:592–593
124. Harkonen S, Kjellstrand C (1977) Exacerbation of diabetic renal failure following intravenous pyelography. Am J Med 63:939–946
125. Krumlovsky F, Simon N, Santhanam S, Del Greco F, Roxe D, Pomarance M (1978) Acute renal failure. Association with administration of radiographic contrast material. JAMA 239:125–127
126. McEvoy J, McGeown M, Kumar R (1970) Renal failure after radiologic contrast media. Br Med J 4:717–718

127. Milman N, Gottlieb P (1977) Renal function after high-dose urography in patients with chronic renal insufficiency. Clin Nephrol 7:250–255
128. Port F, Wagoner R, Fulton R (1974) Acute renal failure after angiography. AJR 121:544–550
129. Tejler L, Ekberg M, Almén T, Holtås S (1977) Proteinuria following renal arteriography. Report of two cases. Acta Med Scand 202:131–133
130. Cohen M, Meyers AM, Milne FJ, Disler PB, Van Blerk PJP (1978) Acute renal failure after use of radiographic contrast media. S Afr Med J 54:662–664
131. Warren SE, Bott JC, Thornfeldt C, Swerdlin A-H, Steinberg SM (1978) Hazards of computerized tomography. Renal failure following contrast injection. Surg Neurol 10:335–338
132. Barrientos A, Gomez-Tejada E, Ruilope LM, Rodicio JL, Leiva O (1978) Fracaso renal agudo inducido por contrastes radiologicos. Actas Urol Esp 2:115–118
133. Byrd L, Sherman RL (1978) Radiocontrast induced acute renal failure: a clinical and pathophysiological review. Medicine (Baltimore) 58:270–279
134. Harkonen S, Kjellstrand CM (1979) Intravenous pyelography in nonuremic diabetic patients. Nephron 24:268–270
135. Berger D (1979) Acute renal failure after intravenous pyelography in patients with diabetes mellitus. Ariz Med 36:889–891
136. Robinson JS, Arzola DD, Moody RA (1980) Acute renal failure following cerebral angiography and infusion computerized tomography. J Neurosurg 52:111–112
137. Older R, Miller J, Jackson D, Johnsrude I (1976) Angiographically induced renal failure and its radiographic detection. AJR 126:1039–1045
138. Swartz RD, Rubin JE, Leeming BW (1978) Renal failure following major angiography. Am J Med 65:31–36
139. Diz-Buxo J, Wagoner R, Hattery R (1975) Acute renal failure after excretory urography in diabetic patients. Ann Intern Med 83:155–158
140. Weinrauch L, Healy R, Leland O (1977) Coronary angiography and acute renal failure in diabetic azotemic nephropathy. Ann Intern Med 86:56–59
141. Gruskin A, Oelitliker O, Wolfish N, Bernstein J, Edelmann C (1970) Effects of angiography on renal function and histology in infants and piglets. J Pediatr 76:44–48
142. Talner L, Davidson A (1968) Effects of contrast media on renal extraction of PAH. Invest Radiol 3:301–309
143. Talner L, Davidson A (1968) Renal hemodynamic effects of contrast media. Invest Radiol 3:310–317
144. Caldicott WJH, Hollenberg NK, Abrams HL (1970) Characteristics of response of renal vascular bed to contrast media: evidence of vasoconstriction induced by renin-angiotension system. Invest Radiol 5:539–554
145. Morris TW, Katzberg RW, Fischer HW (1978) A comparison of the hemodynamic responses to metrizamide and meglumine/sodium diatrizoate in canine renal angiography. Invest Radiol 13:74–79
146. Golman K, Holtås S (1980) Proteinuria produced by urographic contrast media. Invest Radiol [Suppl] 15:61–67
147. Winding O (1977) Foreign bodies in contrast media for angiography. Am J Hosp Pharm 34:705–708
148. Winding O, Grønvall J, Faarup P, Hegedüs V (1980) Sequela of intrinsic foreign-body contamination during selective renal angiography in rabbits. Radiology 134:321–326
149. Holtås S (1978) Proteinuria following nephroangiography. Clinical and experimental findings. Thesis, University of Lund
150. Holtås S, Billstrøm AA, Tejler L (1981) Proteinuria following nephroangiography. Chemical and morphological analysis in dogs. Acta Radiol (Diagn) 22:427–433
151. Krakenes J, Elsayed S, Göthlin J, Farstad M (to be published) Proteinuria after selective nephroangiography in man with three different contrast media. Acta Radiol
152. Holtås S, Almén T, Golman K, Tejler L (1980) Proteinuria following nephroangiography. A study in dog and rat on influence of calcium and magnesium ions in nonionic contrast media. Acta Radiol 21:397–401

153. Holtås S, Almén T, Hellsten S, Tejler L (to be published) Proteinuria following nephroangiography. VI. Comparison between metrizoate and metrizamide in man. Acta Radiol (Stockh)

154. Törnquist C, Almén T, Golman K, Holtøs S (1980) Proteinuria following nephroangiography. VII. Comparison between ionic monomeric, monoacid dimeric and nonionic contrast media in dogs. Acta Radiol (Stockh) Suppl 362:49–52

155. Holtås S, Golman K, Törnquist C (1980) Proteinuria following nephroangiography. VIII. Comparison between diatrizoate and iohexol in rats. Acta Radiol [Suppl] (Stockh) 362:53–56

156. Moreau JF, Diaz D, Sabto J, Jungers P, Kleinknecht D, Hinglais N, Michel JR (1975) Osmotic nephrosis induced by water soluble triiodinated contrast media in man. Radiology 115:329–338

157. Yun CH, Kenney Ra (1978) Structural changes after infusion of manitol in the cat kidney. Renal Physiol 1:283–295

158. Moreau JF, Noel L-H, Droz D (1978) Nephrotoxicity of ioxaglic acid (AG 62-27 or P 286) in humans. Invest Radiol 13:554–562

159. Moreau JF, Droz D, Noel L-H (1978) Nephrotoxicity of metrizamide in man. Lancet:1201

160. Deimling O (1970) Enzymarchitektur der Niere und Sexualhormone. Prog Histochem Cytochem 1:1–50

161. Burchardt U, Mampel E (1974) Das Verhalten der Alaninaminopeptidase-Ausscheidung nach Visotrastapplikation als diagnostischer Test. Z Inn Med 29:853–857

162. Burchardt U, Mampel E, Peters JE, Thulin H (1975) Harnenzymausscheidung nach Gabe nierengängiger Röntgenkontrastmittel. Z Urol 67:807–812

163. Burchardt U, Peters J (1975) Enzyme im Harn nach Applikation hypertoner Lösungen. Z Inn Med 30:248–251

164. Bartels H, Hempfing E-W, Müller-Wiefel D (1975) Der Einfluß der intravenösen Pyelographie auf die Ausscheidung von Leucinarylamidase und γ-Glutamyltranspeptidase im Urin bei Kindern. Monatsschr Kinderheilkd 123:424–428

165. Talner LB, Rushmer HN, Coel MN (1972) The effect of renal artery injection of contrast material on urinary enzyme excretion. Invest Radiol 7:311–316

166. Alexander RD, Berkes SL, Abuelo JG (1978) Contrast media-induced oliguric renal failure. Arch Intern Med 138:381–386

167. Skalpe IO, Evensen A (1973) Toxicity of metrizamide, meglumine iocarmate and sodium metrizoate in selective nephroangiography. Acta Radiol [Suppl] (Stockh) 335:175–185

168. Evensen A, Skalpe IO (1971) Cell injury and cell regeneration in selective renal arteriography in rabbits. Invest Radiol 6:299–307

169. Dibona GF (1978) Effect of anionic and nonionic contrast media on renal extraction of paraaminohippurate in the dog. Proc Soc Exp Biol Med 157:453–455

170. Ziegler TW, Olsen LS (1976) Role of anions in regulating short-circuit current in toad urinary bladder. Proc Am Soc Nephrol 6:604

171. Ziegler TW, Olsen LS (1980) Effect of radiocontrast media on ion transport in the toad urinary bladder. Invest Radiol Suppl 15:51–53

172. Lavaurs G, Riitano F, Anniotti N, Larrieu A, Martin C, Noble JF (1975) Accidents par moyens de contrast iodes hydrosolubles. J Radiol [Suppl] 1:135–136

173. Rothenberger K, Ring J (1979) Das Wiederholungsrisiko von Kontrastmittel-Reaktionen bei der Urographie. Fortschr Med 97:1429–1432

174. Witten M (1975) Reactions to urographic contrst media. JAMA 231:974–977

175. Canigiani G, Deimer E, Wolf G (1974) Über die Injektionszeiten und die Verträglichkeit verschiedener Kontrastmittel bei urographischen und angiographischen Untersuchungen. Röntgenpraxis 27:273–280

176. Dahl SG, Linaker O, Mellbye Å, Sveen K (1976) Influence of the cation on the side effects of urographic contrast media. Acta Radiol [Diagn] (Stockh) 17:461–471

177. Davies P, Roberts MB, Roylance J (1975) Acute reactions to urographic contrast media. Br Med J 2:434–437

178. Coleman WP, Ochner SF, Watson BE (1964) Allergic reactions in 10,000 consecutive intravenous urographies. South Med J 57:1401–1404
179. Penry JB, Livingston A (1972) A comparison of diagnostic effectiveness and vascular side effects of various diatrizoate salts used for intravenous pyelography. Clin Radiol 23:362–369
180. Macht SH, Williams RH, Lawrence PS (1966) Study of 3 contrast agents in 2,234 intravenous pyelographies. AJR 98:79–87
181. Littner MR, Rosenfield AT, Ulriech S, Putman CE (1977) Evaluation of bronchospasm during excretory urography. Radiology 124:17–21
182. Langen JE, Hermans J (1973) Comparative multiclinical studies of iodamide and diatrizoate in excretory urography. Radiology 106:76–86
183. Bhat KN, Arroyave C, Crown R (1976) Reactions to radiographic contrast agents: new development in etiology. Ann Allergy 37:169–173
184. Shehadi WH (1975) Adverse reactions to intravascular administered contrast media. AJR 124:145–153
185. Ansel G (1970) Adverse reactions to contrast agents. Invest Radiol 5:374–384
186. Fischer HW, Doust VL (1972) An evaluation of pretesting in the problem of serious and fatal reactions to excretory urography. Radiology 103:497–502
187. Fisher MMcD (1978) Acute life-threatening reactions to contrast media. Australas Radiol 22:365–371
188. Gorevic P, Kaplan AP (1979) Contrast agents and anaphylactic-like reactions. J Allergy Clin Immunol 63:225–227
190. Pringle H, Maunsell RCB, Pringle S (1905) Clinical effects of ether anaesthesia on renal activity. Br Med J 2:542–544
191. Miles BE, de Wardener HE, Churchill-Davidson HC, Wylie WD (1952) The effect on the renal circulation of pentamethonium bromide during anesthesia. Clin Sci 11:73–79
192. Mazze RI, Schwartz FD, Slocum HC, Barry KG (1963) Renal function during anesthesia and surgery. I. The effects of halothane anesthesia. Anesthesiology 24:279–284
193. Steven K (1974) Influence of nephron GFR on proximal reabsorption in pentobarbital anaesthetized rats. Kidney Int 5:204–213
194. Malvin RL, Wilde WS (1973) Stop-flow technique. In: Orloff J, Berliner RW (eds) Renal physiology. Williams and Wilkins, Baltimore (Handbook of physiology, sect 8, pp 119–143)
195. Barger AC, Herd JA (1973) Renal vascular anatomy and distribution of flow. In: Orloff J, Berliner RW (eds) Renal physiology. Williams and Wilkins, Baltimore (Handbook of physiology, sect 8, pp 249–313)
196. Bastron RD, Deutsch S (eds) (1976) Anaesthesia and the kidney. Grune and Stratton, New York
197. Ahlgren I, Trägårdh B (1973) Renal angiography during halothane anaesthesia in the dog. Acta Anaesthesiol Scand 17:103–107
198. Lyrdal F, Olin T (1975) Renal blood flow and function in the rabbit after surgical trauma. I. An experimental study. Scand J Urol Nephrol 9:129–141
199. Bastron RD, Deutsch S (1976) Post-operative events and renal function. In: Bastrow RD, Deutsch S (eds) Anaesthesia and the kidney. Grune and Stratton, New York
200. Lyrdal F, Olin T (1975) Renal blood flow and function in the rabbit after surgical trauma. II. The role of constriction in the main renal artery and activation of the alpha-adrenergic receptors. Scand J Urol Nephrol 9:142–150
201. Lyrdal F, Olin T (1975) Renal blood flow and function in the rabbit after surgical trauma. III. Effects of temporary occlusion of renal artery. Scand J Urol Nephrol 9:151–160
202. Thapper K (1977) Properties of medical X-ray film. Test methods and optimal values of radiographic contrast and patient irradiation with special reference to iodine-containing contrast media. Thesis, University of Lund

203. Purkiss P, Lane RD, Cattell WR, Fry IK, Spencer AG (1968) Estimation of sodium diatrizoate by absorption spectrophotometry. Invest Radiol 3:271–276
204. Johnson CA, Vickers C (1959) The flask combustion technique in pharmaceutical analysis: iodine-containing substances. J Pharm Pharmacol 11:218–227
205. Foss OP, Hankers LV, Van Slyke DD (1960) A study of the alkaline asking method for determination of protein-bound iodine in serum. Clin Chim Acta 5:301–315
206. Johansen O, Steinness E (1969) Rapid neutron activation method for determination of iodine in milk. J Dairy Sci 53:420–422
207. Johansen O, Steinness E (1976) Determination of iodine in plant material by neutron-activation method. Analyst 101:455–457
208. Moss AA, Kaufman L, Nelson Ja (1972) Fluorescent excitation analysis: a simplified method of iodine determination in vitro. Invest Radiol 7:355–359
209. Grönberg T, Almén T, Golman K, Liden K, Mattsson S, Sjöberg S (1981) Noninvasive determination of kidney function by X-ray fluorescence analysis. Method for in vivo measurements on rabbits. J Phys Biol 26:501–506
210. Leyden DE, Nonidez WK (1977) X-ray fluorescence application to clinical studies. CRC Crit Rev Clin Lab Sci 7:393–422
211. Kaufman L, Shames O, Powell M (1973) An absorption correction technique for in vivo iodine quantitation by fluorescent excitation. Invest Radiol 8:167–169
212. White EA, Korobkin M, Brito AC (1979) Computed tomography of experimental acute renal ischemia. Invest Radiol 14:421–427
213. Brennan RE, Curtis JA, Pollack HM (1979) Sequential changes in the CT number of the normal dog kidney following intravenous contrast administration. I. The renal cortex. Invest Radiol 14:141–146
214. Brennan RE, Curtis JA, Pollack HM, Weinberg I (1979) Sequential changes in CT numbers of the normal canine kidney following intravenous contrast administration. II. The renal medulla. Invest Radiol 14:239–245
216. Pileggi VJ, Henry RJ, Segalove M, Hamill GC (1962) Determination of organic iodine compounds in serum. Clin Chem 8:647–653
217. Jones JE, Shultz JS (1967) Determination of thyroxine iodine content of serum contaminated by organic iodines. A method based on gel filtration. J Clin Endocrinol 27:877–883
218. Roderigues DE, Miranda JF (1967) A method for the quantitative determination of the total concentration of radiopaque agents in plasma. J Pharm Pharmacol 19:161–166
219. Hoch H, Sinnett SL, McGavack TH (1964) The determination of iodine in biological material. Clin Chem 10:799–822
220. Medzihradsky F, Dahlstrom PJ, Hunter TB, Thornbury JR, Silver TM (1975) A simple spectrophotometric procedure for the determination of various contrast media in plasma. Invest Radiol 10:532–535
221. Hegedüs V (1977) Three-dimensioned estimation of renal shape and volume at angiography. Acta Radiol (Stockh) 12:87–99
222. McLachlan MSF, Gaunt A, Fulker MJ, Andersson CK (1976) Estimation of glomerular size and number from radiographs of the kidney. Br J Radiol 49:831–835
223. Moëll H (1961) Kidney size and its deviation from normal in acute renal failure. A roentgendiagnostic study. Acta Radiol [Suppl] (Stockh) 206:1–74
224. Hodson Cj (1961) Physiological changes in size of the human kidney. Clin Radiol 12:91–94
225. Hegedüs V, Faarup P, Nørgaard T, Lønholdt C (1978) Volume changes in the rat renal cortex during urography. Br J Radiol 51:793–798
226. Zubovskij V, Frenkel C, Markova EG (1971) Untersuchung der glomerulären Filtration mit dem radioaktiven Präparaten ^{131}I-Triombrin, ^{51}Cr-EDTA und ^{169}Yb-EDTA. Radiol Diagn (Berl) 12:69–79
227. Barbour GL, Crumb CK, Boyd CM, Reeves RD, Rastogi SP, Patterson RM (1976) Comparison of inulin, iothalamate and ^{99}Tc-DPTA for measurement of glomerular filtration rate. J Nucl Med 17:317–320

228. Bröchner-Mortensen J (1978) Routine methods and their reliability for assessment of glomerular filtration rate in adults. Thesis, University of Copenhagen
229. Favre HR, Wing AJ (1968) Simultaneous ^{51}Cr-edtic acid, inulin and endogenous creatinine clearance in 20 patients with renal disease. Br Med J 1:84–86
229a. Grönberg T, Sjöberg S, Golman K, Mattsson S (1983) Non-invasive estimation of kidney function by X-ray fluorescence analysis. Invest Radiol 18:445–451
230. Malvin RL, Wilde WS, Sullivan LP (1958) Location of nephron transport by stop flow analysis. Am J Physiol 194:135–142
231. Malvin RL, Wilde WS (1973) Stop-flow technique. In: Orloff J, Berliner RW (eds) Renal physiology. Williams and Wilkins, Baltimore (Handbook of physiology, sect 8, pp 119–128)
232. Woodruff MW, Malvin RL (1960) Location of renal contrast media excretion by stop flow analysis. J Urol 84:677–685
233. Engelen AJM (1968) Renal contrast media. Thesis, University of Nijmegen
234. Rennick BR, Moe GK (1960) Stop-flow localization of renal tubular excretion of te-traethylammonium. Am J Physiol 198:1267–1272
235. Zins GR, Weiner IM (1968) Bidirectional urate transport limited to the proximal tu-bule in dogs. Am J Physiol 215:411–417
236. Zins GR, Weiner IM (1968) Bidirectional transport of taurocholate by the proximal tubule of the dog. Am J Physiol 215:840–844
237. Gottshalk CW, Leyssac PP (1968) Proximal tubular function in rats with low inulin clearance. Acta Physiol Scand 74:453–464
238. Gottshalk CW, Lassiter WE (1973) Micropuncture methodology. In: Orloff J, Ber-liner RW (eds) Renal physiology. Williams and Wilkins, Baltimore (Handbook of physiology, sect 8, pp 129–143)
239. De Rouffignac C, Morel F (1969) Micropuncture of water, electrolytes and urea movements along the loops of Henle in psammomys. J Clin Invest 48:474–486
240. Franklin GK, Marchand GR (1976) Study of renal action of diuretics by micropunc-ture techniques. In: Martinez-Maldonado M (ed) Method of pharmacology. Plenum, New York, pp 73–99
241. Burg MB, Grantham JJ, Abranow M, Orloff J (1966) Preparation and study of frag-ments of single rabbit nephron. Am J Physiol 210:1293–1298
242. Kokko JP (1970) Sodium chloride and water transport in the descending limb of Hen-le. J Clin Invest 49:1838–1846
243. Burg MB, Orloff J (1973) Perfusion of isolated tubules. In: Orloff J, Berliner RW (eds) Renal physiology. Williams and Wilkins, Baltimore (Handbook of physiology, sect 8, pp 145–159)
244. Irish JM, Bigongiari LR (1979) Isolated microperfused tubule model to evaluate con-trast media transport in normal and occluded renal tubule segments. Invest Radiol 14:330–333
245. Bárány EH (1972) Inhibition by hippurate and probenacid of in vitro uptake of io-dipamide and o-iodohippurate. A composite uptake system for iodipamide in choroid plexus, kidney cortex, and anterior urea of several species. Acta Physiol Scand 86:12–27
246. Kormano M, Frey H (1980) Toxicity of X-ray contrast media in cell cultures. Invest Radiol 15:68–71
247. Kormano M, Hervonen H (1976) Use of tissue culture to examine neurotoxicity of contrast media. Radiology 120:727–730
248. Mann S, Zeitler E (1975) Verhalten der Serumosmolarität bei hohen Kontrastmittel-dosen im Rahmen der Angiographie. ROFO 122:135–137
249. Schmid HW (1971) Untersuchungen der Toxizität der physikalisch-chemischen Ei-genschaften nach der hämolytischen Aktivität von triiodierten Röntgenkontrastmit-tel-Salzen in wässerigen Lösungen. Pharm Acta Helv 46:210–225
250. Sharratt M, Frazer AC (1963) The sensitivity of function tests in detecting renal dam-age in the rat. Toxicol Appl Pharmacol 5:36–48

251. Kassierer JP (1971) Clinical evaluation of kidney function: tubular function. N Engl J Med 285:499–502
252. Diezi J, Biolliaz J (1979) Renal function tests in experimental toxicity studies. Pharmacol Ther 5:135–145
253. Peters G, Baechtold-Fowler N, Bonjour JP, Chométy-Diezi F, Filloux B, Guidoux R, Guignard JP, Petershaefeli L, Roch-Ramel E, Schelling JL, Hedinger C, Weber E (1972) General and renal toxocity of phenacetin, paracetamol and some anti-mitotic agents in the rat. Arch Toxicol 28:225–269
254. Singer I, Forrest JN (1976) Drug- induced states of nephrogenic diabetes insipidus. Kidney Int 10:82–95
255. Jamison RL, Maffly RH (1976) The urinary concentrating mechanism. N Engl J Med 295:1059–1067
256. Maher JF (1976) Toxic nephropathy. In: Brenner BM, Rector FC (eds) The kidney, vol 2. Saunders, Philadelphia, pp 1355–1395
257. Ling G (1971) Studies on separate renal blood flow and function using a dye-dilution technique and radiochemicals. Scand J Urol Nephrol [Suppl] 8:1971
258. Göthlin J, Olin T (1973) Dye dilution technique with nephroangiography for the determination of renal blood flow and related parameters. Acta Radiol [Diagn] (Stockh) 14:113–137
259. Kety SS (1951) The theory and application of the exchange of inert gas at the lungs and tissues. Pharmacol Rev 3:1–41
260. Conn HL, Anderson W, Arena S (1953) Gas diffusion technique for measurement of renal blood flow with special reference to the intact, anuric subject. J Appl Physiol 5:683–689
261. Zierler KL (1963) Theory of use of indicator to measure blood flow and extracellular volume and calculation of transcapillary movement of tracers. Circ Res 12:464–471
262. Zierler KL (1965) Equations for measuring blood flow by external monitoring of radioisotopes. Circ Res 16:309–321
263. McNay JL, Abe Y (1970) Pressure-dependent heterogeneity of renal cortical blood flow in dogs. Circ Res 27:571–587
264. Idvall J, Aronsen KF, Nilsson L, Nosslin B (1979) Evaluation of the microsphere method for determination of cardiac output and flow distribution in the rat. Eur Surg Res 11:423–433
265. Buckberg GD, Luck JC, Payne DB, Hoffman JIE, Archie JP, Fixler DE (1971) Some source of error in measuring regional blood flow with radioactive microspheres. J Appl Physiol 31:598–608
266. Thorburn GD, Kopald HH, Herd JA, Hollenberg M, O'Morchoe CCC, Barger AD (1963) Intrarenal distribution of nutrient blood flow determined with krypton[85] in the unanesthetized dog. Circ Res 13:290–299
267. Lameire NH, Chuang EL, Osgood RW, Stein JH (1978) Measurement of intrarenal blood flow distribution. In: Martinez Maldonado M (ed) Renal pharmacology. Plenum, New York (Methods of pharmacology, vol 4B, pp 41–75)
268. Pitts FP (1968) Physiology of the kidney and body fluids. Year Book Medical Publisher, Chicago, pp 62–70
269. Mancini G, Carbonara AO, Heremans JF (1965) Immunochemical quantitation of antigens by using single radial immunodiffusion. Immunochemistry 2:235–242
270. Crowle AJ (1973) Immunodiffusion, 2nd edn. Academic Press, New York
271. Balazs T, Hatch A, Zawidzka Z, Grice HC (1963) Renal tests in toxicity studies on rats. Toxicol Appl Pharmacol 5:661–674
272. Nomiyama K, Sato C, Yamamoto A (1973) Early signs of cadmium intoxication in rabbits. Toxicol Appl Pharmacol 24:625–635
273. Nomiyama K, Yamamoto A, Sato C (1974) Assay of urinary enzymes in toxic nephropathy. Toxicol Appl Pharmacol 27:484–490

274. Ellis BG, Price RG, Topham JC (1973) The effect of tubular damage by mercuric chloride on kidney function and some urinary enzymes in the dog. Chem Biol Interact 7:101–113
275. Patel V, Luft FC, Yum MN, Patel B, Zeman W, Kleit SA (1975) Enzymuria in gentamicin-induced kidney damage. Antimicrob Agents Chemoither 7:364–369
276. Stroo WE, Hook JB (1977) Enzymes of renal origin in urine as indicators of nephrotoxicity. Toxicol Appl Pharmacol 39:423–434
277. Baggio B, Favaro S, Antonello A, Borin A, Borsatti A (1978) Phospholipase A_2 in the rat kidney. Subcellular localization and possible physiologic function. Renal Physiol 1:323–328
278. Kinne-Saffran E, Kinne R (1974) Presence of bicarbonate stimulated ATP in the brush border microvillus membrane of proximal tubule. Proc Soc Exp Biol Med 146:751–753
279. Bulger RE, Dobyan D (1978) Morphological techniques for study of the kidney. In: Martinez-Maldonado M (ed) Renal pharmacology. Plenum, New York (Methods of pharmacology, vol 43, pp 1–23)
280. Clark RL, Mandel SR, Webster WP (1977) Microvascular changes in canine renal allograft rejection. A correlative microangiographic and histologic study. Radiology 12:62–67
281. Gade R (1977) Microangiography in the perfusion-fixed rabbit kidney: a single injection technique for the study of the nephron. Invest Radiol 12:348–353
282. Gade R, Gade MF (1978) Microradiography of the collecting ducts in the perfusion fixed rabbit kidney: suggestions for the anatomic basis for the radiographic appearance of cortical striation and intrarenal reflux. Invest Radiol 13:318–324
283. Rebelo AE, Graham EF, Crabo BG, Lillehei RC, Dietzman RH (1974) Surgical preparation, perfusion techniques, and cryoprotectans used in successful freezing of the kidney. Surgery 75:319–331
284. Arborgh B, Bell P, Brunk U, Collins VP (1976) The osmotic effect of glutaraldehyde during fixation. A transmission electron microscopy, scanning electron microscopy and cytochemical study. J Ultrastruct Res 56:339–350

CHAPTER 3

Contrast Media in the Cardiovascular System

C. B. HIGGINS

A. Introduction

This chapter is a review of current knowledge of the cardiovascular effects of contrast media, examining the literature on this subject over the past 1 ½ decades. In the previous encyclopedia on radiocontrast agents [1], ALMEN comprehensively reviewed the published information dealing with the cardiovascular effects of contrast media up to the year 1968. As in other areas of biomedical research the output of scientific papers and new concepts on this subject in the past decade has approached, and on some topics surpassed, the total output prior to this time.

B. Classification of Cardiovascular Actions of Contrast Media

The actions of contrast media (CM) on the cardiovascular system can be conveniently divided into their direct and indirect effects. The direct effects are exerted on the heart (central effects) and on the peripheral circulation and its component regional vascular beds (peripheral effects):

Central
1. Heart rate, rhythm, conduction
2. Contractile state

Peripheral
1. Vasoactivity
2. Reflex activation.

The indirect effects are primarily neurohumoral alterations invoked as compensatory responses to the direct effects (Table 1). Figure 1 is a mechanistic scheme showing the occurrence of the secondary effects of CM.

The effects on the heart consist of electrophysiologic changes and mechanical changes. The former include changes in heart rate, rhythm, conduction, induction of arrhythmias, and various other electrocardiographic changes. The latter include alterations in ventricular pressures and dimensions as well as extent and rate of myocardial contraction. The direct peripheral effects consist of vasodilatation and direct damage to the microvasculature and vascular endothelium.

The indirect effects are those cardiovascular changes which are due to either primary or secondary activation of circulatory reflex responses or due to release

Table 1. Cardiovascular responses to contrast media. [17]

Primary actions	Reflex activation	Secondary responses
↓ Heart rate		
Sinus arrest		
↑ PR interval		
Heart block		
Bundle branch block		
↑ Refractory period (ventricle)		
Ventricular arrhythmias		
Repolarization abnormalities		
↓ Myocardial contractility		
↑ LVEDV ↑ LVEDP	⟶ Intracardiac low pressure receptors	⟶ ?
Peripheral vasodilatation (↓ AP)	⟶ Baroreceptors	⟶ ↑ Heart rate ↓ PR interval ↑ Cardiac output ↑ Myocardial contractility
	Intracoronary stretch receptors	⟶ ↓ HR
	Chemoreceptors	⟶ ↑ Arterial pressure ↓ HR ? Myocardial contractility

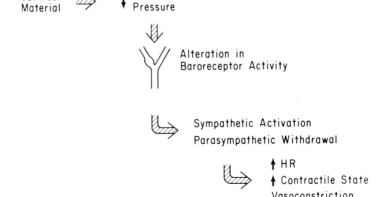

Fig. 1. A mechanistic scheme for some of the secondary effects of contrast media

of neurohumoral and/or vasoactive substances by CM. Although there has been much conjecture regarding the release of vasoactive substances by CM, there is actually little evidence that vasoactive substances play any significant role in the hemodynamic aspect of the cardiovascular response to the administration of CM. This is not to deny that release of vasoactive substances may be of considerable importance in mediating other responses to CM, such as idiosyncratic, i.e., pseudoallergic, reactions. Finally, hemodynamic changes in some regional vascular beds may be mediated through rheological effects of CM.

C. Importance of Experimental Conditions

The results of the various studies dealing with the hemodynamic effects of CM have not always been consonant with each other. A frequent reason for variability of results between studies is differences in experimental conditions. The differences in experimental conditions include species variations, isolated versus intact cardiovascular preparations, conscious versus anesthetized animals, type of anesthesis utilized, and site of injection of CM. Finally, CM may have quantitatively or even qualitatively different effects in the presence of underlying pathologic states compared with the normal state.

I. Influence of the Experimental Model Used for Studying Cardiovascular Effects of Contrast Media

One of the major factors responsible for qualitative and particularly quantitative differences in the cardiovascular effects of CM reported in various studies is the type of experimental model employed. Additionally, hemodynamic responses to any pharmacologic agent may be importantly modified by the anesthetic agent used in the experiments [2, 3]. In particular, reflex responses are substantially attenuated or ablated in the presence of barbiturate anesthetics [2, 3].

The effects of CM on the heart have been evaluated in a variety of experimental preparations including the papillary muscle in vitro [4, 5], isolated heart preparations [6–9], and the intact heart of anesthetized and conscious dogs [10–13].

Perhaps the most frequent experimental preparation used for evaluating the myocardial action of CM over the years has been some type of isolated heart preparation. This experimental model, like the papillary muscle preparation, is not influenced by possible activation of neural and humoral mechanisms. Moreover, preload and afterload can be precisely controlled in the papillary muscle and isolated heart preparations. On the other hand, the extensive surgery needed for this preparation and, in some instances, the artificial nutrient material supplying the isolated heart result in a severely depressed heart. In this model, the effect of CM has been assessed by measuring force development or rate of force development with a strain gauge arch sewn to or a mercury-in-rubber ring placed on the left ventricle (LV). Numerous studies in the isolated heart have revealed profound negative inotropic effects of ionic CM [6–9].

The intact heart provides a less depressed and more physiologic preparation but one in which the influence of preload, afterload, and neurohumoral factors cannot be as precisely controlled. The parameters of contractile state in this preparation are peak $dp/dt - dp/dt$ at a specified level of left ventricular pressure (LVP) (usually 40 or 50 mmHg) and rate of shortening of a minor axis, chord, or segment of the left ventricle. The influence of loading factors on dp/dt measured at a developed LVP of 40 mmHg have been found to be small, and, therefore, changes in this parameter are considered to reflect accurately changes in contractile state (inotropic effects) [14, 15]. Peak dp/dt is more substantially altered by changes in loading factors [14, 15]. However, after direct intracoronary injection of CM, the early changes in this parameter are a reliable indicator of direct myocardial effects, since there is a delay before the CM reaches and affects the peripheral circulation. However, within 6–10 s after injection, changes in these parameters can be expected to be due in part to variations in loading factors and in autonomic neural tone due to the peripheral vasodilatory actions of CM.

In recent years, ultrasonic (piezoelectric) crystals have been implanted in opposition on endocardial surfaces of the left ventricle to monitor dimensional changes in the LV. A dimension gauge measures the instantaneous distance between these crystals on the endocardial surface of the LV and provides a waveform called LV diameter [12, 15]. Differentiation of the LV diameter signal provides the parameter dD/dt (rate of change of LV diameter), which is a reflection of velocity of myocardial contraction. Under specified conditions, an increase or decrease in dD/dt after intracoronary administration of a substance indicates a positive and negative inotropic effect, respectively. Negative inotropic influences usually also cause an increase in end-diastolic and end-systolic diameters and decrease in difference between end-diastolic and end-systolic diameters (extent of contraction). Monomeric ionic CM cause substantial decreases in dp/dt and dD/dt after direct intracoronary administration, which indicates a negative inotropic action in the intact heart [10–12].

It seems clear that the most physiologically relevant data can be expected from experiments in healthy conscious animals. However, very few studies on the cardiovascular effects of CM have utilized conscious animals. The only study comparing the direct effects of CM on the heart of anesthetized and conscious animals showed no important differences between the two experimental states [11]. Moreover, the circulatory responses of conscious man to CM have been found to be qualitatively similar to those observed in anesthetized animals.

II. Influence of the Site of Injection of Contrast Media

The hemodynamic alterations induced by contrast media depend upon the site of administration. The time sequence and intensity of hemodynamic changes after injection of ionic CM into the aortic root and left coronary artery in anesthetized dogs have been investigated [16]. Following selective left coronary artery injection, systolic and diastolic arterial pressures, left ventricular peak systolic pressure, peak dp/dt, and dp/dt at a developed LV pressure of 40 mmHg decreased maximally at 5 s. Following aortic root injection, the arterial and LV systolic changes were biphasic, increasing at 5 s and decreasing at 20 s. The corresponding changes in peak dp/dt and dp/dt_{40} were initial decreases at 5 s and increases above control during the period of hypotension. This study concluded that the cause of the hypotension accompanying injection of ionic CM varies with the site of injection; myocardial depression is the major factor with selective coronary arteriography, while peripheral vasodilatation is the major factor after aortic injection.

Similar results have been observed in somewhat different experimental conditions in the anesthetized dog [17] (Fig. 2). Femoral blood flow was also monitored in these experiments in order to measure any vascular resistance in the limb bed. After selective intracoronary injection, decline in pressures was temporally related to the decrease in parameters of LV contractility (*dp/dt* at a developed LV pressure of 50 mmHg) and preceded the fall in femoral vascular resistance. On the other hand, after intraaortic injection the fall in blood pressure was temporally related to the decrease in femoral vascular resistance.

In a canine model, progressive constriction of the thoracic aorta maintained normal levels of pressure in the ascending aorta while near maximal peripheral vasodilatation was induced [18]. Under this experimental condition injection of CM into the left ventricle caused minimal hypotension while the response in the

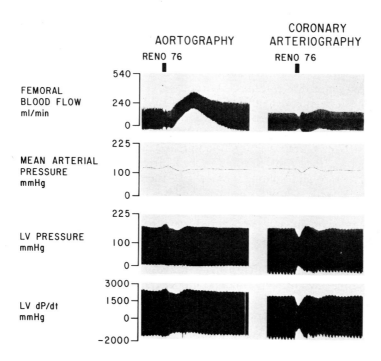

Fig. 2. Experimental tracings depicting the hemodynamic responses to injections of sodium meglumine diatrizoate (Renografin-76) into the aorta (*left*) and left coronary artery (*right*) of the same anesthetized dog. After intraaortic injection the decrease in LV *dp/dt* is delayed and reflects the decrease in arterial pressure as a consequence of peripheral vasodilatation. In contrast, injection into the coronary artery causes an immediate decline in LV *dp/dt* due to direct myocardial depression caused by the ionic CM [17]

same animals without preexisting aortic constriction caused considerable hypotension. Pharmacologic induction of peripheral vasodilatation prior to ventriculography also ablated the hypotensive effect of the CM. The authors concluded that most of the systemic hypotension observed in response to ionic CM during left ventriculography is due to peripheral vasodilatation.

A number of investigations in man [19–24] and experimental animals with intact hearts (as opposed to isolated heart preparations) [19, 25–29] have characterized the hemodynamic response to injection of ionic CM into the left side of the heart and aorta. It was thus observed that with injection into the left-sided chambers, the major changes are increase in left atrial and left ventricular end-diastolic pressures, increases in stroke volume and cardiac output, decrease in systemic arterial pressure, and a small transient decrease in myocardial contractility [19]. These changes are due predominantly to the abrupt increase in volume within the heart and the peripheral vasodilation produced by the hyperosmolal contrast solution. The slight decrease in contractility observed with CM does not ensue until at least five heart beats after the initiation of the intraventricular injection [20, 21, 24, 27].

It has been reported that after injection of ionic CM into the LV or thoracic aorta of dogs, mean left atrial, left ventricular end-diastolic, and pulmonary artery pressure increased and myocardial contractile force decreased [25]. It was also found that the depression in myocardial contractile state induced by CM does not ensue until the sixth to seventh opacified beat during ventriculography [11]. This response differs from the almost immediate depression in contractility after intracoronary injection of ionic CM in conscious and anesthetized dogs.

A biphasic response to the injection of CM into the left ventricle has been noted [26, 27]. Thus, injection of either saline or ionic CM produced an immediate increase in left ventricular end-diastolic pressure and volume, LV peak systolic pressure, stroke volume, ejection fraction, and peak dp/dt [26]. This response was characteristic of the Frank-Starling effect. Thirteen to sixteen beats later, LV end-diastolic pressure and volume increased further, accompanied by a fall in peak dp/dt and LV peak systolic pressure. The later changes were attributed to direct myocardial depression by the CM. Addition of angiotensin II to the ionic CM vitiated the decline in systemic arterial pressure in response to ventriculography and in the absence of hypotensive action the decline in peak dp/dt was not observed [28].

Qualitatively similar biphasic responses to contrast ventriculography have been found in newborn experimental models, after the injection of ionic and to a lesser degree after the injection of nonionic materials into the LV of puppies [30]. Likewise, biphasic alterations were observed after injection of ionic CM into the LV of newborn lambs [31].

The second phase of the hemodynamic response to CM is influenced by activation of baroreceptor and chemoreceptor reflexes [11, 32–35]. Activation of the baroreceptor reflex tends to mollify the late effects of CM since activation of this reflex causes peripheral vasoconstriction and exerts a positive inotropic influence on the LV myocardium [11, 36, 37]. Activation of the chemoreceptor reflex causes complex and variable effects but also tends to cause peripheral vasoconstriction [32–34, 38, 39].

Injection of CM into right-sided cardiac chambers causes less decline in systemic arterial pressure than left-sided or aortic injections and invokes transient but substantial pulmonary arterial hypertension [29]. Injection of ionic and nonionic CM into the right atrium of rabbits elicits biphasic changes in systemic arterial pressure and persistent pulmonary arterial hypertension for approximately 15 s [6].

In dogs, right-sided injections of ionic CM in small volume (1 ml/kg) have been observed to decrease systemic arterial and pulmonary arterial pressure and increase the cardiac output. However, large volumes produced different results: pulmonary artery pressure increased and cardiac output decreased. Hypertonic saline at small and large injectate volumes caused changes similar to those of the larger volumes of CM [19].

Somewhat different responses have been reported to injection of ionic CM (sodium meglumine diatrizoate, 76%) into the pulmonary artery, left atrium, and left ventricle in 43 adult patients [20]. After injection of CM into the pulmonary artery, the only hemodynamic change of statistical significance was an increase in blood flow velocity in the aortic root, while left atrial injection caused only a transient decrease in heart rate initially, followed by an increase in cardiac output. After left ventricular injections there was a small increase in LV end-diastolic pressure followed by a late increase in cardiac output.

The intravenous injection of ionic CM causes initial increases in right atrial and pulmonary artery pressure, followed by systemic arterial hypotension and tachycardia [40, 41]. These effects are similar but less intense than those observed after injection into right-sided cardiac chambers.

In the intact heart of anesthetized dogs, hemodynamic changes induced by pulmonary artery injection of the nonionic CM iopamidol, have been compared with two monomeric ionic CM, meglumine diatrizoate and sodium iothalamate [42]. Iopamidol caused significantly smaller decreases in arterial pressure, peripheral vascular resistance, heart rate, and indices of LV contractile state. At 3–4 min after injection, all three CM increased in LV contractile state as defined by V_{max}. The increase in V_{max} was less for iopamidol.

D. Specific Effects

I. Electrophysiologic Cardiac Effects

Contrast media produce a variety of electrophysiologic alterations both by direct actions on the heart and be *indirect* actions resulting from hypotension and activation of circulatory reflexes [29, 32, 33, 35]. While electrophysiologic alterations occur almost universally during coronary ateriography, important electrophysiologic changes and arrhythmias may also sometimes be induced after intravenous administration of CM for urography [43–45]. The electrophysiologic changes may be classified as: effects of CM on impulse generation, atrioventricular and intraventricular conduction, and atrial and ventricular arrhythmias; and nonspecific changes in electrocardiographic pattern.

1. Impulse Generation

A reduction in sinus rate or sinus bradycardia occurs during coronary arteriography in experimental animals [46–48] and in man [49–56]. The predominant factor responsible for this effect is a direct depressant action of CM on the sinoatrial node [46–48, 56]. Activation of reflexes with the afferent limb originating in the coronary circulation or ventricular myocardium also may contribute to this decrease in heart rate [46, 53, 57–59]. Bradycardia during cerebral angiography ensues as a consequence of the effect of CM on chemoreceptor tissue in the carotid circulation and by a direct action on the cardiovascular center of the brain [43–45].

In another study, infusion of saline, dextrose, sodium diatrizoate (Hypaque 50), meglumine diatrizoate (Hypaque 75M), sodium iothalamate (Angio Conray), and meglumine iothalamate (Conray 60) selectively into the artery to the sinoatrial node in anesthetized dogs caused bradycardia which was partially attenuated by atropine but unaffected by cervical vagotomy [47]. The severity of bradycardia increased with increasing osmolality and infusion rate of the test substances. At high osmolalities, CM caused sinus arrest. Infusion of even normal saline or Ringer's solution at high rates caused bradycardia, indicating that to some extent the bradycardia was due to a nonspecific baroreceptor reflex invoked by a change in tension within the sinoatrial node [60]. These authors concluded that injection of CM into the coronary circulation provokes bradycardia by an action in the sinoatrial node which is related to the osmolality of the solution and the infusion rate. They proposed that this response was in part due to a local intranodal cholinergic mechanism.

A sinus node arterial perfusion system has also been employed to assess the direct effects of sodium meglumine diatrizoate on sinus nodal automaticity in the anesthetized dog [46]. Injection of this CM, as well as other ionic and nonionic solutions, into the isolated circulation to the sinus node, progressively decreased the heart rate, in proportion to increasing osmolality. A linear relationship was demonstrated between the osmolality of ionic solution injected into the sinus node artery and the resulting R–R interval prolongation. The bradycardia in response to administration of CM into the sinus nodal artery was not altered by cholinergic or adrenergic blockade. Injection of CM into the main left and right coronary arteries also caused bradycardia which was partly attenuated by cholinergic blockade. Selective injection of CM into portions of the coronary arterial system other than the sinoatrial nodal artery caused no change in heart rate. These authors concluded that both direct and reflex depression of sinus node automaticity occur with coronary arteriography in the dog. The direct effects are due to the action of hyperosmolality on the sinoatrial node while the indirect reflex effects are mediated by extranodal cholinergic mechanisms.

In another study meglumine/sodium diatrizoate (Renografin-76), metrizamide, and hyperosmolal solutions of saline or dextrose were infused into the arteries supplying the sinoatrial and atrioventricular nodes of the dog [48, 61]. Renografin-76 produced a node-rate-dependent decrease in heart rate (Fig. 3) and increase in atrioventricular conduction time (PR interval) (Fig. 4) when infused into the arteries to the sinoatrial node and atrioventricular nodes, respectively. At

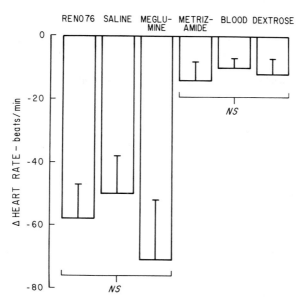

Fig. 3. The maximum changes in heart rate in response to the infusion of various solutions into the artery to the sinoatrial node. There was no significant difference (*NS*) among the changes induced by Renografin-76 (*Reno 76*), saline, and meglumine; and no significant difference among the changes induced by metrizamide, dextrose, and autologous blood [48]

high infusion rates diatrizoate caused sinus arrest and complete heart block. Saline and meglumine solutions equiosmolar with the diatrizoate solution produced similar effects. Infusion of metrizamide and dextrose causes much smaller changes in heart rate and PR interval. The responses to CM were unchanged after cholinergic and adrenergic blockades. These findings indicate that CM have a direct inhibitory effect on sinoatrial automaticity and atrioventricular conductivity, which is dependent on the ionic strength of the CM.

Several studies have assessed the mechanism of bradycardia in man during coronary arteriography [53, 55–59]. After injection of meglumine sodium diatrizoate (Renografin-76) into either the coronary artery supplying the sinoatrial node or the contralateral artery, comparable degrees of slowing of the heart rate (HR) were found in patients. Intracoronary injection of dextrose solution isoosmotic with CM, slowed the HR less. Atropine attenuated the bradycardia response to a greater extent for injections into the coronary artery which did not supply the sinoatrial node. The authors suggest from these results that cardiac slowing during coronary arteriography in man is due partly to stimulation of an intracoronary cholinergic reflex similar to the Bezold-Jarisch reflex and partly to a direct inhibitory action of CM on the sinoatrial node.

Similar finding have been obtained in man [58]. While these two studies report comparable slowing with injection into the right and left coronary arteries, several other investigations in man have found significantly greater reductions in heart rate with injections into the right coronary artery [49, 52, 54].

In patients the decrease in heart rate during coronary arteriography was apparently due to direct and reflex inhibitory influences on the sinoatrial node. In patients in whom the right coronary artery supplied the sinoatrial and atrioventricular nodal arteries, heart rate slowing with left coronary injections was entirely reflex mediated. In these patients, the bradycardia with right coronary arterial injections was due in equal parts to direct and reflex effects [153].

Reportedly during coronary arteriography in man bradycardia and atrioventricular conduction delay did *not* depend upon injection of the coronary artery supplying the specific nodal artery [55].

Other studies in dogs [52] and man [57, 62] indicate that reflex receptors within the coronary circulation stimulated by CM cause bradycardia and hypotension. Left coronary arterial injection of hyperosmotic solutions of polyvinylpyrolidone, ionic CM, sodium chloride, glucose, sucrose, and mannitol produced transient sinus bradycardia and hypotension [59]. The bradycardia was ablated by atropine and reproduced by inflation of a balloon in the coronary sinus. These authors concluded that coronary injection of hyperosmotic solutions causes activation of a reflex originating from stretch receptors in the coronary capillaries and small veins.

It has been reported that bradycardia during coronary ateriography was related to injection of the artery supplying the inferior wall of the left ventricle and not to the injection of the artery supplying the sinoatrial or atrioventricular nodes [57]. The decrease in rate was greater for injections into the dominant coronary artery, which was usually the right coronary. The degree of slowing was greater in normal patients than in those with valvular heart disease and congestive cardiomyopathy. These authors propose that bradycardia during coronary arteriography results from stimulation of receptors located in the inferior wall of the left ventricle. Others have also presented evidence for elicitation of a depressor reflex in the coronary circulation during arteriography in patients, suggesting the possibility of activation of a chemoreceptor reflex during coronary arteriography [62]. Chemoreceptor reflex responses have been elicited with the injection of a variety of substances into the coronary circulation [63].

2. Impulse Conduction

Studies in man [55, 58] and experimental animals [48, 55, 61, 64, 65] have demonstrated a decrease in the rate of atrioventricular conduction during the intracoronary injection of CM (Fig. 4). The delay is for the most part due to prolongation of the AH interval (atrial to His bundle interval).

Effects of left coronary arterial injection of hyperosmolal glucose, sodium meglumine diatrizoate (Renografin-76), sodium/meglumine/calcium metrizoate (Isopaque 370), and metrizamide on the various components of atrioventricular conduction have been studied in anesthetized dogs [64]. Conduction from atrium to the His bundle (AH interval) was delayed after injection of each test solution, but there was no change in the time from activation of the distal His bundle to ventricular activation (HV interval). Metrizamide caused the smallest change in the AH interval. The hyperosmolal glucose solutions also caused a smaller delay than the ionic CM. For the ionic CM, the metrizoate compound caused less pro-

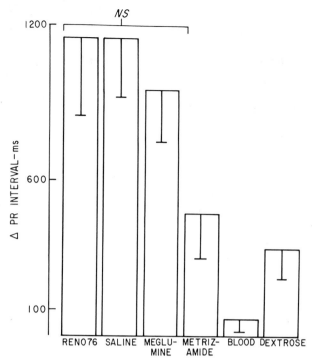

Fig. 4. The maximum changes in "PR interval" in response to the infusion of various solutions into the artery to the atrioventricular node. There was no significant difference (*NS*) among changes induced by Renografin-76 (*Reno 76*), saline, and meglumine. The maximum changes induced by metrizamide and dextrose, while relatively small compared with Renografin-76, were significantly greater ($P < 0.01$) than those induced by autologous blood [48]

longation of the AH interval than the diatrizoate compound. The three CM and the glucose solution caused widening of the QRS complex to a similar extent.

The mechanism of the prolongation of atrioventricular conduction has been examined in anesthetized dogs [65]. Left coronary injection of Tyrodes solution caused no prolongation of the AH interval. The injection of hyperosmolal glucose (15% solution) caused prolongation but to a lesser extent than monomeric ionic CM (sodium meglumine diatrizoate). The authors concluded that conduction delay caused by CM is due to the combined action of hyperosmolality, presence of the nonphysiologic cation, and the nature of the iodine-bearing anion.

Although one study on dogs has shown no change in the AH interval during injection of ionic CM into the left coronary artery [66], prolongation of the AH interval was found in some patients during coronary arteriography [55]. The prolongation was not dependent upon injection of the coronary artery supplying the atrioventricular nodal artery. These authors proposed a vagally mediated reflex inhibition of AH conduction.

His bundle electrograms in patients during coronary arteriography with sodium meglumine diatrizoate (Urografin 76) have revealed prolongation of the

AH interval and no change in the HV interval in all patients following injection of the coronary artery supplying the atrioventricular nodal artery. A similar degree of prolongation was caused by injection of hyperosmolal (20%) glucose solution. These authors concluded that the prolongation of the AH interval during coronary arteriography is the result of a direct osmotic action of ionic CM on the atrioventricular nodal tissue.

The conduction disturbances during coronary arteriography have also been studied in patients with and without preexisting intraventricular conduction delay [69]. Injection of the right coronary, which supplied the atrioventricular nodal artery in all patients, increased the AH interval but did not change the HV interval. Injection of the left coronary artery increased the QRS duration. The responses were similar in patients with an without preexisting conduction abnormalities. Effects on atrioventricular conduction through cholinergic mechanisms were precluded by premedication with atropine. The authors concluded that CM directly inhibits the atrioventricular node but has no effect on intraventricular conduction even in patients with intraventricular conduction abnormalities. The increase in the QRS duration with CM did suggest some delay in conduction in the distal Purkinje system.

Although ionic CM have no detectable effect on the HV interval, inhibitory effects on the Purkinje system have been documented using bipolar electrode catheters to monitor left bundle branch and ventricular cavitary potentials and multipolar electrode needles to minotor subendocardial and subepicardial potentials during coronary arteriography in atropinized, anesthetized dogs [68]. Significant QRS axis changes and/or increased QRS duration were found. They coincided with delays in conduction from the left bundle branch to the subendocardium of the left ventricular myocardium. There was no change in the conduction from the subendocardial to subepicardial myocardium. These authors concluded that ionic CM alters conduction through the distal left ventricular Purkinje system without affecting transmural conduction.

The direct electrophysiologic effects of ionic CM (sodium/meglumine diatrizoate) were studied in isolated canine Purkinje fibers utilizing microelectrode techniques [69]. These studies demonstrated decrease in conduction velocity and maximum rate of depolarization of Purkinje fibers in the presence of ionic CM. Equiosmolal mannitol had no effect on these variables. Both the CM and hyperosmolal mannitol caused increases in the duration of the action potential of the Purkinje fiber. Tyrode solutions with cations (Na^+, Kr^+, Ca^{++}) in a concentration equal to CM had no effect on these parameters. These authors concluded that the increased automaticity and slowed conduction caused by the slow response induced in the Purkinje fibers by CM may cause the serious arrhythmias occurring during coronary arteriography. They hypothesized that hyperosmolality had a minor role, while the chemical properties of the anion and/or of the meglumine ion were the major factors causing this response.

3. Arrhythmias

The most frequent causes of complications and death during clinical coronary arteriography are cardiac arrhythmias, particularly ventricular fibrillation. In the experimental laboratory, the propensity to cause ventricular fibrillation in animals has been used as a measure of CM toxicity. The propensity for ventricular fibrillation is established by a simultaneous change in intraventricular conductivity and rate of local impulse formation. Direct intracoronary injection of CM causes unidirectional block and depression of conductivity, which may predispose to reentry excitation of the ventricle [54]. Contrast medium alters local impulse formation by changing verious phases of the ventricular action potential [70]. Moreover, injection of CM into one coronary artery alters the electrical potential of the myocardium perfused by CM relative to myocardium that is not perfused; this condition in itself predisposes to ventricular fibrillation.

Anesthetized dogs have been used to assess the propensity for ventricular fibrillation caused by several monomeric ionic CM in which sodium ion concentration was varied [71]. Left coronary injection of meglumine diatrizoate and meglumine metrizoate, which contained little or no sodium ions, uniformly caused ventricular fibrillation. The Na^+-rich diatrizoate and metrizoate compounds did not produce a high incidence of ventricular fibrillation. The sodium-rich and sodium-deficient CM caused similar alterations in the ECG. The diatrizoate compounds with both high and low sodium content caused a greater degree of hypotension than the corresponding metrizoate compounds. The sodium-rich materials caused greater hypotension than the sodium-deficient materials. These authors concluded that while replacement of sodium ions with meglumine reduces the hypotensive effects of ionic CM, the propensity for ventricular arrhythmias is lowest with CM containing sodium in concentrations approximating physiologic levels, 140 mEq/liter. The ECG changes were not a reliable reflection of electrophysiologic toxicity.

Several subsequent studies support these observations but suggest the lowest incidence of arrhythmias occurs when the sodium ion concentration in CM is 190 mEq/liter [70, 72–74]. There is a study which is in direct dispute with the evidence present above. It was reported that in dogs rhythm disturbances, including ventricular fibrillation, rose as the sodium concentration of the solution was increased [75]. In this latter study the mildest ECG disturbances and arrhythmias were reported for the pure meglumine diatrizoate or meglumine iothalamate preparations, with intermediate changes observed for sodium meglumine formulations and the most severe changes with pure sodium formulations.

Thus a higher incidence of ventricular arrhythmias has been found in patients in response to coronary arteriography using a diatrizoate compound containing 40 mEq/liter sodium compared with one containing 190 mEq/liter sodium [73]. Injection of the diatrizoate with 40 mEq sodium into the right coronary artery caused ventricular fibrillation in 8 of 18 anesthetized dogs, while injection of the diatrizoate compound with 190 mEq/liter sodium caused fibrillation in only 1 of 15 animals. These authors concluded that the use of a nearly pure meglumine diatrizoate compound for coronary arteriography causes a higher incidence of ventricular fibrillation.

The tendency of various CM to cause ventricular fibrillation has also been evaluated by their addition to the perfusate of the isolated rabbit heart [74]. Introduction of ionic CM without sodium ions into the perfusing solution produced ventricular fibrillation. Ionic CM with sodium concentrations of 118–370 mEq/

liter rarely produced fibrillation. On the other hand, the nonionic CM metrizoate rarely induced fibrillation even though it is virtually devoid of sodium ions.

The mechanism of production of ventricular fibrillation during coronary arteriography has been studied; it provided an explanation for the greater propensity for ventricular fibrillation with CM containing lower concentration of sodium ions [70]: The CM containing 40 mEq/liter sodium ions caused ventricular fibrillation in 78% of anesthetized dogs, while the one with 190 mEq/liter caused fibrillation in only 5% of animals. Recordings of monophasic action potential in response to CM showed prolongation of the time to depolarization with both types of CM. The CM with higher sodium content (190 mEq/liter) also resulted in a prolongation of the phase of repolarization and lengthening of the refractory period. The CM with low sodium concentration caused no prolongation of the repolarization phase. The authors concluded that the failure of the CM with low sodium to displace the vulnerable period of the ventricular myocardial cell combined with the prolonged time of the depolarization might increase the likelihood of occurrence of an independent discharging ventricular focus capable of initiating ventricular fibrillation.

Another study evaluated the effect of intracoronary administration of ionic CM on the ventricular fibrillation threshold of anethetized dogs [71 a]. Renografin-76 and Conray 400 caused transient but substantial decreases in the fibrillation threshold. The fibrillation threshold was found to be lowest at 8–15 s after injection and returned to control by 1 min. Conray 400 lowered the ventricular fibrillation threshold to a greater degree than Renografin-76. Digitalis and ischemia acted synergistically with ionic CM to lower the fibrillation threshold [72 a]. Fibrillation threshold was further lowered by occlusive injections of CM.

Propensity for ventricular fibrillation has been assessed with Renografin-76 and compared with Hypaque 76 after injection into the right coronary artery of anesthetized dogs. Renografin-76 causes fibrillation with a significantly higher frequency than Hypaque 76. The authors attribute the greater fibrillatory influence of Renografin-76 to the presence of chelating agents, such as sodium citrate and sodium edetate, which result in hypocalcemia during coronary arteriography.

Incidence of ventricular fibrillation after the right coronary injection of standard Renografin-76 and Renografin-76 to which 40 mM/liter of calcium ions had been added was found to be significantly reduced [74 a].

ECG changes and ventricular arrhythmias produced by intracoronary injection of monomeric ionic CM [Sodium meglumine diatrizoate (Renografin-76) and sodium meglumine calcium metrizoate (Isopaque 379)] and a nonionic CM (metrizamide) in anesthetized dogs have been studied [75 a]. The nonionic material prolonged the QT and PQ intervals less than the ionic materials. During right coronary injections, metrizamide caused fewer ventricular fibrillations than the diatrizoate compound.

The effects on the ventricular fibrillation threshold of intracoronary administration of two nonionic CM (metrizamide and C545) have been compared with a standard ionic CM (sodium meglumine diatrizoate) [76]. The nonionic material significantly lowered the incidence of the ventricular fibrillation. Since the ventricular fibrillation threshold is a relatively sensitive indicator of the vulnerability to ventricular arrhythmias [77], this study suggests that nonionic CM have a lesser propensity for inducing ventricular fibrillation during coronary arteriography.

The findings of these several studies indicating a lower incidence and tendency for ventricular fibrillation with nonionic materials are curious because nonionic CM solutions are nearly devoid of sodium ions. Apparently, a certain optimal level of sodium ions is needed only in ionic CM to stabilize the myocardium during coronary arteriography, while a low sodium concentration is not deleterious when nonionic materials are used.

In experiments using dogs, injection of CM into the right coronary artery more frequently induced ventricular fibrillation than injections into the left coronary artery [77]. Since the dog has a small right coronary artery with a limited area of distribution, this may be attributable to the higher concentrations of CM in relation to muscle mass achieved during right versus left coronary injections. However, in clinical practice, fibrillation also occurs more frequently during right coronary injections [78], even though man has a greater than 80% frequency of a right dominant coronary circulation. Studies designed to assess the fibrillatory propensity of CM in dogs have most frequently utilized right coronary injections.

The frequency of ventricular fibrillation was evaluated during the intracoronary injection of three ionic CM at progressively larger volumes of CM dogs with normal hearts and in dogs with myocardial infarctions induced by embolization of silastic particles [79]. Increasing volume of CM caused progressive increase in the frequency of ventricular fibrillation. Sodium meglumine diatrizoate (Renografin-76) caused a higher frequency of ventricular fibrillation than similar volumes of iothalamate and metrizoate compounds.

The ventricular fibrillatory potential of two dimeric ionic CM (iocarmate and iozomate) after intracoronary injection in the rabbit has also been tested [80]. For these CM, solutions of sodium meglumine iocarmate containing 260–310 mM/liter sodium and solutions of sodium meglumine iozomate containing 270–380 mM/liter sodium proved least toxic. More arrhythmias were found with a calcium-containing monomeric ionic material than with a sodium meglumine ionic medium.

The effects of several monomeric ionic, dimeric ionic (iozomate), and nonionic CM for alterations in the ECG and frequency of ventricular fibrillation have been assessed by intracoronary injections in anesthetized dogs [81]. Although the number of experiments for each of the CM tested was small, the results suggested that nonionic materials are least toxic, dimeric materials are intermediate in toxicity, and monomeric ionic materials are most toxic.

The arrhythmogenicity of ionic and nonionic CM has been studied in the spontaneously beating isolated rat atria [82]. Three ionic CM induced atrial arrhythmias while metrizamide caused no arrhythmias. With the ionic materials, the greatest depression in atrial contraction rate and highest frequency of atrial arrhythmias occurred with meglumine iothalamate while sodium meglumine calcium metrizoate and meglumine diatrizoate caused less severe effects. A subsequent study found in the same experimental preparation that monomeric ionic CM decreased spontaneous impulse rate, increased sinus node recovery time, decreased atrial excitability, and shortened atrial effective refractory period. These actions were substantially less pronounced with metrizamide [83].

4. Electrocardiographic Changes

While the most profound changes in the electrocardiogram ensue after intracoronary injection of contrast media, lesser changes are also induced by intravenous administration and injection into the left ventricle and ascending thoracic aorta. The major changes after injection into the left coronary artery area shift of the QRS vector to the left and T wave vector to the right, while with injection into the right coronary artery the QRS vector shifts to the right and T wave vector to the left [52].

Electrocardiographic changes induced by injection of several ionic CM into the proximal ascending aorta have been studied [51]. An ECG-toxicity index for comparing CM was thus established, ranking the CM in the following order of ECG-toxicity potential: sodium iothalamate, sodium metrizoate, and sodium diatrizoate. Thus, with the sodium cation, the iodine-containing moiety with greatest toxicity was iothalamate.

In another report, it was shown that a similar degree of ECG toxicity of sodium iothalamate and sodium metrizoate and a substantially lower ECG toxicity index for calcium/sodium metrizoate (Isopaque B) exists [84]. Likewise, myocardial depression was less for the calcium-containing metrizoate.

The electrocardiographic changes induced during clinical coronary arteriography have been reported [49]. Injection into the left coronary artery depressed the ST segment, prolonged the QT interval, and caused a T wave inversion. Injection into the right coronary artery caused prolongation of the QT interval, elevation of the ST segment, and upward peaking rather than inversion of the T wave.

Electrocardiographic changes during selective coronary arteriography using sodium meglumine diatrizoate have been described in 107 patients [54]. Left coronary arterial injection caused a leftward shift in the mean frontal plane QRS vector and a rightward shift in the T wave vector. Right coronary arterial injection caused the mean QRS vector to shift to the right and the T wave vector to shift to the left.

Vectorcardiographic changes during intracoronary injection of sodium meglumine diatrizoate have been analyzed in patients [85]. Injection of CM into either coronary artery caused prolongation of the QRS complex and shift of the QRS vector toward the area of myocardium perfused by the coronary artery injected. With injections into the left coronary artery, the T wave vector increased in magnitude. Similar T wave changes were produced by saline solutions, but minimal or no changes were induced by hypertonic mannitol, Ringer's solution, 5% dextrose, plasma, and hypoxic blood. It was concluded that the T wave changes are caused by regional prolongation of the repolarization process. Delay of the repolarization process and the resulting potential differences in the myocardium may be responsible for reentrant excitation and ventricular arrhythmias.

In another study [86] injection of ionic CM into the left coronary artery of patients caused a transitory electrocardiographic pattern of left anterior hemiblock while injection into the right coronary artery caused the pattern of left posterior hemiblock. It was suggested that these hemiblock patterns resulted from delayed electrical activation of the part of the myocardium irrigated by the opacified coronary artery.

Another group assessed the effects of intracoronary injection of Urografin 60 and Isopaque 290 with and without calcium ions in patients [87]. The most dramatic changes were increases in the T wave amplitude and duration of the QT interval with each CM; Urografin caused the largest increases. The amplitude of the QRS vector was increased and its direction changed to a similar degree by all three materials. There were no differences in the changes caused by Isopaque with and without calcium ions.

Comprehensive analysis of the ECG changes in patients during coronary arteriography with Urografin 60% revealed that these changes consisted of increases in the QRS and QT duration, slight deviation in the ST segment, and shift in the QRS axis in the frontal plane [88]. The QRS and T wave vectors were increased in amplitude and the T wave vector was shifted in a direction opposite the QRS vector. The changes were small or absent in patients with occlusion of major coronary arteries or in those with cardiomyopathies. Injection of the same volume of Ringer's solution evoked no changes, indicating that the instantaneous hypoxia caused by displacement of blood during injections into the coronary arteries was not the cause of ECG changes.

The component of monomeric ionic CM responsible for ischemic electrocardiographic changes during coronary arteriography has been evaluated in dogs and man by comparing the effects of intracoronary injection of CM with those caused by a variety of solutions of different compositions [89]. The momentary displacement of blood in the coronary circulation by the injectate was found to be unimportant, while hypertonicity and the ionic composition of the injectate were shown to be the most critical factors. In particular, if sodium was the only ion present, the electrocardiographic changes were extreme regardless of its concentration. When sodium was absent or balanced with other physiologic cations like calcium, magnesium, and potassium, the electrocardiographic changes were less severe.

The increase in QRS duration during injections of ionic CM into the left coronary artery were found to be greater than those with right coronary arterial injections [67]. The increase in QRS duration and other ECG changes were similar in patients with normal conduction and in those with preexisting bundle branch blocks.

The effects of intracoronary injection of ionic CM have been studied in atropinized, anesthetized dogs [68]. Ionic CM caused increases in QRS interval in all animals but altered the QRS axis in only half of the animals. Based on the results of this study and that described above [67], these investigators suggested that ionic CM inhibit conduction in the peripheral Purkinje system (distal to His branch bundles).

The electrocardiographic effects of left coronary arterial injections of three monomeric ionic CM (diatrizoate, iothalamate, metrizoate) and a nonionic material, metrizamide, have been compared in anesthetized dogs [90]. Metrizamide caused less flattening or inversion of the T wave than the ionic CM. Incongruous with the other studies discussed above, this study reported no changes in the ECG other than the T wave inversion after the injection of either ionic or nonionic CM.

In another study intracoronary injection of Renografin-76 and dextrose solution, equiosmolar to Renografin-76 (1,690 mOsm/liter), caused QRS axis shift and prolongation of the PR, QRS, and QT intervals [13]. On the other hand, a pure saline solution with the same sodium concentration as Renografin-76 (190 mEq/liter) caused marked hemodynamic changes but only minimal changes in the ECG.

A comparative study in patients showed that intracoronary injection of ionic CM with calcium ions (Isopaque 370) caused less change in amplitude of the T wave than ionic material without calcium ions (Renografin-76) [23]. However, other studies [91, 92] have shown no ameliorating effect of calcium on the ECG changes with CM.

II. Hemodynamic Cardiac Effects

1. Hemodynamic Changes During Contrast Ventriculography

The effect of injection of contrast media into the left ventricle has been the subject of a number of investigations in anesthetized animals and conscious man. In spite of anticipated species differences and the potentially complicating influence of anesthesia in the animal experiments, results and conclusions of these studies have been generally similar.

The effects of injection of CM, hypertonic saline, and hypertonic glucose into the left ventricle or aortic root have been studied in canine heart lung preparations and the intact heart of anesthetized dogs [25]. After injection of hyperosmolar sodium chloride or sodium-containing ionic CM (sodium iothalamate), left ventricular end-diastolic, left atrial, and pulmonary artery pressures increased and myocardial contractile force decreased for 10–15 min. The effects were similar for left ventricular and aortic root injections. The sodium-containing CM also caused an initial transient decrease in heart rate, stroke volume, and arterial pressure followed by a longer-lasting increase in stroke volume. Injection of hypertonic glucose or CM containing no sodium (methylglucamine iothalamate) produced no significant cardiovascular changes. After injection of each of the agents, serum osmolality remained elevated for at least 15 min but demonstrated no temporal or quantitative relationship to hemodynamic alterations. These authors concluded that the major determinant of hemodynamic changes was the high sodium concentration of ionic CM. Since they observed a marked depression in LV function in response to sodium-containing ionic CM in the heart lung preparation, they ascribed the changes observed with ionic CM to a direct depressant action on the LV myocardium.

In another study the predominant effects of left ventricular injection of a sodium-containing ionic CM were evaluated in anesthetized dogs [93]. Measurements obtained more than 10 s after injection indicated a substantial decline in arterial pressure and peripheral vascular resistance and rise in heart rate and cardiac output. The peak change in arterial osmolality always preceded the fall in arterial pressure. They attributed these changes to a combination of direct myocardial depression induced by the CM, peripheral vasodilatation due to increase in arterial osmolality, and compensatory reflex changes in autonomic neural tone.

The hemodynamic consequences of left ventriculography with ionic CM (meglumine sodium diatrizoate) have been evaluated in dogs with radiopaque markers implanted near the LV endocardium [26]. In paired experiments the injection of either saline or CM produced an immediate increase in LV end-diastolic pressure and volume, stroke volume, ejection fraction, peak dp/dt, and peak systolic pressure. The transient rises in stroke volume, ejection fraction, and peak dp/dt were interpreted as due to a Frank-Starling effect. Thirteen to sixteen beats after injection of saline, all values returned to control levels; whereas, after injection of CM, left ventricular end-diastolic pressure and volume increased further accompanied by a decrease in peak dp/dt. The late fall in dp/dt was considered to be a consequence of a depression in LV contractile state. Subsequently, at 1 min after injection of CM, peak dp/dt rose and end-diastolic pressure fell. This last change could have been due to a number of factors including reduction in LV afterload (arterial diastolic pressure), increase in adrenergic tone, or hyperosmolality [94].

The early time-related effects of ionic CM in LV dynamics have been determined using high-fidelity LV pressure measurements and cineangiograms of the opacified LV [27]. Force-velocity relations were calculated during isovolumic contraction for each of the first seven opacified beats and 30 min later. Contractility (V_{max}) was unchanged during the first five opacified beats and decreased markedly in the sixth and seventh beats in some animals, in most animals returning to control levels at 30 min. Although mean arterial pressure increased during LV opacification, there was no significant change in parameters of LV contractile state or LV end-diastolic pressure while the ventricle was opacified. These findings suggest that the assessment of LV performance during contrast ventriculography is not importantly influenced by the CM.

Others have observed significant decreases in arterial pressure, LV peak systolic pressure, peak LV dp/dt, V_{ce} (velocity of contractile element), and $-dp/dt$ during left ventriculography with ionic materials (meglumine sodium diatrizoate, 75%) in anesthetized dogs [38]. The addition of angiotensin II to the solution of CM vitiated the decreases in pressure; there was no fall in V_{ce} or peak dp/dt in the absence of the hypotension induced by CM. Only $-dp/dt$, which is considered a reflection of LV relaxation rate [95], decreased with CM before and after the addition of angiotensin II. A preliminary report by the same authors [18] again showed minimal changes in LV dp/dt and LV systolic pressure in canine experimental models when the peripheral vasodilatory action of the CM was obviated by causing near maximal vasodilatation in the control state through thoracic aortic constriction or administration of vasodilators. They concluded that peripheral vasodilatation was the major factor responsible for the decline in systolic pressure and LV dp/dt during ventriculography.

Another study found that left ventriculography with ionic CM caused increases in LV end-diastolic pressure, left atrial pressure, and heart rate; and caused decreases in systemic arterial pressure and hematocrit [19]. Considering that heart rate was elevated at the time of measurement of hemodynamic variables, it is likely that these measurements were obtained later than the first 10 s after the injection when vasodilatation was near maximal and the response included the effect of baroreceptor activation.

A study in patients assessed the hemodynamic changes occurring during the period of left ventricular opacification (2–5 s after onset of injection), with 1 ml/kg 75% sodium meglumine diatrizoate [20]. Left ventricular end-diastolic pressure was the only variable that changed significantly and it increased only slightly. Peak aortic flow velocity, stroke volume, and end-diastolic and end-systolic volumes did not change significantly during this period. The maximal increases in aortic flow velocity, stroke volume, heart rate, and cardiac output occurred at 30 s after injection but these measurements were obtained at 30 s in only two patients. These late changes probably occur as a consequence of or in response to peripheral vasodilatation rather than as a direct effect of the CM on the heart.

Another clinical study found that LV peak dp/dt declined by the fifth beat after the beginning of LV opacification and reached a nadir by the eighth beat in normal patients, along with slight increases in LV end-diastolic pressure and decreases in arterial pressure [21]. Within the initial 10 s after the start of LV opacification in patients with myocardial dysfunction, there were no significant changes in these parameters.

Little change in LV volumes, stroke volume, or ejection fraction has been detected within the first six beats of the injection of ionic CM into the left ventricle of patients [22]. By the seventh beat there were small but significant increases in stroke volume and ejection fraction.

The hemodynamic effects of sodium diatrizoate (Renografin-76) and calcium/sodium/meglumine metrizoate (Isopaque Coronar) for left ventriculography have been compared in normal patients and patients with coronary artery diseases [23]. Both CM caused small decreases in LV peak systolic pressure and increases in cardiac output and LV peak systolic pressure. The changes in the parameters were not significantly different between the two CM. Injection of Renografin-76 into the left coronary artery did cause a significantly greater decrease in heart rate than that caused by Isopaque.

2. Use of Contrast Media as a Stress Test in Coronary Artery Disease

Several studies have examined the use of contrast ventriculography as a stress test for assessing latent myocardial dysfunction in patients with coronary artery disease. One study found that left ventriculography with ionic CM in normal patients usually caused small increases in end-diastolic pressure and increases in stroke work index resulting in an ascending type of ventricular function curve [24]. On the other hand, most patients with coronary artery disease had a greater elevation in end-diastolic pressure but no significant elevation in stroke work index, resulting in a flat or descending type of ventricular function curve. This abnormal response occurred in both patients with coronary artery disease and normal resting hemodynamics and those with depressed resting hemodynamics.

Another study assessed the effect of ventriculography with Renografin-76 on the ventricular function curve of patients with on cardiac disease and patients with severe coronary artery disease [96]. Ventricular function curves (VFC) were constructed by plotting left ventricular end-diastolic pressure (LVEDP) against stroke work index (SWI) before and 3–4 min after a standard left ventriculogram. The increase in output was less and the increase in LVEDP was greater in patients with coronary artery disease. The V_{max} did not change in either group of patients.

Depressed VFCs occurred in patients with coronary artery disease. The authors concluded that depressed curves in coronary artery disease reflect decreased LV compliance in patients with coronary artery disease rather than a greater degree of myocardial depression in response to ionic CM in the presence of coronary artery stenosis.

Atrial pacing and contrast ventriculography have been compared as stress tests for detecting left ventricular dysfunction in patients with coronary artery disease [97]. The ventricular function curves were more frequently abnormal after the stress of contrast ventriculography than during rapid atrial pacing. The authors concluded that the preload stress of CM is more sensitive in detecting abnormal ventricular function in coronary artery disease than atrial pacing.

The hemodynamic effects of three consecutive left ventriculograms were determined in normal patients, patients with cardiomyopathies, and patients with coronary artery disease of various degrees of severity [98]. It was found that systolic and diastolic pressures and maximum dp/dt increased while maximum velocity of contraction remained unchanged after each of the three contrast ventriculograms. No significant differences were observed between the responses of normal patients and patients with diseases causing reduced left ventricular function; between patients with normal and those with increased end-diastolic pressure prior to ventriculography; and between those with slight or severe coronary artery disease. These authors concluded that there is good tolerance to standard ionic CM even in the presence of myocardial dysfunction and severe coronary artery disease.

Left ventricular hemodynamics after coronary arteriography with Renografin-76 have been assessed in normal patients and patients with cardiomyopathies, coronary artery disease, and coronary artery disease with ventricular aneurysms [99]. Larger increases in left ventricular end-diastolic pressure after coronary arteriography were found in patients with coronary artery disease alone and in coronary artery disease with aneurysm. Lesser elevations were observed in normal patients and those with cardiomyopathies. Correlation with the appearance of the left ventriculograms indicated that the largest increase in end-diastolic pressure after coronary arteriography occurred in patients who had the most severe degrees of left ventricular dysfunction.

III. Direct Myocardial Effects

The direct effects of CM on myocardial contraction can be most precisely determined by using either isolated preparations or intact cardiac preparations in which the CM is injected into the coronary artery. In the latter preparation the myocardial effects are observed prior to and can be measured before the onset of systemic hemodynamic changes and reflex activation.

1. Isolated Heart and Isolated Cardiac Tissue

Introduction of CM to the perfusate of the isolated heart generally demonstrates the direct myocardial effects of the material. The responses of the isolated heart to pharmacologic interventions are not modified by reflex or neurohumoral changes; moreover, loading factors on the left ventricle can be controlled. Numerous investigations in the isolated heart have revealed that ionic CM cause transient myocardial depression [6–9, 100].

The effects of various salts of monomeric ionic CM including diatrizoate, iothalamate, and metrizoate on amplitude of contraction have been evaluated by the isolated lapine heart (Langendorff preparation) [100]. CM were injected into the base of the aorta so that most of the CM entered the coronary arteries and perfused the myocardium. Sodium diatrizoate, sodium iothalamate, and sodium metrizoate caused an initial decrease in frequency and amplitude of contraction lasting for 30–60 s followed by a short period of increase in frequency and amplitude. The responses were dose related. Similar responses were observed with contrast solutions composed of mixtures of the sodium and N-methyglucamine salts. The initial severe myocardial depression produced by ionic CM was considered to be due primarily to the cation content while hyperosmolality and high viscosity of the solutions played a minor role. In fact, hypertonic solutions of dextrose caused increases in amplitude of contraction. Addition of increments of calcium ions to sodium metrizoate (Isopaque Na) progressively reduced the severity of myocardial depression and at higher concentrations resulted in a considerable increase in amplitude of contraction. Calcium ions also alleviated the myocardial depression caused by solutions of NaCl. Addition of magnesium ions to CM had no important effect. The authors concluded that calcium ions antagonized the negative inotropic actions of sodium and by this mechanism ameliorated the effect of ionic CM on the myocardium.

The myocardial effects of sodium meglumine diatrizoate (Renografin-76), 5% sodium chloride, and normal saline have been assessed in the isolated perfused canine heart [8]. CM and 5% sodium chloride caused a similar decrease in force of contraction (Walton-Brodie strain gauge arch) and rate of force development of the left ventricle. The depression in contraction was preceded and accompanied by increase in coronary blood flow.

Other similar studies found that the nonionic CM metrizamide caused less decrease in contractile force of the isolated lapine heart than that caused by a variety of monomeric ionic materials [6, 74]. The effects of ionic (meglumine sodium diatrizoate and sodium metrizoate) and nonionic (metrizamide) CM on contractile force have been compared in the isolated lapine heart (Lagendorff preparation) [91]. Metrizamide caused less reduction in contractile force than the diatrizoate and metrizoate compounds. Oxygenated and nonoxygenated metrizamide caused similar effects but metrizamide with cations added in concentrations equivalent to those in plasma caused greater reduction in myocardial contractile force. On the other hand, metrizamide with calcium ions (13,2 mEq/liter) caused only a small decrease in contractile force. Likewise, addition of calcium ions to the metrizoate compound reduced the severity of myocardial depression of this ionic CM. These authors concluded that perfusion of the myocardium by metrizamide affected the left ventricular myocardial function less than the ionic CM which are currently employed for coronary arteriography. The addition of calcium ions to nonionic and ionic CM alleviates their negative inotropic actions.

Another study also compared the effects of monomeric ionic (sodium, meglumine calcium metrizoate), dimeric ionic (meglumine iocarmate), and nonionic (metrizamide) CM on ventricular contractile force of the isolated lapine heart

(Lagendorff preparation) [6]. Perfusion of the coronary arteries with each of the three CM caused decreases in left ventricular contractile force. Metrizamide caused significantly less decrease in force than the same doses of the ionic materials. There was no difference between the effects of the dimeric and monomeric ionic materials. Addition of sodium chloride (145 mEq/liter) to the metrizamide solution significantly increased its depressant effect on contractile force, which again points to the critical role of sodium ions in causing the myocardial depression observed with ionic CM.

The effects of ionic CM (Renografin-76) and 38% sucrose have been studied in the isolated blood perfused canine heart [9]. Continuous infusion of CM (meglumine sodium diatrizoate) or saline into the isolated heart decreased LV systolic pressure and dp/dt for the duration of the infusion. After cessation of the infusion, these parameters rose to above control values. Responses to CM were dose dependent. In this preparation, where ventricular volume was maintained constant, CM caused no change or a slight decrease in end-diastolic pressure, indicating that CM does not diminish ventricular compliance. Infusion of 38% sucrose, a solution which was isoosmotic with the CM, produced a striking increase in LV systolic pressure; the response was dose dependent. This observation indicates that the property of hyperosmolality has no role in the myocardial depression caused by CM. In this regard several studies have revealed that hyperosmolal molecular (nondissociating) solutions have a positive inotropic effect in the isolated heart, although this may not hold at higher osmolalities [94, 101]; and it should be pointed out that the CM injected into the coronary arteries has an osmolality of approximately 1,600–1,800 mOsm/liter, but because it becomes immediately diluted in the coronary circulation, the solution actually contacting myocardial cells probably has an osmolality of less than 600 mOsm/liter [102].

The effects of two nonionic CM (metrizamide and iopamidol) compared with those of three ionic materials (Renografin-60, Renografin-76, Vascoray) have been studied in the isolated murine heart [103]. The three ionic materials caused greater decreases in systolic pressure, heart rate, aortic flow, and minute work than the nonionic materials. Metrizamide did not decrease systolic pressure or minute work, while iopamidol caused small decreases in these parameters.

One group of investigators [7, 5] have used an isolated blood perfused heart preparation in which the coronary perfusion pressure was lowered to approximately 50% of normal in order to attain a model of myocardial ischemia (global ischemia) for comparing the effects of CM on the normal and ischemic myocardium. Meglumine/sodium diatrizoate (Hypaque M-75) caused an initial negative inotropic effect followed by a slight overshoot in contractile force within 10 s after the injection of the CM in the normally perfused state. In the ischemic state the nadir of the contractile force in response to this CM was similar to that in the normal state but the subsequent overshoot was absent and the negative inotropic effect more persistent. Calcium/meglumine/sodium metrizoate (Isopaque Coronar) caused a substantial positive inotropic effect, which persisted several minutes in the normal state. However, during ischemia, this material caused an intital positive inotropic effect followed by a decrease in contractile force at 2 min after injection. They attributed this late decline in contractile force to an intensification of the imbalance in the supply-demand ratio for oxygen and energy within the marginally perfused myocardium after introduction of this positive inotropic agent. In this preparation metrizamide caused only a positive inotropic effect in the normal and ischemic states.

The effects of ionic CM have also been assessed in the feline papillary muscle preparation [4]. Meglumine/sodium diatrizoate and sodium diatrizoate reduced maximal velocity of shortening, maximal isometric tension, and rate of tension development. With equiosmolal solutions, CM has substantially greater negative inotropic effects. The authors concluded that CM have direct negative inotropic effects which are independent of osmolality.

The addition of increasing concentrations of three ionic CM and metrizamide to the nutrient bath of isolated left atrial muscles has been compared for their effects on the amplitude of contraction and work index of the atrial muscles [82]. Ionic CM caused a greater degree of depression of atrial contraction than that caused by metrizamide. The diatrizoate compound caused more severe cardiodepression than the metrizoate and iothalamate compounds.

2. Intracoronary Administration in the Intact Heart

The intracoronary administration of CM causes nearly instantaneous contact of CM with myocardial cells so that the maximum negative inotropic effects of CM are observed within the first 10 s after the start of the injection [10–13, 111] and in normal hearts these negative inotropic changes have dissipated by 20–30 s after injection [104]. Injection of unusually large volumes of CM may slightly prolong this time sequence [81, 105).

GUZMAN and WEST [106] conducted one of the earliest studies on the cardiac effects of intracoronary injection of CM in anesthetized dogs. Myocardial depression was most severe after Urokon and least after Diodrast. The depressant effects of Hypaque, Renografin, and Cardiografin were similar to each other and intermediate between the other two CM. In small doses, all the CM, except Urokon, produced an increased level of myocardial contraction following the initial depressant effect. Each CM also caused increase in coronary blood flow and arterial hypotension.

In another study various CM were injected near the ostia of the coronary arteries at end diastole in dogs with Walton-Brodie strain gauge arches attached to the right ventricle [84]. Iothalamate sodium (Angio Conray 80%) and metrizoate sodium (Isopaque 75%) caused immediate decreases in contractile force and heart rate; the effects of the two CM were similar. Arterial pressures declined at the same time as contractile force. These findings suggested direct myocardial depression by these two monomeric ionic CM. Meglumine/sodium/calcium metrizoate (Isopaque B) at the same doses caused initial myocardial depression of lesser severity followed by a secondary rise in contractile force. Hypertonic solutions of dextrose and saline also caused myocardial depression. The effects of saline were more severe than dextrose, which has a severalfold greater viscosity than saline at equivalent osmolalities. These results suggested that the cation composition of ionic CM was the major factor causing myocardial depression, while hypertonicity and viscosity were less important.

Other studies have compared sodium/meglumine diatrizoate (Urografin 76%) with sodium/calcium metrizoate (Isopaque B 60%) and sodium/meglumine calcium metrizoate (Isopaque Coronar I) during coronary arteriography in patients [107, 108]. No important differences were observed in the severity of hemodynamic effects among the CM. Isopaque B caused greater changes in the ST–T wave changes and arrhythmias than Urografin.

The effects of intracoronary injection of several monomeric ionic CM on cardiac output, left ventricular end-diastolic pressure, and myocardial metabolism have been examined in anesthetized dogs [109]. Despite changes in myocardial metabolites suggesting the presence of ischemia during coronary arteriography, there was no change in left ventricular end-diastolic pressure and, actually, an increase in cardac output after injection of most CM.

The hemodynamic effects of sodium meglumine iodamide with sodium meglumine calcium metrizoate have been compared in patients during coronary arteriography [110]. Injection of iodamide into the left coronary artery caused a greater degree of hypotension than the metrizoate. The study was performed in only 17 patients and no clear advantages were established for either CM.

The effects of intracoronary administration of metrizamide and several monomeric ionic CM on contractile force (strain gauge arch) of the left ventricle have been compared in anesthetized dogs [90]. Sodium/meglumine diatrizoate (Renografin-76) and sodium/meglumine iothalamate (Vascoray) caused greater declines in contractile force, LV systolic pressure, and arterial pressure than metrizamide. Sodium/meglumine/calcium metrizoate (Isopaque 370) caused a decline in these variables similar to metrizamide at the 6-ml dose but caused significantly less depression in force and pressures at the 3-ml dose. It is interesting to note that this study, like a few other early studies evaluating the myocardial actions of metrizamide, reported myocardial depression with metrizamide, albeit less than that with non-calcium-containing ionic materials. On the other hand, more recent reports have shown no change or increases in contractile state with metrizamide and the calcium-enriched metrizoate compound [10, 11, 111].

The hemodynamic effects of ionic and nonionic CM with and without added calcium ions have also been assessed in anesthetized dogs [91]. Following the injection of each CM into the left coronary artery, myocardial contractile force and aortic pressure declined to a nadir within 4–12 s. Metrizamide with added calcium ions (13.2 mEq/liter) caused the least decline in contractile force (8% decrease) and arterial pressure compared with other formulations of metrizamide and ionic CM. Metrizamide without calcium caused a 28% decrease in force and sodium meglumine calcium metrizoate (Isopaque 370) caused a 24% decrease in force. This latter metrizoate formulation composed of low sodium content with calcium ions (Isopaque 370) caused less decline in force compared with metrizoate with low sodium content but without calcium ions. The calcium-free metrizoate compound with low sodium content had a smaller effect on contractile force than the same compound with high sodium content. There was little difference between the calcium-free metrizoate and diatrizoate compounds.

The importance of addition of various concentrations of calcium ions to a diatrizoate compound (Renografin-76) and metrizamide in reducing their effect on peak LV dp/dt and LV contractile force has been assessed in anesthetized dogs

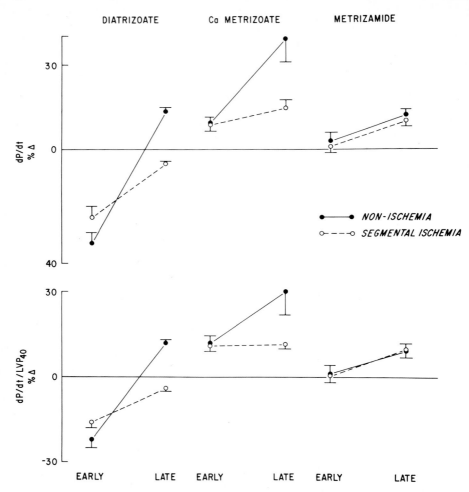

Fig. 5. Percentage changes in parameters of left ventricular contractile state induced by the intracoronary injection of the various CM in a group of 13 anesthetized dogs. The mean values and SEM for the peak changes occurring during the early (3–10 s) and late (10–20 s) observation periods are plotted in each panel [11]

[92]. The optimal amount of calcium for balancing the effects of the CM was found to be approximately 40 mEq/liter for the diatrizoate compound and 10 mEq/liter for metrizamide.

The direct and indirect effects on LV dynamics of intracoronary administration of CM without calcium (meglumine/sodium diatrizoate, Renografin-76), ionic CM with calcium (meglumine/sodium/calcium metrizoate, Isopaque 370), and metrizamide (Amipaque) have been studied in conscious and anesthetized dogs (Fig. 5) [12]. Responses to CM were similar in the conscious and anesthetized animals. The diatrizoate caused early (3–10 s after injection) decreases in isovolumic indices of LV contractile state (peak *dp/dt* and *dp/dt* at an LVP of 40 mmHg) and LV peak systolic pressure, followed by late (10–20 s after injection) increases in these variables. The predominant early and late effects of the calcium metrizoate were increases in these variables. Metrizamide produced no significant early alterations but later induced small increases in these parameters. Beta-adrenergic blockade was associated with attenuation of the positive inotropic effects. Evaluation of the CM during occlusion of the circumflex coronary artery showed no late positive inotropic effects of the diatrizoate compound. The authors concluded that intracoronary administration of meglumine sodium diatrizoate produced direct myocardial depression, followed by enhanced myocardial contractility, which was to a major extent adrenergically mediated. Meglumine/sodium/calcium metrizoate caused direct and adrenergically mediated augmentation in LV contractile state. Metrizamide induced the least alteration in contractile state, which was a slight positive inotropic effect. The adrenergically mediated component of the response may have been due to a combination of activation of circulatory reflexes or release of myocardial catecholamine stores by a local action of the CM. The positive inotropic effects are attenuated or abolished in the presence of a coronary arterial occlusion.

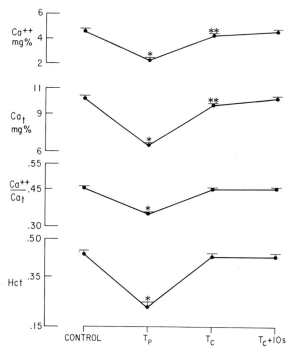

Fig. 6. Time sequence of the alterations in coronary sinus ionic calcium (Ca^{++}), total calcium (Ca_t), ratio of Ca^{++} and Ca_t (Ca^{++}/Ca_t), and hematocrit induced by the intracoronary injection of sodium/meglumine diatrizoate. Changes are shown in the same group of dogs in the normal and acute heart failure states. *, $P < 0.01$; **, $P < 0.05$ [10]

The role of changes in ambient calcium ions in mediating the myocardial depression after intracoronary administration of ionic CM without calcium (meglumine/sodium diatrizoate, Renografin-76) and ionic CM with calcium (meglumine/sodium/calcium metrizoate, Isopaque 370) has been assessed in anesthetized dogs [10]. Blood samples were obtained from the coronary sinus at the time of peak opacification, at the time of CM clearance from the sinus, and 10 s after clearance of the sinus. At the time of myocardial depression and peak opacification of the coronary sinus after injection of the diatrizoate compound, total calcium, ionic calcium, and the ratio of ionic to total calcium (Ca^{++}/Ca_t) decreased (Fig. 6). In the normal state these calcium values returned to control levels within 10 s after clearance of the coronary sinus. In the presence of systemic hypocalcemia and heart failure, the myocardial depressant action of this CM was accentuated (Fig. 7). In the heart failure state the decrease in ionic calcium was greater and more prolonged as was the negative inotropic effect (Fig. 7).

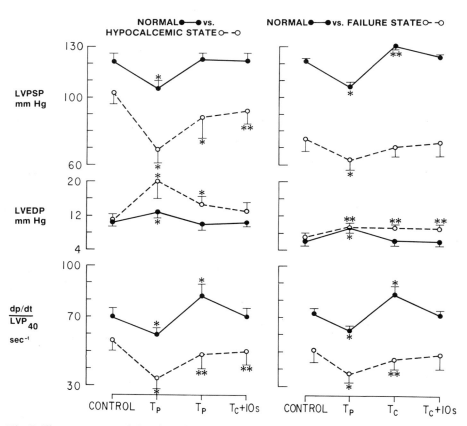

Fig. 7. Time sequence of the alterations in left ventricular (*LV*) hemodynamics in response to sodium meglumine diatrizoate (Renografin-76). Alterations in the normal state are contrasted with those in the hypocalcemic (*left*) and acute heart failure states (*right*). *LVPSP*, left ventricular peak systolic pressure; *LVEDP*, left ventricular end-diastolic pressure. *, $P<0.01$; **, $P<0.05$ [10]

The metrizoate compound containing Ca increased the indices of LV contractile state and increased the concentration of ionic calcium in blood obtained from the coronary sinus. During systemic hypocalcemia and heart failure this CM caused even greater augmentation in LV contractile state than those observed in the normal state.

These results indicated that ionic CM caused myocardial depression which, at least in part, was related to reductions in ambient calcium through a dilutional and binding action. The addition of Ca^{++} to monomeric ionic CM reversed the myocardial depression and produced a transient rise in ambient Ca^{++}.

A recent study in anesthetized dogs identified separate mechanisms for the hemodynamic and electrophysiologic side effects of intracoronary administration of meglumine/sodium diatrizoate (Renografin-76) [13]. The CM and electrolytic solution [with a sodium content (190 mEq/liter) equivalent to Renografin-76] caused arterial hypotension, increase in LV end-diastolic pressure, and decrease in LV dp/dt. Hypertonic molecular solution (dextrose) increased rather than decreased LV dp/dt, but this solution, like the CM, caused a decrease in heart rate, shift of the electrical axis, and prolongation of the PR, QRS, and QT intervals. The addition of calcium ions to the electrolytic solutions partially alleviated but did not prevent the hemodynamic effects, while the addition of calcium ions to Renografin-76 reversed the hemodynamic effects, resulting in a slight elevation in arterial pressure and marked increase in LV dp/dt. The authors concluded that hyperosmolality is responsible for the deleterious electrophysiologic effects of this CM, while the hemodynamic effects are due to excessive sodium ions and hypocalcemia.

The amount of calcium ions added to Renografin-76 in order to alleviate the hemodynamic effects in the latter study was 40 mEq/liter $CaCl_2$. This amount is in agreement with in vitro experiments [112], where 40 mEq/liter titrated the calcium-binding effect of Renografin-76 in vitro. Another study, described above [91], also found that the optimal amount of calcium ions for alleviating the hemodynamic effects of Renografin-76 was 40 mEq/liter.

While the above studies indicate that hypocalcemia has a role in the hemodynamic depression caused by ionic CM, the mechanism by which myocardial hypocalcemia occurs is not entirely clear. Ionic calcium is the component of the total serum calcium which is important in regulating the contractile state; left ventricular contractile state is dependent on competitive interactions between Na^+ and Ca^{++} at active membrane sites and at sites on the contractile proteins [113]. A recent study [11] showed that Ca^{++} levels decline due to a dilutional effect by Renografin-76 as well as disproportionate decreases in the ionic component of the total serum calcium, implicating a Ca^{++}-binding effect as well. CAULFIELD et al. [112] showed that the addition of Renografin-76 to blood in vitro, produces a dose-related decline in Ca^{++} which is counteracted by addition of $CaCl_2$, implying that some component of this CM does bind Ca^{++}. In this regard, Renografin-76 and some other CM contain small quantities of chelating agents, such as sodium citrate and ethylenediaminetetraacetate (EDTA). In addition to Ca^{++} binding by the small quantities of citrate and EDTA, it must be considered that iodine-containing anion itself may bind Ca^{++} or that the CM alters Ca^{++} binding by proteins. An additional mechanism to consider is the non-specific effect that dilution of total calcium has on the proportion of Ca^{++} in biological fluids; dilution of biological fluids with ionic solutions, such as sodium chloride, apparently causes a decline in Ca^{++} activity [114].

The effects of intracoronary administration of various CM in dogs instrumented with pressure gauges in the LV cavity and ultrasonic crystals in opposition on the endocardial surface of the LV [12]. These experiments showed a decrease in peak dp/dt and $-dp/dt$ at a LVP of 50 mmHg in addition to the decrease in peak dp/dt in response to meglumine sodium diatrizoate. These decreases in $-dp/dt$ suggest a decrease in rate of relaxation of the LV. They persisted longer than the decrease in parameters of contractile state. Meglumine/sodium/calcium metrizoate (Isopaque 370) caused increases in peak dp/dt but decrease in $-dp/dt$ at a LVP of 50 mmHg. Metrizamide caused little change in either positive or negative dp/dt. A more persistent effect of ionic CM on $-dp/dt$ is also evident in the published graphs of POPIO et al. [13].

The diatrizoate compound also caused increases in end-diastolic and end-systolic diameters of the LV and proportionate increases in LV end-diastolic pressure. The calcium metrizoate compound and metrizamide caused no significant changes in LV dimensions or end-diastolic pressure. This study indicated that ionic CM induce important changes in LV dimensions and rate of relaxation in addition to their well-known propensity to induce depression in myocardial contraction. The increase in LVEDP observed with ionic materials seems to be due to an increase in LV dimension rather than a decrease in compliance. While the negative inotropic effects of ionic CM are reversed by the addition of calcium ions, the decreases in $-dp/dt$ were not reversed by the addition of calcium ions.

Another study evaluated and compared the effects on left ventricular dynamics of four new CM which have a substantially lower osmolality than standard monomeric ionic materials [111] (Fig. 8). The low osmolality materials studied were the monacid dimer P286 (ioxaglate) and the nonionic materials metrizamide, iopamidol, and P297. In anesthetized dogs instrumented for measurements of isovolumic (peak LV dp/dt) and ejection phase (rate of change of LV dimensions, dD/dt) indices of LV contractile state, responses were assessed in the normal state and during systemic hypoxemia. The monacid dimer P286 caused transient increases in LV end-diastolic and end-systolic dimensions and decreases in LV systolic pressure and parameters of contractile state. These changes were less than those produced by a monomeric ionic material, sodium iothalamate. The alterations in LV function tended to be greater during hypoxemia compared with the normal state. The nonionic CM cause no deleterious effects on LV dynamics in either the normal or hypoxemic states. The nonionic materials actually caused slight increases in parameters of LV contractile state. Other groups have now confirmed the mild positive inotropic effects of the nonionic CM [115, 116].

Another study also found less cardiac depression in the pig after intracoronary injection of the monacid dimer, ioxaglate, compared with the monomeric ionic material, diatrizoate.

The effects of intracoronary injection of iopamidol and ioxaglate (P286) were compared with those of sodium meglumine diatrizoate in anesthetized dogs [116]. Blood samples were also obtained from the coronary sinus for measurement of serum osmolality, and concentrations of calcium, sodium, and potassium ions.

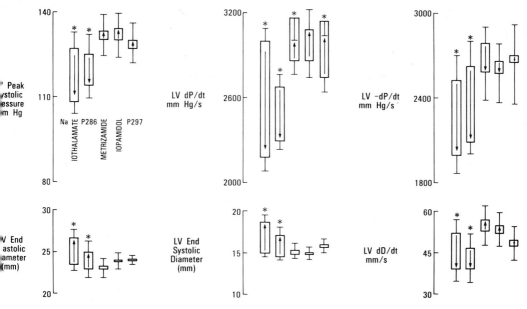

Fig. 8. Block diagrams representing the average changes in various parameters produced by each of five contrast media after intracoronary injection in normal anesthetized dogs. One end of each block indicates the average value and SEM during the control period and the other end the average value and SEM at the peak of the response. The direction of the change is indicated by the *arrow* in each block. ∗, $P < 0.05$ [111]

Ioxaglate caused the maximum and iopamidol caused the least increase in LV end-diastolic pressure. Ioxaglate and the diatrizoate compound induced similar decreases in LV peak *dp/dt*, while iopamidol caused an increase in peak *dp/dt*. Diatrizoate caused a significantly greater increase in osmolality and a significantly greater decline in ionic calcium compared with the other compounds. Sodium was unchanged after ioxaglate but decreased after injection of diatrizoate and iopamidol. The authors concluded that the lesser effects on LV *dp/dt* and ionic calcium levels with ioxaglate and particularly iopamidol offer a potential for lowering the complication rate during coronary ateriography.

The effects of intracoronary injection of sodium/meglumine diatrizoate, ioxaglate (P286), metrizamide, and a new nonionic CM, C-29, were compared in anesthetized dogs [116a]. Ioxaglate, a monacid dimer, has an osmolality similar to the nonionic CM but dissociates into an ionic solution. The two nonionic materials caused essentially no change in left ventricular systolic pressure, peak *dp/dt*, and stroke volume. The diatrizoate compound caused profound decreases in these parameters. Ioxaglate caused significantly less depression in these parameters of LV function compared with diatrizoate but significantly more depression compared with the nonionic compounds. Since the ioxaglate and nonionic CM have a similar osmolality, this study supports the notion that factors other than hyperosmolality are important in causing myocardial depression in response to CM.

The increase in contractile state with nonionic materials in spite of an osmolality nearly two to three times that of normal serum suggested that hyperosmolality per se has no role in mediating the negative inotropic effects of CM. Two papers support the notion that the negative inotropic actions of ionic CM are due to the presence of excess amount of monovalent cations while the hyperosmolality of CM exerts a positive rather than a negative inotropic influence [13, 102].

3. Effects on Ischemic Myocardium and Failing Myocardium

Although coronary arteriography is frequently performed in the presence of regional myocardial ischemia, there is little information available regarding the direct action of various CM on the ischemic myocardium. The blood-perfused isolated canine heart has been employed to assess the effects of sodium/meglumine/calcium metrizoate on contractile force under conditions of normal coronary perfusion and reduced coronary perfusion [5]. In the normally perfused state this calcium-enriched CM produced a positive inotropic effect which persisted for 2 min. However, in the presence of reduced coronary perfusion, this CM caused an initial increase in contractile force between 1 and 2 min after injection and was followed by a small decrease in contractile force. The authors proposed that the late decrease in contractile force was caused by an imbalance in the oxygen supply-demand ratio in the presence of the low and fixed coronary perfusion pressure.

Another recent study used the intact heart of anesthetized dogs to test the effects of sodium/meglumine diatrizoate (Renografin-76), sodium/meglumine/calcium metrizoate (Isopaque), and metrizamide on myocardial contractility of a region of the LV jeopardized by a critical coronary arterial stenosis [117]. In the normal state, diatrizoate initially decreased the parameters of regional myocardial contractile state followed by an increase in contractile state at 10–20 s after injection. In the presence of a critical coronary stenosis the depression in regional contractility was prolonged and the late increase in contractility did not occur. Sodium meglumine calcium metrizoate and metrizamide caused only positive inotropic responses under both the normal and ischemic conditions.

A preliminary report also described a more severe and persistent decrease in regional myocardial contractile force in the area jeopardized by coronary arterial constriction compared with the normally perfused area after intracoronary administration of sodium meglumine diatrizoate [118]. In this study, contractile force was simultaneously monitored in the myocardium perfused by the left anterior descending artery and in myocardium perfused by the constricted circumflex coronary artery.

The negative inotropic influence of standard monomeric ionic CM was also found to be more severe and prolonged in the intact canine heart with acute myocardial failure compared with the normal heart [10]. On the other hand, calcium-enriched ionic CM (sodium meglumine calcium metrizoate) caused a marked improvement in contractile state of the acutely depressed heart.

4. Mechanism of Action of Direct Cardiac Effects

a) Electrophysiologic Effects

The major toxic component of the CM which is responsible for electrophysiologic effects has been shown in most studies to be the hyperosmolality of the solution.

A number of studies in animals and man have revealed that the depression in sinoatrial automaticity [46–48], atrioventricular conduction [48, 58, 65], intraventricular conduction [67–69], and the changes in the electrocardiogram [13] are closely related to the osmolality of the CM and other test solutions. Arrhythmogenicity of CM is related to the sodium content as well as the osmolality of CM [70, 71, 72 a, 73].

Three groups of investigators [46–48] infused CM and hyperosmolal solutions into the sinoatrial nodal artery of anesthetized dogs and found that hyperosmolal solutions had an inhibitory action on sinoatrail automaticity similar to that of ionic CM. A linear relationship was observed between osmolality of the saline injectate and the resulting PR interval prolongation [46].

A study in patients also found bradycardia in response to intracoronary injection of ionic CM and hyperosmolal solutions of glucose or mannitol [58]. The severity of heart rate slowing was greater for Urografin than for the noncontrast solutions. The osmolality of the dextrose and glucose solutions was approximately two-thirds of the osmolality of the CM.

Renografin-76, metrizamide, and hyperosmolal noncontrast solutions have also been infused into the atrioventricular nodal artery of anesthetized dogs [48]. Hyperosmolal ionic solutions as well as ionic CM caused inhibition of atrioventricular conduction. On the other hand, the nonionic CM, which has an osmolality of slightly more than one-third the osmolality of Renografin-76, caused substantially less delay in atrioventricular conduction.

Other studies [64, 65] have injected Renografin 76%, isosmolal Tyrode's solution, isosmolal glucose solution, and hyperosmolal glucose solution into the left coronary artery of dogs while measuring atrioventricular conduction. Large volumes of isosmolal glucose solution caused only a slight delay in atrioventricular conduction while smaller volumes of hyperosmolal glucose solutions and CM caused greater delays in atrioventricular conduction. These findings were interpreted as indicating that hyperosmolality is the major determinant of the prolongation atrioventricular conductivity and that ionic composition also influences this effect. The influence of ionic composition of the solution is supported by the report from the same group [64] indicating that addition of calcium and magnesium ions to Renografin-76 resulted in less prolongation in atrioventricular conduction time. Moreover, they found that a mixture of glucose and Tyrode's solution equal in osmolality to CM caused much less inhibition of atrioventricular conduction than ionic CM. This finding prompted their conclusion that ionic composition as well as hyperosmolality determines the action of CM on atrioventricular conduction.

Atrioventricular conduction has been assessed in patients after intracoronary injection of Urografin, hyperosmolal glucose solution, and isosmolal saline solution [58]. Depression was found in conduction with CM and hyperosmolal glucose solution but not with saline solution. The study concluded tht the prolongation of conduction during coronary arteriography is due to the osmotic effect of CM.

Intracoronary administration of Renografin-76 and hyperosmolal dextrose solution (1,690 mOsm/liter) were found to have similar effects on sinus rate; prolongation of PR, QRS, and QT intervals; and axis shift in dogs [13]. On the other hand, injection of a nearly isosmolal solution with the same electrolytic content as Renografin-76 caused minimal electrocardiographic disturbances. This study concluded that hyperosmolality is responsible for the deleterious electrocardiographic effects of Renografin-76, while excess sodium content or the cationic composition of the CM is not important in this regard.

On the other hand, another study found that both hyperosmolality and cationic composition were not important factors in the slowed conduction through the isolated Purkinje fiber in the presence of ionic CM [69]. It was suggested that the toxic effect on the Purkinje fiber was an inherent chemical property of the diatrizoate molecule or the meglumine ions.

The ventricular arrhythmias induced by ionic CM have been found to be related to the cationic composition of the CM as well as the hyperosmolality of the solution. A marked increase in ventricular fibrillation was found when total sodium content of ionic CM was below normal serum levels [70, 71, 73]. The ideal concentration of sodium ions in ionic CM was found to be approximately 190 mEq/liter. Ionic CM in which the cation is almost solely meglumine caused an increased incidence of ventricular fibrillation compared with a formulation in which sodium ions were present at a concentration of 180 mEq/liter. In this regard it is important to point out that this ideal sodium ion content holds only for ionic CM. While the nonionic CM are virtually devoid of sodium ions, they cause no increased frequently of ventricular fibrillation.

The presence of calcium ions and absence of chelating agents seems also to be important in the mechanism of ventricular fibrillation. The frequency of ventricular fibrillation after right coronary injections in the dog was found to be greater for diatrizoate with calcium-chelating agents than for diatrizoate without chelating agents [73a]. In this regard, a decrease in the frequency of ventricular fibrillation in the same experimental preparation has been observed when Renografin-76 was inriched with calcium ions [74a].

b) Myocardial Contractile Effects

It has generally been held that hyperosmolality of CM is one of the major factors resulting in depression of myocardial contractile state. However, recent studies have suggested that hyperosmolality may actually enhance rather than depress contractile function [9, 13, 102]. The ontracoronary injection of a solution of dextrose equivalent in osmolality to Renografin-76 caused no depression but rather a slight increase in parameters of myocardial contractility [13]. On the other hand, injection of a soline solution with a sodium ion content equivalent to Renografin-76 caused severe myocardial depression.

A recent study described the effects of intracoronary injections of glucose, mannitol, and sodium chloride varying in osmolality from 300 to 1,800 mOsm/liter in dogs [102]. The hyperosmolal solutions of the nondissociating substances, glucose and mannitol, increased parameters of left ventricular contractile state while the ionic solution, sodium chloride, caused myocardial depression. These findings imply that sodium ions are the major factor causing the negative inotropic action of ionic CM and hyperosmolality per se has no role in this regard. This notion gains further support from the finding that nonionic CM with an osmolality more than double that of serum cause a slight positive rather than a negative inotropic effect [111, 116].

The effect of the excess sodium content of CM may be balanced by the addition of calcium ions to ionic CM [10, 92, 100, 104]. The ameliorating effect of the addition of calcium ions to sodium salts of ionic CM demonstrated more than a decade ago [100]. It was also observed that after continued addition of calcium ions, there was reversal of the negative inotropic effect of ionic CM and the appearance of a positive inotropic effect. Subsequent experiments demonstrated a simultaneous rise in calcium ion levels in blood from the coronary sinus and enhanced myocardial contractility after intracoronary injection of a calcium-enriched ionic CM (calcium meglumine sodium metrizoate) [10]. Other recent studies have also directed attention to the importance of Na^+-Ca^{++} ratio imbalance in causing the myocardial depression during coronary arteriography with ionic CM [117, 119, 120].

5. Clinical Evaluation of Contrast Media Used for Coronary Arteriography

The frequency of mortality and complications during coronary arteriography in man has been shown by a multicenter survey to be approximately 0.45% and 4.0%, respectively [121]. The effects of contrast material on the heart are one of the major causes of mortality and morbidity; CM has detrimental effects by inducing asystole, atrioventricular blocks, ventricular arrhythmias, hypotension, depression of myocardial contractility, and electromechanical dissociation [112, 121, 122]. It has been estimated that 25% of complications during angiocardiography are due to CM [123]. These statistics were compiled in the United States during a period when monomeric ionic CM were used exclusively for coronary arteriography.

One early study compared the effects of iodamide (Iodomiron 380) and calcium meglumine sodium metrizoate (Isopaque Coronar) administered alternately to the same 17 patients of coronary arteriography [110]. Both agents caused substantial decline in systolic arterial pressure at approximately 8 s after injection and a decline in heart rate which lasted for 15–20 s. Iodamide caused a significantly greater decreases in systolic arterial pressure (32 mmHg vs 19 mmHg) than the metrizoate compound during left coronary arteriography.

Another study measured heart rate, cardiac output, stroke volume, and left ventricular end-diastolic pressure (LVEDP) in patients after intracoronary injection of sodium meglumine diatrizoate or meglumine sodium calcium metrizoate [23]. At equal iodine concentrations these two CM caused similar increases in LVEDP, stroke volume, and cardiac output. In this, as well as most clinical studies, precise parameters of myocardial contractile state were not measured.

Clinical experience with routine use of meglumine sodium calcium metrizoate (Isopaque Coronar) for coronary arteriography and left ventriculography in more than 2,000 patients has indicated sixteen major complications could possibly be attributed to the CM: a complication incidence of 0.8% for all patients studied [124]. Eleven of the complications were directly due to the effect of CM on the heart. No instances of severe or prolonged hypotension or electromechanical dissociation were reported. The most frequent complications related to CM were ventricular fibrillation, marked bradycardia, and asystole. More than 80%

of complications occurred after injection into the right coronary artery. The frequency of complications directly related to CM in this report was similar or slightly less than those reported for the use of Hypaque 85, Urografin (Renografin-76), and Angio Conray [50, 125].

Meglumine sodium calcium metrizoate (Isopaque Coronar) and metrizamide (Amipaque) were compared for coronary arteriography in a double-blind study in 30 patients [126]. Both CM had an iodine concentrations of 370 mg iodine/ml. Electrocardiographic changes and image quality were similar for the two materials. Metrizamide caused significantly less decrease in diastolic arterial pressure and heart rate, less severe subjective sensations, and a longer transit time through the coronary circulation. A subsequent report extended this comparative study to 130 patients with identical conclusions to the earlier study [127].

A recent study compared the image quality, and electrocardiographic and hemodynamic changes caused by sodium meglumine diatrizoate and metrizamide administered alternately for coronary arteriography in five patients [128]. Image quality and electrocardiographic changes were similar for the two materials. Metrizamide caused no significant changes in heart rate, arterial pressure, stroke volume, or cardiac output. The diatrizoate compound caused a 13% decline in heart rate, a 13% decline in systolic and diastolic arterial pressure, a 20% decrease in stroke volume, and a 30% decrease in cardiac output. These changes commenced within the first few seconds of the initiation of the injection and persisted until 11 s after the injection.

IV. Reflex or Neurally Mediated Circulatory Effects

A number of studies have indicated that angiographic contrast media cause cardiovascular effects through activation of circulatory reflexes. CM can apparently induce reflex responses both by a direct action on afferent receptors and by provoking secondary or compensatory reflex responses as a consequence of their initial effects on the heart and peripheral arterioles. As with any agent that causes sudden vasodilatation and hypotension, systemic administration of CM almost always causes variable degrees of activation of the baroreceptor reflex. In addition to this almost universal involvement of the baroreceptor reflex, CM has been found to provoke a number of other reflex responses directly.

Activation of reflexes in the carotid circulation has been documented in several studies [32–35, 129–133] although the circulatory changes observed after intracarotid injection of CM are contributed to be a direct action on the cardiovascular center in the brain. Early reports [32, 129] noted bradycardia and blood pressure changes after intracarotoid injection of ionic CM (sodium acetrizoate) in anesthetized cats. In most animals, transient hypotension occurred while in a minority of animals hypertension ensued. The bradycardia but not the blood pressure response was abolished by atropinization or bilateral cervical vagotomy. Denervation of the carotid sinus and carotid body did not attenuate the response while preferential intracranial injection accentuated the response. These reports concluded that the circulatory changes provoked by intracarotid injection of ionic CM were due to stimulation of the vasomotor center in the brain and were neurally mediated.

Other studies [130, 131] examined the circulatory changes induced by intra-carotid injection of ionic CM (Renografin 60%, Conray 60%, Angio Conray, and Hypaque 50%) in anesthetized dogs. Injection of CM into the common carotid circulation, internal carotid circulation, or external carotid circulation caused bradycardia and hypotension in most animals. Occasionally, an initial hypertensive peak was observed at the onset of bradycardia. The most severe changes were produced by Hypaque 50%. The bradycardia was abolished by atropine or bilateral vagotomy. These studies concluded that this neurally mediated response was due to a combination of stimulation of receptors in the extra-cranial carotid vessels and the vasomotor center of the brain.

The site of origin of the reflex bradycardia observed during intracarotid injection of ionic CM (sodium acetrizoate 70%, Hypaque 50%, Renografin 60%, Conray 60%, and a dimer of iothalamate) and hypertonic saline solution has been examined in anesthetized dogs [33]. Most CM and hypertonic saline solutions caused asystole or bradycardia upon intracarotid injection; acetrizoate caused the greatest change while the dimer of iothalamate caused no change. This reflex bradycardia was observed upon injection of acetrizoate into the common carotid, internal carotid, external carotid, or lingual arteries or into a closed common carotid arterial sac. The reflex was ablated by vagotomy or cholinergic blockade with atropine. The authors of this study concluded that the receptor sites for this reflex response to CM were situated at multiple sites including the carotid body, within the brain, and in the external carotid circulation.

An early study compared the relative potencies of various CM in causing bradycardia and hypotension after intracarotid injection of CM [132]. The greatest changes were caused by Urokon followed by Hypaque and the least severe effects were observed with Cardiografin [132].

Another study [133] compared the pure meglumine forms with the sodium, meglumine, calcium, and magnesium mixtures of metrizoate and iothalamate for their potency in provoking neurally mediated bradycardia and hypotension after intracarotid injection. The mixtures caused more severe changes than the pure meglumine forms of either compounds.

The circulatory changes after intracarotid injection of meglumine sodium diatrizoate have also been compared with those of metrizamide [134]. Metrizamide caused significantly less bradycardia and hypotension than meglumine sodium diatrizoate.

The intensity of bradycardia and hypotension induced by intracarotid injection of monomeric ionic (Renografin and Conray) and nonionic CM (metrizamide and iopamidol) and hyperosmolal solutions has been assessed in the anesthetized dog [35]. The nonionic CM caused less bradycardia and hypotension than the ionic materials. Metrizamide caused less severe changes than iopamidol. Increasing the osmolality of the mannitol solution progressively intensified bradycardia and hypotension; these responses were minimal until the concentration reached 800 mOsm/liter. The authors of this study concluded that the hemodynamic response caused by intracarotid injection of CM was primarily related to osmolality of the solution and intensified to some degree by the sodium content of the solution.

The effect of injection of meglumine sodium diatrizoate, metrizamide, and nicotine into various portions of the carotid circulation prior to and after selective autonomic blockade and denervation of the carotid body have been studied in anesthetized dogs [34]. Ionic CM and nicotine caused similar biphasic responses consisting of initial decreases followed by increases in heart rate and arterial pressure. Both phases were accompanied by increase in respiratory amplitude. The initial hypotension was not observed when heart rate was maintained constant by cardiac pacing. The initial bradycardia was absent after denervation of the carotid body and cholinergic blockade. The tachycardia was attenuated after ligation of the internal carotid artery and beta-adrenergic blockade. The hypertension persisted after denervation of the carotid body and ligation of the internal carotid artery but was attenuated after alpha-adrenergic blockade. Nonionic CM (metrizamide) caused almost no reflex hemodynamic effects. This study concluded that ionic CM causes complex hemodynamic effects as a consequence of actions on the cardiovascular center of the brain, carotid body chemoreceptors, and chemosensitive tissue in the external carotid circulation. The response was similar to that induced by the classic chemoreflex stimulus, nicotine.

Reflex circulatory alterations are also observed after intracoronary injection of CM in experimental animals [46, 59] and in man [53, 56, 58, 62]. The receptors for these reflexes apparently reside in the coronary circulation, and the reflex responses consist of either hypotension and/or bradycardia.

One study observed transient hypotension, decline in LV dp/dt, and bradycardia after intracoronary injection of hyperosmolal solutions of polyvinylpyrrolidone, sodium chloride, glucose, sucrose, mannitol, and CM (sodium or meglumine diatrizoate) in anesthetized dogs [59]. Identical changes could be reproduced by causing acute coronary venous hypertension through inflation of a balloon catheter positioned in the coronary sinus. The bradycardia was abolished by atropine and the decrease in LV dp/dt averted by beta-adrenergic blockade. Most changes were also attenuated by bilateral cervical vagotomy. These authors concluded that the depressor effects of intracoronary injection of hyperosmolal solutions are due to distention of the coronary sinus and consequent activation of venous stretch receptors.

A reflex mechanism for the bradycardia observed after injection of ionic CM (meglumine/sodium diatrizoate) into the coronary arteries has been detected in anesthetized dogs [46]. CM caused a decline in heart rate which was partially attenuated by cholinergic blockade. This study concluded that after injection of CM into the ostium of the right or left coronary artery, the bradycardia was due to a combination of a direct depressant effect on the sinoatrial node and reflex augmentation in cholinergic activity.

The mechanism of cardiac slowing during coronary arteriography has also been studied in Man [56]. Comparable degrees of slowing were found upon injection of ionic CM (meglumine/sodium diatrizoate) into the right or left coronary artery, regardless of the artery of origin of the sinoatrial nodal artery. Cholinergic blockade with atropine significantly attenuated the degree of heart rate slowing. It was concluded that cardiac slowing during coronary angiography is due primarily to a cholinergic reflex which may be a human counterpart of the Bezold-Jarisch reflex.

Two other studies [53, 58] also found similar degrees of sinus slowing upon injection of CM and hyperosmolal solutions into either the coronary artery supplying the sinoatrial node or the contralateral coronary artery. In the study of FRINK et al. [53] bradycardia was partially attenuated by atropine. These findings were interpreted as indicating a reflex-mediated cholinergic slowing of heart rate in addition to a direct inhibitory effect of CM on the sinoatrial node.

One study [62] measured aortic pressure and forearm blood flow by plethysmography before and during coronary arteriography with Hypaque M-75% and Renografin 75% in patients. Injection of either CM into the left coronary artery caused forearm vasodilatation, which could not be reproduced by injection of comparable volumes of CM into the supracoronary portion of the ascending aorta. After injection of atropine into the brachial artery, the forearm vasodilatation was abolished. This study suggested that coronary arteriography in man stimulates intracoronary or intramyocardial receptors mediating a hypotensive reflex identical to or similar to the Bezold-Jarisch reflex.

The degree of bradycardia found during coronary arteriography in patients has been correlated with injection into the artery supplying the inferior wall of the left ventricle [57]. This suggested that CM activates reflex receptors located in the inferior wall of the left ventricle.

1. Vascular Effects

Contrast medium causes substantial circulatory changes primarily by a direct relaxing effect on arteriolar smooth muscle and to a lesser degree by inducing rheologic changes in the microcirculation. After injection into the general circulation, the vascular effects are predominant and overshadow the cardiac effects, while with selective intracoronary injection of CM the direct myocardial effects are predominant [16, 17]. CM causes vasodilatation and increase in blood flow in all regional vascular beds; however, certain regions respond to CM in a specifically characteristic way.

2. General Circulation and Limb Circulation

The response of the limb circulation to CM is typical of the general systemic circulation. It is characterized by direct vasodilatation. Early studies [135, 136] assessed the direct arterial actions of sodium acetrizoate and sodium diatrizoate in the limb circulation of anesthetized dogs. Incremental vasodilatation was observed with increasing concentration of the CM. This vasodilatation was not reversed by the simultaneous administration of potent vasoconstrictor drugs or by stimulation of sympathetic vasoconstrictor nerves to the limb circulation. the vasodilatation was not altered by a sympathetic neural ablation, or by administration of anticholinergic or antihistaminic drugs. These authors concluded that CM causes vasodilatation by a direct effect. The potency of this effect was partially but not entirely related to the degree of hyperosmolality of the CM. A chemotoxic component was indicated by the finding that sodium acetrizoate had a much more potent vasodilatory action than sodium diatriozate at the same osmolalities. With the weaker vasodilator, sodium diatrizoate, the intensity of the vasodilatory effect was similar to that observed with the sodium chloride solution. Over a wide range of osmolalities, blood flow increased progressively with increasing osmolality of the diatrizoate and saline solutions.

One study [131] compared the effect of injection into the canine femoral artery of ionic CM with the injection of various concentrations of sodium chloride. These experiments quantitated the vasodilatory potency of various CM be relating their effect to that of various concentrations of hypertonic sodium chloride ("equivalent hypertonic sodium chloride solution"). All CM caused increases in femoral blood flow and decreases in femoral vascular resistance. This response was not altered by large doses of atropine on dihydroergotamine or by spinal anesthesia. Increasing osmolality of the CM caused progressive increases in femoral blood flow. Sodium diatrizoate and sodium iothalamate caused greater increases in flow than the corresponding meglumine solutions. Diatrizoate compounds caused greater increases in flow than did the iothalamate compounds.

The effect of proximal aortic injection of four monomeric ionic CM (Renovist, Hypaque 75%, Conray 400, Angio Conray) on aortic and carotid blood flow was studied in anesthetized dogs [137]. Maximum vasodilatation and increase in aortic and carotid flows occurred 30 s after injection. Conray 400 and Angio Conray caused the greatest increases in blood flow.

A number of earlier reports [138, 139] have described the influence of hyperosmolality in increasing blood flow in the limb circulation. HADDY [140] demonstrated the effect of increasing the concentration of specific cations on vascular resistance in the isolated forelimb vascular bed. Infusion of increasing concentrations of sodium or magnesium ions caused vasodilatation, while infusion of calcium ions caused vasoconstriction. These findings are consistent with the notion that vasodilatation in response to ionic CM is contributed to by the hyperosmolality and the cation content of the CM.

One study [141] estimated blood flow and venous tone in the legs using venous occlusion plethysmography during lumbar abdominal aortography in ten patients with suspected peripheral vascular obstructive disease. Several monomeric ionic CM and physiologic saline were studied. Blood flow increased to a similar extent in the extremities of both patients with and without obstructive disease. Flow increased in all patients by 20 s after injection, reached a peak between 30 and 70 s, and had dissipated by 2 min after injection. There was no appreciable difference in the increase in blood flow in response to Urografin 60%, Urografin 45%, Angiografin 60%, Isopaque 60%, or Urografin 75%. Physiologic saline caused a small and less sustained increase in flow compared with the CM. The CM also caused decreases in venous tone over the same time frame.

Subsequently, the effects of repeated injection of Conray 60 (methylglucamine iothalamate) into the femoral artery were studied in anesthetized dogs [142]. The peak increase in femoral blood flow was highly variable among dogs; it ranged from 27% to 1,000% of baseline flow and decreased in one dog. There was essentially no change in aortic blood pressure. In 12 of 15 animals repeat injections of CM had no cumulative effect on blood flow; baseline levels of femoral blood flow were attained within 4 min after each injection.

The vasodilatory potency and mechanism of action of several CM and hyperosmolal solutions on the isolated hind limb circulation have been evaluated in anesthetized dogs [143]. Sodium and meglumine forms of iodopamide, acetrizoate, diatrizoate, iothalamate, and equiosmolal sodium chloride caused distinct vasodilatation. Equiosmolal solutions of glucose and methylglucamine chloride caused only slight vasodilatation. Sodium iodipamide caused the greatest vasodilatation. The vasodilatation in response to CM was ablated by cholinergic blockade (atropine, 2 mg/kg). The vasodilatation was unaffected by pretreatment with ganglionic blockers, alpha- or beta-adrenergic blockers, or histaminergic blockers.

The effects on femoral blood flow of a nonionic CM, metrizamide (Amipaque), have been compared with those of ionic CM in anesthetized dogs [144]. After direct injection into the femoral artery, metrizamide caused less increase in femoral blood flow than the ionic materials. However, considering that the osmolality of metrizamide is about one-third that of most of the ionic materials tested, the vasodilator effect was greater than expected and not proportional to its lower osmolality. Observation of behavioral responses of unanesthetized rats during peripheral arteriography showed that ionic CM cause a greater intensity of pain than nonionic media. Sodium salts were more painful than meglumine salts. Pain was attributed primarily to the osmotic pressure of the media.

3. Renal Circulation

The response of the renal vascular bed to CM is similar to those of other regional vascular beds, but some components of the response are unique to the renal circulation. Controversy has existed in characterizing this response. To a major extent, the controversy has arisen as a consequence of temporal and frequency variations, in sampling the response by direct continuous measurements of renal blood flow (flowmeters) used in some studies and indirect intermittent measurements (dye dilution and inulin clearance techniques) employed in others.

One study [145] measured renal blood flow by the dye dilution technique in anesthetized dogs and patients after renal arterial injection of sodium diatrizoate (Urografin 60%). In dogs and patients, intrarenal injection of CM was followed by renal vasoconstriction. No dose-response relationship for this vasoconstriction was observed. Vasoconstriction dissipated within 5–10 min. During the 1st min after injection of CM, inulin and PAH clearance increased. This report concluded that the primary site of vasoconstriction was at the level of postglomerular arterioles. Since the dye dilution technique used in the study cannot detect rapid changes in renal blood flow and the first flow measurement was not obtained until 30–45 s after injection of CM, a transient vasodilation in the kidney could not be detected with this methodology.

Other researchers have [146] employed rapidly repeated dye dilution techniques to measure renal blood flow in anesthetized dogs before and after direct renal arterial injection of three monomeric ionic CM and hypertonic saline solution. Sodium diatrizoate, meglumine diatrizoate, meglumine iothalamate, and hypertonic saline solutions each caused a decrease in renal blood flow. The first measurement of renal blood flow was obtained 1 min after injection of the test solution. The authors concluded that the predominant response to CM in the renal circulation is a reduction in renal blood flow. They suggested that the major factor causing this response was the hyperosmolality of the solution.

Renal blood flow after renal arteriography was continuously measured with electromagnetic flowmeters in anesthetized dogs [147]. They detected a large initial transient increase in renal blood flow within the first minutes after injection of ionic CM followed by a late decrease in renal blood flow. These authors concluded that direct renal arterial injection of CM caused a biphasic alteration in renal blood flow which was not appreciated in some earlier investigations because of the limitations of the dye dilution technique for measuring instantaneous changes in flow and for measuring flow of blood laden with CM.

In another study [148] renal vascular resistance after direct renal arterial injection of ionic CM was also assessed in two experimental models. In the canine kidney perfused with a pump at a constant flow rate sodium diatrizoate 50%, sodium iodopyracet 45%, hyperosmolal saline solution, and hyperosmolal urea solution caused a biphasic change in perfusion pressure. In a second group of animals with intact renal circulation, continuous measurement of renal blood flow with an electromagnetic flowmeter revealed a triphasic response with two separate phases of increased resistance occurring between 15 s and 6 min after injection of CM. In both preparations the predominant change caused by ionic CM and other hyperosmolal solutions was a prolonged increase in renal vascular resistance.

The effects of direct renal arterial injection of meglumine diatrizoate, meglumine iothalamate, and sodium diatrizoate and other hyperosmolal solutions on renal vascular resistance have been compared in anesthetized dogs using electromagnetic flowmeters [149]. An initial transient vasodilatation was noted followed by a more prolonged period of vasoconstriction (Fig. 9). Phenoxybenzamine blocked the hemodynamic response to norepinephrine and 5-hydroxytryptamine but failed to alter the response to CM. On the other hand, the vasoconstriction caused by the bolus injection of angiotensin, CM, and other

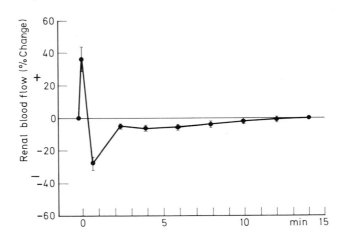

Fig. 9. Biphasic renal blood flow response to meglumine diatrizoate. The mean ±SEM is shown at various time intervals after the injection of CM into the renal artery. An initial transient vasodilatation of less than 30 s was followed immediately by a more prolonged period of vasodilatation [149]

hyperosmolal solutions was completely abolished during angiotension tachyphylaxis. This study concluded that the vasoconstrictor response to CM apparently is related to the hypertonicity which in some manner activates the renin-angiotensin system.

Renal vein renin activity and renal blood flow after renal arterial injection of sodium meglumine diatrizoate have been measured in anesthetized dogs [150]. Measurement of blood flow with an electromagnetic flowmeter revealed an initial increase in renal blood flow followed by a decrease in renal blood flow; both the peak increase and decrease in flow occurred within the 1st min after injection. Hyperosmolal solutions of saline caused similar biphasic responses. The time sequences for vasoconstriction and increase in renin activity were different; the increase in renin activity occurred after the time of maximal renal vasoconstriction. Moreover, in some experiments renin activity did not increase but renal vasoconstriction did ensue after injection of CM. The authors concluded that CM caused alterations in renal blood flow and renal plasma renin activity but that the decrease in renal blood flow may have preceded the increase in plasma renin activity. Hyperosmolality of the CM and other solutions was the primary factor renal hemodynamic alterations.

A recent preliminary report [151] described the use of angiotensin antagonist Saralasin, in an attempt to ablate the renal vasoconstrictive response to intrarenal injection of ionic CM (Renografin-76) and other hyperosmolal solutions. Saralasin did not abolish the late decline in renal blood flow induced by CM. Mannitol 5% solution, which is freely filtrable, caused similar changes to those caused by Renografin-76. Dextran, which is *not* freely diffusible, caused no late decline in renal blood flow. The authors of this report concluded that the late decrease in blood flow was not mediated by angiotensin but might have been due to rapid filtration of the CM into the renal parenchyma. The authors further suggested that the resultant acute increase in hydrostatic pressure within Bowman's capsule might have contributed to the decrease in blood flow by compression of the glomerular capillary tuft.

Another study also examined the mechanism of the biphasic renal vascular response to CM after systemic and renal arterial administration of CM [152]. The initial vasodilatation was not blocked by atropine and was reproduced by the injection of hyperosmolal saline. The late renal vasoconstrictor response was not blocked by bilateral cervical vagotomy or by alpha- or beta-adrenergic blockade; however, it was blocked by prior extracellular fluid expansion and after the responsiveness of the kidney to angiotensin II had been blocked. These authors concluded that the initial vasodilatation is a direct effect of hyperosmolality while the late vasoconstriction is due to activation of the renin angiotensin system.

Several studies [153, 154], exploring the effects of osmolality on renal vascular resistance, have indicated that hyperosmolal solutions other than CM also cause a biphasic change in vasoactivity. Infusion of hyperosmolal solutions of dextrose, saline, and urea decreased resistance in the renal, as well as the limb and coronary vascular, beds. Cessation of the infusion of saline or urea was followed by a rise in resistance in the renal vascular bed. These findings support the notion that the renal hemodynamic response to CM is to a major extent due to the hyperosmolality of the solution.

The renal hemodynamic effects of four iothalamate-based monomeric and dimeric CM (sodium or meglumine iocarmate) have been studied anesthetized dogs using electromagnetic flowmeters [155]. A biphasic response was observed with all four CM. The early renal vasodilatation was similar for monomeric and dimeric CM but was significantly larger with meglumine than sodium-containing materials. The later vasoconstriction was significantly greater for monomeric than for dimeric materials. The sodium salt of the iothalamate dimer (iocarmate) caused the least vasoactive changes of the four CM.

One study [156] assessed renal size, blood flow, urine flow rate, renal blood volume, and mean renal transit time in anesthetized dogs after direct renal arterial injection of meglumine iothalamate and sodium iothalamate in anesthetized dogs. All changes were similar for the two CM. Each produced a small initial and transient decreases in renal size followed by a prolonged increase in size.

During renal enlargement urine flow increased while mean transit time and renal vascular volume decreased. Renal blood flow increased immediately, reached a peak at 30 s, and remained elevated for 5–7 min after injection. There was essentially no vasoconstrictor response observed in these experiments.

The renal vascular effects of ionic CM (meglumine sodium diatrizoate), nonionic CM (metrizamide), hyperosmolal saline, and isosmolal saline after direct renal arterial injection were compared in anesthetized dogs [157]. All solutions caused a biphasic response with an initial fall followed by a rise in renal vascular resistance. The initial fall in resistance was similar for metrizamide and the diatrizoate compound. However, the increase in resistance was approximately twice as great for the diatrizoate compound. This study concluded that nonionic CM caused less alteration in renal hemodynamics than ionic materials.

Renal blood flow after cardiac angiography in normal children and in children with congenital heart disease has been evaluated using the radioactive xenon flow technique [158]. In the small number of normal children that were studied, no decrease in either outer or inner cortical blood flow was detected after angiography. In children with congenital heart disease, there was a significant decrease in outer cortical blood flow after angiography with monomeric ionic CM.

4. Splanchnic Circulation

Early studies revealed that CM can have a variable effect on intestinal blood flow depending upon whether the direct vascular effects or rheologic changes are predominant. Such studies [135, 136] measured intestinal blood flow after direct arterial injection of CM. They found that CM induced an increase in flow which was greater and longer lasting with sodium acetrizoate than with sodium diatrizoate. On the other hand, some other studies revealed that ionic CM transiently reduced mesenteric blood flow by inducing red-cell aggregation and increasing viscosity [159, 160]. Few studies exist regarding the splanchnic vascular response to CM.

Direct microscopic visualization of the mesenteric vascular response to ionic CM and saline after injection into the thoracic aorta revealed that all ionic CM caused adhesion of white blood cells to vascular endothelium [161]. This white-cell adhesion was considered a sign of endothelial injury. A cetrizoate and dio-done compounds caused more severe changes than diatrizoate compound.

Superior mesenteric blood flow (electromagnetic flowmeter) and systemic arterial pressure have been measured in anesthetized dogs before and after injection of several ionic CM into the superior mesenteric artery of anesthetized dogs [162]. Hypaque 50%, Renografin 75%, and Conray 60% caused an immediate increase in superior mesenteric blood flow and decrease in resistance which peaked at 20–24 s and returned toward preinjection levels at 15 min. Hypaque M-90% and Urokon sodium 70% caused an initial decrease in flow for 10–30 s followed by a secondary rise to a peak of 80–150 s.

The changes in total and segmental mesenteric vascular resistance in response to meglumine/sodium diatrizoate (Renografin-76) have been measured in anesthetized dogs [163]. The CM caused an initial transient increase in total and segmental resistance followed by a greater and more persistent decrease in total and segmental resistance.

The alterations in hepatic arterial blood flow after hepatic arterial injection of CM (Renografin-60), blood, and saline have been evaluated with electromagnetic flowmeters in anesthetized dogs [164]. Hepatic arterial blood flow increased within 6 s after the start of the injection of all three fluids. The increase in blood flow persisted for longer with the CM. The increase in flow was maximum at 6–17 s and returned to baseline levels 3 min after injection.

5. Carotid Circulation

Injection of CM into the carotid circulation causes vasodilatation similar to that observed in other regional circulatory beds. In addition, it causes systemic hemodynamic changes consisting of alterations in heart rate, blood pressure, and systemic vascular resistance (this response is discussed in the section on reflex and neurally mediated effects).

An early study [165] observed the circulatory effects of the injection of acetrizoate and diatrizoate into the carotid circulation. This study was one of the first to document vasodilatation in the carotid circulation after intracarotid injection of ionic CM. Both ionic CM caused vasodilatation in the carotid circulation.

A subsequent study [131] also observed increases in carotid blood flow after injection of ionic CM into the common carotid artery. Injection into the middle cerebral artery or common carotid artery after ligation of the external carotid artery did not cause vasodilatation. This study concluded that ionic CM causes increase in flow after injection into the common carotid artery due to vasodilatation in the external carotid circulation.

Carotid blood flow has been measured with electromagnetic flowmeters in patients after intracarotid injection of 50% meglumine/sodium diatrizoate [166]. This CM caused increases in internal carotid blood flow and decreases in carotid vascular resistance.

Cerebral blood flow after intracarotid injection of Urografin 76% was also measured in patients using the radioactive xenon clearance technique [167]. Contrast medium caused a 15% increase in flow at 1 min and an 8% increase 3 min after injection. Flow was at baseline levels by 5 min after injection.

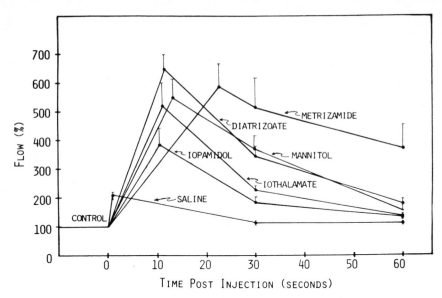

Fig. 10. Time sequence of the changes in carotid blood flow in response to the injection of various CM into the common carotid artery [35]

The effects of intracarotid injection of sodium iothalamate, meglumine sodium diatrizoate, iopamidol, metrizamide, and hypertonic mannitol on carotid blood flow and resistance have been compared in anesthetized animals [35]. The carotid vasodilatation was greatest with metrizamide and diatrizoate and least with iopamidol (Fig. 10).

6. Coronary Circulation

Numerous studies have documented that CM causes increase in coronary blood flow with vasodilatation. Pharmacologic agents that alter coronary blood flow do so by a direct vascular effect or indirectly by changing myocardial oxygen requirements resulting in a metabolically mediated change in blood flow. CM are known to act by the former mechanism in all vascular beds including the coronary. Since ionic CM cause profound alterations in the mechanical determinants of myocardial oxygen requirements, they probably affect coronary blood flow by the latter mechanism as well.

An early study [168] used a rotameter to measure coronary blood flow in dogs in response to intracoronary injection of saline, Renografin 76%, and Urokon 70%. CM caused an initial brief decline in coronary blood flow followed by a larger and more sustained increase in flow.

More recently coronary blood flow was measured with the xenon 133 precordial clearance method in dogs at various times after intracoronary injection of Hypaque M-75% [169]. There were variable changes in flow in the first 25 s and almost uniform increases in flow at 25–50 s after intracoronary injection of the CM.

Total coronary blood flow was measured in isolated hearts of rabbits by timed measurements of coronary vernous drainage after injections of several ionic CM into the aortic root [25]. Sodium iothalamate caused a substantial decrease in coronary blood flow in the first minutes followed by a slight increase in flow at 3 min after injection. On the other hand, hypertonic glucose and methylglucamine iothalamate caused increases in coronary blood flow which persisted for at least 10 min after injection.

Coronary blood flow has been measured in patients during coronary arteriography by the Xenon 133 washout technique [170]. Coronary blood flow rose in all patients 1 min after intracoronary injection of Renografin 76% and remained elevated at 5–7 min. Blood flow responses in patients with coronary artery disease were no different from normal subjects.

Others have measured coronary blood flow with ^{131}I-antipyrine and simultaneously sampled blood gases, pyruvate, and lactate in coronary sinus blood before and after intracoronary injection of several ionic CM in anesthetized dogs [109]. All ionic CM increased coronary blood flow and some decreased the fractional extraction of lactate, decreased lactic acid uptake, and increased the lactate-pyruvate ratio and free fatty acid uptake of the myocardium.

Coronary blood flow was also measured in the isolated perfusion canine heart during the response to Renografin-76 [8]. Coronary blood flow increased substantially while coronary arteriovenous oxygen and potassium did not change significantly.

Electromagnetic flowmeters have been used to measure coronary blood flow in dogs during the response to intracoronary injection of meglumine sodium diatrizoate, metrizamide, and metrizamide with added calcium ions [171]. The increase in flow with metrizamide was smaller than the increase with the diatrizoate compound or metrizamide with added calcium ions. The increase in coronary blood flow due to metrizamide with added calcium ions was similar to that due to the diatrizoate compound.

Coronary vascular resistance along with the hematocrit, protein, and osmolality of blood from the coronary sinus have been measured during and after coronary arteriography with meglumine sodium diatrizoate in anesthetized dogs [172]. There was an initial transient increase in resistance during injection of CM followed by vasodilatation lasting for 2 min. During opacification of the coronary arteries, there was a marked decrease in hematocrit and protein, and rise in osmolality of blood from the coronary sinus.

In one report coronary sinus oxygen content, myocardial oxygen consumption, and coronary blood flow were monitered in dogs and myocardial oxygen consumption was measured in patients during coronary arteriography [173]. Coronary vasodilatation was accompanied by an increase in coronary sinus oxygen content and no significant increase in myocardial oxygen consumption. These findings suggest that the vasodilatation caused by CM was a direct vascular effect rather than a consequence of a rise in myocardial oxygen requirements.

CM (Hypaque M-75%) has been used to assess the coronary flow reserve at various levels of coronary artery stenosis in anesthetized dogs [174, 175]. In the absence of stenosis, CM increased flow to four times the resting baseline value; the increase in flow peaked at 6 s and lasted for 3 min. The degree of augmentation of blood flow after injection of CM started to decline with 45%–50% stenosis and disappeared at approximately 90% stenosis.

The changes in coronary blood flow in response to intracoronary injection of Renografin 76% have been studied in patients using the thermodilation technique for continuous measurement of coronary sinus blood flow [176]. Coronary flow increased in response to left coronary ateriography in all patients but the increase was significantly greater in patients with normal coronary arteries compared with those with obstructive disease of the left coronary artery.

The increase in coronary blood flow in anesthetized dogs after intracoronary injection of Urografin-76 has been compared with the increase induced by 10 s of coronary occlusion [177]. The increase in flow with CM was accompanied by an increase in coronary sinus pO_2 and was almost equivalent to that caused by 10 s of coronary occlusion.

Coronary blood flow and myocardial perfusion have been measured after intracoronary injection of meglumine sodium diatrizoate in patients [178]. Myocardial blood flow increased approximately 50% after CM and returned to baseline levels after 5 min.

The vasodilatory potency of intracoronary injection of ionic CM has been compared with several potent vasodilator drugs in anesthetized dogs [179]. Meglumine sodium diatrizoate increased coronary arterial conductance 2½-fold while infusion of ATP and/or papaverine caused a sevenfold increase in conductance. This study showed that bolus injection of ionic CM does not approach the level of maximum possible coronary vasodilatation.

Several studies [180–182] assessed the changes in myocardial subcellular structures and electrolytes after perfusion of the coronary arteries of the isolated guinea pig heart with several ionic CM and the nonionic material, metrizamide. Some of the nonionic and the ionic CM caused a shift of sodium from the extracellular to the intracellular space. On the other hand, Conray 60 caused a shift of sodium out of the myocardial cells. Electron microscopic autoradiographic studies of the guinea pig myocardium after Urografin showed no change in myocardial subcellular structure but swelling of the mitochondria and myofilaments with Angiografin. No change in subcellular elements was observed in samples of human myocardium obtained after coronary arteriography performed at the time of cardiac surgery. In general, most ionic CM caused a decrease in intracellular potassium and increase in sodium [180]. The nonionic material, metrizamide, caused increase in intracellular potassium and decrease in sodium [182].

7. Microcirculation and Vascular Endothelium

Early studies [159, 160, 183] showed that angiographic CM caused intravascular clotting due to aggregation and agglutination of red blood cells. This phenomenon was thought to be related to hyperosmolality of both contrast and noncontrast solutions.

Another study [184] evaluated the effects of meglumine sodium diatrizoate on the microcirculation after topical application to the submucosal surface of the hamster cheek pouch. Topical application of the CM produced crenation of red blood cells and intravascular sludging. The crenation and sludging were rapidly reversed by washing the submucosal surface with physiologic saline. They concluded that these potential obstructive and ischemic actions of CM are related predominantly to hyperosmolality.

The actions of Urokon 70%, Hypaque M-90%, Renografin 76%, and Renovist on the microcirculation of the canine mesentery have been studied using in vivo high-speed cinemicroangiography [185]. It was observed that the severity of changes was related to increasing osmolality of the CM. There were major alterations in red blood cells consisting of crenation and spherocyte formation, producing marked decrease in capillary cellular flow. It was proposed that this phenomenon may contribute to resistance to blood flow on the microcirculation after administration of CM.

Direct microscopic observation has also been used to determine the effects of ionic CM on the microcirculation of the bat wing [186]. Topical application of ionic CM and hyperosmolal solutions of saline or mannitol halted normal spontaneous intravascular aggregation of red blood cells. The intensity of this effect was found to be directly related to the osmolality of the solutions.

The effects of monomeric CM (sodium metrizoate) and glucose have been compared with those of solutions consisting of polymers of the same contrast moiety and glucose (dextran) in the microcirculation of the bat wing [187]. The reduction in osmolality of the polymeric solutions was accompanied by a decrease in the severity of the effects on the microcirculation after topical application.

The mechanism of the toxic microcirculatory action of ionic CM and vital dyes has been assessed by direct in vivo microscopic observation of the bat wing [188]. Methylene blue halted spontaneous contraction in lymphatic vessels at a molar concentration 1,000 times lower than the concentration of CM required to cause this effect. Moreover, this effect was more rapidly reversed for CM than for the vital dyes. Because of these differences between the vital dye and CM, the authors proposed a different mechanism of action of the two classes of substances. They proposed that the toxic microcirculatory effects of CM were due to hyperosmolality while the effect of vital dyes was a direct chemotoxic action on intracellular enzymes.

The effect of topical application or submucosal injection of a number of ionic CM has been evaluated on the microcirculation of the hamster cheek pouch using intravital microscopy with microphotographic recording of structures and microcinematographic registration of flow patterns [189]. Application of each of the CM initially caused slowing and finally cessation of flow in venules, arterioles, and capillaries. They also caused collection of white blood cells along vessel walls, indicating local endothelial damage. Higher concentrations of ionic CM caused more rapid cessation of flow and slower recovery of microvascular motion. These authors concluded that the cessation of microcirculatory flow in the presence of ionic CM is due to both endothelial damage and alterations in red blood cell characteristics.

The effects of multiple CM on the microcirculation of the canine mesentery have been compared [190]. Urokon 70%, Hypaque M-90%, Renografin 76%, and Renovist were injected into the isolated ileocolic artery while normal and high-speed cinemicroangiograms were obtained. The most severe effects were caused by Urokon and repeated injections of CM caused cumulative toxic effects.

Progressive alterations in red blood cell morphology and evidence of endothelial damage were related to increasing osmolality.

The microcirculatory effects of several ionic (Isopaque Coronar, Angiografin, and Conray) and nonionic (Compound 6, Compound 18, and metrizamide) CM have been compared [191]. At all iodine concentrations nonionic CM caused less depression of spontaneous contractile activity of venous and lymphatic vessels and slowed the flow rate of red blood cells through capillaries. The authors concluded that the lower osmolality of nonionic CM was responsible for reduced vascular toxicity of these materials.

The effects of intraarterial injection of CM (Hypaque 50%, and Conray 60%) on the permeability of microvessels in the rat's cecal mesentery have been examined using direct microscopic observation [192]. Changes in vascular permeability were assessed by accumulation of intraarterially injected colloidal carbon black particles. There was no significant increase in permeability of normal microvessels after CM but changes in permeability were observed in damaged and occluded vessels.

The effects of ionic CM were also evaluated on normal and inflamed venous endothelium [193]. It was found that CM produce more extensive and severe inflammatory changes in vessels which had prior endothelial damage. These changes consisted of red blood cell aggregation and fibrin formation.

The endothelial damage on the murine aorta has been determined after contact with monomeric ionic, dimeric ionic, and nonionic CM [6]. Dimeric ionic and nonionic CM caused less damage than monomeric ionic materials but there was no perceptible difference in the actions of dimeric ionic and nonionic materials.

The influence of varying the cation content in solutions of ionic and nonionic CM on the endothelial toxic action has been evaluated in the microvasculature of the bat wing [194]. Buffered saline solutions containing sodium, potassium, calcium, magnesium, chloride, and bicarbonate ions caused no effect on venous contractile activity, while solutions of meglumine metrizoate, metrizamide, and glucose prepared at the same osmolality as the buffered saline solution stopped spontaneous venous contractile activity within 5–10 min after topical applications. The authors of this study concluded that solutions without an optimal cation content cause microcirculatory toxicity. Solutions with suboptimal anion content caused a less deleterious effect than those with suboptimal cation content. CM (sodium metrizoate) to which sodium ions, potassium, calcium, and magnesium ions were added had the least deleterious action on vasomotion. The authors concluded that the inhibitory action on vasomotion is related to hyperosmolality and ionic composition. The most favorable CM in this regard should be a nonionic one containing physiologic concentrations of sodium, potassium, calcium, and magnesium.

The microcirculatory effects of meglumine metrizoate and metrizamide in the ear chamber of rabbits after intraarterial injection have been compared [195]. After injection of CM, microcirculation was slowed followed by a phase of arteriolovenular shunting and poor capillary perfusion. No significant difference was observed between the toxic effects of meglumine metrizoate and metrizamide.

Plasma histamine concentration and microvascular changes have been assessed in the exteriorized omentum of rabbits after intraarterial injection of hypertonic saline solution, methylglucamine iodipamide (Cholografin), and methylglucamine diatrizoate (Hypaque 60) [196]. Both CM caused decline in arteriolar pressure, decrease in red blood cell velocity, sticking of white blood cells to endothelium, and increase in plasma histamine levels. Increased rather than decreased vasomotion in small arterial vessels was also noted. Hypertonic saline solutions did not produce these effects or caused only mild transient changes in the microcirculation. These findings suggested that hyperosmolality of CM may be associated with initial microhemodynamic changes, but it is not the sole cause of long-lasting changes or cellular damage. The release of histamine was not temporally related to changes in the microvessel diameter.

E. Summary

Contrast media cause a multitude of alterations in function of the cardiovascular system. These alterations are predominantly due to direct actions of the CM on the heart and vasculature and, to a lesser extent, these changes are reflex mediated. Ionic CM cause direct depression of cardiac electrophysiologic and contractile function. Electrophysiologic effects are related to hyperosmolality and the contractile effects are due mainly to the cationic content of the CM. Nonionic CM cause milder electrophysiologic alterations and enhance rather than depress myocardial contraction.

Both ionic and most nonionic CM cause vasodilatation in the peripheral circulation. This is a direct effect which is predominantly related to the hyperosmolality of the solutions and to a lesser degree to the cation content and chemical nature of the iodine-bearing moiety. The hemodynamic responses of the carotid and renal vascular beds to CM are unique compared with other regional circulations.

References

1. Almen T (1971) Toxicity of radiocontrast agents. In: Knoefel PK (ed) Radiocontrast agents. Pergamon, Oxford, p 443 (International encyclopedia of pharmacology and therapeutics, vol 2)
2. Price HL (1960) General anesthesia and circulatory homeostasis. Physiol Rev 40:187
3. Peiss CN, Manning JW (1964) Effects of sodium pentobarbital on electrical and reflex activation of the cardiovascular system. Circ Res 14:228
4. Spann JR Jr, Mason DT, Beider GD, Gold HK (1969) Myocardial effects of angiographic dye (Abstr). Am J Cardiol 23:140
5. Serur JR, Als AV, Miner-Green N, Paulin S (1980) Comparative effects of three radiographic contrast agents in isolated normal and ischemic canine hearts. Invest Radiol 15:5196
6. Almen T, Aspelin P (1976) Cardiovascular effects of ionic, monomeric, ionic dimeric, and nonionic contrast media. Invest Radiol 10:557
7. Als AV, Serur JR, LaRaia PJ, et al. (1978) Differential effects of sodium meglumine calcium metrizoate on the inotropic state of normal and ischemic myocardium. Radiology 128:499
8. Wolf GL, Gerlings ED, Wilson WJ (1973) Depression in myocardial contractility induced by hypertonic coronary injections in the isolated perfused dog heart. Radiology 107:655
9. Lipton MJ, Higgins CB, Wilea AAN, et al. (1978) The effect of contrast media on the isolated perfused canine heart. Invest Radiol 13:519

10. Higgins CB, Schmidt W (1978) Alterations in calcium levels of coronary sinus blood during coronary arteriography in the dog. Circulation 58:512

11. Higgins CB, Schmidt W (1978) Direct and reflex myocardial effects of intracoronary administered contrast materials in the anesthetized and conscious dog: comparison of standard and newer contrast materials. Invest Radiol 13:205

11a. Higgins CB, Bookstein JJ (1977) Comparative hemodynamic effects of coronary vasodilators and contrast material on the normal and ischemic canine myocardium. Determination of the optimal agent for clinical augmentation of coronary blood flow. Invest Radiol 12:299

12. Newell JD, Schmidt W, Higgins CB (1979) Effects of intracoronary administration of contrast materials on left ventricular dimensions and rate of relaxation. Invest Radiol 14:233

13. Popio KA, Ross AM, Oravec JM, Ingram JT (1978) Identification and description of separate mechanisms for two components of Renografin cardiotoxicity. Circulation 58:520

14. Braunwald E, Ross JJ, Sonnenblick EH (1976) Mechanisms of contraction of the normal and failing heart. Little, Brown, Boston

15. Mahler F, Ross JJ, O'Rourke RA, Covell JW (1975) Effects of changes in preload, afterload, and inotropic state on ejection and isovolumic phase measures of contractility in the dog. am J Cardiol 35:626

16. Chahine RA, Raizner AE (1976) The mechanism of hypotension following angiography. Invest Radiol 11:472

17. Higgins CB (1980) Overview and methods used for the study of the cardiovascular actions of contrast materials. Invest Radiol 15:S188

18. Shaw DD, Wolf GL, Kraft L, Baltaxe HA (1977) The role of peripheral vasodilatation and direct myocardial depression in the systemic hypotensive response to ventriculography. Invest Radiol 12:424 (Abstr)

19. Freisinger GS, Schaefer J, Crilley JM, Gaertner RA, Ross RS (1965) Hemodynamic consequences of the injection of radiopaque material. Circulation 31:730

20. Hammermeister KE, Warbasse JR (1973) Immediate hemodynamic effects of cardiac angiography in man. Am J Cardiol 31:307

21. Karliner JS, Bouchard RJ, Gault JH (1972) Hemodynamic effects of angiographic contrast material in man. Br Heart J 34:347

22. Vine DL, Hegg TD, Dodge HT, Stewart DK, Frimer M (1977) Immediate effect of contrast medium injection on left ventricular volumes and ejection fraction. A study using metallic epicardial markers. Circulation 56:379

23. Baltaxe HA, Sos TA, McGrath MB (1976) Effects of the intracoronary and intraventricular injections of a commonly available vs. a newly available contrast medium. Invest Radiol 11:172

24. Cohn PF, Horn HR, Teichholz LE, Kreuler TH, Herman MV, Jorlen R (1973) Effects of angiographic contrast medium on left ventricular function in coronary artery disease. Am J Cardiol 32:21

25. Gootman N, Rudolph AM, Buckley NM (1970) Effects of angiographic contrast media on cardiac function. Am J Cardiol 25:59

26. Mullins CB, Leshin SJ, Mierzwiak DS, Alsobrook HD, Mitchell JH (1972) Changes in left ventricular function produced by the injection of contrast media. Am Heart J 83:373

27. Behar VS, Waxman WB, Morris JJ Jr (1970) The effects of a contrast medium (sodium iothalamate, 80%) on left ventricular function. Am J Med Sci 60:202

28. Shaw DD, Wolf GL, Wilson WJ, Trevisani T (1975) The effect of angiotension II during ventriculography in dogs with normal coronary arteries. Radiology 115:717

29. Krovetz LJ, Mitchell BM, Neumaster T (1967) Hemodynamic effects of rapidly injected hypertonic solutions into the heart and great vessels. Am Heart J 74:453

30. Kelley MJ, Higgins CB, Schmidt WS, Newell JD (1980) Effects of ionic and nonionic contrast agents on left ventricular and extracellular fluid dynamics during angiocardiography in an infant model. Invest Radiol 15:335

31. Romero TE, Higgins CB, Kirkpatrick SE, Friedman WF (1977) Effects of contrast material on dimensions and hemodynamics of the newborn heart: a study in conscious newborn lambs. Invest Radiol 12:510
32. Lindgren P, Tornell G (1958) Blood pressure and heart rate responses in carotid angiography with sodium acetrizoate. Acta Radiol (Stockh) 50:160
33. Lynch PR, Harrington GJ, Michie C (1969) Cardiovascular reflexes associated with cerebral angiography. Invest Radiol 4:156
34. Higgins CB, Schmidt W (1979) Identification and evaluation of the contribution of the chemoreflex in the hemodynamic response to intracarotid administration of contrast materials in the conscious dog: comparison with the response to nicotine. Invest Radiol 14:438
35. Morris TW, Francis M, Fischer HW (1979) A comparison of the cardiovascular responses to carotid injections of ionic and nonionic contrast media. Invest Radiol 14:217
36. Vatner SF, Higgins CB, Franklin D, Braunwald E (1971) Extent of carotid sinus regulation of the myocardial contractile state in conscious dogs. J Clin Invest 50:1116
37. Higgins CB, Vatner SF, Eckberg DL, Braunwald E (1972) Alterations in the baroreceptor reflex in conscious dogs with heart failure. J Clin Invest 51:715
38. Downing SE, Remensnyder PP, Mitchell JH (1962) Cardiovascular responses to hypoxic stimulation of the carotid bodies. Circ Res 10:676
39. Comroe JH Jr (1964) The peripheral chemoreceptors. In: Fenn W, Rahn H (eds) Respiration. American Physiological Society, Washington, D.C., p 557 (Handbook of physiology, vol 1)
40. Fischer HW (1968) Hemodynamic reactions to angiographic media. A survey and commentary. Radiology 91:66–73
41. Amundsen AK, Amundsen P, Muller O (1956) Blood pressure and heart rate during angiocardiography, abdominal aortography, and arteriography of the lower extremities. Acta Radiol (Stockh) 45:452
42. DiDonato M, Bongrani S, Cucchini F, Baldi G, Fappani A, Colla B, Visioli O (1979) Cardiovascular effects induced by the injection of a new nonionic contrast medium (iopamidol): experimental study in dogs. Invest Radiol 143:309
43. Berg GR, Hutter AM, Pfister RC (1973) Electrocardiographic abnormalities associated with intravenous urography. N Engl J Med 289:87
44. Stanley RJ, Pfister RC (1976) Bradycardia and hypotension following use of intravenous contrast media. Radiology 121:5
45. Stadalnik RC, Vera Z, Da Silva O (1977) Electrocardiographic response to intravenous urography: prospective evaluation of 275 patients. AJR 129:825
46. White CW, Eckberg DL, Inasaka T, Abboud FM (1976) Effects of angiographic contrast media on sinoatrial nodal function. Cardiovasc Res 10:214
47. Adams DF, Paulin S (1968) Effects of radiographic contrast media in selective injections into the sinus node artery. An experimental study in dogs. Radiology 91:719
48. Higgins CB (1977) Effects of contrast media on the conducting system of the heart. Mechanism of action and identification of toxic component. Radiology 124:599
49. Benchimol A, McNally EM (1966) Hemodynamic and electrocardiographic effects of selective coronary arteriography in man. N Engl J Med 274:1217
50. Banks DC, Rafferty EB, Oram S (1970) Evaluation of contrast media used in man for coronary arteriography. Br Heart J 32:317
51. Brown TG Jr (1967) Cardiovascular actions of angiographic media. Angiology 18:273
52. Coskey RL, Magidson O (1967) Electrocardiographic response to selective coronary arteriography. Br Heart J 29:512
53. Frink RJ, Merrick B, Lower HM (1975) Mechanism of bradycardia during coronary angiography. Am J Cardiol 35:17
54. MacAlpin RN, Weidner WA, Kattus AA, Hanafee WN (1966) Electrocardiographic changes during selective coronary cineangiography. Circulation 34:627
55. Nakhjavan FK, Smith AM, Dratch MB, Goldberg H (1974) His bundle electrogram during coronary arteriography in man: studies at spontaneous and constant heart rates. J Electrocardiol 7:101

56. Eckberg DL, White CM, Kioschos JM, Abboud FM (1974) Mechanisms mediating bradycardia during coronary arteriography. J Clin Invest 54:1455
57. Perez-Gomez F, Garcia-Aguado A (1977) Origin of ventricular reflexes caused by coronary arteriography. Br Heart J 39:967
58. Abe S, Itoh M, Unakami H, Kobazashi T (1976) Sinus slowing produced by intracoronary arterial injections of hyperosmotic solutions in man. Am Heart J 91:339
59. Carson RP, Lazzara R (1970) Hemodynamic responses initiated by coronary stretch receptors with special reference to coronary arteriography. Am J Cardiol 25:571
60. James TN, Nadeu RA (1963) Sinus bradycardia during injections directly into the sinus node artery. Am J Physiol 204:9
61. Higgins CB, Feld GK (1976) Direct chronotropic and dromotropic actions of contrast media: ineffectiveness of atropine in the prevention of bradyarrhythmias and conduction disturbances. Radiology 121:205
62. Zelis R, Caudill C, Baggette K, Mason DT (1976) Reflex vasodilation induced by coronary angiography in human subjects. Circulation 53:490
63. Daves GE, Comroe JH Jr (1954) Chemoreflexes from the heart and lungs. Physiol Rev 34:167
64. Tragardh B, Bove AA, Lynch PR (1974) Cardiac conduction abnormalities during coronary arteriography in dogs: reduced effects of a new contrast medium. Invest Radiol 9:340
65. Tragardh B, Bove AA, Lynch PR (1977) Mechanism of production of cardiac conduction abnormalities due to coronary arteriography in dogs. Invest Radiol 11:563
66. Nakhjavan FK (1973) Recording of His bundle and left bundle potentials during left coronary arteriography in the dog. J Electrocardiol 6:45
67. Langou RA, Sheps DS, Wolfson S, Cohen LS (1977) Intraventricular conduction during coronary arteriography in patients with pre-existing conduction abnormalities. Invest Radiol 12:505
68. Sostman HD, Simon AL, Langou RA (1977) Localization of the conduction delay occurring during coronary arteriography. Invest Radiol 12:128
69. Miller D, Lohse J, Wolf G (1976) Slow response induced in canine Purkinje fiber by contrast medium. Invest Radiol 11:577
70. Simon AL, Shabetai R, Lang JH, Lasser EC (1972) The mechanism of production of ventricular fibrillation in coronary angiography. AJR 114:810
71. Paulin S, Adams DF (1971) Increased ventricular fibrillation during coronary arteriography with a new contrast medium preparation. Radiology 101:45
71a. Wolf GL, Kraft L, Kilzer K (1978) Contrast agents lower ventricular fibrillation threshold. Radiology 129:215
72. Hildner JF, Scherlag B, Samet P (1971) Evaluation of Renografin M76 as a contrast agent for angiocardiography. Radiology 100:329
72a. Wolf GL (1980) The fibrillatory propensities of contrast agents. Invest Radiol 15:5208
73. Snyder CF, Formanek A, Frech RS, Amplatz K (1971) The role of sodium in promoting ventricular arrhythmia during selective coronary arteriography. AJR 113:567
73a. Violante MR, Thomson KR, Fischer HW, Kenyon T (1978) Ventricular fibrillation from diatrizoate with and without chelating agents. Radiology 128:497
74. Almen T (1973) Effects of metrizamide and other contrast media on the isolated rabbit heart. Acta Radiol [Suppl] (Stockh) 335:216
74a. Thomson KR, Violante MR, Kenyon T, Fischer HW (1978) Reduction in ventricular fibrillation using calcium enriched Renografin 76. Invest Radiol 13:238
75. Gensini GG, DiGiorgi S (1964) Myocardial toxocity of contrast agents used in angiography. Radiology 82:24
75a. Tragardh B, Lynch PR (1978) ECG changes and arrhythmias induced by ionic and nonionic contrast media during coronary arteriography in dogs. Invest Radiol 13:233
76. Kilzer K, Mulry BS, LeVeen R (1980) New angiographic agents that are less fibrillatory. Invest Radiol 15:416
77. Moore EN, Spear JF (1975) Ventricular fibrillation threshold. Its physiological and pharmacological importance. Arch Intern Med 135:446

78. Ross RS, Gorlin R (1968) Coronary arteriography. Circulation [Suppl 3] 37:67
79. Frech RS (1975) Toxicity studies of coronary arteriographic media in dogs. Invest Radiol 10:323
80. Carter AM, Olin T (1976) Ionic composition and cardiotoxicity of dimeric contrast media at injections into the coronary arteries of rabbits. Acta Radiol [Diagn] (Stockh) 17:433
81. Bjork L, Eldh P, Paulin S (1977) Nonionic and dimeric contrast media in coronary angiography. Experimental investigation in dogs. Acta Radiol [Diagn] (Stockh) 18:235
82. Refsum H, Passwal M (1978) Arrhythmogenic and cardiodepressive effects of contrast media on isolated rat atria. Invest Radiol 13:444
83. Refsum H, Hotvedt R (1979) Cardiotoxic effects of contrast media on isolated rat atria (Abstr). Circulation [Suppl 2] 59/60:162
84. Brown TG, Hoppe JO, Borisenok WA (1967) Cardiovascular studies of Isopaque B and other radiopaque media. Acta Radiol [Diagn] [Suppl] (Stockh) 270:58
85. Smith RF, Harthorne JW, Sanders CA (1967) Vectorcardiographic changes during intracoronary injections. Circulation 36:63
86. Fernandez F, Scebat L, Lenegre J (1970) Electrocardiographic study of left intraventricular hemiblock in man during selective coronary arteriography. Am J Cardiol 25:1
87. Eie H, Grendahl H, Nordvik A, Muller C (1972) Electrocardiographic changes during selective coronary angiography. Acta Radiol [Diagn] (Stockh) 12:554
88. Grendahl H, Eie H, Nordvik A, Muller C (1972) Electrocardiographic changes during selective coronary arteriography. Acta Med Scand 191:493
89. Ovitt T, Rizk G, Frech RS, Cramer R, Amplatz K (1972) Electrocardiographic changes in selective coronary arteriography: the importance of ions. Radiology 104:705
90. Tragardh B, Lynch PR, Vinciguerra T (1975) Effects of metrizamide, a new nonionic contrast medium, on cardiac function during coronary arteriography in the dog. Radiology 115:59
91. Tragardh B, Almen T, Lynch B (1975) Addition of calcium or other cations and oxygen to ionic and nonionic contrast media. Effects on cardiac functions during coronary arteriography. Invest Radiol 10:231
92. Tragardh B, Lynch PR, Vinciguerra T (1976) Cardiac function during coronary arteriography with calcium-enriched diatrizoate and metrizamide. Invest Radiol 11:569
93. Bristow JD, Porter GA, Kloster FE, Griswold HE (1967) Hemodynamic changes attending angiocardiography. Radiology 88:939
94. Wildenthal K, Mierzwiak DS, Mitchell JH (1969) Acute effects of increased serum osmolality on left ventricular performance. Am J Physiol 216:898
95. Karliner JS, LeWinter MM, Mahler F, Engler R, O'Rourke RA (1977) Pharmacologic and hemodynamic influences on the rate of isovolumic and left ventricular relaxation in the normal conscious dog. J Clin Invest 60:511
96. Brundage BH, Cheitlin MD (1974) Ventricular function curves from the cardiac response to angiographic contrast: a sensitive detector of ventricular dysfunction in coronary artery disease. Am Heart J 88:281
97. Brundage BH, Farr JE (1977) Comparison of contrast medium and atrial pacing as tests of ventricular function in coronary artery disease. Br Heart J 40:250
98. Kober G, Schroder W, Kaltenbach M (1978) Der Einfluß intrakardialer Kontrastmittelinjektionen auf die Hämodynamik des linken Ventrikels. Z Kardiol 67:474
99. Gensini GG, Dubiel J, Huntington PP, Kelley AE (1971) Left ventricular end-diastolic pressure before and after coronary arteriography. The value of coronary arteriography as a stress test. Am J Cardiol 27:453
100. Salvesen S, Nilsen PL, Holtermann H (1967) Ameliorating effects of calcium and magnesium ions on toxicity of isopaque sodium. Acta Radiol [Suppl] (Stockh) 270:30
101. Wildenthal K, Skelton GL, Coleman HN III (1969) Cardiac muscle mechanics in hyperosmotic solution. Am J Physiol 217:307
102. Newell JD, Higgins CB, Kelley MJ, Treen CE, Schmidt WS, Haigler F (1980) The influence of hyperosmolality on left ventricular contractile state. Disparate effects of nonionic and ionic solutions. Invest Radiol 15:363

103. Sink JD, Wechsler AS, Pellom GL, Thompson WM (1979) Effects of B-15,000 (iopamidol), a new nonionic contrast agent, on cardiac function of the isolated rat heart. Invest Radiol 14:508
104. Higgins CB (1980) Effects of contrast materials on left ventricular function. Invest Radiol 15:5220
105. Kaftori JK, Paulin S (1974) The effect of pH on the toxicity of diatrizoate in selective coronary arteriography. An experimental study in dogs. Invest Radiol 9:351
106. Guzman SV, West JW (1959) Cardiac effects of intracoronary arterial injections of various roentgenographic contrast media. Am Heart J 58:597
107. Jacobsson B, Paulin S (1967) Experiences with different contrast media in coronary angiography. Acta Radiol [Suppl] (Stockh) 270:103
108. Jacobsson B, Paulin S (1967) Experiences with different contrast media in coronary arteriography. Acta Radiol [Suppl] (Stockh) 270:194
109. Oppenheimer MJ, Ascanio G, Henny CG, Caldwell E, Vineiguerra T (1973) Metabolic and cardiovascular effects of selective intracoronary injections of contrast media. Invest Radiol 8:13
110. Kaude JV, Lunderquist A, Persson S, Arnman K (1974) Selective coronary angiography with iodamide. A comparison of myocardial toxicity of two contrast media. Angiology 25:449
111. Higgins CB, Sovak M, Schmidt W, Kelley MJ, Newell JD (1980) Direct myocardial effects of intracoronary administration of new contrast materials with low osmolality. Invest Radiol 15:39
112. Caulfield JB, Zir L, Harthorne JW (1975) Blood calcium levels in the presence of arteriographic contrast material. Circulation 52:119
113. Langer GA (1973) Heart: excitation-contraction coupling. Annu Rev Physiol 35:55
114. Moore EW (1969) Studies with ion exchange calcium electrodes in biological fluids: some applications in biological research and clinical medicine. In: Durst RA (ed) Ion specific electrodes. Nat Bur Stand U.S. Spec Publ 314:215
115. Latrou J, Bergin M, Cardinal A (1978) Action of contrast media solutions on cardiac hemodynamic parameters during coronary angiography in the pig. Ann Radiol (Paris) 21:261
116. Thomson KR, Eviel CA, Fritzche J, Beness GT (1980) Comparison of iopamidol, ioxaglate, and diatrizoate during coronary arteriography in dogs. Invest Radiol 15:234
116a. Tragardh B, Lynch PR (1980) Cardiac function during left coronary ateriography in canines with ioxaglate, nonionic compounds, and diatrizoate. Invest Radiol 15:449
117. Green CE, Higgins CB, Kelley MJ, Newell JD, Schmidt WS (1981) Effects of intracoronary administration of contrast materials on left ventricular function in the presence of severe coronary artery stenosis. Cardiovasc Radiol 4:110–116
118. Yamazaki H, Banka VS, Bondenheimer MM, Helfant RH (1979) Differential effects of Renografin 76 on ischemic and non-ischemic myocardium (Abstr) Circulation [Suppl 2] 59:244
119. Zipfel J, Baller D, Karsch KR, Reutrop P, Hellige G (1980) Decrease in cardiotoxicity of contrast media in coronary angiography in addition of calcium ions. Combined experimental and clinical study. Clin Cardiol 3:178
120. Wolpers HG, Baller D, Ensink FBM, et al. (1981) Influence of contrast media on calcium in blood. Cardiovasc Radiol 4:8
121. Adams DF, Abrams HL (1979) Complications of coronary arteriography: a follow-up report. Cardiovasc Radiol 2:89
122. Bourassa MG, Noble J (1976) Complication rate of coronary arteriography. A review of 5,250 cases studied by percutaneous femoral technique. Circulation 53:106
123. Swan HJ (1968) Cooperative study on cardiac catheterization. Complications associated with angiocardiography. Circulation [Suppl 3] 37:81
124. Nitter-Hauge S, Enge I (1976) Metrizoic acid (isopaque coronar) used in man for coronary angiography. Radiology 121:537
125. McIntosh HD (1968) Cooperative study on cardiac catheterization. Arrhythmias. Circulation [Suppl 3] 37:27
126. Enge I, Nitter-Hauge S, Andrew E, Levorstad K (1977) Amipaque. a new contrast medium in coronary angiography. Radiology 125:317

127. Enge I, Nitter-Hauge S, Levorstad K, et al. (1979) Amipaque in coronary angiography. Diagn Imaging 48:219
128. Ludwig JW (1979) Use of metrizamide in coronary arteriography. Diagn Imaging 48:223
129. Lindgren P (1959) Carotid angiography with tri-iodobenzoic acid derivatives: a comparative experimental study of the effects on the systemic circulation in cats. Acta Radiol (Stockh) 51:353
130. Hilal SK (1966) Hemodynamic responses in the cerebral vessels to angiographic contrast media. Acta Radiol (Stockh) 5:211
131. Hilal SK (1966) Hemodynamic changes associated with intra-arterial injection of contrast media. Radiology 86:615
132. Fischer HW, Eckstein JW (1961) Comparison of cerebral angiographic contrast media by their circulatory effects. AJR 86:166
133. Cornell SH, Fischer HW (1967) Comparison of mixtures of metrizoate and iothalamate salts with their methylglucamine solutions by the carotid injection technique. Invest Radiol 2:41
134. Fischer HW, Kurland C, Burgener FA (1977) Cardiovascular responses to metrizamide and meglumide sodium diatrizoate in cerebral angiography (Abstr). Invest Radiol 12:440
135. Lindgren P (1970) Hemodynamic responses to contrast media. Invest Radiol 5:424
136. Lindgren P, Tornell G (1958) Blood circulation during and after peripheral arteriography: experimental study of the effects of Triurol (sodium acetrizoate) and hypaque (sodium diatrizoate). Acta Radiol (Stockh) 49:425
137. Gonzales LL, Stieritz D (1966) Cardiovascular responses to injection of contrast medium into proximal aorta. Radiology 86:1070
138. Marshall RJ, Shepherd JT (1959) Effect of injections of hypertonic solutions on blood flow through the femoral artery of the dog. Am J Physiol 197:951
139. Mellander S, Johansson B, Gray S (1967) The effect of hyperosmolarity on intact and isolated vascular smooth muscle: possible role of exercise hyperemia. Angiologica 4:310
140. Haddy FJ (1960) Local effects of sodium, calcium, and magnesium upon small and large blood vessels of the dog forelimb. Circ Res 8:57
141. Delius W, Erikson V (1969) Effect of contrast medium in blood flow and blood pressure in lower extremities. AJR 107:869
142. Mottram RF, Lynch PR (1970) Circulatory effects of repeated intraarterial injections of Conray 60. Invest Radiol 5:534
143. Coel MC, Lasser EC (1971) A pharmacologic basis for peripheral vascular resistance changes with contrast media injections. AJR 111:802
144. Almen T, Tragardh B (1973) Effects of nonionic contrast media on the blood flow through the femoral artery of the dog. Acta Radiol [Suppl] (Stockh) 335:197
144a. Speck U, Siefert H-M, Klesik G (1980) Contrast media and pain in peripheral arteriography. Invest Radiol 15:S335
145. Aperia A, Broberger O, Ekengren K (1968) Renal hemodynamics during selective renal angiography. Invest Radiol 3:389
146. Talner LB, Davidson AJ (1968) Renal hemodynamic effects of contrast media. Invest Radiol 3:310
147. Sherwood T, Lavender JP (1969) Does renal blood flow rise or fall in response to diatrizoate? Invest Radiol 4:327
148. Chou CC, Hook JB, Hsieh CP, et al. (1971) Effects of radiopaque dyes on renal vascular resistance. J Lab Clin Med 78:705
149. Caldicott WJH, Hollenberg NK, Abrams HL (1970) Characteristics of response of renal vascular bed to contrast media. Evidence for vasoconstriction induced by renin-angiotension system. Invest Radiol 5:539
150. Katzberg RW, Morris TW, Burgener FA, Kamm DE, Fischer HW (1977) Renal renin and hemodynamic response to selective renal artery catheterization and angiography. Invest Radiol 12:381

151. Katzberg RW, Meggs LG, Hollenberg NK, Abrams HL (1980) Investigations into the decrease in renal blood flow following selective angiography (Abstr). Invest Radiol 15:429
152. Norby LH, Bibona GF (1975) The renal vascular effects of meglumine diatrizoate. J Pharmacol Exp Ther 193:932
153. Gazitua S, Scott JB, Chou CC, Haddy FJ (1969) Effects of osmolarity on canine renal vascular resistance. Am J Physiol 217:1216
154. Gazitua S, Scott JB, Swindall B, Haddy FJ (1971) Resistance responses to local changes in plasma osmolality in three vascular beds. Am J Physiol 220:384
155. Russel SB, Sherwood T (1974) Monomer/dimer contrast media in the renal circulation: experimental angiography. Br J Radiol 47:268
156. Dorph S, Sovak M, Talner LB, Rosen L (1977) Why does kidney size change during urography? Invest Radiol 12:246
157. Morris TW, Katzberg RW, Fischer HW (1978) A comparison of the hemodynamic responses to metrizamide and meglumine/sodium diatrizoate in canine renal arteriography. Invest Radiol 13:74
158. Gruskin AB, Auerbach VH, Black IFS (1974) Intrarenal blood flow in children with normal kidneys and congenital heart disease: changes attributable to angiography. Pediatr Res 8:561
159. Read RC, Meyer M (1959) The role of red cell agglutination in arteriography complications. Surg Forum 10:472
160. Johnson JH, Knisely MH (1962) Intravascular agglutination of the flowing blood following the injection of radiopaque contrast media. Neurology (Minneap) 12:560
161. Sutherland GR, Rasensen O (1967) The effects of intra-arterial injections of radiographic contrast media on the mesenteric circulation of rats. Clin Radiol 18:200
162. Siegelman SS, Warren A, Veith FJ, Boley SJ (1970) The physiology response to superior mesenteric angiography. Radiology 96:101
163. Sovak M, Rosch J, Lakin RC (1975) Vasodilators in the canine mesenteric circulation. Invest Radiol 10:595
164. Itzchak Y, Groszmann RJ, Glickman MG (1978) The effect of hepatic arterial injection of contrast medium, blood, and saline on hepatic artery flow. Invest Radiol 13:528
165. Kagstrom E, Lindgren P, Tornell G (1958) Changes in cerebral circulation during carotid angiography with sodium acetrizoate (Trirol) and sodium diatrizoate (Hypaque). An experimental study. Acta Radiol (Stockh) 50:151
166. Tindall GT, Greenfield JC Jr, Dillingham W, Lee JF (1965) Effect of 50 percent sodium diatrizoate (Hypaque) on blood flow in the internal carotid artery in man. Am Heart J 69:215
167. Herrschaft H, Gleim F, Schmidt H (1974) Effects of angiographic contrast media on regional cerebral blood flow and haemodynamics in man. Neuroradiology 7:95
168. Talbert JL, Joyce EE, Sabiston DC Jr (1959) The effect of intra-arterial injection of radiopaque contrast media on coronary blood flow. Surgery 46:400
169. Carson R, Wever WJ, Wilson WS (1969) Effect of selective coronary arteriography on myocardial blood flow in the intact dog. Am J Med Sci 257:228
170. Kloster FE, Friesen WG, Green GS, Judkins MP (1972) Effects of coronary arteriography on myocardial blood flow. Circ Res 46:438
171. Tragardh B, Lynch P, Tragardh M (1976) Coronary angiography with diatrizoate and metrizamide. Comparison of ionic and nonionic contrast media effect on coronary blood flow in dogs. Acta Radiol (Stockh) 17:69
172. Lehan PH, Harman MA, Oldewurtel HA (1963) Myocardial water shifts induced by coronary arteriography (Abstr). J Clin Invest 42:950
173. Griggs DM Jr, Nakamura Y, Leunissen RLA, Kasparian H, Novack P (1966) Effects of radiopaque material on phasic coronary flow and myocardial oxygen consumption. Clin Res 14:247
174. Gould KL, Lipscomb K, Hamilton GW (1974) Physiological basis for assessing critical coronary stenosis. Am J Cardiol 33:87

175. Gould KL, Lipscomb K (1974) Effects of coronary stenoses on coronary flow reserve and resistance. Am J Cardiol 34:48
176. Bassan M, Ganz W, Marcus HS, Swan HJC (1975) the effect of intracoronary injection of contrast medium upon coronary blood flow. Circulation 51:442
177. Yamazaki H, Aya S, Horikawa M, Matsumura N, Nakamura Y (1975) Effects of radiopaque material on coronary vascular reserve. Jpn Heart J 16:57
178. Scheibel RL, Moore R, Korbuly D, Ovitt TW, Payne JT, Trexa N, Amplatz K (1975) Regional myocardial blood flow measurement in the evaluation of patients with coronary artery disease. Radiology 115:379
179. Bookstein JJ, Higgins CB (1977) Comparative efficacy of coronary vasodilatory methods. Invest Radiol 12:121
180. Lohr VE, Makoski HB, Fiebach O (1972) Contrast tolerance during angiography, with special reference to blood electrolyte changes. ROFO 116:367
181. Lohr E, Reidemeister JC, Popitz G, Otto H, Timmermann J (1977) Myocardial response to contrast media: effects on electrolyte metabolism and subcellular structures. Invest Radiol 12:135
182. Lohr E, Timmermann J, Reidemeister JC, Popitz G (1978) Metabolic action and cellular structure of the myocardium during coronary angiography. Cardiovasc Radiol 1:15
183. Read RC, Vick J, Meyer MW (1959) Influence of perfusate characteristics on the pulmonary vascular effects of hypertonic solutions (Abstr). Fed Proc 18:124
184. O'Connor JF, Sitzman SB, Dealy JB (1967) Vascular injury due to topical application of cardiovascular contrast medium in the hamster cheek pouch. Radiology 89:20
185. Derrick JR, Brown RW, Livanec G, Bond JP, Guest MM (1968) Experimental effects of selective arteriography on the microcirculation. Am J Surg 116:712
186. Almen T, Wiedeman MP (1968) Application of contrast media to the external surface of the vasculature. Effects on microcirculation in the bat wing. Invest Radiol 3:151
187. Almen T, Wiedeman MP (1968) Application of monomers and polymers to the external surface of the vasculature. Effects on microcirculation of the bat wing. Invest Radiol 3:408
188. Almen T, Standertskjold-Nordenstam N (1969) Effects of dyes on microvasculature of the bat wing in vivo. Invest Radiol 4:63
189. Branemark PI, Jacobsson B, Sorensen SE (1969) Microvascular effects of topically applied contrast media. Acta Radiol [Diagn] (Stockh) 8:547
190. Brown RT, Youmans CR Jr, Livanec G, Derrick JR, Bond TP, Guest MM (1968) Cinemicrographic observations of the effects of contrast media on the microcirculation. Vasc Surg 2:109
191. Almen T (1973) Application of non-ionic and ionic contrast media to the external vessel surface. Acta Radiol [Suppl] (Stockh) 335:239
192. Tuma RF, Ritchie WGM, Wiedeman MP (1974) Effects of intra-arterially injected contrast media on microvessels in the rat's cecal mesentery. Invest Radiol 9:273
193. Ritchie WGM (1975) The effect of contrast media on normal and inflamed canine venous endothelium (Abstr). Br J Radiol 48:945
194. Almen T (1976) Effects on venous vasomotion from the ionic content of contrast agent solutions. Acta Radiol [Diagn] (Stockh) 17:439
195. Ekeland A, Uflacker R (1978) Effect of meglumine metrizoate and metrizamide on the microcirculation. Acta Radiol [Diagn] (Stockh) 19:969
196. Endrich B, Ring J, Intaglietta M (1979) Effects of radiopaque contrast media on the microcirculation of the rabbit omentum. Radiology 132:331

CHAPTER 4

Basic Methods
of Investigative Cardiovascular Radiology

M. Sovak and C. B. Higgins

A. Introduction

Experimental cardiovascular radiology is a tool for the investigation of morphological and functional problems. Its methods are derived from interdisciplinary improvizations. Clinically oriented investigators are trained to define a problem and the possible ways and means to solve it; often, however, they encounter considerable difficulty in finding a description of the indispensable laboratory know-how. Sometimes these vital pieces of information are preserved only by oral tradition or are scattered throughout the literature. Unfortunately, the amount of written information has become so discouragingly voluminous that it may be tempting, rather than going through a timce-consuming and difficult search, to start experimenting by trial and error. Improper choice of laboratory animals and research techniques can in this way endanger the validity of a laborious study.

It is not the purpose of this chapter to review all that has been achieved by experimental cardiovascular radiology. Instead, this text attempts to present a synopsis of basic experimental techniques which are particularly applicable to the field and refer the reader to appropriate methodology that can be retrieved readily from the literature. Therefore, choices of reference are dictated not by the scientific merit or the extent of the results, but by their methodological relevance.

B. Contrast Media

Contrast media (CM) and experimental cardiovascular radiology have been engaged in a useful dialogue. CM assists research by visualization of cardiovascular structures, while in turn cardiovascular radiology plays an important role in pharmacologically evaluating the contrast media.

The currently used new generation of CM are discussed elsewhere in this text. For the researcher it is important to know that all CM affect the circulation in some way [1–4], which may or may not be compatible with the objectives of the experimental protocol. In varying degrees, all ionic materials decrease myocardial contractility, sinoatrial modal automacity, and atrioventricular nodal conductivity. They are also potent vasodilators. We found that among the ionic CM, a monovalent dimer [1] (ioxaglate) has the least effects. Nonionic CM affect the peripheral circulation and mycardial performance only slightly by their tendency to increase heart contractility. The colloidal Thorotrast, which due to its radioactiv-

---

1 P286, Hexabrix, Laboratoires Guerbet, France

ity is acceptable only in acute animal studies (see also Chap. 9), has the least effects on myocardial function.

I. Pharmacological Evaluation of Radiographic Contrast Media

Efforts to lower the toxicity of CM even further than the present state-of-the-art continuously result in the development of new products. For intravascular CM, vascular testing in animals has been shown to be a reliable way of predicting clinical toxicity. Also, myocardial responsiveness to even minute disturbances of its milieu can serve as a sensitive indicator of the overall toxicity of the tested CM.

Methods used in evaluation of CM toxicity have been extensively reviewed [5]. Although radiology has been committed more or less to the investigation of a single class of drugs, we are still far from knowing precisely the exact mechanisms of their toxicity, to which the plethora of methods amply attests.

The interactions of such mechanisms are also extremely complex. In general, the eliciting factors have been identified as toxicity of the triiodinated, substituted benzene moiety and/or, in the ionic compounds, of the cation; further, as electrical charge, and hyperosmolality of the aqueous solutions. At molecular level, CM interact with proteins, inhibiting their normal functions [6]. Recently, it was discovered that CM activate the serum complement systems, which initiates a cascade reaction leading to disturbances in blood coagulation and in immunological systems [7, 8].

Prior to using the more sophisticated experimental machinery for the evaluation of a new compound, the systemic toxicity should be determined. This can best be done by intravenous injection in a small rodent, i.e., by establishing the lethal dose, LD_{50}. The derangement of the cardiovascular system is most frequently the cause of LD_{50} death. LD_{50} is dependent not only on the total amount of drug tested, but also to a great extent on the concentration of its solution and the speed of injection. For comparison among the laboratories, it is important to adhere to a standardized method [9].

A simple preliminary way to study the myocardium is to use a modified Langendorff's perfused rabbit heart preparation [10]. This technique requires that clamped-off heart and lungs be rapidly removed en bloc from an animal anesthetized with a short-acting barbiturate. The ascending aorta is catheterized and perfused with Krebs' solution to which glucose and sucrose and/or dextran have been added. The solution is saturated with oxygen/carbon dioxide and the tested drug is injected into the perfusate or into the coronary arteries/aortic root. It is important, with selective injections, to match the flow of the perfusate, in order *not* to introduce an additional variable. Changes in the heart's contractility can be measured with a strain gauge or with a mercury-in-rubber ring, standard in plethysmography. ECG from two surface electrodes can also be registered. This preparation has the advantage of simplicity and high reproducibility. Also, it eliminates the effects of complex in vivo cardioperipheral reflexes. An ideal radiographic CM should not affect myocardial performance at all, but even with the mos innocuous CM, depression of contractility and rhythm disturbances are seen.

The drug's effects on the myocardium can be examined in the intact heart of either anesthetized or conscious animals. CM are injected in a standard manner

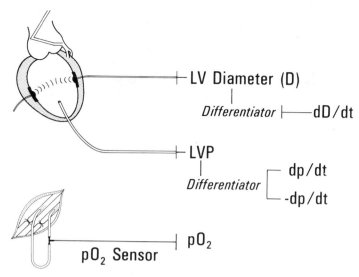

Fig. 1. Experimental model used for evaluating the effects of the intracoronary administration of CM on global left ventricular (*LV*) function. The catheter is inserted in the LV apex and ultrasonic crystals are implanted on opposing endocardial surfaces of the LV chamber. A sensor is used to continuously monitor pO_2 of blood flowing through a femoral arteriovenous fistula circuit

into the major coronary artery and changes of various parameters are registered. For studies of myocardial function in dogs, the injection is made into the left coronary artery since this artery supplies most of the myocardium. Since there is virtually an infinite number of parameters which can be followed, it will depend upon the ingenuity of the investigator to provide an experimental design based on formulation of pertinent questions and delineation of proper methods to obtain relevant answers.

In recent years, we have utilized the experimental model shown in Fig. 1. Tracings depicting the response to CM are shown in Fig. 2. A brief description of this preparation may be useful to those interested in initiating such studies:

Via a left thoracotomy, two ultrasonic crystals to measure the distance changes were placed in apposition on endocardial surfaces of the left ventricle (LV) through myocardial stab wounds. Fluid-filled catheters or solid-state pressure gauges were inserted in the aorta and LV. A modified Judkins left coronary artery catheter was inserted into the left femoral artery and advanced into the left coronary artery. Contrast materials were manually injected in a 3-ml bolus over a 2-s period during fluoroscopic observation.

During the control period and during responses, continuous records were obtained of LV pressure and its positive and negative first derivative, dP/dt and $-dP/dt$, and LV diameter and its derivate, dD/dt, at paper speeds of 2 mm/s and 50 mm/s. The parameter dD/dt was determined at an isolength point during the control period and during the hemodynamic responses to injected contrast media.

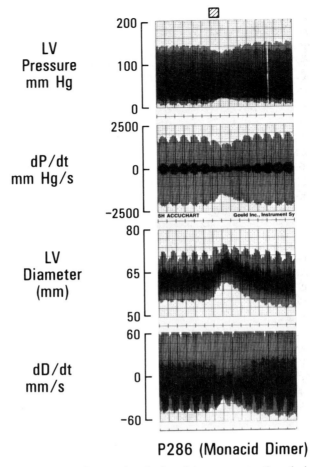

P286 (Monacid Dimer)

Fig. 2. Experimental tracings from a dog during the response to the administration of the monacid dimeric CM P286 (Hexabrix, Guerbet Laboratory) into the left coronary artery. The time and duration of injection are indicated by the *hatched box* at the top. Since the dimension decreases from diastole to systole, the parameter *dD/dt* is a negative or downward deflection. A decline in the rate of change of dimension (*dD/dt*) is indicated by a decrease an amplitude of the downward deflection

The effects of CM on cardiac rate and conduction may involve a direct inhibitory effect on the specialized tissue of the conducting system or be secondary to reflexes elicited from baro- and chemoreceptors located in the heart itself and/or in the vessels. The direct effects can be studies by injecting the drugs into arteries which directly supply the components of the cardiac conduction system. Both the artery to the sinoatrial (SA) node and to the atrioventricular (AV) node can be isolated and directly catheterized [1] (Fig. 3). A brief description of the experimental model used in our laboratory for this purpose is contained in the next paragraph.

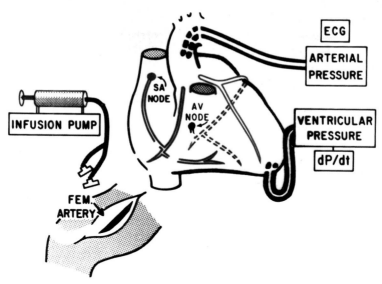

Fig. 3. Experimental model used to assess the direct effects of CM on the SA and AV nodes. CM is infused through catheters inserted into the arteries to the SA and AV nodes. The infusion pump is connected to an external perfusion circuit between the femoral artery and the artery to the sinoatrial node or the artery to the atrioventricular node

The artery to the SA node, which arises as a distal branch of the right coronary artery, is isolated and directly catheterized; so is the atrioventricular nodal artery, which arises from the distal circumflex coronary artery. Circulation to the SA and AV nodes can be maintained by an extracorporeal circuit from the same animal's femoral artery. However, this may be superfluous, since results in animals undergoing autoperfusion did not differ from the results in those with interrupted circulation to the node. The identity of the SA and AV nodal arteries can be confirmed at the start of each experiment by noting sinus arrest and bradycardia or varying degrees of heart block, respectively, after the injection of 1.0 µg acetylcholine into these arteries. The ECG is obtained from standard limb leads in order to measure heart rate and PR interval. When second degree or complete heart block occurs, the "PR interval" is computed as the interval from the P wave following the QRS complex to the next succeeding QRS complex.

During the control period (1 min) and during the infusion of CM and other solutions into the SA and AV nodal arteries, continuous records are obtained of ECG, left ventricular pressure (LVP) and its first derivative (dP/dt), and arterial pressure (AP). The duration of each infusion is 2 min. All solutions are infused at of 0.2, 0.4, 0.8, and 1.6 ml/min. All solutions are maintained in a water bath at the dog's body temperature, since varying temperatures of perfusate can cause changes in heart rate.

Correlation of metabolism of the heart muscle, morphological changes of myocardial cells, and myocardial function in response to CM has been accomplished in a dog model in which hemodynamic variables were measured and simultaneous blood samples obtained for analysis [11]. A similar preparation has

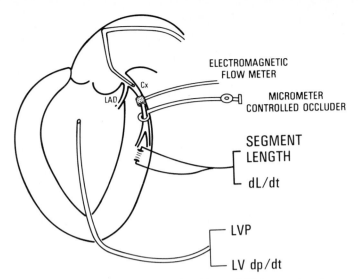

Fig. 4. Experimental model used to compare the effects of CM on regional myocardial contractile function in the normal state and in a state of regional ischemia. Regional contractile function is assessed by a pair of miniature ultrasonic crystals implanted in the myocardial wall in the distribution of the circumflex coronary artery. Regional myocardial ischemia is produced by narrowing the circumflex coronary with a micrometer-controlled constricting ring

been used in order to correlate changes in myocardial contractile state with calcium levels in the coronary sinus blood (Fig. 4).

Most studies evaluating the cardiovascular effects of CM have used normal anesthetized dogs. However, coronary arteriography is frequently performed in the presence of regional myocardial ischemia. We have developed an experimental model for comparing the contractile effects of CM in the normal state and in the presence of a critical coronary arterial stenosis. The experimental model is shown in Fig. 4, and a brief description of it follows:

Using a left thoracotomy, a polyethylene catheter is placed in the outflow portion of the through a small apical incision. The catheter tip is placed in the outflow portion of the LV in order to prevent catheter entrapment; this is confirmed by fluoroscopic observation. The proximal circumflex coronary artery is dissected free, and a 2.0- or 2.5-mm electromagnetic flow probe is snugly fitted around the artery, avoiding kinking and/or constriction, while maintaining a good wall-probe contact. Two ultrasonic piezoelectric crystals are placed in the area of the myocardium destined to become ischemic during coronary artery stenosis. The crystals are separated by a distance of approximately 1 cm. A modified Judkins coronary artery catheter is introduced into the right femoral artery and manipulated under fluoroscopic control so that the tip enters and remains wedged in the circumflex coronary artery (Cx).

The electromagnetic flow meter is calibrated in vitro using known flow rates of saline through a segment of excised vessel. During experiments, electrical zero is referenced to mechanical zero flow, induced by occlusion.

Left ventricular pressure can be measured with a strain gauge manometer (Statham P23Db) and differentiated by an R-C electronic circuit to give LV dP/dt. The ultrasonic crystals and dimension continuously measure the transit time of acoustical impulses traveling at approximately 1.5×10^6 mm/s between the two 5-MHz crystals. This provides a measure of the instantaneous distance between the crystals (segment length) after calibration with signals of known time duration. Thereby, the length of a regional myocardial segment is continuously recorded during each cardiac cycle. Differentiation of the segment length (L) signal by an R-C electronic circuit provides a measure of the velocity of contraction of the myocardial segment (dL/dt).

Calibration of the dimension gauge is performed by substituting signals of known duration from a calibrated pulse generator. A voltage proportional to transit time is recorded and calibrated in terms of crystal separation. Left ventricular pressure, dP/dt, segment length, and dL/dt are recorded on a multichannel strip chart recorder during a 30-s control period and during the response to intracoronary injection of CM.

Following injections of CM in the normal state, an occluding ligature is placed around the proximal Cx and gradually tightened until an inital increase in end-diastolic segment length (EDL) or end-systolic segment length (ESL) or a decrease in dL/dt occurs. Effects of CM are thus assessed in the presence of such "critical" coronary artery stenosis.

The effects of CM on microcirculation can be studied in standard physiological models which involve observations on the vessels in the wing of a bat [12], a rabbit's ear chamber [13], or a hamster's cheek pouch [14].

The numerous studies performed in the field of cardiovascular testing of CM are extensively reviewed in the *Encyclopedia of Radiographic Contrast Materials* [5] and the *Symposium on Contrast Media Toxicity* [15]. Pharmacological testing should ultimately result in explaining the reasons for a drug's effect on a specific organ. Only by also studying the organ function at cellular and molecular levels can this be achieved. Further elucidation of the mechanisms of CM toxicity should have considerable impact on the design of new compounds.

C. Experimental Cardioradiographic Visualization

For experimental purposes, unconventional CM may be considered. When relative inertness is the objective in an acute experiment, Thorotrast (colloidal solution of thorium dioxide) is the medium of choice. Minimum effects are produced by new nonionic materials such as metrizamide, iopamidol or iohexol, or certain experimental media [16, 17]. As a negative CM, carbon dioxide can be used. Even when large amounts of this gas are injected into the heart, its function is affected but minimally [18].

Intravascular clots can be opacified by injection of microparticles which have affinity for fibrin and adhere to the surface of the thrombus. Tantalum powder injected i.v. in small quantities can be used for this pupose [19]. A bovine osseous alkali-processed gelatin (8%–9% w/v) can be dissolved in 60% solutions of standard CM. Upon warming to 40°–50 °C, a gel is formed which injected at 38 °C adheres to the endothelium of the cardiovascular system [20]. The washout of this

adhesive CM from the vascular walls is relatively slow; thus, opacification is prolonged and areas of stagnant flow are indicated. This phenomenon can be utilized
in selective opacification of heart valves [21, 22], contour-outline of otherwise
nonopacified cardiac cavities, or prolonged opacification of terminal vessels.

For the study of blood flow patterns and/or velocity, particulate CM can be
used in conjunction with fluorography. Iodized oils (Ethiodol, Lipiodol) injected
slowly through a small catheter will form droplets in the blood stream. This approach is feasible where effects of oil microembolization are negligible (i.e., in the
portal vein and its branches [23, 24]. Nonembolizing, soluble contrast particles
are gelatin droplets imbued with CM [25, 26].

Structures can be permanently visualized by implantation of inert markers.
These can be injected as a slurry of barium sulfate or metallic tantalum powder;
metallic screws can be inserted into the tissues [27]; fine silver chains can be affixed
to moving and pliable structures [28]. It is also conceivable that small amounts
of surgical glue (cyanoacrylate) mixed with an opaque marker can be injected.

D. Choice of Experimental Animals

A wide variety of cardiophysiological studies can be conducted on practically any
animal. Circulation in creatures as exotic as the spider [29], iguana [30], snake [31
a, b], crocodile [32], and fish and amphibians [33] has been studied; often with the
help of radiology. Ducks and seals are routinely used for research on effects of
diving [34]. Such studies may be of interest to comparative physiology, but when
the results are to be applied to human cardiophysiology, the choice of experimental animals is usually limited to a narrower range, i.e., rabbit, cat, dog, pig, calf,
and infrahuman primate.

An animal model of a human disease should resemble the human condition
as closely as possible. Although this may seem an obvious prerequisite, a large
body of research carried out with the intention of applying experimental results
to clinical practice has been conducted in animals chosen more for convenience
than for model suitability. In planning experimental protocols, a comparative
animal physiology text should be consulted. Much useful data can be found in
Comparative Cardiology [35], *Biology Data Book* [36], *Handbook of Biological
Data* [37], *Handbook of Physiology* [38], and *Laboratory Animals* [39]. The physiology of the baboon was the subject of a separate monograph [40]. A thorough
review of veterinary hematology, which has become a large and complex field, is
also available [41].

I. Infrahuman Primates

Infrahuman Primates are expensive, and because of the epidemiological risks involved, their mode of use is restricted. They are, however, indispensable as models
of human arteriosclerosis, especially of the heart (see Sect. C), and may be important when human morphology is to be closely simulated. Their cost and upkeep
make them very expensive for routine cardiophysiological-pharmacological experiments.

The anatomy and physiology of the monkeys is the subject of several monographs [40, 42–46]. A well-referenced review on anesthesia in infrahuman primates is also available [47].

II. Cats

Cats are useful for cardiological research, but although they are otherwise comparable to the rabbit as an experimental animal, their cost is several times higher and they are more difficult to handle. There appear to be large variations in the blood pressure of normal cats. The comparative cardiology of the cat has been studied [48] and a detailed anatomical atlas is available [49].

III. Calves

Calves are more frequently considered for testing of cardiosurgical techniques and compatibility of implanted materials, and as models of congenital heart diseases (see Sect. C). The cardiophysiology of the calf [35] and its cardioradiographic [50] and systemic [51] anatomy have been reviewed. It is important to bear in mind when studying the calf's azygoz-hemiazygoz vein system that it is similar to that of the pig but different from that of dog and man. In calf, the hemiazygoz system is predominant. It drains the left thoracic wall and enters the anterior mediastinum at the level of the left hilar vessels to join the coronary sinus of the heart. The azygoz system is rudimentary. It drains only part of the right thoracic wall and empties into the cranial caval vein. A catheter placed into the right atrium can easily enter this vessel; fluoroscopically, the catheter seems to be lodged into a branch of the pulmonary artery.

In the following, the most accessible and easily manageable animals, i.e., rabbit, pig, and dog, will be considered in more detail.

IV. Rabbits

Rabbit has the obvious advantage of easy handling and low cost. It is ideal when a standardized animal model is needed and can be used in physiological and pharmacological studies in which the small size of its organs is not a limitation.

Because of its reproducible responses and narrow range of weight variations, the *isolated and perfused rabbit heart* is used for testing of drugs. The small physical size of the rabbit limits extensive surgical procedures and supraselective catheterization of small vessels. Intubation of the rabbit is extremely difficult and controlled ventilation generally requires tracheostomy. Mechanical ventilation may be avoided for noncomplex thoracic operations by performing a medial sternotomy and carefully confining the operation to the mediastinum so that a pneumothorax is avoided.

Rabbits intended for long-term experiments should be screened for coccidiosis, which in young animals is a relatively common disease, characterized by diarrhea and eventual dehydration.

Anatomy has been extensively reviewed in an atlas [52]. Physiological data of the rabbit can be found in *Biology of the laboratory rabbit* [53], which is the most comprehensive reference guide to the experimental use of this animal. Another source of extensive information is *Laboratory animals* [39].

V. Pigs

The pig has certain characteristics which make it a very useful animal for cardiovascular investigation. With the exception of the infrahuman primates, the anatomy of the pig most closely resembles that of the human [54]. Compared with the dog, the pig has the advantage of rapid growth. Thus, lesions such as aortic coarctation can be produced operatively in piglets to be fully developed and ready for study only a few months later. The pig is cheap and readily available and there is a consistent physiological uniformity within the species. Its rapid growth may be a disadvantage for long-term experiments. However, with the development of the so-called miniature swine, long-term studies have become feasible.

Anatomy of the pig is described in detail in a standard text [54]. Here we will mention only the most important features.

The pig's right lung consists of four lobes, the fourth being the intermediate one. The heart is in the midline and its base-apex axis lies almost parallel to the sternum. The porcine cardiovascular system is similar to that of man and other mammals. There are, however, a few important differences: (a) Unlike dog, the pig's left coronary system does not have the extensive collateral connection with the right coronary system [55]. In this respect, however, the pig's heart circulation resembles human and consequently lends itself better to the studies of altered coronary circulation [56]. The ostium of the right coronary artery, unlike that of the dog, is relatively wide and funnel shaped. Consequently, this vessel can be catheterized without severely compromising its blood flow [10].

Another important difference is a large ostium of the coronary sinus which makes it easily accessible to catheterization via the right atrium [57]. While the dog and man have a rudimentary hemiazygoz and prominent azygoz venous systems, the opposite is true in pigs. Its prominent azygoz vein joins the great cardiac vein or empties directly into the right atrium.

Young piglets have a prominent ductus arteriosus which can be easily catheterized. The vessels of young pigs are more fragile than those of dogs.

The pig's chest configuration is important for thoractomy. Although median sternotomy gives good exposure of the heart, it is not, unless absolutely necessary, the approach of choice for long-term experiments. The clavicules articulate with each other behind the manubrium sterni and good exposure requires incision into this joint. Healing of mid-sternal thoractomy takes longer compared with approaching through the lateral wall of the chest.

Unlike other animals, the pig does not manifestly go through the excitation phase of barbiturate anesthesia. Since they are prone to stop breathing, especially if the drug is given too rapidly, it is advisable to intubate the animal as soon as possible. This is best done with the animal supine on the table with head extended downwards, while an assistant opens the pig's mouth and extends the tongue. A tracheal tube is inserted using a laryngoscope. The insertion must be swift and under direct visual control since pigs are especially prone to develop laryngospasm. Remedies such as blowing oxygen or spraying xylocaine on the vocal cords are usually futile. Thus, in the case of laryngospasm it is best not to lose any more time, but perform tracheotomy as quickly as possible.

Porcine physiology is extensively reviewed in a comprehensive reference describing various methods applicable to cardiovascular research in both pigs and miniature pigs, and listing normal values of blood gases, blood volume, blood volume in relation to body weight, cardiac output, blood pressure, pulse rate, etc. [58]. The hematology of the pig is dealt with in a specialized review [41].

1. Catheterization: Implantation of Chronic Catheters

For chronically indwelling venous catheters, the external jugular vein of the central ear vein [59] can be used. Small-diameter silastic catheters are preferable to polyethylene ones because of their low thrombogenicity. Even with both external jugular veins occluded, it does not affect the animal since the thrombosis remains localized. The catheters can be tunneled under the skin to emerge and can be anchored in the region of the posterior neck. Unlike dogs, pigs are prone to scratch that region by rubbing and catheters must therefore be protected by a leather harness.

2. Acute Catheterization

Larger blood samples can be rapidly withdrawn from the cranial caval vein of an anesthetized animal by percutaneous puncture from the region above the right sternoclavicular joint.

The umbilical artery can be catheterized directly in a newborn piglet. However, the artery tends to obliterate very rapidly and more than 48 h after the birth it must be searched for via a paramedian incision below the umbilicus [60]. The heart can be most conveniently catheterized from the vessels of the neck, i.e., the interior or exterior jugular veins and carotid arteries. The vessels of the groin can be easily exposed in young and miniature pigs but may be difficult to localize in older animals.

VI. Dogs

The dog is the easiest and most manageable experimental animal, responding to most stimuli in a manner similar to man, and is therefore popular for model studies. The one major drawback of the dog is the difficulty in achieving uniformity within the experimental series. Ideally, in a comparative study, only one breed of dog should be used since the physiological differences within a group of "mongrels" may be considerable. Consequently, the investigator will have to decide whether his protocol is meaningful without a series of standardized experimental animals.

As a general rule, hounds, bassets, and beagles are best suited for cardiac experimentation. Collies and related breeds should be avoided since their vessels are more fragile and their hearts more prone to develop arrhythmias upon direct manipulation. In standardized experiments, beagles are probably the most widely used. The anatomy and some physiological experimental techniques in this breed have been reviewed extensively [6]. Much of the valuable information contained in that book can be applied to related breeds, however. The hematology of the dog has been the subject of a thorough review [41].

Anatomy has been reviewed in detail elsewhere [62]; hence only the most important features will be mentioned here.

No gross differences exist between the numerous breeds, but the thoracic structures of the dog differ substantially from those in humans.

The canine *thoracic cavity* has a triangular, pyramidal shape. Diaphragmatic cupoles are high, resulting in a rather sharp angle between the thoracic wall and the diaphragm, especially in the anterior portion of the thorax. The level of the diaphragm's attachment to the rib cage is more caudal than in man. This must be remembered in order to avoid inadvertent production of the pneumothorax during laparotomy. The left lung has three lobes: apical, cardiac, and diaphragmatic. The apex of the apical lobe usually has a curved-beak shape, which in the sagittal plane projects behind the manubrium sterni. The right lung is larger than the left and is divided into apical, cardiac, intermediate, and diaphragmatic lobes. The right apical lobe is in the form of a casquet which covers the upper third of the right heart.

The *pericardium* is loosely attached to the diaphragm and sternum in the mediastinal sagittal plane, thus being fairly mobile.

Heart position in the thoracic cavity varies greatly in different breeds. In those with a relatively wide thorax such as hounds, greyhounds, bassets, and beagles, the heart apex is in the left side of the thorax and its base-apex axis is thus placed similarly to man's. In dogs with a narrow thorax the apex may be behind the sternum and the base-apex axis of the heart is almost parallel to the spine and the axis of the sternum in the sagittal plane. In certain breeds, especially the brachycephalic ones, it is not unusual to find the apex in the right side of the thorax.

Thoracotomy. Access to the heart is best achieved through the left fourth or fifth intercostal space. When a rib-spreader is used costotomy is not usually necessary. In contradistinction to man, the mediastinum contains only esophagus, trachea, and heart with the great vessels, and the supporting tissue is all but nonexistent. Therefore, although the pleura divides the dog's thorax into two cavities, the high pliability of the mediastinum is the reason why a unilateral pneumothorax always means a collapse of both lungs. The sternum is an important strain-bearing component of the canine thoracic cage. For this reason, mid-sternal thoracotomy is not the access of choice in long-term experiments because healing can be compromised.

The radiographic anatomy of the canine heart has been extensively studied [63 a, b]. In different breeds there is considerable variation in the shape of the cardiac silhouette and its relation to the thoracic organs both in lateral and posteroanterior radiography. The left anterior lateral aspect of the canine heart roughly corresponds to the anterior aspect of the human heart. The position of the dog's great vessels is variable in relation to the cardiac silhouette. Thus, the aortic arch may be almost totally superimposed over the other cardiac structures while the relationship of the ascending and descending aorta may also vary greatly. Within the left cardiac border the pulmonary artery is the structure showing greatest pulsation at fluoroscopy.

In younger dogs the pulmonary arteries as well as the aortic arch may be obscured by a prominent thymus. The position and number of pulmonary veins (usually six) may also vary considerably. The azygoz vein is almost parallel to the aorta and joins the posterior aspect of the cranial caval vein close to the right atrium.

During repeated radiographic examinations, it should be recalled that due to the high pliability of he mediastinum and pericardium the heart position is not fixed and great variations may occur.

Detailed descriptions of the anatomy of dog's heart are available [64–66]. The anatomy of the dog's *heart valves* is similar to that of pig and man except that canine valves contain some blood vessels in their base, close to their attachment to the annulus fibrosus. Also, the edges of the valves are more irregular than in man and in addition to the large cusps, both mitral and tricuspid valves may have small accessory leaflets. The chordae tendinae anchor the mitral valve to two papillary muscles while the tricuspid valve is attached to four papillary muscles. The relative contribution by the cusps to the total area of the mitral or tricuspid valve may vary considerably [67].

The aortic valve is situated on the basis of the aortic bulb, arising from the three aortic sinuses. There are left, right, and posterior semilunar cusps. In the center of the outer border of each cusp is a nodulus which permits close conformation and adaptation of the cusps during the diastolic phase. The valve of the pulmonary artery also consists of left, right, and central semilunar cusps located at the base of the trunk of the pulmonary artery.

In lateral radiography, the plane of mitral annulus projects into the fifth intercostal space (i.s.) or overlaps the sixth rib, perpendicular to its axis. The plane of the aortic valve is in the fourth i.s. and almost parallel with the fourth rib, over which it may be superimposed. The plane of the pulmonary valve projects into the third i.s. and that of the tricuspid valve into the fourth i.s. Both are nearly perpendicular to the ribs.

The mitral valve sound can be best heard in the fifth left intercostal space and the tricuspid valve in the fourth right. Sounds of the aortic pulmonary valves are most prominent in the fourth left intercostal space [68].

The cardiac conduction system consists of the SA node, intraatrial bundle, AV node, common bundle of His with its left and right branches, and the terminal Purkinje fibers. The SA node is located where the ventral aspect of the cranial caval vein joins the right auricle. The AV node is located in the interatrial septum and can be best approached from the right atrium. From the AV node the common bundle of His originates, running anteriorly and caudally, and divides at the level of the fibrous base of the heart into the right and left bundles of His. These bundles are located in the interventricular septum immediately under the endocardium. They end in a complex system of Purkinje fibers in the outer wall of both ventricles [68–72].

The ECG of the dog is similar to that of man, but not identical. The conduction patterns are different and should an inference from the dog study be made to a human condition, it is advisable to consult the appropriate references [68, 73].

The normal impulse arises from the SA node and is conducted into the AV node to reach the ventricular myocardium through the bundle of His. The ventricular depolarization starts with the caudal portion of the interventricular septum, spreading thereafter into the outer walls and apex and finally into the parts of the ventricle close to the heart base and the cranial part of the interventricular septum [73]. The resting heart rate in conscious dogs is extremely variable, ranging from 70 to 160 beats/min in dogs of 15–30 kg. In smaller breeds it is not unusual to find 180 beats/min as a normal resting frequency. Puppies have a normal rhythm of approximately 220 beats/min. In average dogs, veterinary medicine considers frequencies under 70 beats/min as bradycardia and above 160 beats/min as tachycardia [68].

Coronary Vessels. The anatomy of the canine coronary system has been the subject of a separate study [14]. The differences between the coronary systems of dog and man are great enough that, should a close simulation be desired, other experimental animals must be chosen. The main differences are:

1. The myocardium of the dog is supplied preponderantly by the left coronary artery.
2. The interventricular septum is supplied mostly by the single septal ventral artery, a branch of the ventral interventricular artery or of the left common coronary artery [75].
3. The left and right coronary arteries communicate through a large net of anastomoses found most abundantly near the heart apex, in the outer layer of the myocardium [76]. Other communications between the right coronary artery and other parts of the coronary system are the right and left auricular arteries, the ventricular lateral branches of the right coronary artery, and the anterior descending branch of the left circumflex coronary artery.
4. The main atrial branch of the right coronary artery usually supplies the SA node via the SA node artery, although the node may also be supplied by a branch from the internal mammary artery. Because of this variability and the large number of anastomoses between the right and left coronary systems, it is practically impossible to deprive completely the SA node of its blood supply [77].
5. The AV node is supplied only by branches from the left coronary and septal arteries; their ligation produces an AV block [78].

Arising from the right aortic sinus, *the right coronary artery* is smaller than the left. It supplies mainly the outer wall of the right ventricle and part of the right atrium. Reportedly, in 20% of all dogs, an accessory right coronary artery can be found originating in the right aortic sinus [79]. The main right coronary artery divides into four to nine ventricular branches. *The left coronary artery* arises from the left aortic sinus dividing into ventral, interventricular and left circumflex arteries. Occasionally these two vessels may arise directly from the left aortic sinus. The left circumflex artery gives off 4 to 11 ventricular branches, the main ones being the left marginal, dorsal interventricular, and central interventricular. The ventral septal artery arises from the left common coronary artery in 19% of dogs; in 49% it branches off the central interventricular; from the aorta in 5%; from the circumflex in 1%; and in 27% it can be one of three terminal branches of the left coronary artery. The cranial portion of the ventral septal artery runs close under the endocardium of the right ventricle. The caudal part runs in the middle of the septum toward the papillary muscles. The sometimes multiple dorsal septal artery originates from the left circumflex, supplying in part the atrial septal wall and the region of the AV node. In older dogs it is not unusual to find intimal proliferation in those larger coronary vessels which are exposed to the largest motion [80].

The coronary veins in general accompany the arteries but may be double. In veterinary anatomical terminology the veins are not named according to the corresponding artery, which may lead to confusion. All veins eventually end in the coronary sinus, which is usually cranially from the circumflex branch of the left coronary artery, and empties into the caudal part of the posteromedial aspect of the right atrium, in the vicinity of the junction of the caudal caval vein. In the sinuses ostium, a small semilunar valve can sometimes be found, which may be a potential obstacle during catheterization.

The lymphatic system of the dog's heart has been extensively described [81, 82], but is omitted from standard dog anatomy textbooks. This study may be important, especially in view of the recently recognized important role of lymphatics in the pathophysiology of myocardial infarction. Briefly, lymphatic vessels of the heart can be divided into cardial, myocardial, and epicardial plexuses. They communicate through many lymphatic channels whose course in general follows the cardiac vessels. Ultimately united into a single cardiac lymphatic, they carry the lymph to the pulmonary artery via an ingress on the artery's anterior surface. The myocardial lymph flow has been studied in detail in [82].

E. The Laboratory for Cardiovascular Contrast Media Research

Minimum requirements include one large room, an adjacent preparatory area, a separate area for X-ray equipment control, and an easily accessible dark room. In the laboratory itself the design should provide for free movement and flexibility. All furniture and apparatus should be as mobile as possible and any heavy equipment should be located only after the traffic patterns have been determined. The layout should not serve to accommodate the technology, but to adapt it to the normal patterns of human locomotion. A laboratory assembled without consideration to the human form and function induces stress, which, while perceived only subconsciously, negatively influences the work.

If the laboratory can house only one single plane X-ray unit, it is advisable to suspend the X-ray tube from a ceiling crane which can be moved across the entire room. The image intensifier and film changer should be suspended on movable stands which permit their use both in horizontal and vertical positions for fluorography or radiography in either of the two planes. With overhead X-ray tubes, scattered radiation is higher than with tubes mounted under the table, but this can be easily counteracted by careful collimation and use of lead-containing curtains suspended around the tube.

C-arm-mounted X-ray equipment for both fluoroscopy and fluorography is also useful. The C-arm unit should be constructed so that the rotational movement is counterbalanced and the arm can be manually turned. The vertical movement can be accomplished using simple electrohydraulics.

X-ray tables should have adjustable height both for surgery and magnification radiography, using electrohydraulics whenever possible.

The basic animal radiographic techniques are described elsewhere [83]. Since multiple exposures are required in cardiac experimentation, the X-ray tube must have a high-speed rotating anode equipped with two focal spots (preferably 0.3 and 1.2 mm). Another tube with a very small focal spot (50–100 μm) for magnification radiography should be available as accessory equipment. A good image intensifier is a necessity; most of the work can be done with a 6″ screen. The fluoroscopical system should be televised. It is possible to improvise the fluorovideo chain inexpensively by using a standard Plumbicon-tube TV camera and a TV monitor.

Video recording systems are finding increasing application for cardiodynamic studies. Improvement of video signal processing plays a significant role in experimental angiography and will certainly be affected by CM developments. Although the resolution of most video is still limited, video is inexpensive to operate; with continuous development in the field, higher frame registration rates are becoming feasible. Most usually, the frame rate is limited to a standard of 30/s.

Since cardiac morphological studies largely depend upon resolving the movement of fast-moving structures, *cinefluorographic equipment* is a necessity. All clinical units operate with a pulsed X-ray, bu in animals filming can be carried out with continuous exposure since radiation is not a hazard. Avoiding the X-ray-pulsed unit saves money both in purchase and upkeep cost. With the availability of high-resolution films and absence of time pressure in clinical situations, a 16-mm film system is advisable. Even the standard 16-mm films [*Plus-X, Tri-X* (Kodak)] yield high-quality images when developed for fine grain at low temperatures and slow speed. Compared with 35-mm films, 16-mm films can be more easily analyzed and are more economical. In the 16-mm system when high resolution is needed, certain color films offer an alternative to black and white by being virtually grainless. Although most cinceradiography in a cardiac lab can be carried out at speeds of less than 100 frames/s, it is advisable to have the capability of filming at higher speeds. High-speed 16-mm cameras originally developed for military reconnaisance (for example, Teledyne Camera Systems, Arcadia, CA) are available at a fraction of the cost of cameras offered by X-ray companies for clinical use. They are capable of maintaining highly precise filming rates ranging from 1 to 500 frames/s. The shutter mechanism of such cameras has a great advantage over the previously used rotating prism film transport since it allows more light per frame to reach the film. The so-called ultrafast lenses of F 0.9 and less are expensive but not superior to the standard lenses of F 1.1–1.3 based on the light transmission measurements.

Cineradiography can be applied to studies of blood-flow patterns [84], measurement of left ventricular performance [85, 86], and movement of cardiac structures [21, 22]. The filming rates are determined by what information the investigator wishes to obtain. To resolve in detail the patterns of the heart valve's movement at a heart rate of 70–80 beats/min, a filming rate of over 200 frames/s must be used. On the other hand, for left ventricular volumetry using a biplane system, volume curves with less than 5% error can be generated at filming speeds of 15 frames/s because of the low frequency content of the recording [87]. A study using a computer data reduction system has shown that left ventricular volume, left ventricular length, and left ventricular pressure are all low-frequency signals. Filming speeds of 60 frames/s are therefore adequate for reconstruction of their continuous curves [88].

Biplane X-ray Apparatus. Although single-plance cinefluorography can yield a reasonable approximation of the true size of cardiac cavities in motion [89], precise reconstruction of the tree-dimensional space can be obtained only from two perpendicular, simultaneous recordings.

Equipment for Cine Analysis. A cardioradiographic laboratory should have a capability of frame-by-frame analysis. Projection apparatus based on rotating prism is designed primarily for clinical applications and is rather expensive. For research, where flexibility is of importance, an overhead projector (Vanguard, Inc.) or a modified standard 16-mm projector (Athena, L & W Photo, Inc. Van Nuys, CA) capable of frame-by-frame film transport is more economical and versatile; it can also be used with a sound track.

Correlation Systems. A way of synchronizing physiological parameters with the cinefluorography recordings is needed in order to correlate the dynamical and morphological aspects of heart function. At low filming speeds, i.e., 24 frames/s, a reasonably accurate correlation can be achieved using good paper recorders with a marker signal simultaneously recorded on the paper and on the film. With higher filming speeds it is necessary to record the tracings of the parameters directly on the fluoroscopically exposed film. Oscilloscope can be attached directly to the camera, allowing projection of the tracing through an optical system using a side lens, to the back of the film [90]. If a biplane X-ray system is used, both films have to be time coded for future analysis. This can be achieved by a time-code generator which marks both films simultaneously during the run.

Instead of modifying the camera, it is possible to project the displayed traces into the camera's aperture via a modified light distributor of the image intensifier. The physiological parameters converted into their digital form can be displayed simultaneously with the traces on each of the cine frames [91]. Such arrangement allows precise correlation and accelerates the film evaluation process.

When a video rather than a cine recording system is used, the correlation is simple. The input of the video recorder's audio channels can be electronically divided into three bands each by a frequency modulator (Vetter Co., Rebersburg, PA). In this way, up to six parameters can be recorded simultaneously with the video image on the same tape.

Magnification Radiography. To visualize small structures, some form of magnification is needed. A full account of this technique including photographic enlargement, direct magnification radiography, microradiography of specimens, and in vivo microradiography is available [92]. Briefly, photographic enlargement is limited by the resolution of the radiogram. A standard radiogram can be magnified about ten times without great loss of detail [93]. Industrial films with very fine grain emulsions increase the resolution, but require longer X-ray exposure. Some of the newer fine emulsion films developed for mammography and also the newer aerial reconnaisance films offer an improvement in their contrast-to-grain size ratio. Such films are better suited for optical (photographic) magnification than the standard X-ray films.

The degree of direct *geometrical magnification* achieved by decreasing the focus-to-object distance is limited by the size of the focal spot. Every focal spot except an infinitely small one will produce some penumbra, thus imposing a limit on how close the object can be to the tube. The closer the object is to the focus and the larger the focal spot, the larger the image penumbra and thus the less sharp the image edges. A large focal spot, however, may be indispensable if the object is moving and a short exposure required to avoid image blurring. Another factor which influences the image quality is scattered radiation generated by the X-rayed object. If the object is close enough to the film for the scattered radiation to reach the image, blurring will occur. Scattered radiation can be absorbed by grids, but stationary grids decrease the image quality, and moving grids of the reciprocating type are too slow for very short exposures. Using a 100-cm distance focus-to-film and 33-cm object-to-focus distance technique, little of the scatter radiation will reach the film; however, a rotating circular grid (Cook, Inc., Indianapolis, IN) [94, 95] further enhances the image quality.

Radiography with a 0.3-mm focal spot and a twofold geometrical magnification results in doubling of the line pair resolution compared with a 1-mm focal spot [96]. Unfortunately, most of the 0.3-mm tubes on the market do not have a sufficiently high capacity to allow the short exposure required for radiography in larger animals. Tubes with focal spots under 0.3 mm with high-speed rotating anodes and heat capacity close to 8,000 watts are now available [97]. Even so, X-ray exposure has to be relatively long, which poses a limitation on image sharpness in radiography of rapidly moving objects. In cardioradiography it is possible to ameliorate this condition by tying the exposure to a given part of the cardiac cycle [98 a, b]. Most of the automatic injectors are, or can be, equipped with appropriate intercalative programmers. For large magnification in smaller animals, or for magnification fluorography, a very small focal spot (50–100 µm) tube can be used.

Field Emission X-Ray Apparatus (Field Emission Corp., McMinneville, OR). This offers a useful and economical alternative to visualization of rapidly moving structures in smaller animals without image blurring caused by motion [99]. The end-emission X-ray tube is energized for approximately 30 ns by a condensor discharge; at a tube-film distance of 20–24 ins. and 150–180 kV, excellent chest radiographs in dogs and pigs can be produced. These ultra-short bursts of X-rays can be repeated at a rate of 20/s. The exposures can be triggered by physiological recording apparatus.

Computed tomography (CT) has added a new dimension to the field. A fast-scanning CT can be a useful tool in the study of cardiac morphology, while dynamic CT scanning is an efficient tool for investigation of CM pharmacokinetis (see Chap. 10, this volume).

Automatic Injectors. Programmable injectors are indispensable when injection is to be made at a certain point in the cardiac cycle. Manual, simple air, or motor-operated "one-shot" injectors will suffice for most of the work.

Recording of Physiological Parameters. Physiological recording equipment purchased with insufficient technical information often later causes much unhappiness. Elaborate medicoclinical terminology often makes it easy to forget that what are basically needed are only preamplifiers, amplifiers, filters, and possibly integrating and derivating circuits. The investigator should primarily decide what he needs, i.e., which biosignals he wants to record, what range amplification is required, and how the signals will be electronically manipulated. Excellent experimental physiological equipment can be purchased inexpensively from the general electronics market and smaller companies specializing in animal instrumentation.

When purchasing amplifiers, the most important factors to be considered are:

1. Degree of amplification.
2. Possible interference of the power source.
3. Shielding against the interference of other apparatus, especially the X-ray generators.
4. Quality and ranges of filtration. Filters are indispensable and a selective net frequency filter is desirable. Stepwise frequency bandpass filters are accurate, but filtration based on a frequency cutoff is difficult to calibrate.
5. Versatility: The unit must have inputs and outputs to be used as a module. Extra signal outputs are required so that additional monitors (oscilloscopes) can be connected. "Engineered systems" made not to allow combination with any other manufacturer's apparatus have no place in the experimental laboratory.

Oscilloscopes should be of the storage type and be able to accommodate at least four to six channels. The channels should have low-gain amplifier capability and be able to record correlation of different high-frequency biosignals. Instant photography of the screen is useful as well. Clinical "display scopes", i.e., "monitoring equipment", have a limited use in the laboratory.

Recorders use plain, plastic-coated, heat- or UV-sensitive, or photographic paper. In the latter system the signal is reduced by an oscilloscopic beam, giving an extremely fast frequency response, but the disadvantage is the time-consuming development of the paper. UV-sensitive papers are not light-permanent and bleach out with time. Frequency response of pen recorders suffices for most applications; recorders using pressurized ink are generally superior to systems based on gravity or capillary ink flow. There is no advantage to recorders which use a heated stylus and heat-sensitive paper if their frequency response is not superior to inks systems or if they are not substantially cheaper. Certain heat-sensitive papers are also touch sensitive, which under laboratory conditions can prove to be a major nuisance.

Electromagnetic tape recorders are very useful for recording long experiments with the possibility of later editing such tape on an oscilloscope and writing out the relevant portions on a paper recorder. Multichannel recorders built especially to register biological signals simultaneously are expensive. In both experimental and clinical laboratories, signals can be recorded economically and precisely with a good standard stereo casette type recorder used in conjunction with frequency modulators (Vetter Co., Rebersburg, PA). The frequency modulator makes it possible to record three analog signals on each of the two standard stereo audio channels. Thus, simultaneous recording of up to six parameters is feasible; or, three parameters and an audio channel can be utilized. The inexpensive casette tapes have a running time capacity of up to 1 h on each side. Certain stereo casette systems allow doubling the time by halving the speed.

F. Cardiovascular Catheterization

Angiographic techniques have been developed to the point where in principle anything can be catheterized. The only limitations are size of catheter, dexterity of the investigator, and resolving power of the radiographic system.

Catheterization of the mammalian heart and its vessels can be conveniently accomplished either through direct insertion of the catheters upon thoracotomy or via the vessels of the neck of groin. Since the normal pressure in the thorax is negative (-5 mmHg), thoracotomy increases the right atrial pressure, which affects the cardiac performance. Thus thoracotomy should be avoided and indirect catheterization of the heart and its vessels should be carried out from the periphery whenever possible.

Compared with man, femoral arteries of dog and pig are surrounded by a relatively thin layer of fasciae. Thus, in long-term experiments the percutaneous approach (Seldinger) is preferable, but following the retraction of the catheter, prolonged compression of the punctured artery is necessary. Because of vessel fragility, exchange of percutaneously introduced catheters may lead to seepage-bleeding around the puncture, with ensuing hematomas which can mar the entire experiment.

Therefore, when the experiment is of short-term nature, it is more advantageous to catheterize the vessels by a cut-down under direct vision. The vessels of the groin and neck are easily accessible to arteriotomy or venotomy. In dogs, the scalpel is preferable to the elctric knife for a cut-down in the groin region. The vessels are so close to the skin they may take part in the electrical circuit and burst.

Femoral arteries of dogs, pigs, or rabbits can be tied off with no damage to limb circulation. These animals have plentiful collateral arterial systems which supply the pelvic limb in absence of the main femoral artery. In addition to the femoral artery and its branches, the leg's vascular supply arises from the superficial circumflex iliac and caudal gluteal arteries. The *femoral vein* is not essential for free drainage of blood from the limbs. *The external jugular vein* of dog or pig is especially well suited for catheter access to the heart. It is located laterally on the neck, crossing the sternocleidomastoid muscle at various heights, depending upon the breed, but always lying subcutaneously. In dogs, if the vein is not immediately visible it can be made prominent by applying pressure on the neck, simulating a tight collar, above the manubrium sterni. In pigs this is feasible only in younger animals of approximately 20–40 kg weight. In larger pigs the external jugular vein is buried in fat and may be difficult to find. In such cases it is advisable to extend the incision, reach the lateral aspect of trachea, and catherize the internal jugular vein instead.

In mammals *the common carotid artery* and *the internal jugular vein* closely follow the posterolateral aspect of the trachea. It can be easily reached by a lateral or mid-neck incision. The lateral approach, however, is preferable since by blunt splitting of the plethysma muscle and blunt entry into the paratracheal space these vessels can be approached rapidly and bloodlessly. The portion of common carotid artery between the thoracic inlet and the inferior thyroid artery does not usually give out branches and it is in this portion that arteriotomy is most conveniently carried out. In dogs, the internal jugular vein is smaller than the external jugular vein, but not so in pigs and rabbits.

The left ventricle can be approached either retrogradely via the aorta or from the left atrium. In transaortic catheterization with relatively large and/or stiff catheters, a loop at their end should help to cross the aortic valve. Alternatively, the left ventricle as well as *left atrium* can be catheterized via the external jugular vein and puncture of the interatrial septum [100]. This human cardiological technique was adapted to the anatomy of dogs and pigs [101]. The original Ross needle for humans is too long, flexible, and curved for a puncture in dogs or pigs; a short, stiff stylet is preferable. It is remarkable that even after experiments of long duration with several exchanges of large-diameter catheters no shunt is created in surviving animals [102]. This may be explained by the structure of the mammalian interatrial septum which contains several layers of myofibrils running in different directions. A contraction of these fibrils seals off a puncture very efficiently. The scar takes but a few days to form.

Access to the left heart via the external jugular vein and interatrial septal puncture is extremely useful and will be described here in some detail. With the animal supine, the external jugular vein is approached by skin incision where the vein crosses the sternocleidomastoideal muscle. A segment 3 cm in length is exposed, the cranial end is tied off, and a free snare is placed on the caudal end. Prior to the venotomy the snare is gently pulled up to prevent an accidental air embolus should the pressure in the right atrium be negative. A catheter with a slightly curved tip is introduced into the caudal caval vein through the venotomy under the control of lateral beam fluoroscopy. After flushing with heparinized saline, the curved tip is pointed toward the spine and the catheter is slowly retracted. In pigs, the catheter will tend to enter the ostium of the coronary sinus. Passing the junction of the caudal caval vein with the right atrium, the tip of the catheter is seen "climbing up" the promontorial torus intervenosus (intervenous tubercle) (see Figs. 5, 6). At that point the AV node is stimulated and extrasystolies occur. On further retraction, the tip of the catheter falls from the torus posteriorly.

A stylus which has been made to fit the tip of the catheter and which has about 30° curvature is passed inside the catheter and turned, while still in the catheter, toward the atrial septum at an angle of approximately 45° to the sagittal plane. With the tip pointing directly against the septum, the stylus is advanced beyond the tip, and the catheter with the stylus punctures the septum. When both the stylus and the catheter enter the left atrium, the catheter is threaded over the stylus further into the left atrium, the catheter is threaded over the stylus further into the left heart, the stylus is retracted, and the catheter is flushed. Using a flexible tip guide wire, catheters can be exchanged. With this technique, the puncture site lies cranially high in the septum. In dogs, puncture can be carried out of the fossa ovalis, but then only via the caudal caval vein. Such an approach carries no obvious advantage.

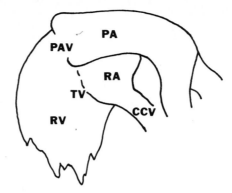

Fig. 5. Semischematic outline of opacified right ventricle (*RV*), tricuspid valve (*TV*), right atrium (*RA*), caudal caval vein (*CCV*), pulmonary artery (*PA*), and pulmonary artery valve (*PAV*) in left lateral projection

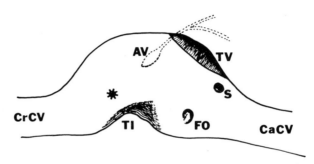

Fig. 6. Schematic outline of the right side of the interatrial septum in the dog. In the pig, the relative position of structures is similar, but the ostium of the coronary sinus is wider. *, approximate site of the puncture; *CrCV*, cranial caval vein; *TI*, torus intervenosus ("crista interveniens"); *FO*, fossa ovalis; *S*, sinus venosus; *AV*, atrioventricular node; *TV*, ostium of the tricuspid valve; *CaCV*, caudal caval vein

The pulmonary artery (PA) can be catheterized via the caval veins. It can be entered more conveniently from the caudal than the cranial caval vein. Very much as in humans, the technique is based on passing a slightly curved catheter into the right ventricle, subsequently formed into a loop. To enter the PA, the bow of the loop has to be "knocked" across the pulmonary valve, and the catheter straightened by a gentle retraction.

The right ventricle and right atrium can be catheterized via either of the caval veins. The coronary sinus and the azygoz and hemiazygoz veins can all best be entered via the external jugular vein with a curved catheter.

Coronary arteries can be opacified by a nonselective technique using a pigtail catheter placed into the aortic bulb. Selectively they can be catheterized with a small-diameter slightly curved catheter, which can be introduced from the femoral or carotid arteries. Slight modification of the curve of the Judkin's left coronary catheter allows for relatively simple selective catheterization of the left coronary artery of larger dogs (over 20 kg).

Supraselective catheterization of coronary branches is difficult, mainly because the catheters interfere with the blood flow. If the size of the main vessel permits, the catheter can be lodged into its ostium and another catheter (a thin polyethylene catheter, stiffened with wire) is passed beyond its tip and wedged into a coronary branch. The larger catheter is then retracted to the aorta. Further retraction is almost impossible without dislodging the small-size catheter. It is important to keep the friction between the two catheters as low as possible by applying a thin film of silicon oil on the surface. The supraselective approach may require heparinization of the animal.

In short-term experiments, thin stainless steel 18-gauge tubing can be employed for catheterization of the left coronary artery, causing minimal interference with the coronary blood flow [103]. The steel tubing should be slightly curved, and furnished with a flexible plastic tubing tip. Under fluoroscopic guidance with the tip pointing posteriorly, the tubing assembly is passed from the right common carotid artery to the ascending aorta. Pulsations felt on the tubing mean that the tip has reached one of the aortic leaflets. With clockwise rotation, the tip enters the ostium of the left coronary artery. If the protocol design precludes a test injection of a CM, the catheter's position can be ascertained by taking a pressure recording. A characteristic coronary pressure tracing indicates the tip's position in the coronary vessel.

It is more difficult to enter the ostium of the right than the left coronary artery from the common carotid artery. Generally, the right canine coronary artery is more difficult to catheterize and although it is usually possible to introduce a catheter into the ostium, interference with the blood flow usually ensues. Unlike the gradually narrowing left coronary artery in the dog or right coronary artery in the pig, the proximal portion of the dog's right artery has a cylindrical shape. A simple technique for catheterization of rabbit's coronary arteries has been developed [104].

Catheters used in experimental work are in principle the same as those used clinically. In dogs and pigs exceeding 25 kg, Judkins' coronary catheters can be utilized. In other animals, variability of the morphology makes demands on the improvisational talents of the investigator. Polyethylene thermoplastic materials are preferred.

Catheters intended for high-speed injections should have side holes to prevent jet injury to the cardiovascular structures, and catheters introduced for blood sampling should be relatively large with numerous side holes to allow free withdrawal even if the catheter is adjacent to the vascular wall.

All catheters are to a greater or lesser extent thrombogenic. During any catheterization, thrombi develop on the surface of the catheters. This occurs in clinical situations and even more so in the dog, whose clotting system is more easily activated. Upon retraction of the catheters the thrombi strip and remain in the terminal vessel. In humans, they are subject to rapid dissolution provided the fibrinolytic system functions normally. In animal experiments, however, the thrombi may compromise the protocol. Thus, the investigator has a choice of occasionally flushing the catheters with heparinized saline in a concentration of

5,000 IU (42 mg) heparin/liter or, since this is not always effective, of fully heparinizing the animal with 50 IU/kg (1 IU = 0,0084 mg). One should always be able to account for the total amount of heparin injected over a period of time. With diligent flushing, the animal can become inadvertently overheparinized. Total heparinization may result in bleeding from the operative wounds and be otherwise undesirable. Heparin can be inhibited by intravenous infusion of protamine sulfate (1–15 mg/mg heparin). It is also possible to make the catheters nonthrombogenic in vivo for several hours by rubbing into their surface a precipitated heparin-benzalconium complex [105].

Practically any connector or stopcock is prone to trap a tiny air bubble when connected. At a trial withdrawal, this bubble does not usually appear in the syringe. When multiple injections into a terminal vessel are made, the accumulated air microemboli may produce adverse effects.

Percutaneous vascular occlusion can be produced by induction of thrombosis or by injection of an occluding material. All methods require wedging of the delivery catheter into the vessel to be obstructed. Further slowing of the blood flow can be achieved by occluding the draining venous channels. Thrombosis can be produced by impeding the blood flow over an extended period. Instantaneous thrombosis of small vessels can be produced by injection of most organic solvents. Small vessels or capillaries can be occluded with glass microbeads or Sephadex beads (polymerized dextrans, Pharmacia, Sweden). A rapid embolism of small vessels with ensuing thrombosis can be produced with a fine mesh ion-exchange resin.

Larger vascular structures can be occluded by injection of fluid silicon rubber, which rapidly polymerizes in situ and which is well tolerated over a long period even years [106]. Occlusion by combination of instantaneous thrombosis with foreign body is achieved by rapid injection of an organic adhesive, isobutyl 2-cyanoacrylate [107]. Such surgical glue can be made opaque with admixed metal powder or Pantopaque. Thrombosis selectively damaging to the endothelium can also be produced with electrical current. This can be achieved by passing into the target vessel a slightly curved catheter containing a wire with a tip blunted by dipping into liquid soldering metal. DC current at 50 V and 10 mA applied for 15–20 min will produce the intimal injury [108].

G. Animal Models of Cardiovascular Pathological States

Models of pathological states should closely resemble the human condition and their production should be convenient. A number of models can be produced by surgery. Principles of experimental surgery in the dog and generally applicable to pigs are outlined elsewhere [109]. The following is a brief review of other methodology.

Arteriosclerosis (AS). Experimental production of AS is a vast topic and has been extensively reviewed [110]. AS can be induced by diets, catecholamines, thyroid hormones, mineralocorticoids, renal interventions, various organic chemicals, antigens, etc. There are many variations of each of the numerous approaches. Efforts to develop a suitable animal model of AS have focused on those animals in which the disease occurs naturally, or can be induced easily, such as in rabbits, dogs, and pigs as well as in infrahuman primates.

Rat and various avian species are highly susceptible to the development of AS; the turkey is known for producing dissecting aortic aneurysms. Experimental AS in these species is described elsewhere [122].

The rabbit is a classical model for experimental AS. Although AS occurs naturally only in certain strains. AS can be produced in any rabbit breed by cholesterol and fat feeding. Diet hypercholesterolemia may range from 10 to 40 times the normal [111]. The lesions first occur in the aortic arch but their appearance differs from those in humans. Ulceration and thrombus formation occurs only with extensive additional manipulations such as injections of catecholamines and vitamin D [112]. Diet-induced rabbit AS is marked by extensive lesions in small myocardial vessels while epicardial arteries are little affected. Development of myocardial infarcts is unusual.

AS closely resembling human lesions can be produced by the synergistic effect of cholesterol and fat feeding with allergic injury [113]. The rabbit, unlike the dog, is insensitive to allylamine, but i.v. injections of carboxy-methyl-cellulose will elicit hyperlipermia, hypercholesterolemia, and arterial lesions [114].

A rapid method for production of prominent lesions in the thoracic and abdominal aorta employs acute hypoxia [115]. In a tight box, rabbits are exposed to nitrogen, which they inhale until convulsions appear. Thirty seconds later they are given air. This is carried out daily for 3 weeks to produce lesions that closely mimic the Monckeberg type of human disease. These changes are possibly attributable to the release of catecholamines rather than to hypoxia nevertheless, the method is extremely efficient in producing a workable model.

Dogs, in general, are not the animal of choice as a model of a human type of sclerosis due to their resistance.

To develop AS lesions in the dog by means of a cholesterol-rich diet requires suppression of thyroid activity [116]. Intravenous infusions of large doses of epinephrine or norepinephrine produce endocardial and valvular hemorrhages and necrotic changes in small arteries, but calcifications in the aorta do not develop [117]. Acute hypoxia is not a feasible method in dogs.

Intravenous chronic injections of nonionic surface active agents such as Triton produce marked arteriosclerotic lesions of the coronary vessels [118]. Chronic i.v. injections of polyvinyl alcohol produce atheromatic lesions in the aorta and in smaller arteries [119]. Necrotizing arteritis with fibrinoid necrosis of the media and periarteritis can be produced in dogs by intravenous injection of allylamine and methylcellulose [120]. This method is relatively easy and the lesions develop rapidly.

The *pig* is a suitable animal for induction of AS. In the Pitman-Moore breed (miniature pig) atherosclerosis often occurs naturally. Production of atheromatosis by cholesterol feeding is a convenient method [121, 122]. Use of hypoxia, catecholamines, allylamine, methylcellulose, or polyvinyl alcohol have not been reported in the pig, presumably because the induction of the disease by dietary means is so simple.

Cats are difficult to use as AS models. Occasionally plaque lesions can develop in the aorta of a domestic cat fed with a high cholesterol diet [123].

Infrahuman Primates. Since it became apparent that certain primates fed atherogenic diets produce AS lesions very closely resembling the human condition, they have been used extensively in comparative studies involving AS. This is especially true for AS of cerebral and myocardial arteries. It is because of the readiness with which the primate develops arteriosclerosis by dietary means that other methods of induction have not gained popularity.

The *rhesus monkey (Macaca mulatta)* is particularly well suited for AS studies since natural hypercholesterolemia occurs even with a normal diet, upon confinement in a cage [124]. The rhesus is known to be useful as a model of atherosclerotic changes in peripheral arteries. In contradistinction to lower mammals such as rabbit, arteriosclerotic lesions of the coronary arteries are prominent in the epicardial branches and the incidence of myocardial infarction is high [125]. Severe AS lesions can be produced in the rhesus monkey in periods ranging from 6 to 15 months with a combination of radioiodine thyroid suppression and cholesterol feeding [126]. According to one study, the feeding regime of the rhesus monkey may include a daily dose of 3 g cholesterol and 30 g butter suspended in warm water. This diet results in hypercholesterolemia ranging from 250 to 600 mg%, and over a period ranging from 3 to 6 months results in the development of AS lesions. A diet producing serum cholesterol levels of only 250 mg% suffices to produce some arteriosclerotic changes in 3–4 months. This can be greatly accelerated by arterial injuries inflicted, for example, with a freezing probe [127, 128]. Another experimental way to produce AS is by administration of toxic doses of vitamin D [129]. Occasionally, an individual rhesus monkey is found resistant to the development of AS by dietary means.

Subcutaneous injections of isoproterenol produce severe cell changes in the heart muscle of the rhesus but no gross AS pathology results.

The distribution of AS lesions in the rhesus monkey is very similar to that in man, and even the sequence in which the lesions appear follows the human pattern. Thus, the changes appear in the abdominal and thoracic aorta, aortic arch, iliac arteries, carotid sinuses, and the proximal portion of the coronary arteries. With hypercholesterolemia extending for 17–65 months, atheromata can be found in the circle of Willis, in the mesenteric, celiac, splanchnic and femoral arteries, and in the more distal segments of the epicardial coronary arteries. No atheromata develop in the coronary myocardial branches [130].

The *squirrel monkey (Simiri sciurea)* sometimes also develops spontaneous arteriosclerosis. The animal's responsiveness to a high cholesterol diet is, however, very variable [131].

The *capuchin monkey (Cebus)* shows large age- and sex-related differences in response to dietary manipulation. In principle, diet-induced AS leads to lesions mainly in the aorta and in the carotid arteries, at bifurcations. While old *cebus* monkeys show lesions in the coronary vascular bed, young ones do not. No AS lesions occur in the cerebral arteries [132].

The *chimpanzee (Pan troglodytes)* is extremely expensive. An atherogenic diet usually leads to hypercholesteremia and atherosclerosis closely resembling the human disease. It appears, however, that the degree of AS is determined more by the stress of captivity than by diet alone [133].

The metabolism of cholesterol in the *baboon (Papio anubis)* closely resembles that of man, and the animal is therefore well suited for production of AS by dietary means. The baboon has personality characteristics similar to the typical young patient with coronary disease, and the very competitive nature of the male baboon is "... not too unlike that sometimes seen in the human executive class..." [134]. Thus, the animal is also very well suited for production of myocardial necrosis by exposure to excessive stress.

Takayasu's arteritis can be produced in rabbits by long-term administration of isologous aortic extracts or human sera with antiaortic antibodies [135].

Arterial aneurysms in animals may be found as a by-product of atherosclerosis. Isolated aneurysms in otherwise normal vasculature can be produced by an operative technique.

Arterial aneurysms in animals may be found as a by-product of atherosclerosis. Isolated aneurysms in otherwise normal vasculature can be produced by an operative technique [136]. In our experience, repeated injections of collagenases and/or steroids into the wall of the canine femoral artery is unreliable. On the other hand, injections of 3% $AgNO_3$ invariably produced wall necrosis, sometimes resulting in formation of an aneurysm.

Myocardial Infarction (MI). Methods of production in animals have been extensively reviewed [137]. Arteriosclerosis in animals is not suitable as a model of MI. Even with severe coronary sclerosis, incidence of spontaneous myocardial infarction in animals is very low and the occurrence unpredictable.

The most frequently used procedure has been *ligation of the coronary artery*. After ligation, irreversible damage occurs, usually after 30–45 min. The outcome of this procedure, however, is somewhat unpredictable as to size of the infarct. Also, an acute ligation may be fatal. A better approach is a gradual decrease of the coronary flow. This can be achieved with snares placed around the coronary arteries [138], by implantation of ameroid rings (a hygroscopic compressed casein plastic of a predictable degree and rate of swelling [139], or cuffs which at a later date can be inflated for a predetermined period of time. At the time of thoracotomy, chronic flow probes can be placed on the coronary artery so that the degree of occlusion can be precisely monitored [140, 141]. The effect can be produced also by a transcatheter implantation of an Ivalon sponge. The latter elegant technique is based on the expandability of Ivalon in blood and has the substantial advantage of allowing occlusion at a preselected site in a closed-chest dog [142].

Although the dog may be more convenient to handle, the resemblance of the coronary anatomy of the pig to man should make the pig the preferred animal [148]. In normal pig, unlike dog, there are no anastomoses of hemodynamic significance between the left and right coronary arterial system. Another difference pertains to the postocclusion interarterial anastomoses, which in dog's heart develop predominantly in the epicardial region. In pig, subendocardial and endomural anastomoses prevail [144].

MI and large hemorrhages in the myocardium can be produced by ligature of the coronary veins. The procedure is frequently fatal. Another approach to the MI model is implantation of various thrombogenic materials into coronary arteries resulting in the development of thrombotic occlusion [145]. These techniques require anesthesia and thoracotomy. Animal mortality is low due to the slow change of coronary perfusion.

If the protocol calls for monitoring various physiological parameters for a very limited period of time, or if thoracotomy must be avoided, a closed-chest approach in a lightly anesthetized animal is preferable. Percutaneous coronary catheterization allows selective injections of various embolizing materials. Selective catheterization of branches of the coronary system can be accomplished with a thin polyethylene catheter (PE 160) introduced through a larger diameter catheter placed percutaneously into the coronary ostium (Sect. F).

A small amount of formaldehyde or mercury can be injected to produce almost immediate myocardial necrosis [146]; the latter has the advantage of being a stable radiographic marker. Infarction can also be readily produced by intracoronary injection of hexachlorotetrafluorobutane, a sclerosing agent [147]. Under fluoroscopic control, small stainless steel cylinders can be introduced into the coronary artery via the carotid artery [148]. A technique exists for embolization of a preselected myocardial site by i.v. injection of iron particles which are directed by a magnet placed outside the body [149]. Wire conductors can be introduced via catheters to induce thrombosis upon their heating or passage of electrical current [150]. Glass or plastic beads can also be injected [151]. Nonradiopaque, radiopaque gelfoam, or Ivalon pledgets can be injected into the coronary artery.

The technique should be selected depending upon the objectives of the protocol. Methods obstructing small vessels and/or having a direct toxic effect on the myocardium in scattered and largely unpredictable locations may have to be avoided. When the occlusion is practically immediate, collateral circulation cannot develop and the average acute mortality in such experiments is rather high. Death is usually caused by ventricular arrhythmias as a result of a sudden potassium egress from the damaged myocardium [152].

Experimental Ventricular Fibrillation. Pharmacological methods which produce a reversible ventricular fibrillation but damage the myocardium permanently should be avoided. A convenient and satisfactory method is electric shock [153].

Experimental Pericarditis. Injection of sodium hypochlorite into the pericardium in a short time produces pericarditis marked by adhesions and hemorrhage [154]. Constrictive pericarditis can be produced by various fibroplastic agents such as asbestos, talc, sodium morrhuate, cellophane, and assorted acids and alkalis deposited either freely into the pericardium or into a localized pouch [155]. The technique can be based either on thoracotomy or, more conveniently, on a percutaneous (Seldinger) approach [156].

In the supine animal, under fluoroscopic control (preferably with a lateral beam) a 16- to 18-gauge needle is inserted by a subxiphoid puncture into the pericardium close to the cardiac apex. No substantial damage will occur should the needle pierce the myocardium in this region. Attempts to enter the pericardial sac closer to the heart base, however, may damage the more vulnerable structures, sometimes resulting in tamponade. Manipulation in the apical region should be minimized. It is advisable to advance a fine-tip catheter over the needle into the pericardial cavity. A standard venepuncture set can be conveniently used for this purpose.

Endomyocardial fibrosis and endocardial fibroelastosis can be produced by obstructing the lymphatic outflow of the myocardium. This method is, however, not completely reliable [157].

Experimental Heart Block. Right bundle branch block can be produced upon thoracotomy by introducing an iridectomy scalpel into the auricle of the right atrium and incising the septal endocardium of the right ventricle at the basis of the anterior septal papillary muscle. *Left bundle block* can be produced by incision of the left anterior ventricular wall and a horizontal stab into the septum about 5 mm below the aortic valve [158].

Blocks of varying degrees can be produced percutaneously by puncture of either of the septa followed by injection of a small amount (½ ml) of a standard monomeric water-soluble CM through the puncture cannula, producing a transient block. The CM persists in the septum for several minutes and its position can be verified by opacification of the heart cavities.

Permanent damage to the AV node can be inflicted with formaldehyde. About 0.1 ml 40% solution can be injected either using a Ross needle (preferably shortened), under fluoroscopic guidance, via the external jugular vein [159], or by thoracotomy and transatrial injection [160]. The latter approach has a higher rate of success. Ligation of the arteries supplying the AV node is technically difficult and has no advantage over the other methods.

Wolff-Parkinson-White Syndrome. Ventricular fused beat can be produced in dog by atrial pacing and stimulation of various sides of ventricles. This manipulation will grossly simulate the pathological QRS complex of the ECG seen in the human Wolff-Parkinson-White syndrome [166].

Cardiac Hypertrophy. Induction of cardiac hypertrophy can be rapid (within several days) or slow (over several months). The rapid form can be produced by obstructing the outflow of the ventricles. This can be achieved by constricting the aorta or pulmonary artery and can sometimes be combined with monolateral pulmonectomy and/or administration of thyroid hormone or sympathomimetic drugs. A slowly increasing cardiac hypertrophy can be produced by anemia, nutritional deficiencies, hypoxia, myocardial ischemia, and continuous massive stress [162].

Chronic congestive heart failure (see also discussion of pulmonary stenosis) can be produced in practically any animal by gradual constriction of the pulmonary artery, preferably with an inflatable rubber cuff so that the degree of stenosis can be regulated [163]. The controlled increase of stenosis is important for gradual development of *right-ventricular hypertrophy*. It can also be done by implanting rings around, the pulmonary artery of a newborn dog, pig, or calf. A model which has low operative mortality and good postoperative progress involves avulsion of the anterior leaflet of the tricuspid valve and gradual pulmonary stenosis produced by an implanted hydraulic occluder placed at the base of the pulmonary artery [164]. A model for reversible long-term overload of the right ventricle using a removable band on the pulmonary artery in cat has been reported [165].

Left ventricular hypertrophy (LVH) can be conveniently produced by partial destruction of the aortic valve, carried out via the right common carotid artery using a straight stylet passed through a catheter positioned into the anterior aortic sinus. Upon piercing the semilunar cusp, insufficiency is immediately marked by the appearance of a strong diastolic murmur. LVH can also be produced by placing a constricting ring on the ascending aorta of young puppies or piglets [166] or it can be induced by surgically producing subcoronary stenosis [167]. A reproducible model of chronic, stable LVH can be obtained by banding the ascending aorta of 7- to 8-week-old puppies [168] or piglets. A gradient of 15–20 mmHg is achieved in 3 months. The animals are usually asymptomatic and later die of ventricular arrhythmias. It is difficult to produce LVA in dog by inducing mitral insufficiency. We have observed only a very minimal hyperthrophy of the left ventricle in dogs with a regurgitant flow as high as 50% of the cardiac output during 2 years of unrestricted movement, after an operatively produced mitral insufficiency.

Perfusion pulmonary hypertension can be produced by chronic overperfusion. The model requires resectioning of the apical and intermedial lobes of the left lung, division of the left pulmonary artery at its origin and anastomosis to the side of the ascending aorta, beyond the arch [169].

Congenital Heart Disease. Although animals exhibit a wide variety of congenital cardiovascular defects similar to man, their occurrence is largely unpredictable and practically impossible to achieve by genetic manipulations. There are a number of procedures which can result in some kind of congenital heart disease (CHD) by exposing the pregnant animal or the embryo to a teratogenic agent. Techniques include mechanical manipulation, hypoxia, hypercapnea, uterine vascular clamping, X-ray irradiation, vitamin A deficiency or A hypervitaminosis, riboflavin deficiency, folic acid deficiency, use of actinomycin, ribonuclease, thalidomide, and tissue antisera [170]. One anomaly which can be obtained with reasonable reproducibility is the transposition, induced by trypan blue, of the great vessels in rats [171]. By selective breeding, certain cardiac malformations can be produced in dogs, a lengthy and unreliable procedure [144]. A large variety of CHDS can be caused during fetal growth by teratogenic sera. Given to pregnant animals such as rats, they can produce situs inversus, single ventricle, truncus arteriosus, various transpositions, interventricular septal defects, and abnormalities of the ascending aorta [172].

Transposition of the great vessels, and ventricular and atrial septal defects must be produced by surgical means including thoracotomy. The lamb fetus is remarkably tolerant to surgical procedures in utero and is therefore well suited for the production of various models of CHD [173].

Septal defects in grown-up animals require excision of a large portion of the septum. With an instrument designed to excise a portion of the interatrial septum in a dog, via the external jugular vein, defects of up to 0.8 cm^2 were found at autopsy, but no functional shunt could be produced in vivo. The canine interatrial septum thus must contract to reduce or close a defect.

Models of Coarctation of the Aorta and Poststenotic Dilation in the Great Vessels. Models can be produced with relative ease by operatively placing rings on the vessels of interest. The rapid growth of piglets will lead to a relatively tight stenosis in 2–3 months [174]. The procedure can also be performed in lamb fetus in utero [173] and in calf.

Ductus Arteriosus. The hemodynamics of a patent ductus arteriosus can be conveniently studied in puppies [175], sheep or goat fetuses [176], or newborn pigs [177].

Models of the heart valves diseases should simulate as closely as possible the congenital or acquired human condition. Congenital stenotic valvular malformations in man mainly concern the pulmonary valve. Defects of other valves are almost invariably acquired. A model of the acquired disease can be produced by experimental endocarditis or by production of the hemodynamically significant valvular defect in otherwise normal hearts. Although the former approach closely resembles the human pathological picture, it is time-consuming and the results are unpredictable. Moreover, the animals are prone to succumb rapidly to heart failure. *Experimental endocarditis* can be produced in the laboratory mammal by severing the valves and infecting the animal with a microbial agent [56, 178, 179]. Carditis and simultaneous glomerulonephritis can be produced by streptococcal infection in dogs in whom a large AV fistula has been operatively produced [180]. The combination of the bacterial agent with anoxia further accelerates development of endocarditis, resulting primarily in aortic and mitral valvular vegetations. Chronic valvular changes closely resembling those of human rheumatic carditis can be produced by ultrasound at a dosage of about 1 megacycle at 5 W/cm^2 applied to a valve for 5–20 min [181]. With such nonspecific procedures, it is impossible to predict whether insufficiency, stenosis, or both will develop. A stable, chronic, hemodynamically significant model of pure stenosis or pure insufficiency can only be produced operatively.

Mitral valve insufficiency can be produced by left thoracotomy and introduction of a sharp instrument into the left auricle to cut the cordae tendinae. This approach has the drawback of leaving the valve itself intact. It is possible to excise a portion of the valve under direct vision, but this requires rather complicated surgical instrumentation.

The mitral valve can be approached percutaneously in intact animals via interatrial septal puncture using a specially constructed valvulectome (Kifa, Solna, Sweden). Following puncture of the interatrial septum from the external jugular vein (see Sect. F), a guide wire is passed into the left ventricle and left in situ. The valvulectome is threaded on the guide wire and advanced, under fluoroscopic control, transseptally into the mitral ostium. Pressures can be measured and CM injected through this instrument, which allows excision of a portion of the valvular leaflet in a semilunar shape (area approximately 0.45 cm^2). This method is facile and has a very low mortality [102].

Mitral stenosis. Open-heart surgery and suturing of the leaflets is a difficult procedure with high postoperative mortality due to the unpredictability of the magnitude of stenotic obstruction and the resulting pulmonary edema. A closed-heart approach is based on invagination of the left atrial appendage, to which a cylindrical-shaped sponge has been sewn, into the mitral orifice [182]. Another operative method uses a heavy mattress suture placed across the mitral ring and

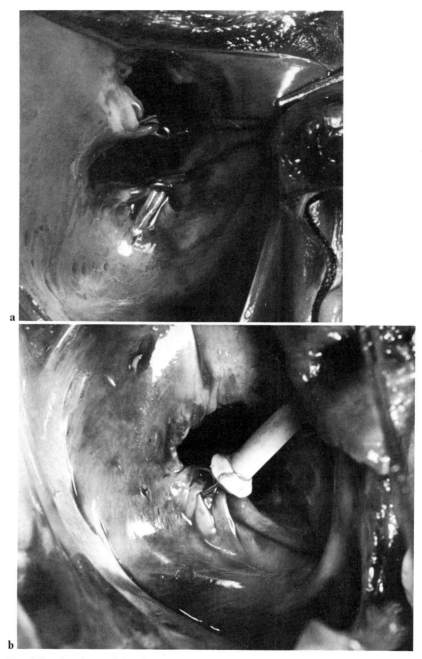

Fig. 7. a Mitral ostium of the dog seen from the left atrium. The chordae tendinae of each of the leaflets are caught by hooks on threads. A postmortem specimen. **b** Coaptation of the hooks by advancing a catheter over the threads

tied over buttons [183]. This approach may, however, compromise the vascular supply and deform the inlet portion of the left ventricle.

A radiological operative method in dogs or pigs involves only the valve. After left thoracotomy, a purse-string suture is placed on the left atrial appendage. Small hooks made from threaded atraumatic needles with silk are grasped by a needleholder which is introduced into the mitral ostium through an opening in the atrial appendage. The purse string controls the bleeding. Using lateral fluoroscopy, with the animal in a supine position, the hooks are maneuvered to catch the chordae tendinae close to the commissures on both leaflets of the valve (Fig. 7a). With the hooks in place, the silks are threaded into a catheter which, upon advancement, coapts the leaflets and controls the valve mobility and the valvular area (Fig. 7b). Retraction of the catheter restores the normal valvular area and function.

Tricuspid Valve. In principle the techniques used for the mitral valve can be applied to the tricuspid valve.

Pulmonary Valves. Insufficiency can best be produced by excision of the leaflets under direct vision. The approach is relatively simple [184].

Pulmonary stenosis can be produced by painting the leaflets with a strong acid under direct vision [184]. The development of hypertrophy of the right ventricle is dependent upon the age at which the stenosis becomes hemodynamically significant. Thus, pulmonary stenosis produced at birth results in large hypertrophy of the right ventricle with blood pressures reaching the systemic levels. This is not possible in older animals [185].

Pulmonic artery stenosis can best be produced in a gradual manner using an inflatable cuff implanted around the artery [186].

Infundibular pulmonic stenosis can be produced in newborn animals by sutures run through both posterior and anterior portions of the right ventricle, through the area of the crista supraventricularis [187]. Ductus arteriosus must be ligated.

Aortic valve insufficiency can be produced by piercing or cutting the aortic leaflets with instruments introduced via the common carotid artery. Since unprotected instruments can damage the arteries during their passage, it is advisable to introduce them through a catheter. A sharp stylet can be passed through after a stiff catheter has been firmly lodged against the chosen aortic cusp and its position fluoroscopically verified.

Aortic stenosis can be produced only by surgical means including aortotomy upon establishing an auxilliary coronary perfusion.

Experimental pulmonary embolism can be produced by a number of methods. Microembolism can be produced by injecting a 30% saline suspension of barium sulfate (0.2 ml/kg) into the right atrium of the dog, directly into the pulmonary artery, or one of its branches [188]. Macroembolism can be produced by obstruction of the entire pulmonary artery or of its branches. The artery can be temporarily obstructed by a catheter with a detachable balloon tip which is maneuvered to the desired position, inflated, detached, and left in situ.

Thromboembolism requires production of thrombi either in vitro or in one of the veins of the body. Thrombi simulating the clinical situation can be made in one of the peripheral veins and left in situ for 1 week to organize. In pig or dog, sufficiently long segments of femoral veins are not easily accessible and the thrombi produced therein are relatively small. A clamped caval vein will yield large thrombi. Total caval obstruction below the renal veins is well tolerated in dogs, pigs, and rabbits. The procedure, however, requires laparotomy and the release of developed thrombi is often difficult.

A better choice is the external jugular veins, which are easily accessible and have a reasonably large capacity. Silk snares are placed on an exposed venous segment filled with blood, and removed 1 week later. Cohesive thrombi can also be rapidly produced by injection of thrombin (50 IU in 0.2 ml) into an isolated vein segment. Upon removal of the snares, the thrombus is forced toward the heart by digital propulsion.

It is also possible to make thrombi ad hoc using the autologous blood clotted by thrombin in small plastic syringes. Upon their retraction, the thrombi are suspended in saline and injected directly into the external jugular vein via a syringe with a large-diameter funnel-shaped nozzle.

Long, worm-like radiopaque emboli can be made in vitro from a concentrated gelatin solution allowed to gel and soaked in CM [189].

Various tracers can be added into the preformed clots: in the lungs, barium sulfate or tantalum powder is useful for radiography, and isotopic tracers ^{131}I- or ^{125}I-labeled fibrinogen or ^{99}Te are useful for scanning [190].

Thrombi introduced into the right heart circulation of a supine animal will tend to lodge unpredictably. Unilateral distribution, however, can be achieved by positioning the animal. Most of the thrombi are directed toward the dependent side. Both in dogs and pigs embolization of one entire lung by large emboli usually fails to affect cardiopulmonary hemodynamics significantly, while rabbits are always affected by such a procedure [191, 192].

Pulmonary air embolism can be produced by injecting air through catheters into the pulmonary circulation [193]. Injection into peripheral veins may fail to produce pulmonary obstruction because some of the air may remain trapped in the structures of the right ventricle. Fat embolism can be produced by peripheral intravenous injections [194].

Experimental thrombosis can be produced in veins, arteries, and heart by mechanical, chemical, or electrical methods, causing endothelial injury and favoring subsequent development of a clot. For radiographic investigation of venous thrombosis in rabbit, caval veins are the area of choice; in dogs or pigs, femoral, external jugular, iliac, or caudal caval veins are suitable. The approach should not require extensive surgery and should produce a gradually growing thrombus.

Mechanical methods consist of severance of the endothelium by crushing or clamping of the vessel, insertion of silk threads soaked in thrombin and left in situ, or "brushing" of the vessel lumen with a bronchoscopy brush introduced via a vascular catheter.

Chemical methods employ injection of 0.1 ml 2% $AgNO_3$, 10% formaldehyde, thrombin, etc. into the vessel wall using a fine cannula.

Electrically, thrombosis can be produced with a blunt-tipped conducting wire introduced via a vascular catheter and serving as an electrode. A standard surgical coagulation apparatus setting can be used as an AC power source, but a DC current is preferable in that there is less likelihood of the electrode burning through the vessel wall. The method is useful for total thrombotic occlusion, but is unreliable for production of mural thrombi since the electrode contact with the endothelium varies.

References

1. Higgins CB, Feld GK (1976) Direct chronotropic and dromotropic actions of contrast media: ineffectiveness of atropine in the prevention of bradyarrhythmias and conduction disturbances. Radiology 121:205–209
2. Higgins CB, Schmidt W (1978) Direct and reflex myocardial effects of intracoronary administered contrast materials in the anesthetized and conscious dog. Comparison of standard and newer contrast materials. Invest Radiol 13:205–216
3. Sovak M, Ranganathan R (1980) Stability of nonionic water-soluble contrast media: implications for their design. Invest Radiol 15:S323–S328
4. Sovak M, Siefert HM, Ranganathan R (1980) Combined methods for assessment of neurotoxicity: testing of new nonionic radiographic media. Invest Radiol 15:248–253
5. Knoefel PK (ed) (1971) Radiocontrast agents. International encyclopedia of pharmacology and therapeutics, vol 76. Pergammon, New York
6. Lasser EC (1968) Basic mechanism of contrast media reactions. Theoretical and experimental considerations. Radiology 91:63–65
7. Lasser EC, Kolb WP, Lang JH (1974) Contrast media activation of serum complement system. Invest Radiol 9:6A
8. Lang JH, Lasser EC, Kolb WP (1976) Activation of serum complement by contrast media. Invest Radiol 11:303–308
9. Salvesen S (1973) Acute toxicity test of metrizamide. Acta Radiol [Suppl] (Stockh) 335:5–13
10. Almen T (1973) Effects of metrizamide and other contrast media on the isolated rabbit heart. Acta Radiol [Suppl] (Stockh) 335:216–222
11. Oppenheimer MJ, Ascanio G, Henny GC, Caldwell E, Vinciguerra T (1973) Metabolic and cardiovascular effects of selective intracoronary injections of contrast media. Invest Radiol 8:13–21
12. Harrington GJ (1968) In vivo microangiography. In: Felson B (ed) Roentgen techniques in laboratory animals. Saunders, Philadelphia, p 230–233
13. Branemark P-I, Lindstrom J (1963) A modified rabbit's ear chamber: high-power, high-resolution studies in regenerated and preformed tissues. Anat Rec 145:533–540
14. Fulton GP, Lutz BR (1957) The use of the hamster cheek pouch and cinephotomicrography for research on the microcirculation and tumor growth, and for teaching purposes. Boston Med Q 8:13–19
15. Symposium on contrast media toxicity (1970) Invest Radiol 5 (6):373–569
16. Speck U, Mutzel W, Mannesmann G, Pfeiffer H, Siefert HM (1980) Pharmacology of nonionic dimmers. Invest Radiol Suppl 15:S317–S322
17. Sovak M, Ranganathan R, Haghighi N (1981) New nonionic intravascular contrast media. Invest Radiol 16:421
18. Oppenheimer MJ, Durant TM, Stauffer HM, Stewart GH III, Lynch PR, Barrera F (1956) In vivo visualization of intracardiac structures with gaseous carbon dioxide. Cardiovascular-respiratory effects and associated changes in blood chemistry. Am J Physiol 186:325–334
19. Dumont AE, Acinapura A, Martelli AB, Biris L (1972) Radiopacification of intravascular clot by intravenous injection of tantalum particles. Invest Radiol 7:56–60
20. Sovak M, Lang JH (1972) Polymeric additives to angiographic contrast medium: development of an adhesive contrast material. Invest Radiol 7:16–23
21. Sovak M, Lynch PR, Stewart GH (1973) Movement of the mitral valve and its correlation with the first heart sound. Invest Radiol 8:150–155
22. Heckman JL (1973) High-speed cineradiography of the canine aortic valve. PhD thesis, Temple University, Philadelphia, Pa.

23. Sovak M, Oigaard A, Kardel T, Dabb R (1971) Radiological assessment of portal vein blood flow; description of method and application. Invest Radiol 6:146–151
24. Sovak M, Soulen RL, Reichle FA (1971) Blood flow in the human portal vein. Radiology 99:531–536
25. Mygind T, Sovak M, Oigaard A, Christensen O, Jarlov A (1970) Soluble contrast particles for radiographic analysis of blood flow. Determination of cardiac output in dogs. Invest Radiol 5:1–12
26. Sovak M, Lynch PR, Mygind T (1970) Improved technique for production of particulate contrast medium. Invest Radiol 5:566–569
27. Carlsson E, Milne ENC (1967) Permanent implantation of endocardial tantalum screws: a new technique for functional studies of the heart in the experimental animal. J Can Assoc Radiol 19:304–309
28. Rushmer RF, Finlayson BL, Nash AA (1956) Movement of the mitral valve. Circ Res 4:337–342
29. Sherman RG, Pax RA (1970) The spider heart. In: Kerkut GA (ed) Experiments in physiology and biochemistry, vol 3. Academic, New York, pp 351–364
30. Tucker VA (1966) Oxygen transport by the circulatory system of the green iguana (*Iguana iguana*) at different body temperatures. J Exp Biol 44:77–92
31. Johansen K, Hol R (1959) Circulation in the three-chambered snake. Circ Res 8:823–828
31a. Johansen K, Hol R (1960) A cineradiography of the snake heart. Circ Res 8:253–259
32. Greenfield LJ, Morrow AG (1961) The cardiovascular hemodynamics of Crocodilia. J Surg Res 1:97–103
33. Johansen K (1965) Cardiovascular dynamics in fishes, amphibians, and reptiles. Ann NY Acad Sci 127:414–442
34. Elsner R (1972) Comparative circulatory studies of diving and asphyxia. Adv Exp Med Biol 22:69–80
35. Whipple HE (ed) (1965) Comparative cardiology. Ann NY Acad Sci 127:1–875, art 1
36. Altman PL, Dittmer DS (eds) (1964) Biology data book. Fed Am Soc Exp Biol, Washington DC
37. Spector WS (ed) (1956) Handbook of biological data. Saunders, Philadelphia
38. Hamiton WF (ed) (1963) Handbook of physiology Sect 2, vol 2, circulation. American Physiology Society, Washington DC
39. Cass JS (1971) Laboratory animals. An annotated bibliography of information resources covering medicine-science (including husbandry) technology, 3rd compilation. Hafner, New York
40. Vagtborg H (ed) (1965) The baboon in medical research, 2nd edn. University of Texas Press, Austin
41. Schalm OW, Jain NC, Carroll ES (1975) Veterinary hematology, 2nd edn. Lea and Febiger, Philadelphia
42. Hartman CG, Straus WL Jr (eds) (1961) The anatomy of the rhesus monkey. Hafner, New York
43. Fisher EW, Dalton RG (1959) Cardiac output in cattle. Nature 183:829
44. Frick H (1960) Das Herz der Primaten. Hofer H, Schultz AH, Stark D (eds) Primatologia. Karger, Basel, pp 163–272 (Handbook of primatology, vol III/2)
45. Platzer W (1960) Das Arterien- und Venensystem. In: Hofer H, Schultz AH, Stark D (eds) Primatologia. Karger, Basel, pp 273–287 (Handbook of primatology, vol III/2)
46. Chase RE, DeGaris C (1938) Arteriae coronariae (cordis) in the higher primates. Am J Phys Anthropol 24:427–448
47. Domino EF, McCarthy DA, Deneau GA (1969) General anesthesia in infrahuman primates. Fed Proc 28:1500–1509
48. Tashjian RJ, Das KM, Palich WE, Hamlin RL, Yarns DA (1965) Studies on cardiovascular disease in the cat. Ann NY Acad Sci 127:581–605
49. Crouch JE (1969) Text atlas of cat anatomy. Lea and Febiger, Philadelphia
50. Brogden BG, Bartley TD, Schiebler GL, Shanklin DR, Krovetz LJ, Lorincz AE (1964) Cardiovascular radiology in calves. Angiology 15:496–504

51. Sisson S, Grossman JD (1953) Anatomy of the domestic animals. 4th edn. Saunders, Philadelphia
52. Barone R, Pavaux C, Blin PC, Cuq P (1973) Atlas d'anatomie du lapin. Masson, Paris
53. Weisbroth SH, Flatt RE, Kraus AL (eds) (1974) The biology of the laboratory rabbit. Academic, New York
54. Mount LE, Ingram DL (1971) The pig as a laboratory animal. Academic, London
55. Christensen GC, Campeti FL (1959) Anatomic and functional studies of the coronary circulation in the dog and pig. Am J Vet Res 20:18–26
56. Akbarian M, Salfeder K, Schwarz J (1964) Experimental histoplasmic endocarditis. Arch Intern Med 114:784–791
57. Altland PD, Highman B (1956) Effects of high altitude exposure on dogs and on their susceptibility to endocarditis. Fed Proc 15:3
58. Bustad LK, McClellan RO (eds) (1966) Swine in biomedical research. Proceedings, symposium at the Pacific Northwest Laboratory, Richland, 19–22 July 1965. Battelle Memorial Institute, Richland
59. Anderson DM, Elsley FWH (1969) A note on the use of indwelling catheters in conscious adult pigs. J Agric Sci 72:475–477
60. Brogden BG, Criley JM, Rowe RD (1968) Cardiovascular techniques in large animals. In: Felson B (ed) Roentgen techniques in laboratory animals. Radiography of the dog and other experimental animals. Saunders, Philadelphia, p 186
61. Andersen AC (1970) The beagle as an experimental dog. Iowa State University Press, Ames
62. Miller ME, Christensen GC, Evans HE (1964) Anatomy of the dog. Saunders, Philadelphia
63a. Rhodes WH, Patterson DF, Detweiler DK (1960) Radiographic anatomy of the canine heart, part I. J Am Vet Med Assoc 137:283
63b. Rhodes WH, Patterson DF, Detweiler DK (1963) Radiographic anatomy of the canine hart, part II. Am Vet Med Assoc 143:137–148
64a. Thomas CE (1957) The muscular architecture of the ventricles of hog and dog hearts. Am J Anat 101:17–58
64b. Thomas CE (1959) The muscular architecture of the atria of hog and dog hearts. Am J Anat 104:207–236
65. Yokoyama HO, Jennings RB, Wartman WB (1961) Intercallated discs of dog myocardium. Exp Cell Res 23:29–44
66. Robb JS (1965) Comparative basic cardiology. Grune and Stratton, New York
67. Frater RWM, Ellis FH Jr (1961) The anatomy of the canine mitral valve. J Surg Res 1:171–178
68. Ettinger SJ, Suter PF (1970) Canine cardiology. Saunders, Philadelphia, p 102
69. Hoffman BF (1969) Atrioventricular conduction in mammalian hearts. Ann NY Acad Sci 127:105–112
70. James TN (1962) Anatomy of the sinus node of the dog. Anat Rec 143:251–265
71. James TN (1964) Anatomy of the A-V node of the dog. Anat Rec 148:15–25
72. Baird JA, Robb JS (1950) Study, reconstruction and gross dissection of the atrioventricular conducting system of the dog heart. Anat Rec 108:747–758
73. Hamlin RL, Smith ER (1960) Anatomical and physiological basis for interpretation of the electrocardiogram. Am J Vet Res 21:701–708
74. Kazzaz D, Shanklin WM (1950) The coronary vessels of the dog demonstrated by colored plastic (vinyl acetate) injections and corrosion. Anat Rec 107:43–59
75. Bertho E (1964) A comparative study in three dimension of the blood supply of the normal interventricular septum in human, canine, bovine, porcine, ovine and equine hearts. Dis Chest 46:251–262
76. Blair E (1961) Anatomy of the ventricular coronary arteries of the dog. Circ Res 9:333–341
77. Meek WJ, Keenan M, Theisen HJ (1929) The auricular blood supply in the dog. I. General auricular supply with special reference to the sino-auricular node. Am Heart J 4:591–599
78. James TN (1961) Anatomy of the coronary arteries. Harper and Row, New York

79. Moore RA (1930) The coronary arteries of the dog. Am Heart J 5:743–749
80. Boucek RJ, Fojaco R, Takashita R (1964) Anatomic considerations for regional intimal changes in the coronary arteries. Anat Rec 148:161–169
81. Baum H (1918) Das Lymphgefäßsystem des Hundes. Arch Wiss Prakt Tierheilkd 44:521–650
82. Robert JT (1969) Arteries, veins, and lymphatic vessels of the heart. In: Luisada AA (ed) Cardiology: an encyclopedia of the cardiovascular system, vol 1. McGraw Hill, New York, pp 85–118
83. Felson B (ed) (1968) Roentgen techniques in laboratory animals. Saunders, Philadelphia
84. Ohlsson NM (1962) Left heart and aortic blood flow in the dog. Precision motion analyses of high speed (270 frames/sec.) cinefluorographic recordings. Acta Radiol [Suppl] (Stockh) 213:1–80
85. Bove AA, Lynch PR (1970) Measurement of canine left ventricular performance by cineradiography of the heart. J Appl Physiol 29:877–883
86. Bove AA, Lynch PR (1970) Radiographic determination of force velocity length relationship in the intact dog heart. J Appl Physiol 29:884–888
87. Freeman E, Ziskin MC, Bove AA, Gimenez JL, Lynch PR (1970) Cineradiographic frame rate selection for left ventricular volumetry. Radiology 96:387–392
88. Bove AA, Ziskin MC, Freedman E, Gimenez JL, Lynch PR (1970) Selection of optimum cineradiographic frame rate relation to accuracy of cardiac measurements. Invest Radiol 5:329–335
89. Santamore WP, DiMeo FN, Lynch PR (1973) A comparative study of various single-plane cineangiocardiographic methods to measure left ventricular volume. IEEE Trans Biomed Eng 20:417–421
90. Giminez JL, Stewart GH, Lynch PR, Stauffer HM (1968) High speed (540/sec.) biplane cineradiography. Invest Radiol 3:51–55
91. Sovak M, Shakleford E, Dearing LM, Lasser EC (1973) A new system of precise correlation of physiological parameters with a cineradiogram. Proc Soc Photo Opt Instrum Eng 43:243–245
92. Greenspan RH (1968) Magnification techniques. In: Felson B (ed) Roentgen techniques in laboratory animals. Saunders, Philadelphia, pp 218–224
93. Margulis AR, Carlsson E, McAlister WH (1961) Angiography of malignant tumors in mice. Acta Radiol (Stockh) 56:179–192
94. Bookstein JJ, Powell TJ (1972) Short target film rotating grid magnification. Radiology 104:399–402
95. Amplatz K (1967) Simple Bucky diaphragm for high speed angiography. Invest Radiol 2:387–390
96. Bookstein JJ, Voegeli E (1971) A critical analysis of magnification radiography. Radiology 98:23–30
97. Greenspan RH, Simon AL, Ricketts HJ, Rojas RH, Watson JC (1967) In vivo magnification angiography. Invest Radiol 2:419–431
98a. Simon AL, Greenspan RH (1965) Magnification coronary arteriography, part I, normal. Clin Radiol 16:414–416
98b. Simon AL, Greenspan RH (1966) Magnification coronary arteriography, part II, experimental pathology. Clin Radiol 17:89–91
99. Hugh AE, Lynch PR, Bove AA, Stauffer HM (1969) Use of short exposure field emission x-ray apparatus in physiological research. J Appl Physiol 26:489–491
100. Ross J Jr (1959) Transseptal left heart catheterization. A new method of left atrial puncture. Ann Surg 149:395–401
101. Petersen KO, Harrington G, Ohlsson NM, Ascanio G, Oppenheimer MJ (1965) Technic of transseptal catheterization of the left atrium pulmonary veins, and left ventricle in the dog. Radiology 85:658–662
102. Sovak M, Mygind T (1968) Experimental mitral insufficiency. A new radiologic closed chest operative method. Invest Radiol 3:292–295
103. West JW, Kobayashi T, Guzman SV (1958) Coronary artery catheterization in the intact dog. Circ Res 6:383–388

104. Carter AM, Olin T (1973) Selective catheterization of the coronary arteries in the rabbit. Invest Radiol 8:350–353
105. Amplatz K (1971) A simple non-thrombogenic coating. Invest Radiol 6:280–289
106. Doppman JL, Zapol W, Pierce J (1961) Transcatheter embolization with a silicone rubber preparation. Invest Radiol 6:304–309
107. Dotter CT, Goldman ML, Rosch J (1975) Instant selective arterial occlusion with iso-butyl-2-cyanoacrylate. Radiology 114:227–230
108. Phillips JR (1973) Transcatheter electrocoagulation of blood vessels. Invest Radiol 8:295–304
109. Murat J (1972) Précis de chirurgie expérimentale abdominale et thoracique chez le chien. Masson, Paris
110. Selye H (1970) Experimental cardiovascular diseases, part I. Springer, Berlin Heidelberg New York
111. Prior JT, Kurtz DM, Ziegler DD (1961) The hypercholesteremic rabbit. Arch Pathol 71:672–684
112. Constantinides P (1965) Experimental atherosclerosis in the rabbit. In: Robert JC, Straus R (eds) Comparative atherosclerosis. Harper and Row, New York, pp 276–290
113. Minick CR, Murphy GE, Campbell WG Jr (1965) Experimental induction of athero-arteriosclerosis by the synergy of allergic injury to arteries and lipid-rich diet. I. Effect of repeated injections of horse serum in rabbits fed a dietary cholesterol supplement. J Exp Med 124:635–651
114. Stehbens WE, Silver MD (1966) Arterial lesions induced by methyl cellulose. Am J Pathol 48:483–501
115. Lorenzen I, Helin P (1967) Arteriosclerosis induced by hypoxia. Acta Pathol Microbiol Scand 69:158–159
116. Schenk EA, Penn I, Schwartz S (1965) Experimental atherosclerosis in the dog. A morphologic evaluation. Arch Pathol 80:102–109
117. Selye H (1961) The pluricausal cardiopathies. Thomas, Springfield
118. Scanu A, Orientel P, Szajewski JM, Page IH (1960) Atherosclerotic lesions produced in dogs by prolonged administration of triton-WR-1339. Circulation 22:685–686
119. Hueper WC (1941) Experimental studies in cardiovascular pathology. III. Polyvinyl alcohol atheromatosis in the arteries of dogs. Arch Pathol 31:11–24
120. Bloor CM, Lowman RM (1963) Experimental coronary arteriography. The distribution and extent of allylamine induced vascular lesions in the dog. Radiology 81:770–777
121. Moreland AF, Clarkson TB, Lofland HB (1963) Atherosclerosis in "miniature" swine. I Morphologic aspects. Arch Pathol 76:203–210
122. Moreland AF (1965) Experimental atherosclerosis of swine. In: Roberts JC, Straus R (eds) Comparative atherosclerosis. Harper and Row, New York, pp 21–24
123. Manning PJ, Clarkson TB (1970) Diet-induced atherosclerosis of the cat. Arch Pathol 89:271–278
124. Morris MD, Fitch CD (1968) Spontaneous hyperbetalipoproteinemia in the rhesus monkey. Biochem Med 2:209–215
125. Clarkson TB (1972) Animal models of arterosclerosis. Adv Vet Sci Comp Med 16:151–173
126. Younger RK, Scott HW Jr, Butts WH, Stephenson SE Jr (1969) Rapid production of experimental hypercholesterolemia and atherosclerosis in the rhesus monkey. Comparison of five dietary regimes. J Surg Res 9:263–271
127. Taylor CB (1966) Experimental pathology of atherosclerosis and myocardial infarction in rhesus monkeys. In: Bajusz E, Jasmin G (eds) Methods and achievements in experimental pathology, vol 1. Karger, New York, pp 355–384
128. Cox GE, Trueheart RE, Kaplan J, Taylor CB (1963) Arteriosclerosis in rhesus monkeys. Arch Pathol 76:166–176
129. Kent SP, Vawter GF, Dowben RM, Benson RE (1958) Hypervitaminosis D in monkeys. A clinical and pathologic study. J Pathol 34:37–59

130. Taylor CB (1965) Experimental atherosclerosis in the subhuman primate. Acta Cardiol (Brux) [Suppl] 11:238–275
131. Lofland HB Jr, Clarkson TB, Bullock BC (1970) Whole body sterol metabolism in squirrel monkeys (*Saimiri sciureus*). Exp Mol Pathol 13:1–11
132. Schaper W, Vandesteene R (1967) The rate growth of interarterial anastomoses in chronic coronary artery occlusion. Life Sci 6:1673–1680
133. Vastesaeger MM, Delcourt R (1965) L'atherosclerose experimentale du chimpanze. Recherches preliminaires. Acta Cardiol (Brux) [Suppl] 11:283–297
134. Groover ME (1965) Experimental arterial lesions in the baboon. In: Vagtborg H (ed) Baboon in medical research. University of Texas Press, Austin, pp 525–529
135. Ueda H, Saito Y, Morooka S, Ito I, Yamaguchi H, Sugiura M (1968) Experimental arteritis produced immunologically in rabbits. Jpn Heart J 9:573–582
136. Kerber CW, Buschman RW (1977) Experimental carotid aneurysms: I. Simple surgical production and radiographic evaluation. Invest Radiol 12:154–157
137. Selye H (1958) The chemical prevention of cardiac necrosis. Ronald, New York
138. Rushmer RF (1964) Initial ventricular impulse. A potential key to cardiac evaluation. Circulation 29:268–283
139. Litvak J, Sideridea LE, Vineberg AM (1957) The experimental production of coronary artery insufficiency and occlusion. Am Heart J 53:505–518
140. Bloor CM (1972) Pathophysiology of acute myocardial infarction in conscious dogs. In: Bloor CM (ed) Comparative pathophysiology of circulatory disturbances. Plenum, New York, pp 347–358 (Advances in experimental medicine and biology, vol 22)
141. Hood WB Jr, Joison J, Kumar R, Katayama I, Nieman RS, Norman JC (1970) Experimental myocardial infarction. I. Production of left ventricular failure by gradual coronary occlusion in intact conscious dog. Cardiovasc Res 4:73–83
142. Zollikofer C, Castende-Zuniga W, Vlodever Z, Rysavy J, Gomes AS, Amplatz K (1981) Experimental myocardial infarction in the closed-chest dog: a new technique. Invest Radiol 16:7
143. Lumb G, Singletary H (1961) High intraventricular septal infarcts in pig and dog. Fed Proc 20:103
144. Patterson DF (1968) Epidemiologic and genetic studies of congenital heart disease in the dog. Circ Res 23:171–202
145. Gage AA, Olson KC, Chardack WM (1956) Experimental coronary thrombosis in the dog. Ann Surg 143:535–543
146. Pisa Z, Hammer J (1961) Experimental myocardial infarction in closed chest dogs with selective embolisation of the coronary vascular bed. Exp Med Surg 19:1–8
147. Levitt J, Oppenheimer MJ (1968) Central neural organization of an automatic reflex following cardiac necrosis. Circulation [Suppl] 38:(6)127
148. Nakhjavan FK, Shedrovilzky H, Goldberg H (1968) Experimental myocardial infarction in dogs. Description of a closed chest technique. Circulation 38:777–782
149. Elzinga WE, Kaufman WM, Upright DE, Powell D (1969) A new animal model – myocardial infarction. Physiologist 12:215
150. Salazar AE (1961) Experimental myocardial infarction. Induction of coronary thrombosis in the intact closed chest dog. Circ Res 9:1351–1356
151. Agress CM, Rosenberg MJ, Jacob HI, Binder MJ, Schneiderman A, Clark WG (1952) Protracted shock in the closed chest dog following coronary embolization with graded microspheres. Am J Physiol 170:536–549
152. Harris AS (1966) Potassium and experimental coronary occlusion. Am Heart J 71:797–802
153. Leeds SE, MacKay ES, Mooslin K (1951) Production of ventricular fibrillation and defibrillation in dogs by means of accurately measured shocks across exposed heart. Am J Physiol 165:179–187
154. Beck CS (1929) The effect of surgical solution of chlorinated soda (Dakin's solution) in the pericardial cavity. Arch Surg 18:1659–1671
155. Isaacs JP, Carter BN II, Haller JA Jr (1952) Experimental pericarditis, the pathologic of constrictive pericarditis. Bull John Hopkins Hosp 90:259–300

156. Christensen EE, Curry GC, Bonte FJ (1967) Technique for percutaneous indwelling catheterization of the pericardium and the production of pericardial effusions in dogs. Invest Radiol 2:391–393

157. Miller AJ, Pick R, Katz LN (1964) The importance of the lymphatics of the mammalian heart: experimental observation and some speculations. Circulation 29:485–487

158. Erickson RV, Scher AM, Becker RA (1957) Ventricular excitation in experimental bundle branch block. Circ Res 5:5–10

159. Fisher VJ, Lee RJ, Christianson LC, Kavaler F (1961) Production of chronic atrioventricular blocks in dogs without thoracotomy. J Appl Physiol 21:1119–1121

160. Steiner C, Kovalik ATW (1968) A simple technique for production of chronic complete heart block in dogs. J Appl Physiol 25:631–632

161. Ueda H, Harumi K, Mashima S, Kuroiwa A, Sato C, Yamamoto M, Iguchi K, Murao S (1974) Experimental production of ventricular complex simulating A, B, and C types of WPW syndrome. Jpn Heart J 15:503–516

162. Norman TD (1962) The pathogenesis of cardiac hypertrophy. Prog Cardiovasc Dis 4:439–463

163. Bishop SP, Cole CR (1969) Ultrastructural changes in the canine myocardium with right ventricular hypertrophy and congestive heart failure. Lab Invest 20:219–229

164. Higgins CB, Pavelec R, Vatner SF (1973) Modified technique for production of experimental right-sided congestive heart failure. Cardiovasc Res 7:870–874

165. Cooper G, Satava RM (1974) A method for producing reversible long term pressure overload of the cat right ventricle. J Appl Physiol 37:762–764

166. Rogers WA, Bishop SP, Hamlin RL (1971) Experimental production of supravalvular aortic stenosis in the dog. J Appl Physiol 30:917–920

167. Iyengar SRK, Charrette EJP, Iyengar CKS, Lynn RB (1973) An experimental model with left ventricle hypertrophy caused by subcoronary stenosis in dogs. J Thorac Cardiovasc Surg 66:823–827

168. O'Kane HO, Geha AS, Kleiger RE, Abe T, Salaymeh MT, Malik AB (1973) Stable left ventricular hypertrophy in the dog. Experimental production, time course, and natural history. J Thorac Cardiovasc Surg 65:264–271

169. Friedman PJ, Harley RA, Liebow AA (1972) Comparative pathophysiology of pulmonary hypertension. Development of a model. In Bloor CM (ed) Comparative pathophysiology of circulatory disturbances. Plenum, New York, pp 205–249

170. Patterson DF (1967) Animal models of congenital heart disease, with special reference to patent ductus arteriosus in the dog. In: Animal models for biomedical research. Proceedings of symposium, publication no 1594. National Academy of Sciences, Washington DC, pp 131–156

171. Monie IW, Takacs E, Warkany J (1966) Transposition of the great vessels and other cardiovascular abnormalities in rat fetuses induced by trypan blue. Anat Rec 156:175–190

172. Barrow MV, Taylor WJ (1971) The production of congenital heart defects with the use of antisera to rat kidney, placenta, heart and lung homogenates. Am Heart J 82:199–206

173. Haller JA Jr, Suzuki H, El Shafie M, Shaker IJ (1973) Intrauterine production of coarction of the aorta with normal birth and survival. J Pediatr Surg 8:171–174

174. Kline JL, Gimenez JL, Maloney RJ (1962) Post-stenotic vascular dilation: confirmation of an old hypothesis by a new method. J Thorac Cardiovasc Surg 44:738–748

175. Patterson DF, Detweiler DK (1967) Hereditary transmission of patent ductus arteriosus in the dog. Am Heart J 74:289–290

176. Kaplan N, Rudolph AM (1969) Physiologic studies of pulmonary circulation and ductus arteriosus of sheep and goat fetuses. Invest Radiol 4:68–82

177. Rowe RD, Folger GM Jr, Bor I, Criley JM (1964) Cineangiographic demonstration of changes in caliber of the ductus arteriosus in newborn swine breathing high and low oxygen mixtures. Circulation [Suppl 3] 30:149–150

178. Robinson JJ (1951) Attempts to produce rheumatic carditis in laboratory animals by the means of streptococcic injury. Arch Pathol 51:602–616

179. Walker WF, Hamburger M (1959) A study of experimental staphylococcal endocarditis in dogs. I. Production of the disease, its natural history and tissue bacteriology. J Lab Clin Med 53:931–941
180. Lillehei CW, Shaffer JM, Spink WW, Bobb JRR, Wargo JD, Visscher MB (1951) Role of cardiovascular stress in the pathogenesis of endocarditis and glomerulonephritis. Observations including method of experimental production utilizing arteriovenous fistulas. Arch Surg 63:421–434
181. Reeves MM, Dick HLH, McCawley EL (1969) Effects of ultrasound on the canine mitral valve. Med Res Eng 8:16–17
182. Vasko JS, Elkins RC, Fogarty TJ, Morrow AG (1967) The experimental production of chronic mitral valvular obstruction. J Thorac Cardiovasc Surg 53:875–880
183. Ferrin AL, Adams WL, Baronofsky ID (1951) Evaluation of experimental methods of producing functional mitral stenosis. Surg Forum 2:206–211
184. Kay JH, Thomas V (1954) Experimental production of pulmonary stenosis. Arch Surg 69:651–656
185. Frater RWM, Rothman D, Yuan S, Silver L, Weber C, Amirana M, Wexler H (1968) Experimental pulmonary stenosis created at birth. Surgery 64:322–331
186. Bishop SP, Cole CR (1969) Production of externally controlled progressive pulmonic stenosis in the dog. J Appl Physiol 26:659–665
187. Sabiston DC Jr, Williams GR (1954) The experimental production of infundibular pulmonic stenosis. Ann Surg 139:325–329
188. Nadel JA (1965) Alveolar duct constriction after barium sulfate microembolism. In: Sasahara AA, Stein M (eds) Pulmonary embolic disease. Grune and Stratton, New York, pp 153–161
189. Standertskjöld-Nordenstam C-G, Tähti E, Harjola, P-T, Scheinin T (1969) Preparation of elongate radiopaque gelatin emboli. Invest Radiol 4:396–397
190. Cade JF, Hynes DM, Garnett ES, Regoeczi E, Hirsh J (1974) Hot clot scan – a method for the accurate identification of experimental pulmonary emboli. Invest Radiol 9:32–36
191. Marshall R, Sabiston DC, Allison PR, Bosman AR, Dunnill MS (1963) Immediate and late effects of pulmonary embolism by large thrombi in dogs. Thorax 18:1–9
192. Raffer PK, Montemurno R, Scudese V, Sherr S (1972) Experimental production and recovery of pulmonary fat emboli in dogs – origin of the fat. Surg Forum 22:446–448
193. Dahlgren SE, Josephson S (1970) Pulmonary air embolization in the dog: postmortem findings. Acta Pathol Microbiol Scand [A] 78:482–488
194. Sherr S, Gertner SB (1974) Production and recovery of pulmonary fat emboli in dogs. Exp Mol Pathol 21:63–73

CHAPTER 5

Contrast Media for Imaging
of the Central Nervous System

M. Sovak

A. Introduction

The desire to image the brain and spinal cord has been motivated by two major
needs: to depict the pathology and to assess the pathophysiology of the structures
which, after the First World War, became amenable to surgical interventions. The
development of contrast media (CM) has brought increasingly safer compounds,
which are increasingly devoid of side effects and capable of visualizing both the
vasculature and the cavities of the CNS. Computed tomography (CT) further extended the diagnostic capabilities of CM. Thus, a CT-localized contrast enhancement indicates the barrier breakage since water-soluble CM normally do not pass
the blood-brain barrier CT also revived the use of negative CM (i.e., intrathecal
nonopaque gases) and prompted experimentation with freely diffusable positive
contrast-enhancing agents exhibiting general affinity for the lipids of the CNS. Inhalation of 70% xenon increases the density of the gray matter by 12 HU and that
of the white matter by 20 HU; it provides excellent visualization of both brain [1]
and spinal cord [2]. The disadvantages of xenon, i.e., its high cost and systemic
and anesthetic effects, may well be outweighed by its potential for detecting
pathological conditions of the CNS and regional blood flow disturbances. New
high-resolution CT scanner systems capable of rapid serial data collection are
making dynamic studies possible [3, 4].

As an alternative to xenon, iodoantipyrine has been tested in dogs in doses of
approximately 60 mg/kg. Intravenous injections resulted in a contrast enhancement ranging from 1 to 5 HU, while bolus injection into the common carotid artery gave substantial enhancement of the brain with a preference for gray matter
[5]. The authors encountered low aqueous solubility of the test compounds. The
high hydrophobicity of iodoantipyrine is presumably responsible for the passage
into the CNS, but also for the high toxicity. Further research should attempt to
design a biologically inactive compound capable of passing the blood-brain barrier. This may prove difficult, since only lipophilic substances can pass an intact
blood-brain barrier, and from a lipophilic compound biological activity in the
CNS can be expected.

Isotopes have long since been integrated into the neurodiagnostic armamen-
tarium. An important achievement is positron imaging based on entrapment of
2-[^{18}F]-2-deoxy-D-glucose, a compound which competes readily with glucose for
cerebral uptake. Once in the cell, the compound is phosphorylated to a 6-phos-
phate which, while being slowly metabolized, provides in conjunction with a posi-

tron-emission tomographic scanner information not only about CNS morphology but also about regional metabolism [6].

Nuclear magnetic resonance (NMR) tomography is emerging as a noninvasive imaging method free of ionizing radiation and affording image reconstruction along multiple axes with clinically negligible energy exposure [7, 8]. Although a number of atoms like Na or P can be used, the most practical NMR-scanning technology is based on imaging of protons, specifically the protons' density and behavior in the magnetic field. Because of the relatively low water content of the CNS and preponderance of lipids, which are known to affect the proton relaxation times, CNS structures image well on NMR tomograms. There seems to be no obvious need for CM in the normal CNS. On the other hand, albeit with varying degrees of specificity, pathological processes have been shown to alter the NMR signal [9]. Possibly the specificity in detecting the pathology could be enhanced by compounds known to increase the proton-generated NMR signal. It is also conceivable that the morphological information could be increased if substances selectively enhancing or suppressing the NMR signal were utilized. Nuclear magnetic resonance CM could perhaps depict a breakage of the blood-brain barrier and/or reflect dynamic flow changes. Molecules known to affect the proton signal, i.e., paraffinic, ferromagnetic, and paramagnetic compounds, are being considered, the Gd 3^+/DTPA/bismeglumine complexes so far showing the greatest promise [10, 11].

The following text reviews the state of the art of the positive contrast media for neuroradiography, principally focusing on developments of the past decade. Contrast media for cerebral and spinal cord angiography and for the subarachnoid space will be addressed separately. Sources of methodology applicable to investigative neuroradiology in the CM field are summarized in Chap. 6.

In reviewing the voluminous literature, it appeared appropriate for the purpose of this book to focus on work significant for the improvement of CM design. For most new CM, opinions in the literature are becoming increasingly critical; this text focuses on recent reactions in the hope of provoking the reader's criticism and of stimulating further research toward a totally biologically inert and economical CM.

B. Angiographic Contrast Media in Neuroradiology

In spite of recent advances in computed tomography, cerebral angiography (CA) retains its value in the diagnosis of an extensive spectrum of vascular and neural tissue diseases. The diagnostic potential of CA was first realized by Moniz, who in 1927 injected strontium bromide by direct carotid puncture.

After much experimentation, techniques of neuroangiography have reached a stage of well-established routine; the methodology is the subject of extensive reviews [12–16].

CNS angiography was first attempted with percutaneous puncture and/or surgical exposure of the common carotid artery. The method was later refined by the introduction of selective external and internal carotid punctures and simultaneous bilateral carotid puncture. Although the latter method reduces the number of exposures and enables a comparison of the hemodynamics of both injected sites to be made, it has not been generally recommended, due to the ischemia and toxicity of CM.

Unlike the carotid artery, direct approach to the vertebral artery is more difficult. Technical failures, complications ranging from thrombosis of the artery to the development of an arteriovenous fistula, subintimal injection of the CM, and inadvertent entry into the subarachnoid space were all reported. Because of these hazards, vertebral angiographies are often performed via the subclavian artery, or more often by a retrograde brachial artery approach. Biocompatible and maneuverable intravascular catheters, reliable CM delivery instrumentation, and modern fluoroscopy make the approach to the cerebral circulation from distant periphery possibly. Thus, not only brachial but also femoral arteries are widely used as points of entry. In venography, techniques of access to the orbital, cavernous superior sagittal sinus directly or in the jugular vein have been developed.

Techniques of spinal cord arteriography (SCA) have also been reviewed in detail [17–19]. Typically, SCA is performed using a catheter introduced via a femoral or axillary artery. In SCA, even more so than in cerebral angiography, CM's toxicity plays an important role. To some extent, the toxicity can be potentiated by the injection technique. The nonselective technique of aortic injection limits the CM toxicity but its diagnostic information is also limited. Selective injections into the spinal cord arteries are highly informative but they carry a risk of serious sequelae caused both by CM toxicity and ischemia. Therefore, selective injection of current ionic monomers has not evolved into a routine radiological examination.

Spinal cord phlebography (SCP) is a safer technique, but it has a different diagnostic value. The first SCPs were obtained by injection of CM into the processus spinosus or the body of a vertebra. The method was superseded by catheterization of the epidural veins, which has the advantage of opacifying the epidural venous plexus bilaterally. Lesions located within the intradural space and the spinal cord cannot be demonstrated by spinal phlebography, however. Lumbar and cervical techniques of SCP are most commonly used; transfemoral lumbar epidural phlebography has been described in a monograph [20]. The method has also been recommended as a screening procedure before myelography, as an alternative in the diagnosis of herniated disks not demonstrated by myelography. With the advent of CT technology, the relevance of SCP for disk disease diagnosis has diminished considerably.

I. Current Ionic Contrast Media

1. Cranial Angiography

After some initially disastrous results, MONIZ produced the first clinical radiograms using 25% sodium iodide. Shortly thereafter, a colloidal thorium dioxide suspension (Thorotrast) was developed and heralded as an innocuous, nontoxic vascular contrast medium. Although devoid of acute neurotoxicity in cerebral angiography, Thorotrast produced serious late sequelae due to the retention in the RES and to the emanating α-radiation (see also Chap. 9).

Even before Thorotrast was removed from clinical use, a number of iodine-containing compounds were developed and used in cranial angiography (CA) in spite of their relatively high toxicity. The pharmacology of these compounds (iodopyracet, methiodal sodium and sodium iodomethamate, acetrizoate, and diprotrizoate) is now only of historical interest [21, 22] and so is an attempt to utilize emulsified iodinated poppyseed oil as an angiographic agent [23].

Currently, the most extensively used agents for CA are diatrizoate, iothalamate, metrizoate, and ioglicinate, which, as sodium and/or methylglucamine salts or mixtures with added calcium or magnesium, have been comparatively studied extensively. The mechanisms of neurotoxicity of these ionic monomers were studied adequately to permit formulation of a design theory of an improved CM, which in turn yielded nonionic metrizamide, followed by a second generation of nonionic CM.

The effects of ionic CM on the brain circulation are similar to those in other vascular beds. Since many side effects stem from alteration of blood rheology, a great deal of attention has been given to the interaction of CM and erythrocytes. Originally, it was believed that CM affect the microcirculatory blood flow by causing erythrocyte aggregation. The subject is well reviewed elsewhere [21]. It was, however, demonstrated that hypertonic solutions, by extracting the intracellular water, change the erythrocyte morphology while making the cells rigid.

When intravascular erythrocytes flowing in CM were observed in vivo, aggregation occurred. The erythrocytes became more rigid, which was explained by increased hemoglobin concentration, resulting from the loss of water, which in turn decreased the cellular flexibility normally needed for unhindered passage of the erythrocytes through the capillaries. Experiments with human erythrocytes led to the conclusion that the CM effects on their morphology are a combination of hypertonicity and chemotoxicity of CM, the smallest changes being induced by the most hydrophilic CM whose tonicity was as close to that of blood as possible [21].

Ionic CM affect the neural structures directly and they also elicit a secondary array of systemic hemodynamic responses. Such responses in turn evoke a number of compensatory reactions which render the pharmacodynamic picture even more complex [24–33].

Intracarotid injection of CM produces vasodilation, primarily of the external carotid bed. The injection, however, also results in bradycardia and hypotension. As mentioned above, CM increase the blood viscosity, transiently decreasing the bolus passage through the cerebral circulation. Some discrepancies can be found in the literature describing effects of CM on the brain circulation. Often, they were caused by the experimental design's inability to control fully the interplay of various autoregulative mechanisms governing local and systemic hemodynamics. Because of the autoregulation, effects of CM on cerebral blood flow (CBF) are of importance. CBF is remarkably stable even when potent adrenergic manipulation is attempted or profound functional shifts of the cerebral regional flow occur. Thus, injection of norepinephrine into the common carotid artery produces vasoconstriction in the external, but not in the internal, carotid vascular beds. It is well known that regional blood flow in the brain of conscious humans studied with the ^{133}Xe method is considerably different for various motoric and mental activities; yet the total CBF remains the same. Vasomotor reflexes do not participate to any great extent in the regulation of CBF although both vasoconstrictor and vasodilator fibers are found in the cerebral vasculature. On the other hand, the brain arteries are sensitive to the plasma levels of carbon dioxide, whose decrease elicits vasoconstriction.

Another regulatory mechanism maintaining CBF constancy is the Cushing reflex: Increasing systemic blood pressure results in an increase of the intracranial pressure. Within the physiological range, the rise in intracranial pressure parallels the rise in systemic blood pressure.

The cardioinhibitory center located in the nucleus ambiguous may produce reflex bradycardia while the vasomotor center in the medulla oblongata may produce vasoconstriction/dilation of the peripheral vasculature by affecting the peripheral vascular resistance.

When CM are injected into the cerebral circulation, it must be surmised that they act not only on the brain vasomotor centers, but also on the baro- and chemoreceptors in the cranial vasculature. Hyperosmolality clearly affects the baroreceptors, but there is some evidence that the baroreceptors in the carotid sinuses normally influencing the systemic blood pressure and the heart rate might also be activated or reactivated by the chemotoxicity of the CM. Further, it is quite possible that some responses to CM are mediated by the chemoreceptors within the carotid circulation.

A number of ingenious experimental designs have attempted to unravel this complexity by isolating the potential factors. It was debated whether the bradycardia and hypotension reflexes are mediated by the receptors located in the carotid circulation [25–27], or also by a vasomotor brain center [29, 30]. The former studies noted that the bradycardia could be abolished by atropine or by lateral vagotomy.

Originally, it was thought that the site of origin of both the bradycardia and the hypotensive reaction was only the internal carotid system [31]. Both chemotoxicity and hyperosmolality of the CM solutions were considered eliciting factors. Thus, when sodium acetrizoate, sodium diatrizoate, meglumine iothalamate, and a mixture of sodium and meglumine diatrizoates (Renografin) were compared with Dimer-X and a hypertonic saline solution, it was found that acetrizoate, the most hydrophobic and thus most chemotoxic of the CM tested, caused the greatest change, while Dimer-X, a less hypertonic and more hydrophilic medium, produced no significant change [25].

Another study has shown that with increased osmolality of test mannitol solutions, bradycardia and hypotension increased. The intensity of bradycardia and hypotension produced by the hypertonic diatrizoate and iothalamate meglumine salts was greater compared with the less hypertonic metrizamide and/or iopamidol. Interestingly, metrizamide produced less changes than iopamidol, possibly because of metrizamide's lower osmolality at equal iodine levels. Since chemotoxicity of metrizamide and iopamidol is known to be lower than that of ionic monomers and since it was realized that solutions of low chemotoxicity but high osmolality could mimic the effects of the ionic CM, the mechanism of vascular neurotoxicity was attributed primarily to the high osmolality of the CM solutions. It was also noted that sodium potentiated the neurotoxic effects [27].

Further light on the question of the origin of the reflectoric response was shed by a study which compared meglumine sodium diatrizoate with metrizamide and/ or nicotine in canine carotid circulation before and after autonomic blockade and denervation of the carotid body. Cholinergic blockade, denervation of the carotid body, and cardiac pacing all abolished the usual initial bradycardia and hypotension. Nicotine produced a similar response. The authors concluded that the hemodynamic effects of CM result from a composite action on the cardiovascular brain centers and on the receptors in the carotid body and in the external carotid bed [26]. Another study confirmed that the vasomotor effects of diatrizoate and iothalamate originating from the external carotid bed and the vasomotor center of the brain were due to the CM chemotoxicity. Thus, repeated CM intracarotid injections elicited convulsions with frequency reproducibly characteristic for any given compound [28]. This effect could not be elicited with other hypertonic solutions [32, 33].

Efforts to localize the origins of the reflex were further extended by studying injection into the lingual, internal, and external carotid, and common carotid arteries, and closed common carotid arterial sac, using vagotomy or atropinization. This study supported the conclusion that the responses to CM were elicited from the periphery of the external carotid bed, from the carotid body, and from the brain [25].

Ionic CM are epileptogenic when in direct contact with the neurons, either via a subarachnoid injection or when injected into the brain circulation followed by diffusion from the capillaries. That can happen only if the blood-brain barrier (BBB) is severely damaged. The damage to the BBB by vascular ionic CM can be demonstrated by detection of extravasated tracers such as Trypan blue injected following angiography in animals. The method has been refined by employing $[^{197}Hg]Ac_2$, a small molecular tracer [35].

To maintain the nearly constant environment of the CNS neurons, necessary for their normal function, the BBB acts as a selective filter. Thus, exchange across the cerebral capillaries differs from that in other capillary beds. The BBB allows certain substances to pass the barrier at rates increasing with the compounds' lipophilicity and decreasing with their molecular size.

The anatomical site of the BBB is primarily the tight junctions linking the endothelial cells of the capillaries. CM injure the BBB of the arterioles as well as the venules of the cerebral circulation [36]. It has been claimed that the endothelial junctions could be opened indirectly by serum complement activated by CM [37] but it is now generally thought that hyperosmolality is the primary cause of opening the junctions [38, 39]. Once CM penetrate into the environment of the neurons they can exert their chemotoxicity on the neurons, thus eliciting a spectrum of adverse effects.

There is a voluminous body of literature on the toxicological comparisons of the three most extensively used ionic monomers, diatrizoate, iothalamate, and metrizoate, which, including enumeration of the sometimes conflicting findings, has been exhaustively reviewed elsewhere [22]. The evidence permits the conclusion that the effects of the ionic monomeric CM are not substantially different, that methylglucamine salts of either of the monomers are less toxic than the sodium-containing compounds, that addition of small amounts of calcium and magnesium ions decreases the toxicity, and that both hyperosmolality and chemotoxicity are responsible for CM toxicity. The advantage of ionic dimers over monomers appears marginal [22].

A number of adverse effects of clinical applications of CM in cranial circulation have been noted. Functional changes, such as electroencephalographic disturbances, have been described [40] as well as serious complications such as cortical blindness [42, 42]. Postangiographically occurring neuropsychiatric symptoms which culminated in the onset of GTS (Gilles de la Tourette Syndrome) suggested to the authors that the syndrome, previously thought to be purely psychogenic, may well be of organic origin [43]. A transient global amnesia was also reported [44]. An analysis of over 4,000 cerebral angiograms has shown an incidence of 13.6% of transient complications, of which 3.1% were of the neurologic-psychiatric type, mostly in younger patients and/or when a diffuse cerebrovascular disease was present [45].

Another study compared iothalamate and diatrizoate. Analysis of 5,000 cerebral angiograms revealed that the complication rate attributable to CM did not differ for Conray 60 and Renografin 60; however, when the injection volume was increased beyond the standard dose, the complication rate did not increase with Conray 60 while it did with Renografin 60 [46].

The pain produced by Conray 60, Renografin 60, and Renografin-M-60 was assessed in 40 subjects undergoing cerebral angiography. A subtraction technique was utilized to record the extent of the head movement, which the authors attributed to pain. From this and the subjective pain rating it was concluded that Conray 60 produced less pain than the other CM [47].

2. Spinal Cord Angiography

Because of the different physiology and anatomy of the spinal cord, spinal cord angiography (SCA) is, a more risky procedure than CA. The vasculature of the spinal cord is a complex system of surface and parenchyma arterial nets interconnected by intermedullary anastomoses. Knowledge of the segmental distribution of the spinal cord vasculature is important for angiographic procedures, both diagnostic and therapeutic. Comprehensive treatises of the topographic and radiographic anatomy of the spinal vasculature are available [17–19]. Because of the subtlety of the vasculature structures and CM toxicity, spinal cord angiography developed only relatively recently as a valuable procedure. Injuries to the spinal cord by angiography arise from catheter interference with the spinal blood flow. The resulting ischemia in turn potentiates the chemotoxicity of CM, sometimes inducing plegias [17, 18].

The hemodynamics of the spinal cord are, like those of the brain, governed by a complicated autoregulatory system which protects the parenchyma against sudden changes in perfusion. Akin to the cerebral circulation, oxygen and acidobasic balance affect the flow but the autoregulation maintains the spinal blood flow (SBF) within the narrow area even when the systemic blood pressure changes considerably [48, 49]. Since mechanical impediment of regional blood flow by trauma is one of the major causes of spinal cord damage, methods to measure SBF were developed. Techniques previously established for determination of the cerebral blood flow (^{133}Xe, fluorescent indicators, ^{14}antipyrine, [^{3}H]nicotine, and ^{14}C iodoantipyrine [49, 50]) are all applicable for SBF determination.

Experimental spinal cord trauma in the dog, its effects on SBF and CNS functions, and its therapeutic possibilities have been studied extensively [51–53]. More research is needed to establish the value of early diagnosis in traumatic vasculature deficiency for surgical or interventional therapy. Selective catheterization, use of nontoxic CM, and selectively delivered drugs could be useful. In this respect, vasoactive substances known to affect the spinal circulation may find application. Intraarterial papaverine, nitroglycerine, a combination of raubasine with dihydroergosistine (Iskedyl), and YC-93 have been found applicable [54–56].

Akin to the cerebral vasculature, the endothelial cells and their tight junctions of the spinal cord arteries form a blood barrier which protects the milieu of the neurons. Destruction of the barrier by a chemotoxic and/or hypertonic agent makes the neurons extremely vulnerable. It has been shown that neuronal damage increases with increased dose of ionic CM. These experiments indicated that toxicity increases not only with increased dose but also with increased concentration, even if blood flow is unaffected by selective catheterization [57, 58]. The Brown-Séquard syndrome and complete paraplegias were described after unintentional ingress of large amounts of ionic monomeric CM into the spinal cord arteries, mainly via the thoracic aorta, the artery of Adamkiewicz and the superior dorsal radiculomedullary arteries [59–62].

II. Newer Nonionic Monomers and Monovalent Dimer in Neurovascular Use

It was expected that the first nonionic medium, metrizamide, would improve carotid angiography qualitatively and quantitatively. A comparison of metrizamide and meglumine metrizoate (Isopaque Cerebral) showed, however, the same frequency of complications for both compounds; nevertheless, metrizamide did produce significantly less discomfort in selective external carotid angiography [63]. Other studies, both in animals and humans, have consistently shown an overall superiority of metrizamide over the ionic monomers [64, 65]. When temporary deterioration of EEG and the length and extent of bradycardia were used as criteria, metrizamide proved less toxic than meglumine metrizoate [65].

A review of 479 CNS angiographies accomplished in ten separate studies comparing metrizamide with ionic media conclusively demonstrated that metrizamide caused significantly less discomfort, mainly pain and heat sensation, than the ionic media. This difference was particularly evident in selective and supraselective carotid injections. Metrizamide caused fewer EEG and electromyograph (EMG) changes, but some studies disagreed on metrizamide's potential to elicit bradycardia and hypotension. Compared with meglumine iothalamate, metrizamide had the same cerebral circulation time (CCT), but showed a shorter CCT when compared with metrizoate (Isopaque Cerebral). Significantly, SCA performed without general anesthesia with metrizamide produced no adverse reactions [66]. The extent of clinical use of metrizamide as an intravascular CM has unfortunately been limited by its high cost.

In an effort to obtain an improved but more economical alternative, Guerbet laboratories developed a monovalent ionic dimer (ioxaglate, Hexabrix). In a clinical vascular study, the compound was found to produce significantly less heat sensation and overall discomfort than meglumine iothalamate [67]. This can be attributed primarily to the compound's relatively lower osmolality, since the overall hydrophobicity of ioxaglate is similar to the ionic monomers. Recent experience with Hexabrix is reviewed in Chap. 3 and the Introduction.

The second generation of nonionic monomers is eminently applicable to cerebral angiography. Iohexol (Nyegaard Co), tested by experimental carotid angiography in animals, caused only minimal damage to the BBB, to an extent similar to ioxaglate [68].

Injection of iohexol into the common carotid artery of rats, however, produced some disturbances of motor coordination and occasionally proved epileptogenic. There was no statistically significant difference found between iohexol and metrizamide at concentrations of 370 mgI/ml, at six dose levels [69]. Iohexol was compared with metrizamide in selective vertebral angiography in rabbits using 280 and 350 mg I/ml. The injection was continued until a convulsion occurred or until a maximum of 10 ml was injected. Both iohexol and metrizamide were found substantially less toxic than metrizoate, but iohexol's toxicity was inferior to that of metrizamide [70]. The authors speculated that the higher osmolality of iohexol could possibly explain the finding. In contrast, injection into the common carotid artery of rabbits found iohexol substantially less injurious to the BBB than metrizamide [68].

Clinical studies of iohexol in CA have been consistent in demonstrating iohexol's superiority over ionic agents, but they also indicate that this nonionic agent is far from being inert [71–74]. By direct comparison with metrizamide, it is apparent that the incidence of pain with iohexol is greater than with metrizamide [72, 75]; results of cerebral [76] and peripheral [77] angiographic trials with iopamidol [77] suggest that vascular pain is essentially absent. Yet, the hydrophilicity of metrizamide is lower than that of iohexol and/or iopamidol (which are nearly equal). The observation thus further supports the idea that vascular pain is attributable to hyperosmolality [78], the critical threshold being 650–750 mOsm. Iopamidol also shows superiority to ionic agents in lumbar epidural venography [79] and cerebral angiography [80]. An agent of similar toxicity and osmolality to iopamidol, iopromide, is reportedly comparable to the other nonionic CM [11, 81, 82].

Recently, a nonionic dimer iodecol (Schering) has been tested by excessive-dose carotid angiography in rabbits. While iopamidol, metrizamide, and iopromide (350 mg I/ml) all produced a similar incidence of side effects, including intracerebral vasospasm, iodecol proved comparatively more toxic. Inasmuch as iodecol, with an osmolality of 380 mOsm, does not induce vasospasm, it is possible that the higher toxicity is attributable to an effectively higher dose delivered to the CNS [82].

An ideal CM for CNS angiography does not yet exist. An ideal CM would have to be more hydrophilic than the best ones at present to be completely inert, and have osmolality at diagnostically useful concentrations under the pain threshold; since satisfying these requirements would mean high viscosity, CM based on benzene chemistry will remain a compromise.

C. Intrathecal Contrast Media

With the advent of the first successful neurosurgical operations in the early twenties, the need for imaging of the pathological morphology of the perispinal, pericerebral, and intracerebral cavities became a clinical necessity.

The techniques of entry into the spinal subarachnoid space (SAS) were developed early. DANDY and JOCOBAEUS used a spinal puncture to produce the first air encephalo- and myelograms [83–85]. Techniques of air delivery and percutaneous approach into the SAS at the lumbar, cervical, and cranial levels were established. The scope of myelography and encephalography is reviewed in specialized monographs [86–88]. In principle, the techniques have remained unchanged until the present.

A number of modifications have taken place, mainly to extend the diagnostic yield. One such technique is lumbar epidurography, which utilizes the Seldinger approach for insertion of a catheter through the sacral notch to make a selective nerve root injection. The indication for this method is an equivocal result of standard myelography or suspicion of disk herniation in patients with adhesive arachnoiditis. The method was originally developed in dogs [7], but was soon applied to patients [90, 91].

For elucidation of syndromes of the cauda equina roots, radiculosaccography can be employed [92]. Diskography is considered a useful adjunct to myelography when the diagnosis has not been equivocal and in selecting patients for fusion of cervical disks [93]. With the latest advances in CT and NMR imaging, the invasive techniques supplementary to myelography may lose their importance.

Some investigators attempted to increase the diagnostic yield by a double contrast technique. Air in combination with metrizamide was used in monkeys [94] and oxygen and metrizamide in clinical double contrast ventriculography [95]. The authors considered the method superior to CT in the diagnosis of obstructive hydrocephalus, small central tumors, and intraventricular cysts. A combination of intrathecally applied water-soluble media and CT was also found useful [96].

The question of relative contribution of the technique to the CM side effects became pertinent when CM received systematic pharmacological evaluation. It became recognized that every puncture of SAS carries with it the risk of inadvertent hemorrhage from a vascular tear, which can have serious consequences. Blood has been shown to be a potentiating agent in Pantopaque arachnoiditis [97]. Another risk is accidental transsection and withdrawal of a nerve filament [98]. Removal of large amounts of CSF can, in patients with CSF kinetics impeded by a pathological process, dislodge the CNS structures. This life-threatening adverse reaction, as well as a desire for a better diagnostic yield, prompted development of positive contrast myelographic media to replace air or other gas myelography. Even in patients with unaltered kinetics, large withdrawal of CSF acts as a stimulus for increased production and/or resorption, and almost invariably induces headaches.

The incidence of postmyelography headaches has been reported as low as 29% and as high as 62% [99–101]. Although originally attributed to the CM, it has been shown that the headaches, to some extent, correlate with the leakage of CSF at the puncture site [102]. A surgical repair of the leaking spinal cord envelopes causes the headaches to disappear [103]. Studies using isotopes have demonstrated that leakage of CSF into the epidural space coincides with headaches [100, 104], and some studies have been related size of the cannulas to headache incidence [99, 100, 105–107].

For this reason, some authors recommend the use of 22-g or 25-g cannulas; it seems, however, that the most important preventive factor is a proper technique for accurate insertion of the needle into the subarachnoid space, to prevent meningeal tears [100]. The headaches of the postlumbar puncture (so-called "postlumbar puncture syndrome") can most probably be classified as "traction headaches": due to the disturbed balance of CSF pressure, tension develops to partially displace and stretch the brain envelopes, activating the pain-sensitive receptors.

The myelography postlumbar puncture syndrome is to a large extent also attributable to the toxic effects of myelographic CM. Both oily and water-soluble CM can induce a meningeal reaction, which manifests itself by headache, nausea, vomiting, and neck stiffness [108, 109]. The postmyelography headache is thus not only a result of the puncture, but also of the meningism. A study has shown that intrathecal corticoids diminish or abolish the headache after myelography with iodophendylate [110]. Steroids cannot be used routinely with water-soluble ionic CM: when injected into the subarachnoid space at the time of myelography, the steroids did not diminish the incidence of the acute side effects and, in fact, potentiated the development of late arachnoiditis [111–113].

A potentially important observation on the occurrence of headache was made in a clinical study which compared two intrathecal CM, metrizamide and iopamidol. The overall frequency of side effects was similar for the two CM. The authors, however, found a correlation between headache frequency and the rate of elimination from the SAS: the higher the rate of elimination, the more frequent the headaches [114]. A parallel finding is that iocarmate, a much more toxic CM than the nonionic metrizamide, ioglunide, iohexol, and iopamidol, appears in higher concentration in the serum of monkeys injected intrathecally than nonionic media [115]. The rate of excretion is determined by the molecular structure of CM, and also by the positioning of the intrathecally injected subject [116].

The question of prophylaxis of postmyelographic headaches is still open. Related considerations were the subject of a separate study [117]. Preliminary experience with tiapride, an agent stimulating CSF production [118], suggests that further research is needed with this drug as a possible way of alleviating the postlumbar puncture headache.

A great deal of attention has been given to the effects of hydration on possible development of late arachnoiditis after intrathecal water-soluble CM. The problem has been studied in hydrated and dehydrated monkeys. Dehydrated animals had a lower CM concentration in the blood than hydrated animals, permitting the conclusion that the hydration slowed elimination of CM from the SAS [119].

In a series of 100 patients divided into hydrated and nonhydrated groups, hydration significantly reduced headaches and vomiting after metrizamide myelography. A study employing meglumine iocarmate in monkeys indicated a lower incidence of both seizures and arachnoiditis in the hydrated animals [120, 121]. It remains to be investigated whether the beneficial effect of hydration is indeed attributable to the faster elimination rate of the CM. As mentioned above, a higher rate of CM elimination from the SAS did not correlate with a lower incidence of headaches when metrizamide and iopamidol were compared in a double-blind study [114].

Since the introduction of Pantopaque, there has been no unified opinion about the removal of the CM after the procedure; some radiologists, especially in Great Britain, have preferred not to remove Pantopaque. On the other hand, substantial evidence has accumulated favoring CM removal from the patient. For example, in a case of chronic, severe urticaria and intermittent anaphylaxis which was found to be mediated by an anti-iophendylate IgE, removal of iophendylate from the SAS brought about almost complete relief [122]. Even in metrizamide myelography, CM removal has resulted in reducing the incidence of headache and nausea [123].

To alleviate the side effects of CM, premedication with Valium has been suggested for iocarmate, but it has not gained general acceptance [124]. Neuroleptic drugs have been shown to potentiate the epileptogenicity of metrizamide. This peculiar interaction between a CM and neuroleptic drugs was first described in experimental corticography and cisternography in dogs. The animals showed strong epileptic activity [125]. During metrizamide myelography in a patient taking chlorpromazine, a grand mal seizure occurred [126]. At present it is general practice to exclude neuroleptics for at least 2 days before myelography with metrizamide. It should be investigated whether nonionic media other than metrizamide would also exhibit such an unusual synergistic effect.

An ideal CM for the intrathecal space should be a completely biologically inert material, easily deliverable and rapidly excretable; it should mix with the CSF to outline the fine structures and crevices. These criteria can be at least theoretically approximated in a water-soluble nonionic, highly hydrophilic material forming aqueous solutions isotonic with CSF even at high concentration levels, like the recently described iotrol [127, 128]. For the best diagnostic yield, a CM should also be sufficiently viscous to remain initially as a bolus at the injection site [129]. Both isotonicity with CSF and higher viscosity prevent early dilution when the CM is being maneuvered along the spinal canal.

I. Intrathecal Visualization

The intrathecal space and brain cavities were first radiographically visualized by replacing CSF with air, resulting in a successful demonstration of CNS pathology in patients. The search for a positive CM was far more complicated, but the results also more rewarding. Pneumoencephalography has been almost totally replaced by modern positive CM. The initial stage of this development was thoroughly reviewed in the *Encyclopedia of Contrast Media* [93]; the following text will only summarize the subject to maintain the continuity. Although considered obsolete by most investigators, oily CM continue to be used clinically, and their pharmacology will therefore be reviewed more thoroughly.

The first radiopaque substances tested were inorganic compounds containing thorium, silver, bismuth, and/or iodine; studies now only of historical interest report on their effect in animals. Even the relatively less harmful compounds, Collargol (colloidal silver) and potassium iodide, were shown to be extremely toxic in the SAS of the dog [130].

In the 1920s, iodinated poppyseed oil (Lipiodol) was introduced in France for intrathecal treatment of epidemic encephalitis and sciatica. The rationale for the use of Lipiodol was the expected beneficial effect of iodine gradually released from the iodinated oil. Later, Lipiodol was employed as a radiographic CM by SICARD and FORESTIER. The idea of application of Lipiodol as a myelographic agent originated from an accidental subarachnoid injection which reportedly caused no ill effects. Within 4 years, the authors published a series of 500 patients with varying spinal cord and spinal column pathology, established the technique of epidural, intraventricular, and subarachnoid injections, and laid the basis for radiographic interpretation of spinal pathology [131]. This work established Lipiodol as a medium of choice for the next decade although it became generally recognized that Lipiodol could produce paraesthesias and pain in the lower extremities, headache, fever, and arachnoiditis. The toxicology of Lipiodol was the subject of several studies [132–134]. In diagnostic neuroradiology, the story of Lipiodol represented a quantitative leap which has maintained its momentum to the present; albeit Lipiodol is no longer used as a myelographic medium.

Attempts to modify Lipiodol by mixing it with olive oil or using partially chlorinated/iodinated poppyseed or peanut oils resulted, especially when emulsified, in high toxicity upon injection into the ventricles and/or the spinal subarachnoid space of dogs [135]. Today it is our understanding that emulsification of an essentially hydrophobic material, while creating a large surface contact area with the body, increases the exposure to the substance, thus potentiating its noxious binding to the biomacromolecules. The resulting perturbance of normal functions of such molecules induces toxicity.

In 1928, thorium dioxide in a colloidal suspension was introduced as a universal contrast material (see also Chap. 9). The history of Thorotrast was the subject of a number of publications and it also was reviewed extensively [86]. Although originally considered an ideal CM devoid of any significant toxicity, it was clear from the beginning that, due to its particulate and nonbiodegradable nature, Thorotrast could not be eliminated from the body. It was not until the 1950s that Thorotrast was finally completely abandoned, but even today patients are occasionally encountered who present with neoplastic and other lesions resulting from the long-term alpha-irradiation by the radioactive thorium.

In the subarachnoid space, Thorotrast was found to damage the ependymal lining of the ventricles and induce chronic inflammation with accumulation of macrophages in the perivascular spaces of the subependymal areas as well as around the choroid plexus [137]. For a while it was suspected that the meningeal reactions were caused by the dextrins contained in the Thorotrast colloidal preparations, and, as a remedy, forced drainage of the perispinal space was recommended after myelography [138]. Nevertheless, reports of clinical cases of nerve root irritation and damage manifesting itself by leg weakness, sensory loss, and fecal incontinence continued to appear [139].

Inasmuch as some of the adverse effects of Thorotrast were known by the early 1930s, efforts were made to develop a water-soluble CM. In 1931, an aqueous solution of sodium salt of iodo-methane-sulfonic acid (Abrodil) was introduced as CM for retrograde pyelography [140]. The medium was used extensively in the SAS, especially in Scandinavia, but it required a spinal anesthesia and had to be confined strictly to the lumbosacral region because of its high degree of acute neurotoxicity. To some extent, the toxicity was caused by the release of iodine. Although several times more stable than in the iodized oils, the aliphatic I–C bond of water-soluble Abrodil could not withstand the in vivo deiodinating mechanisms.

Reasoning that a substance naturally found in the body should be biologically acceptable as an intrathecal CM, some investigators developed and tested suspensions of diiodothyrosine and polymerized diiodothyrosine. These opaque amino acids were successfully kept in suspension in vivo by gelatin and resorbed totally from the subarachnoid space, but severe side effects were encountered in the small trial series of patients, and the medium was abandoned [141, 142]. Other suspensions like acetrizoic acid in soybean oil, ethyl iopodate in glucose, and 2,3,5,6-tetraiodohydroquinone-diethyl ether were considered but they did not leave the experimental stage [143].

Efforts of the investigators thereafter reverted toward improvement of myelographic oily CM, with the goal being development of an oily fluid inert in acute application like Lipiodol, but stable and easily eliminated from the subarachnoid space. In 1942, STRAIN developed ethyliodo-phenylundecylate (iodophenylate), a stable oily compound with a firm I–C aromatic bond [143]. This new compound, Pantopaque, was almost immediately accepted as a suitable medium for visualization of the subarachnoid space. Early experiments in canines have indicated that doses simulating clinical use were resorbed from the SAS within a year. Compared with Lipiodol, and additional advantage to the stability was the high fluidity of Pantopaque, enabling it to be easily maneuvered from the spinal canal into the cranial cavities.

Myelography with Pantopaque was reviewed extensively [142–144], but because of its continuing clinical use, in some countries it seems reasonable to reiterate here the main aspects of Pantopaque application.

Pantopaque has both advantages and disadvantages: the main advantage is a nearly complete lack of acute neurotoxicity. The medium is chemicophysically stable, water insoluble, and thus immiscible with the cerebrospinal fluid. It also has extremely slow action and elimination pharmacokinetics, and is almost devoid of immediate biological activity, which makes cisternography or myelography a relatively safe acute procedure.

The disadvantages are several. Due to its high hydrophobicity and consequent high surface tension Pantopaque forms globules in the aqueous milieu of CSF. Therefore, this CM cannot depict the fine crevices accurately. Since it cannot be diluted by the CSF, radiodense Pantopaque often obscures small lesions. For this reason, derivatives containing less than the standard 30.5% iodine have been tested clinically. A 22.5% I-containing Pantopaque, in spite of a slightly higher viscosity, was found in cervical and thoracic spinal regions diagnostically superior to regular Pantopaque [145]. Nevertheless, further development of this medium has not been pursued, partly because of other oily media alternatives and partly because of the efforts to develop water-soluble CM suitable for intrathecal use.

The most frequently encountered acute side effects of Pantopaque myelography are backache and headache, ranging from 29% to 46% of cases. A number of studies, however, ascertained that these headaches are predominantly attributable to the interference with the CSF kinetics by spinal puncture rather than to the CM [131, 135].

Convulsions with Pantopaque are an extremely rare complication. One study identified a focal seizure disorder [146]. In another case, following myelography and a laminectomy, convulsions occurred in a patient; intracranial CM and resulting encephalopathy were the suspected cause of the seizures [147]. Acute visual loss after Pantopaque myelography was also reported and attributed to chemotoxicity [148]. A late loss of vision in conjunction with optic nerve disease also occurred [149].

A rare complication, diabetes insipidus, was thought to be elicited by a mechanical irritative effect on the hypothalamohypophyseal area by unresorbed droplets of supracellar Pantopaque [150].

Intravasation leading to pulmonary embolization has also been encountered. It was noted that this is particularly prone to occur when the injection is carried out at the L5–S1 level [151]. A number of cases have been reported [151, 152] and the subject has been reviewed [153].

An irritative effect of iodophendylate on the ependymal lining leading to occlusion of the foramina of MAGENDI and LUSCHKA by granulation tissue producing obstructive hydrocephalus has been described [154]. The chemotoxicity of Pantopaque has been found to be overly manifest in demyelinating processes. Thus, an increase of adverse reactions in patients with multiple sclerosis has been reported [155].

Occasionally, complication of myelography with iodophendylate involves an immunological mechanism. Meningitis and urticaria have been reported in patients exposed to Pantopaque; since the patients underwent intradermal testing with Pantopaque prior to myelography, the authors suspected sensitization [156]. Chronic urticaria and intermittent anaphylaxis have also been reported [122].

The truly serious sequelae of Pantopaque result from chronic inflammation of the CNS envelopes. The actual frequency of the inflammatory reaction has never been determined since only a minority of the patients who develop arachnoiditis also develop clinical symptoms. Even when this happens, it is usually after a long interval, sometimes of many years. Occasionally, arachnoiditis (in the absence of symptoms) can be demonstrated in patients restudied radiographically. There is nevertheless reason to suspect that the incidence is quite high. One study analyzed 100 patients with lumbosacral arachnoiditis documented by surgery or unequivocal myelography. The contribution of Pantopaque to the development of arachnoiditis was judged quite significant [157]. Although predominantly occurring in the lumbosacral area, constrictive arachnoiditis in the thoracic region was reported after Pantopaque myelography, unrelated to any trauma [158].

The reason for the late occurrence of side effects has been the subject of much speculation. It is known that Pantopaque increases the CSF proteins and induces lymphocytosis, which is indicative of sterile inflammation. This, however, has not been found to correlate with the development of late arachnoiditis. One possibility is that inflammation develops as a result of Pantopaque breakdown. The breakdown products could be toxic. That Pantopaque decomposes in vivo to some extent is evident since elevated serum protein-bound iodine was found after intrathecal injection [159]. Iodophendylate also affects CSF fractions [160]. An alternative mechanism of toxicity was proposed by the authors, who found minute fragments of glass in the vials of commercial Pantopaque and suspected that these fragments could enter the intrathecal space with the CM and cause an inflammatory reaction [161].

The fibrocytic-stimulating effect of Pantopaque found an application in interventional radiology: a number of investigators ascertained that injection of Pantopaque into renal cysts induces a proliferative process often resulting in the cyst's obliteration [162–164].

Arachnoiditis has been produced in a number of experimental animals. A model utilizing monkeys was particularly successful [163]. In rats, intraventricular iodophendylate caused enlargement of the ventricles; accumulated macrophages containing the CM were attached to the ependymal lining [164]. Other studies have also utilized rats [167, 168]. Electron microscopy of the meninges of rats and dogs demonstrated moderate cellular damage and multilayered proliferation of the ependymal epithelium [169].

Perfluorooctyl bromide (described in more detail in Chap. 9) was also tested in myelography. When injected into dogs, this remarkably acutely inert compound was well tolerated in animals which received up to 1 ml/kg intrathecally. Although not miscible with CSF due to its low viscosity, perfluorooctyl bromide provided better structure delineation than Pantopaque. Because of its chemical structure, akin to the inert plastic material Teflon, the compound cannot be excreted rapidly [170]. Experimental myelography in rabbits has shown that retained perfluorocarbons produce extensive arachnoiditis within a short period [171].

In view of the difficulties encountered with unexcretable oily materials, it is not surprising that a number of investigators attempted development of improved media. One approach addressed the problem of design and synthesis of oily materials which could be eliminated from the subarachnoid space at a fast rate. An extensive project resulted in preparation of a large number of carbonates, carbamates, and esters obtained from iodinated aromatic alcohols [172]. Studies of the structure-toxicity relationship found that carbonates were more rapidly eliminated than Pantopaque while having an acceptably low viscosity, and some of these compounds also demonstrated a surprisingly low toxicity in mice, determined by the intraperitoneal lethal dose [173].

As mentioned previously, the water-soluble salt of iodosulfonic acid (Abrodil, Methiodal) has been used in Scandinavia for lumbar myelography. In the 1960s, enough evidence of the toxicity of Methiodal accumulated to stimulate experimentation with an alternative, the aromatic monomers [174]. Unfortunately it was some years after the withdrawal of Methiodal that the evidence of high-frequency arachnoiditis secondary to this CM emerged [175, 176]. The acute side effects were recognized early. It was reported that Methiodal directly affected the spinal cord and the nerve roots [177]. Tonic and clonic spasms of lower extremities were frequently reported, often with escalation to frank epileptic seizures. Temporary loss of reflexes, paralysis of the extremities, paresis of the urinary bladder, and impotence were reported in a number of cases [178–185].

Similar acute side effects, albeit of a relatively low frequency, were expected for meglumine iothalamate. After long-term observations, the potential of iothalamate to produce arachnoiditis was shown to be far lower than that of Methiodal [186]. The new ionic medium thus replaced Methiodal completely in the visualization of the lumbar intrathecal space [111]. Although diatrizoate had also been considered, iothalamate was shown to have a lower seizure-inducing potential than diatrizoate [187, 188].

With time, evidence has accumulated that melgumine iothalamate was also prone to induce serious acute complications [189]. Although its epileptogenic potential has been recognized, some authors have used meglumine iothalamate in ventriculography [190–192]. Neurotoxicity of meglumine iothalamate has also been studied experimentally. Epileptogenicity has been demonstrated in rabbits [193]. Iothalamate in canine ventriculography produced chronic inflammatory changes in the ventricular lining, though not in the brain tissue [194]. The adverse reactions to iothalamate were in part attributed to hyperosmolarity [195]. A comparative study of iothalamate meglumine, iophendylate, and metrizamide in cerebral ventriculography in the rat identified the toxicity of iothalamate [166].

In patient studies arachnoiditis was reported [196, 197]. Also, when intracranial pressure was measured at the time of isovolumetric instillation of meglumine iothalamate into the lateral ventricules, a marked pressure increase in excess of 40% was recorded and attributed to the CM [198]. In cats, iothalamate was found to cause cardiovascular disturbances, motor hyperirritability, and convulsions in experimental myelography [199]. Epileptogenicity of iothalamate was also studied in rabbits, by comparison with other CM. Meglumine iothalamate has shown lower epileptogenicity, as measured by the EEG average maximum amplitude and duration of spike activity, than metrizoate, diatrizoate, Methiodal, and Dimer-X [200].

In an effort to decrease the osmolality of the iothalamate solutions, two iothalamate molecules were coupled [201]. The ionic dimer iocarmate (Mallinckrodt Inc.), under the name of Dimer-X, was quickly introduced into myelography. A number of studies have initially shown the dimer's superiority to the monomeric ionic media [202–204]. Myelography with iothalamate was recommended without spinal anesthesia, in contradistinction to the previously used Methiodal, but it was Dimer-X that attained general use in Europe without any anesthesia whatsoever [205]. Essentially no ill effects were found in a review of 1,702 myelograms [206]. Another study found Dimer-X acceptable in 500 myelograms [207].

Experimental studies in animals have, however, warned of the dimer's potential for adverse effects. Epileptogenicity following injection into the cranial intrathecal space was reported in rats [208]. Morphological changes in cats' ventricles were found [209], and the arachnoiditis-eliciting potential of Dimer-X otherwise documented [175, 210, 211]. Experimental study in monkeys demonstrated moderate to severe arachnoiditis with Dimer-X.

In an effort to reduce its arachnoiditis potential, a steroid was added to iocarmate, but, paradoxically, the steroid proved to potentiate development of arachnoiditis [180, 212–216]. The ineffectiveness of intrathecal methylprednisolone was also ascertained in experimental studies in the monkey [112]. In reviewing 3,000 clinical myelograms, arachnoiditis was found to be a frequent complication [217]. Paralysis following radiculography of the cauda equina syndrome was also reported [218, 219].

The epileptic potential of Dimer-X was then recognized both in animal studies [200] and in a clinical series, including 355 lumbar myelograms [220]. The authors of the latter article found that diazepine had a therapeutic effect on the paroxysms and have consequently recommended use of phenothiazines. When a new generation of CM, especially the nonionic materials, appeared, Dimer-X was used as a standard of excellence in almost every comparative study. There are several references available which summarize such information [221–223].

Dimer-X has been removed recently by FDA from the trade in the United States due to the occurrence of a single but fatal overdose accident.

The dimeric concept has been tested by the development of another ionic dimeric compound with a longer connecting bridge (PhDZ59B by Pharmacia, Sweden) [224]. The material was compared with meglumine iothalamate in canine myelography. In the same study, the dimer was also compared with iocarmate in monkeys and in rats. The compound showed only marginal advantage over iocarmate and iothalamate in monkeys and dogs while rabbits and rats showed low tolerance to all media tested. The authors also identified increased pressure in the SAS as a contributing factor to the side effects [225].

A number of triiodobenzoate derivatives containing various amino acids in the side chain have been synthesized (Schering AG, Berlin) [226]. One of the compounds containing serine has shown a surprisingly low neurotoxicity in preliminary tests and was therefore developed as a myelographic agent, Myelografin. In a comparative study with Dimer-X and metrizamide, the double-blind protocol included comparison of clinical side effects, EEG and EMG, as well as CSF changes after radiculography. The frequency of leptomeningeal arachnoiditis found at operation was lower for Myelografin than for Dimer-X, but the frequency of the acute side effects was comparable among the three media tested [227]. Myelografin, however, produced transitory root irritation [228], in contrast to metrizamide [229]. A study of 200 patients who underwent lumbar myelography with Myelografin nevertheless found a low incidence of side effects [230]. Similar results have been achieved by others [229].

A quantitative improvement in myelography was achieved with the development of metrizamide by ALMEN. ALMEN realized that most of the neurotoxic manifestations could be reduced if a nonionic hydrophilic contrast medium forming solutions of osmolality close to that of CSF was synthesized. In a nonionic agent, i.e., a molecule which would be solubilized by polar functional groups, and not by a salt formation, the need for an osmolality-increasing cation could be eliminated. Moreover, the charge (known to be a neurotoxic factor) could be removed [231]. The chemicophysical properties of metrizamide, its synthesis, stereochemistry, and physical characteristics have been reviewed in great detail [221–223]. More information on the chemistry of metrizamide can be found in Chap. 1 of this volume.

Metrizamide is not stable in aqueous solutions due to the vulnerability of the sugar portion of its molecule which is subject to a hydrolytically mediated rearrangement [232]. Metrizamide is isotonic with CSF at 180 mg I/ml. At 280 mg I/ml, it has an osmolality of 450 mOsm, while at the same iodine concentration iocarmate has an osmolality of about 1,040 mOsm, and that of the ionic monomers is about 1,450 mOsm. Compared with CSF, the osmolality of diagnostic metrizamide is thus less than twice the physiological value (Table 1).

Acute intravenous and intrathecal lethal dose determination in mice has established the superiority of metrizamide to any other contrast medium known at present [233]. In an effort to predict the effects of metrizamide in man, extensive studies in laboratory animals have been undertaken. The toxicity of metrizamide to the brain capillaries was tested by injection into the carotid artery of guinea pigs, followed by ^{32}P. The same study tested CNS cellular changes and the epileptogenic potential after pericerebral injection. Virtual absence of tissue reaction after subarachnoid injection, only minimal damage to the blood-brain barrier, and no seizures after subarachnoid injection of 0.1 ml 280 mg I/ml were reported in these experiments. The author concluded that by extrapolation, up to 10–15 ml metrizamide could be clinically injected without irritative effects [240]. As will be shown below, such extrapolation is not necessarily valid.

Injecting relatively large doses of metrizamide and/or iocarmate into anesthetized or unanesthetized rabbits found that metrizamide in contrast to iocarmate had only a slight depressive effect on the central nervous system [235]. Experimental lumbar myelography in cats revealed that metrizamide only minimally affected the cardiovascular parameters. Also, pressure in the urinary bladder utilized as a secondary indicator of spinal toxicity increased only minimally compared with iocarmate and/or iothalamate [199]. Metrizamide was also tested by occipital injection in rabbits in comparison with iocarmate, iothalamate, and another experimental Nygaard product, Compound 18, N-(3-acetamido-5-N-methyl acetamino-2,4,6-triiodobenzoyl)-2-amino-2-deoxy-D-glucitol (Table 1, Introduction). Changes in respiratory rate, arterial blood pressure, and excitability demonstrated the superiority of metrizamide. The authors observed immediate postinjection pressure increase in the cisterns, but found no difference among the CM or correlation with the side effects except for flattening of cortical EEG activity whenever pressure rose above 40 mmHg [236]. Suboccipital injection of metrizamide in cats did not reveal epileptogenicity for metrizamide [237]. Using a direct approach through a burr hole into the right frontal horn, the ventricular system of cats was injected. With this test, strong epileptogenicity was demonstrated for meglumine iothalamate and meglumine iocarmate. At a low dose level, no abnormalities were seen with metrizamide, but at 3 ml 280 mg I/ml some slowing of the EEG and spikes were observed; three out of eight cats died [238]. Neurotoxicity of CM in general is lower upon application to the ventricles rather than to the cortex. This study has indicated, in contradistinction to the earlier reports, the possible epileptogenic potential of metrizamide.

Metrizamide injected into the caudal sac of cats did not affect the amplitude or latency of the somatosensory evoked potentials while the ionic CM did. Neither did metrizamide and the concurrently tested Compound 18 increase motor neuron excitability [239]. This study left open the question of whether metrizamide penetrates less into the CNS, or whether, although it penetrates as well as the other media, it is inherently less chemotoxic.

The effect of CM on spinal reflexes in the cat has been studied by measuring electrically evoked cortical spinal responses and segmental spinal reflexes. Following intrathecal administration in cats anesthetized with alpha-chloralose, methylglucamine diatrizoate showed a pronounced increase in both cortical spinal responses and segmental spinal polysynaptic reflexes. Methylglucamine iothalamate increased the amplitude of these reflexes to a lesser degree while metrizamide showed no consistent effect [240].

An important study was conducted with rabbits instrumentalized with a chronic catheter placed operatively into the cisterna magna. Compared with iocarmate, which was tested concurrently, metrizamide produced no convulsions or pain reaction but did produce a transient ataxia 5–10 min after the injection. The ataxia was interpreted as the depressant effect of metrizamide on the motor centers. In the absence of epileptogenicity (the protocol did not include EEG), the neuromuscular depression would have been masked by anesthesia. It can be concluded from the results of this study that a depressive effect on the motor centers is one of the main pharmacologic effects of metrizamide [241]. This conclusion is also supported by an unpublished study [242]. Metrizamide produced fewer neurological deficits than equiosmolar sodium chloride, suggesting that disturbances of the electrolytic balance in CSF are an important toxicologic factor and that for this reason nonionic substances should be preferable to ionic ones.

Injected into the lumbar subarachnoid space of cats in doses up to 175 mg I/kg, metrizamide did not cause disturbance of EMG while hypertonic sucrose did [243]. This study thus demonstrated that hyperosmolality is another important toxicological factor and that tonicity of CM in the intrathecal space should be as close to CSF as possible.

Injection into the cisterna magna in young baboons with the CM spilling over the hemispheres produced tonic/clonic convulsions in a concentration of 300–400 mg I/ml [244]. Although in two cases droperidol and fentanyl were used for premedication, no drugs were utilized in the other seizure-suffering animals. It is, therefore, unlikely that in this study the neuroleptic drugs were the reason for the convulsion. Rather, these experiments suggest that with more developed CNS, the epileptogenic potential of metrizamide increases. The interaction of metrizamide with neuroleptic drugs has also been shown to occur in rabbits [161].

Assessing the potential of metrizamide for eliciting arachnoiditis in patients has been the subject of a number of experimental studies. We have mentioned above that iocarmate proved to induce arachnoiditis after lumbar myelography; yet preclinical testing in animals of iocarmate gave no indication that this might happen. In a number of experimental models, investigators attempted to produce arachnoiditis with intrathecal metrizamide [166, 246, 247].

The effects of metrizamide on the meninges have been studied by suboccipital injection in rats. Only a small change in the CSF protein content and cell count was found in the majority of the animals. There were no histological changes in the meninges of cats killed 48 h after the injection [248]. A slight increase in cell count was also found following ventriculography in a dog [249]. Whether such small increases in cell count are significant is doubtful since injection of isotonic, hypertonic saline and/or metrizamide at 300 mg I/ml into the cisterna magna of a rhesus monkey elicited similar cell count increases as a result of all injections. Histological investigation of the CNS of rabbits after injection into the cisterna magna revealed no changes attributable to the metrizamide injection of 300 mg I/ml, 0.5 ml/kg [250]. One particular study distinguished itself by simulating the clinical myelography. The investigators pointed out that only subhuman primates having a cauda equina structure similar to that of humans would make a suitable model. *Macaca fascicularis* monkeys were anesthetized and lumbar puncture performed at L3–L4 level with a 22-gauge spinal needle, 0.2 ml/kg 300 mg I/ml metrizamide was injected, and the monkeys were placed in a sitting position for 16 h. Repeat myelograms were performed after 12 weeks, then the dural sacs were investigated histologically. Using this model and both histologic and myelographic assessment, some arachnoiditis was found after both metrizamide and/or iopamidol, but substantially less than after iocarmate [213]. These results correlated well with the previously reported extensive work carried out by the same group of investigators [120, 121, 251–254]. The question of arachnoiditis was aptly reviewed in a monograph [255]. It should be noted that the adhesive arachnoiditis in the monkey experiments was produced with concentrations substantially higher than those normally used in a clinical situation. Most clinicians tend to accept lower concentrations, since CM hyperosmolality was identified as a toxicity factor in myelography [254, 360]. Another group of investigators attempted to produce arachnoiditis in a dog model. Although all animals were anesthetized with pentobarbital, all five dogs injected with 300 mg I/ml metrizamide developed multiple grand mal seizures 30–45 min postinjection. Arachnoiditis with multifocal distribution throughout the cervical cord envelopes was found in these animals. In the absence of subarachnoid hematomas, considering that the injection was carried out by cisternal puncture, the authors concluded that in dogs the high concentration of metrizamide elicited arachnoiditis. On the other hand, in the same model 170 mg I/ml concentration of metrizamide did not elicit neurofunctional deficits except in one dog, and there was no arachnoiditis [256].

Subacute reactions to intrathecal metrizamide were studied in rabbits which were injected with 300 or 200 mg I/ml metrizamide and/or meglumine iocarmate or iothalamate. The animals were studied by histology and electron microscopy. All animals showed subpial edema and inflammatory reaction of the superficial brain leptomeninges, subarachnoid space, and arachnoid granulation. The severity decreased with time. Like the preceding study in dogs, these findings indicate that 300 mg I/ml, although diagnostically desirable in certain patients and certain areas, carry an increased risk of adverse reactions [257].

The fate of metrizamide upon injection into the subarachnoid space has been the subject of a number of detailed studies [257a]. As a comparative baseline, the routes and rates of excretion of radiocontrast ionic agents were used [258, 259]. Thus, metrizamide was found to have a biological half-life identical to that of diatrizoate [260]. The volume distributions of metrizamide and its excretion from the organism have been studied extensively [261]. After intravenous or suboccipital injection of ^{125}I-labeled metrizamide, 95.6%–98.3% of the dose was recovered in urine and feces within 48 h in rabbits and cats. In rats, the extrarenal clearance was found to be more than twice as high as in rabbits. In rabbits, after 4 h 52.8%

of the dose was recovered in urine. Another study using a pharmacokinetic model determined that the rates are constant for absorption and excretion as well as distribution. Thus, during the first 3 h after the injection, over 99% of the absorbed dose disappeared from the CSF [262]. In humans, following subarachnoid injection, less compound has been recovered [263]. The biological half-life of metrizamide in CSF is about 4 h, which is not different from that of ionic CM.

Following injection into the intrathecal space, metrizamide is absorbed by the arachnoid proliferations and passed into the blood. Due to the circulation of CSF, some CM is distributed within the entire intrathecal space. Using autoradiography, a study of the passage of metrizamide through the arachnoid granulations has been conducted [264].

Elimination of CM from the subarachnoid space has also been studied by computed tomography. The authors concentrated on the two basic elimination mechanisms, i.e., diffusion through the meningeal membranes and transport through the CSF pathways. They found that diffusion predominates with CM of low molecular weight while arachnoid absorption is the main mode of elimination of larger molecular weight CM [265]. An extremely careful distribution study of metrizamide and diatrizoate using ^{125}I-labeled substances found, in a model employing ventriculocisternal perfusion by artificial CSF, profiles of radioactivity through the cerebral gray matter. The authors concluded that metrizamide passed through the gray matter by simple diffusion, that it was largely distributed in the extracerebral fluid, and that it did not move back across the blood-brain barrier to any great extent [266]. Absorption of metrizamide from the SAS of rabbits following injection into the lumbar area showed that most of the CM was absorbed from the area of injection. The study found that, in rabbits, the absorption from the SAS of the spine is different, depending upon the area into which CM has been deposited [267].

Although it has been demonstrated by these studies that most metrizamide is resorbed through the arachnoid granulations, elimination through the capillary endothelium and the choroid plexus has not yet been investigated.

It has been shown by CT that metrizamide increases the gray matter density [268, 269]. Penetration of metrizamide apparently occurs in both normal and abnormal states of the CSF dynamics [270]. A number of reports indicated that the incidence of the side effects of metrizamide depends not only upon the dose but also upon the site [271–280]. Significantly, a study of 25 patients found that maximum penetration into the gray matter correlated with the peak of adverse reactions, including headache, nausea, perceptual aberrations, and EEG abnormalities [281]. Severe reactions were shown to occur more often with cervical than with lumbar myelography [282], and in those patients who had a high metrizamide concentration in the cranial CSF side effects occurred with high frequency [283].

Penetration of metrizamide into the CNS tissue can be expected since the extracellular space and subarachnoid space of the brain are continuous. Since molecules solvated in the CSF can migrate freely [284], the migration of metrizamide is determined only by the rate of diffusion, CSF flux within the compartment, and the rate and route of elimination [285]. A study of the penetration of intrathecally injected CM concluded that penetration was unavoidable and independent of molecular size and osmolality. The degree of persistence of the examined compounds in the CNS correlated with their neurotoxicity. Since CM chemotoxicity is based upon interaction with large biomacromolecules, it can be speculated that the slowly clearing CM somehow affect the gel filling the extracerebral brain tissue space. The gel is formed principally by mucopolysaccharides; their alteration would conceivably change the gel's physical properties and possibly impede the CSF flow [286].

The first clinical reports on metrizamide were enthusiastic. Excellent results of 100 lumbar myelographies were reported with only minor side effects, occasional transient changes in EEG, and moderately increased total white-cell count and protein levels in the CSF [287]. From a series of 650 patients it was concluded that metrizamide was safe in lumbar myelography [288]. Other series came to a similar conclusion [289–291].

With increased clinical use, evidence of the side effects of metrizamide began to accumulate. Careful registration of the EEG after lumbar myelography in 79 patients revealed a 16% transient preponderance of slow wave activity. In this series, no epileptiform discharges were observed [192]. An array of side effects ranging from headache (the most prominent) to neck pain, stiffness of the neck, nausea, vomiting, dizziness, tinnitus, blood pressure decrease, collapse, fever, radicular pains, paresthesias, fasciculation, myoclonus, mental disorders, and epileptic seizures have since been reported. Headache occurring with various frequencies has been reported. In a study of 100 patients, headache also occurred in 31.9% [293] and in 38% of 117 patients, compared with 32% with Pantopaque [108]. In a series of 200 myelograms, headache occurred in 62% and vomiting in 38% [101]. Analysis of 215 patients showed side effects in 67%; 39% were moderate or severe [290]. Analysis of a series of 439 myelographies differentiated early headaches attributable to the lumbar puncture and late headaches attributable to metrizamide. The frequency of the latter was 27%; meningeal irritation was seen in 5%, sometimes in a severe form mimicking aseptic inflammation. Spinal irritation and epileptic fits were rare. Frequently occurring after cervical myelography, which was performed with higher doses of metrizamide than those diagnostically needed for lumbar myelography, were acute psychoorganic syndromes [294]. Occurrence of such mental disorders was also noted in CT with metrizamide when the CM rose above the tentorial level [285]. On the other hand, when metrizamide was confined only to radiculographies, a series of 600 patients showed only minor side effects and no serious complications [295].

The occurrence of mental disorders, especially after cervical myelographies, has been confirmed by a number of studies. Organic psychosyndromes were reported in 6 out of 18 patients, occurring 10 h after lumbar myelography. Psychometric methods have demonstrated impaired memory and depression; hypo- and areflexia were seen in four patients. There was no correlation between EEG changes or reflex abnormalities and the organic psychosyndrome, which completely disappeared 5 days after myelography [296]. Eight cases of cognition disorders were also described [297]. Chemotoxicity of metrizamide was suspected in cervical myelopathy [298] and electromyelographic abnormalities following myelography [299]. The effects of metrizamide on spinal CNS can apparently be potentiated by impeded CSF circulation; i.e., spinal irritation in kyfoscoliosis was described [300]. *Asterixis* was also found [301]. As an unusual combination, aseptic meningitis, arachnoiditis, communicating hydrocephalus, and Guillain-Barré syndrome were described [302]. Although the risk of arachnoiditis from metrizamide was suspected [303], none was found in 90 patients studied by repeated myelography [304, 305].

The subject of cervical myelography with metrizamide has been reviewed, based predominantly on the experience in the Scandinavian countries [306].

In a series of 260 cervical myelograms performed by lumbar injection, headache occurred in 47% and vomiting in 27%. EEG disturbances occurred in 20% of the patients, but only one patient showed grand mal seizures and mental confusion. The dose used was 10 ml containing 250 mg I/ml [307].

In a series of 102 patients with cervical myelography with 270 mg I/ml (average dose = 6 ml), cervical myelography was performed with special precautions preventing the ingress of the CM into the cranial space. Headache and nausea appeared in 20% of the patients and in one case, visual hallucinations were reported. There was no case of severe neurological deficits [308].

The discrepancy between the results of this and the previous studies is possibly explainable by the technique. When metrizamide is injected via lumbar puncture, it reaches the upper cervical area in a somewhat diluted state. Cervical injections of metrizamide, dictated by diagnostic necessity, use CM concentrated to hyperosmolal levels and are more prone to introduce metrizamide into the cranial space.

EEG disturbances following myelography, cisternography, and ventriculography have been described. Two types of EEG abnormalities have been recognized: theta waves during the following day, considered to be without clinical significance; and paroxyms of delta waves or spikes occurring minutes or a few hours after the myelography. This type of EEG abnormality was considered more serious: one of these patients developed epileptic seizures [309].

Metrizamide represents a qualitative leap in the development of an intrathecal CM. It has all but replaced Pantopaque in lumbar and thoracic myelography and to a great extent it has been used for cervical and cranial opacification of the CNS cavities. It has been the general consensus both in Europe and in the United States that the need to reconstitute metrizamide solutions prior to the examination, and to accept some acute side effects, is a small price to pay for a low risk of chronic late arachnoiditis. On the other hand, intracranial application of metrizamide which requires higher than CSF isotonic concentrations increases the risk of serious acute side effects, presumably elicited by a combination of hypertonicity and chemotoxicity of the material.

In an effort to produce a compound superior to metrizamide, investigators designed a number of both ionic and nonionic compounds. Ionic monomers P-94, P-115, and P-182 (developed by Guerbet labs) were all shown to have an epileptogenic threshold inferior to nonionic CM in a model using *guinea pig* and injections into the anterior fossa while the EEG is recorded. Ionic dimer P-193 and a trimer P-291 were also tested. The trimer P-291 had an epileptogenic threshold about twice as high as ioserinate (Myelografin, Schering AG), but even this compound's epileptogenicity was judged about three times worse than that of nonionic monomers. Nonionic monomers P-232 and P-236 were epileptogenically akin to the ionic monomers. Nonionic dimer P-308 was more epileptogenic than nonionic monomers P-277 and P-297, but since P-277 produced inflammatory reactions, only P-297 (ioglunide) was considered for further development by the manufacturer (Guerbet Labs.). Tested by pericerebral injection of 0.3 ml 400 mg I/ml solution, metrizamide produced no changes in the EEG while P-297 produced no seizures but slow waves and spikes. In the same study, another nonionic monomer, iopamidol (Bracco Ind.), systematically induced seizures [310].

Ioglunide, akin to metrizamide, is nonionic material whose water solubility is achieved by attaching gluconic acid to the triiodoaniline by an amide linkage. Comparative investigation of metrizamide and P-297 under conditions of autoclaving showed decomposition and/or rearrangement of the sugar residue in metrizamide, while in P-297 the entire sugar substituent was cleaved of the triiodoaniline moiety [311]. Iogluconide therefore must, akin to metrizamide, be lyophilized, and solutions must be made prior to their use.

Testing ioglunide in pigtail monkeys by lumbar myelography showed no more changes in the arachnoid after ioglunide than were found with metrizamide and for control animals injected with autologus CSF [303]. Neurotoxicity of ioglunide was also tested in *Macaca mulatta* and in the cat. Intrathecally injected medium (280 mg I/ml, 2.5 ml) into nonanesthetized monkeys produced no convulsions after a single injection of iogluconide or metrizamide. A second injection of the same amount of metrizamide led to generalized convulsions in five out of eight experiments. By comparison, ioglunide induced convulsions in only one animal, and that to only a moderate degree. Two animals showed spike activities in their EEG and one animal developed a unilateral tremor. In the cat model, the evoked cortical spinal responses have shown no significant change in the threshold level both after ioglunide, metrizamide, and/or hypertonic sodium chloride, although there was a threefold increase with meglumine iothalamate. Interestingly, meglumine iothalamate did not affect the amplitude while hypertonic sodium chloride produced a significant decrease and metrizamide and/or P-297 a slight decrease of this parameter. The authors concluded that ioglunide had a lower epileptogenicity than metrizamide and they attributed this property to incresed hydrophilic properties of ioglunide.

Elimination of ioglunide from the intrathecal space has been studied in *Macaca* monkeys. The compound is transported slowly into the basal cisterns and eliminated rapidly into the serum and urine. No significant differences in excretion were found compared with metrizamide or iopamidol [115].

The concept of "reversed amide linkage" utilized in ioglunide was also part of the chemical synthesis program at Mallinckrodt Laboratories. HOEY suggested a systematic testing of other linkages, i.e., ureide, carbamate, dipeptide, and esters to link a variety of smaller sugars to the triiodobenzene moiety. Compared with the amides, the ester carbamate and dipeptide series generally gave compounds of high aqueous solubility, but also higher toxicity. Generally, they were also less stable than the amides or "reversed amides". Neurotoxicity of the novel molecules was tested by intracerebral and intracisternal LD_{50}s in rodents. All compounds, including metrizamide used as a control, were epileptogenic when injected intracerebrally in mice while no epileptogenicity was seen following intracisternal application in rats. The authors introduced a new toxicological index by relating the intracerebral LD_{50} to the intracisternal LD_{50} in a ratio. This index suggested low acute CNS toxicity of one of the derivatives, MP-1013, the keto-gulonamido-bis-dihydroxypropyl compound. All compounds for a given iodine concentration had higher osmolality than metrizamide but when compared at a concentration of 300 mg I/ml, osmolalities did not correlate with intracisternal LD_{50}s or the convulsive potential [312].

II. New Developments in Intrathecal Contrast Media

An experimental compound utilizing the linkage of the sugar moiety by a hindered glycolytic bond has been synthesized. Because of steric problems, only two iodines were introduced on the ring of the diiodotriglucosylbenzene. The compound proved extremely hydrophilic and nontoxic (i.v. LD_{50} in mice in the range of 34 g/kg) [313]. Although the compound was highly water soluble and stable, it was not further developed because of its low iodine content.

Another attempt in our laboratories to produce highly hydrophilic, stable, nonionic CM employed sugars attached to the triiodophenyl moiety by an ether bond. Based on this concept, two series of compounds containing one or two sugar residues were synthesized. Benzyl and phenyl-hexosyl ether-based nonionic radiocontrast media were used as model compounds to determine the toxicological significance of the methylene group [314]. As a further improvement, a method was devised to convert bis-glucose-3-yl ether into a bis-arabinos-2-yl ether, which increased the iodine content. The lowest neurotoxicity was achieved with a 1,3 bis-hexose-ether with a glycolyl-amide on the C5 position. In a series of comparative experiments, compound DL-2-98 proved to be substantially less toxic than metrizamide, statistically indistinguishable from iopamidol, and stable under autoclaving conditions [315, 316].

Because of the synthetic complexity of the sugar derivatives, investigators have been looking into the possibility of using other hydrophilic, water-solubilizing substituents. The use of aminopropanediol (aminoglycerol) to solubilize acyl-amino-triiodoisophthalic acids by amidation of the carboxylic functions was suggested at an early stage [317]. Although some of these compounds proved toxicologically promising, none at them matched the low toxicity of metrizamide. Further, because of unresolved solubility problems, the compounds were not developed for clinical use; however, this experience served as a launching stage for design of nonionic compounds containing small amine-hydroxyalkyls instead of sugars.

There was an additional reason, apart from problems of stability and viscosity, for replacing sugars in the nonionic CM synthesis with less complicated hydroxyl-containing moieties: during the synthesis of the first batches of metrizamide, pyrogens were detected in the sample which had induced a high leukocyte count in the CSF of experimental animals. Of interest for the subarachnoid space is that the authors found the sensitivity toward the pyrogens about 1,000 times higher upon intraventricular than upon intravenous injection [313]. The problem was solved by modifying the production process.

Working originally with antibiotics, FELDER and PITRE at Bracco Industries developed a series of 5-hydroxyacylamino-triiodosophthalic acid derivatives solubilized by amidation with various aminoalcohols. They obtained high water solubility with the 1,3-dihydroxypropyl-amide group, by using serinol. (Serinol can be derived, by chemical reduction, from the amino-acid serine.) When lactic acid was substituted on the C5 position, extremely interesting solubility data emerged. By a mechanism which is still poorly understood and contrary to accepted theories, the L-lactic acid proved to solubilize the compound far more than the D,L form. Further, it was found that the anhydrous form was more solubizing than the monohydratic form of L-lactoyl. Iopamidol at 300 mg I/ml has a higher osmolality than metrizamide, but its viscosity is substantially lower (see Table 1). Iopamidol proved to be stable under the conditions of autoclaving and presented the first nonionic nonsugar-containing material that could be dispensed in solution [318–320].

Table 1. Physical properties of pharmaceutically developed nonionic CM at a concentration of 300 mg I/ml (37 °C)

	Osmolality (mOsm/kg)	Viscosity (cps)	Mol wt.
Metrizamide	470	7.1	789
Iopamidol	615	4.5	777
Iohexol	690	6.1	821
Iotrol	310	9.1	1,629

Preclinical data indicated that the compound has a lower systemic toxicity than metrizamide, the i.v. LD_{50} in mice being in the range of 20 g I/kg. It was found to be rapidly eliminated from the cisterns of anesthetized dogs, giving blood peak levels between 1 and 2 h postinjection [321]. The medium was found to be rapidly eliminated into the serum and urine upon injection into the lumbar subarachnoid space, akin to metrizamide or iocarmate. It was also found to be slowly transported into the basal cisterns [115]. Using a guinea pig model, adapted for direct delivery of CM into the anterior fossa of the skull base, and concurrently registered EEG, iopamidol produced seizures while metrizamide produced no changes and ioglunide produced slow waves and spikes. The maximal amount of 400 mg I/ml solution that could be injected without inducing seizures (of iopamidol) was approximately 3.7 times smaller than that for metrizamide. Using the same approach in a *Macaca* monkey, iopamidol was compared with iocarmate and metrizamide by a lumbar intrathecal injection. Twelve weeks later, after additional myelography, the presence or absence of arachnoiditis was studied. Using both histological and myelographic scores, it was concluded that iopamidol has a low arachnoiditis-eliciting potential, compared with metrizamide [210].

When iopamidol was injected into the common carotid arteries of guinea pigs, and autoradiography of the brain tissue with ^{32}P was carried out, minimal effects on the blood-brain barrier were found [322].

Iopamidol was found to elicit only minimal cardiovascular responses when compared with other nonionic and ionic CM [323]. Low neurotoxicity was reported in animal experiments [324]. Testing iopamidol by injection into the cisterna magna in rabbits and computerized analysis of EEG has shown iopamidol affecting the EEG spectrum energy less than metrizamide [325]. Iopamidol also proved superior to metrizamide by scoring neurofunctional deficits following injection through an implanted cannula in nonanesthetized rats [326], and by aversion conditioning of rats [327]. Using a method of behavioral research capable of quantification of an induced aversion to a drug, a high degree of conditioned aversion was obtained against metrizamide while conditioning with iopamidol was low. Acute neurotoxicity of iopamidol following subarachnoid injection was the subject of a separate study [328]. The relatively high resistance of iopamidol to deiodination was ascertained [329]. The studies on metabolism of iopamidol in the dog, rabbit, and man were published [330].

In order to assess the excitative and/or depressive effect of new nonionic CM, metrizamide, iopamidol, iohexol, and ioglunide (P-297) were injected by slow infusion into the cisterna magna of nonanesthetized rabbits. The study demonstrated that iopamidol caused less depression than metrizamide with 1 ml/kg 370 mg I/ml. Iohexol caused less depression than metrizamide and the differences between P-297 and metrizamide were not significant. In contradistinction, P-297 and iopamidol both caused less excitation than metrizamide. Interestingly, saline produced severe convulsions when injected in volumes of between 0.6 and 0.9 ml/kg while Ringer's solution did not. This finding supports the notion that perturbation of the electrolyte balance in CSF induces epileptogenicity [331]. In Europe, iopamidol was introduced early into clinical use. In a double-blind study conducted in 100 patients using 9 ml of solutions isotonic with CSF, iopamidol was tested against metrizamide. Headache was the most common symptom correlating with the excretion rate. The authors found that iopamidol was eliminated faster than metrizamide and headache frequency was also higher. There were no convulsions observed in either of the groups and the overall incidence of side effects was similar for both CM [114]. Cervical myelography with iopamidol was reported in a series of 65 patients; no neurodeficits were encountered, although headache frequency was 37% [129]. Numerous clinical studies have found iopamidol a medium superior to metrizamide but not inert in the intrathecal space [332–336].

The technology for synthesis of the key substituent in iopamidol, the originally esoteric serinol, has advanced to the degree that serinol can now be synthesized in large quantities, but the cost of this CM is still several times that of ionic CM. Other laboratories synthesized a number of derivatives containing aminopropanediols (see Chap. 1). At the Nyegaard Company in Norway these efforts resulted in a number of compounds [337]. Compound 593 is N,N'-bis(1,3-dihydroxy-2-propyl)-5-[N-(2-hydroxy-ethyl)acetamido]-2,4,6-triiodoisophthalamide. In an analogous molecule, C-29, serinol was replaced with 2,3-dihydroxypropyl, i.e., aminoglyceryl, in an effort to arrive at a substantially cheaper compound. Because of solubility problems, another derivative of C-29 was obtained, by introducing an additional hydroxyl group. The new derivative, N,N'-bis(2-3-dihydroxypropyl)-5-[N-(2,3-dihydroxypropyl   acetamino)]-2,4,6-triiodoisophthalamide was further developed as iohexol. This approach increased the molecular weight to 821 compared with 789 for metrizamide, decreasing the iodine content to 46.4%. In aqueous solutions, the molecules of iohexol do not associate like those of metrizamide, so that at 300 mg I/ml iohexol has an osmolality of about

690 mOsm. On the other hand, at the same concentration, iohexol is less viscous than metrizamide. A detailed comparison of osmolality, viscosity, molecular weights, and iodine concentrations of these compounds is available [338] (Table 1).

Using $^{197}HgAc_2$ and trypan blue as markers for evaluation of injury to the blood-brain barrier upon carotid injection in rabbits, in one test with statistically significant results iohexol was superior to metrizamide, and in another indistinguishable. From this experiment, it can be surmised that the higher osmolality of iohexol is possibly compensated for by its low chemotoxicity [339]. The systemic intravenous toxicity tested in mice (i.v. LD_{50}) is reported as a low 23–25 g I/kg. The i.v. LD_{50} in rats is in the range of 12–15 g I/kg, statistically not different from that of metrizamide or between male and female animals [340].

Neurotoxicity of iohexol was assessed in rats by intracisternal, intracerebral, and intracarotid injections. Interestingly, the intracisternal tolerance of iohexol was significantly higher than that of metrizamide, while intracerebral administration showed a lower tolerance of iohexol. The authors noted, nevertheless, than when animals were scored for hyperexcitability and motor discoordination or the mortality rate, iohexol was the better tolerated medium. No statistically significant difference was found between iohexol and metrizamide upon intracarotid injection [341]. In a previously quoted study, iohexol was tested in nonanesthetized rabbits by injection into the cisterna magna. The authors developed an index for convulsive activity and depressive and excited states. Iohexol caused less excitation than metrizamide and/or iopamidol while iohexol and iopamidol caused less depression than metrizamide. Iohexol caused less depression than P-297 and metrizamide at higher dose levels, and there was no significant difference between iopamidol, P-297, and metrizamide [331]. Low systemic toxicity can also be expected on the basis of recent in vitro experiments. Iohexol in comparison with metrizamide and ioxaglate had the lowest binding to plasma proteins, least inhibition of lysozyme, and the smallest tendency to liberate histamine from mast cells. Also, the serum complement system and morphology of erythrocytes were affected to a lesser degree by iohexol than by metrizamide [342–348]. Recent clinical studies suggest that iohexol, although far from being inert, is superior to metrizamide [346, 347]. An analog of iohexol, experimental compound MP-328, recently announced by Mallincrodt Inc., also shows promise as an intrathecal agent [348].

During the search for a CM isotonic with CSF, the concept of nonionic dimers has been explored based on the following considerations: to be sufficiently radiopaque, the iodine content of the molecule should be between 45% and 50% of the molecular weight. This requirement cannot be reconciled with the demand of isoosmolarity in a single triiodobenzene molecule, except theoretically in compounds containing iodine both in cationic and anionic parts of a salt [349]. Since charge confers high neurotoxicity on compounds in the intrathecal space, only nonionic compounds can be considered. A number of nonionic dimers have been synthesized [350, 352]. The first nonionic dimers utilizing amino-glycerol and/or serinol as substituents of a dimerized triiodoisophthalic acid were shown by intracerebral injection in rats to have a neurotoxicity lower than that of metrizamide [351]. In that study, in the absence of epileptogenic activity, the effective dose for eliciting sedation was in the range of 40 mg I/kg for metrizamide, and

95 mg I/kg for the experimental dimer. When lack of motor coordination and epileptogenicity were used as criteria for the determination of ED_{50}, injection of CM into the diencephalon of a rat gave an average of 56.7 mg I/kg for metrizamide and 67.9 mg I/kg for iohexol [341]. Using the same technique, an average value of 158 was found for iopamidol and 219 for iotrol [127] (Table 2), a nonionic dimer developed at the University of California in San Diego [128].

Table 2. Neurotoxicity in experimental animal models of nonionic CM intended for intrathecal space

	Neural deficit scores (intraventricular injection in rats) (300 mg I/kg)	Intracisternal LD_{50} in rats (mg I/kg)	Diencephalic injection ED_{50} in rats (mg I/kg)
Metrizamide	N/A (death)	310 (252–385)	60.1 (47.2– 73.7)
Iopamidol	22.00 ± 0	1,056 (974–1,193)	158.2 (128.2–212.4)
Iohexol	8.20 ± 3	1,025 (954–1,113)	67.9 (50.4– 84.4)
Iotrol	1.66 ± 2	1,133 (1,066–1,278)	219.0 (194.5–245.1)
Iogulamide	N/A	850	N/A
MP-328	N/A	1,050	N/A

The LD_{50} values vary depending upon a number of genetic and environmental factors as well as techniques used. Therefore, only approximate ranges are given

Iotrol contains D,L-amino-tetritols as water-solubilizing and detoxifying substituents. Small amounts of D-amino-erythritol and L-amino-threitol are found in nature, but had never been synthesized before the development of D,L-amino-tetritols. L-amino-erythritol and D-amino-threitol are unknown. A new synthetic approach makes these compounds economically available in large quantities [128, 352, 353]. Incorporation of these bases into a number of monomeric and oligomeric structures resulted in a number of nonionic compounds of high stability, water solubility, and low toxicity, both for intravascular and intrathecal use [127, 128, 354].

Several dimers were synthesized and tested for intrathecal use. It became apparent that the structure of the bridge connecting the two triiodoisophthalic moieties was of importance for the water solubility: The dimers containing D,L-amino-erythritol or D,L,-amino-threitol and a malonyl bridge between the amino groups of the isophthalic moieties proved less water soluble than an analogous compound containing the N-methyl amino group. This experience supports the notion that introduction of steric variability into a molecule often increases its water solubility.

The type of the dimerizing bridge also proved to affect the toxicity. The longer bis-glycolyl bridge increased the neurotoxicity, as measured by intraventricular injection through a chronically implanted cannula in nonanesthetized rats, and scoring for neurofunctional deficits [127]. Whether the increased toxicity is attributable to the lengthening of the bridge and, thus, to an increase in distance between the triiodinated moieties or to the character of the bridge itself remains uncertain. The bis-glycolyl bridge has a slightly higher hydrophobicity when compared with the malonyl bridge (see below). The dimer DL-3-117 (iotrol) containing the malonyl bridge and D,L-amino-threitol has been subjected to a number of tests, which are reviewed elsewhere [127]. Additional testing, both preclinical and clinical, has also been conducted. Aversion conditioning in rats, a psychophysiological method, was established previously as a valuable pharmacological tool (for details see Chap. 6). In principle, rats, when exposed to an agent-eliciting malaise given at the same time as a novel-tasting substance is ingested, will reject such an agent in the future. By pairing the experience of injection of a number of CM into the chronically cannulated lateral ventricles of awake rats, preference/avoidance data were obtained. The degree of aversion is gleaned from the differences in consumption of flavored water, accounting for a controlled flavor and a controlled injection. In this sensitive test, which is capable of detecting much more subtle manifestations of toxicity than the standard methods, a 22.5 mg I/kg dose induced aversion only in metrizamide-injected rats, while at the 45 mg I/kg dose the new dimers did not induce aversion whereas iopamidol and metrizamide did [327].

An elegant technique for testing neurotoxicity, applied to comparative evaluation of metrizamide, iopamidol, iohexol, and iotrol, utilizes in vitro slices of rat hippocampus and registration of field potentials from the pyramidal cell layers [355]. In this model, ionic agents synaptically induce repetitive negative spikes indicative of epileptogenicity. In principle, nonionic agents and/or hyperosmolar solutions of sucrose were found to depress the amplitude. In this test, iotrol almost had no effect on the amplitude while metrizamide, iopamidol, and iohexol produced definite depression; metrizamide evoked mild epileptic activity [356]. This study also established hyperosmolality of nonionic myelographic CM as an important factor of their neurotoxicity. A previously described technique [357] was used to compare iotrol with iohexol by intracisternal injection in nonanesthetized rabbits. Iotrol produced more excitation, but less depression than iohexol [358]. In another study, the technique was only slightly modified by increasing the injection rate to achieve a rapid ingress of highly concentrated CM (300 mg I/ml) into the brain SAS. Also, the animals were temporarily obnubilated with ether. In groups of six rabbits, Ringer's solution gave no neural deficits, while iohexol produced considerably more excitation (including epileptic fits in two animals) and depression than iotrol [353]. This study complemented the preclinical pharmacological profile of iotrol [358].

In a study using a monkey model, nonionic media were injected into nonanesthetized animals via a chronically implanted catheter into the subarachnoid space at L1–S2 level. Following inversion and radiographically controlled spread of the CM over the hemispheres (300 mg I/ml, 0.5 ml/kg), eight-channel EEG was carried out and EEG spectrum analysis performed by a computer. For each medium (metrizamide, iopamidol, iohexol, and iotrol), four studies were carried out. In this sensitive model (*Macaca cynomolgus*), epileptic activity was invariably elicited with metrizamide. Iopamidol was less epileptogenic, but all animals showed increase in low frequencies. Iohexol produced an overall depression and an occasional preponderance of the low-frequency spectral component, but no spikes. Iotrol induced no adverse effects [359]. The validity of this experimental model was vindicated by the clinical tests of iotrol [353, 360].

It can be expected that in future the availability and quality of high-resolution X-ray and NMR scanners will improve to the extent that some indications for myelography will be eliminated, especially those concerning lumbar disk pathology. On the other hand, there is probably going to be a continuing need for a nontoxic medium for cranial and cervical use also in conjunction with CT. Research in this area should concentrate on the development of an agent which would enter the CSF from the blood stream.

References

1. Coin CG, Coin JT (1980) Contrast enhancement by xenon gas in computed tomography of the spinal cord and brain: preliminary observations. J Comput Assist Tomogr 4:217–221
2. Pullicino P, du Boulay GH, Kendall BE (1979) Xenon enhancement for computed tomography of the spinal cord. Neuroradiology 18:63–66
3. Keltz F, Hilal SK, Hartwell P, Joseph PM (1978) Computed tomographic measurement of the xenon brain-blood partition coefficient and implications for regional cerebral blood flow: a preliminary report. Radiology 127:385–392
4. Drayer BP, Gur D, Solfson SK, Cook EE (1980) Experimental xenon enhancement with CT imaging: cerebral applications. AJR 134:39–44
5. Drayer B, Coleman E, Bates M et al. (1980) Non-radioactive iodoantipyrine enhanced cranial computed tomography: preliminary observations. J Comput Assist Tomogr 4:186–190
6. Phelps ME, Kuhl DE, Mazziotta JO (1981) A metabolic mapping of the brain's response to visual stimulation: studies in humans. Science 211:1445–1448
7. Hawkes RC, Holland GN, Moore WS, Worthington BS (1980) Nuclear magnetic resonance imaging – an overview. Radiography 40:253–255
8. Partain CL, James EA, Watson TF et al. (1980) Nuclear magnetic resonance and computed tomography. Radiology 136:767–770
9. Herfkens R, Davis PL, Crooks LE et al. (1981) NMR imaging of the abnormal live rat and correlation with tissue characteristics. Radiology 141:211–218
10. Hoey GB, Adams MD, Robbins MS, Dean RT, White DH, Rizzole RR, Monzyk MA, Bosworth ME, Wolf GL (1984) Factors in the design of NMR imaging agents. Invest Radiol 19:S150
11. Speck U, Gries H, Klieger E, Mutzel W, Press WR, Weinmann HJ (1984) New contrast media developed at Schering AG: first experience. Invest Radiol 19:S144
12. Huber P (1982) Cerebral angiography. Thieme-Stratton, New York
13. Krayenbuhl HA, Yasargil MG (1968) Cerebral angiography. Lippincott, Philadelphia
14. Osborn AG (1980) Introduction to cerebral angiography. Harper & Row Hagerstown
15. Newton TH, Potts DG (eds) (1974) Radiology of the skull and brain. Angiography, vols 2, 3. Mosby, St. Louis
16. Abrams HL (1971) Angiography, 2nd edn. Little Brown, Boston
17. Djindjian R (1970) Angiography of the spinal cord. University Park Press, Baltimore
18. Doppman JL, Di Chiro G, Ommaya A (1969) Selective arteriography of the spinal cord. Green, St. Louis
19. Perovitch M (1981) Radiological evaluation of the spinal cord. CRC Press, Boca Raton
20. Theron J, Moret J (1978) Spinal phlebography. Springer, Berlin Heidelberg New York
21. Knoefel PK (ed) (1971) Radiocontrast agents. Pergamon, New York (International encyclopedia of pharmacology and therapeutics, sect 76, vol 2)

22. Newton TH, Potts DG (eds) (1974) Radiology of skull and brain. Mosby, St. Louis
23. Masy SI (1950) Expérience personnelle avec le di-iodostéarate d'éthyle dans l'artério-graphie. Acta Radiol 34:350–356
24. Ulano HB, Ascanio G, Rice V, Ohern R, Houmas E, Oppenheimer MJ (1970) Effects of angiographic contrast media and hypertonic saline solutions on cerebral venous outflow in autoregulating brains. Invest Radiol 5:518–533
25. Lynch PR, Harrington GJ, Michie C (1969) Cardiovascular reflexes associated with cerebral angiography. Invest Radiol 4:156–160
26. Higgins CB, Schmidt WS (1979) Identification and evaluation of the contribution of the chemoreflex in the hemodynamic response to intracarotid administration of contrast materials in the conscious dog: comparison with the response to nicotine. Invest Radiol 14:438–446
27. Morris TW, Francis M, Fischer HW (1979) A comparison of the cardiovascular responses to carotid injections of ionic and nonionic contrast media. Invest Radiol 14:217–223
28. Hilal SK (1974) Cerebral hemodynamics assessed by angiography. In: Newton TH, Potts DG (eds) Radiology of the skull and brain. Mosby, St. Louis, pp 1067–1085
29. Lindgren P, Tornell G (1958) Blood pressure and heart rate responses in carotid angiography with sodium acetrizoate. Acta Radiol 50:160–174
30. Lindgren P (1959) Carotid angiography with tri-iodobenzoic acid derivatives: a comparative experimental study of the effects on the systemic circulation in cats. Acta Radiol 51:353–362
31. Lindgren P, Tornell G (1958) Blood pressure and heart rate responses in carotid angiography with sodium acetrizoate (Triurol): an experimental study in cats. Acta Radiol 50:160–174
32. Hilal SK (1966) Hemodynamic responses in the cerebral vessels to angiographic contrast media. Acta Radiol [Diagn] (Stockh) 5:211–231
33. Hilal SK (1966) Hemodynamic changes associated with intra-arterial injection of contrast media. Radiology 86:615–633
34. Broman T, Olsson O (1948) The tolerance of cerebral blood vessels to a contrast medium of the diotrast group. Acta Radiol 335:25–44
35. Gonsette RE (1973) Biologic tolerance of the central nervous system to metrizamide. Acta Radiol [Suppl] (Stockh) 335:25–44
36. Casady RL, Kitten GT, Gradley IM, Sterrette PR (1978) Sites of cerebrovascular injury induced by radiographic contrast media. Am J Anat 153:477–482
37. Gonsette RE (1978) Animal experiments and clinical experiences in cerebral angiography with a new contrast agent (ioxaglic acid) with a low hyperosmolality. Ann Radiol (Paris) 21:271–273
38. Rappaport SI, Thompson HK, Bidinger JM (1974) Equiosmolal opening of the blood-brain barrier in the rabbit by different contrast media. Acta Radiol [Diagn] (Stockh) 15:21–32
39. Waldron RL, Bridenbaugh RB, Dampsey EW (1974) Effect of angiographic contrast media at cellular level in the brain: hypertonic vs. chemical action. Am J Roentgenol 122:469–476
40. Lundervold A, Engeset A (1969) Electroencephalographic and electrocardiographic studies of complications in cerebral angiography. Acta Radiol [Diagn] (Stockh) 9:399–406
41. Labauger R, Cailar J, Xhardez M et al. (1968) Cortical blindness after cerebral angiography: reversibility under hyperbaric oxygen therapy. Rev Neurol (Paris) 118:283–289
42. Studdard WE, Davis DO, Young SW (1981) Cortical blindness after cerebral angiography. A case report. J Neurosurg 54:240–244
43. Bleeker HE (1978) Gilles de la Tourette syndrome with direct evidence of organicity. Psychiatr Clin (Basel) 11:147–154
44. Wales LR, Nov AA (1981) Transient global amnesia: complication of cerebral angiography. AJNR 2:275–277

45. Kachel R, Ritter H, Schiffmann R, Schumann E (1980) Complication following cerebral angiography: report on 4,181 cerebral angiographies. Zentralbl Chir 105:504–512
46. Mani RL, Eisenberg RL (1978) Complications of catheter cerebral arteriography analysis of 5,000 procedures. III. Assessment of arteries injected, contrast medium used, duration of procedure, and age of patient. AJR 131:871–874
47. Dempsey PT, Goree TA, Jimenez TP, McCord GM (1975) The effect of contrast media on patient motion during cerebral angiography. Radiology 115:207–209
48. Kindt GW (1971/72) Autoregulation of spinal cord blood flow, cerebral blood flow and intracranial pressure. Eur Neurol 6:19–23
49. Sandler AN, Tator CH (1976) Review of the measurements of normal spinal cord blood flow. Brain Res 118:181–194
50. Ohno K, Pettigrew KD, Rapaport SJ (1979) Local cerebral blood flow in the conscious rat as measured with ^{14}C-antipyrine, ^{14}C-iododantipyrine and ^{3}H-nicotine. Stroke 10:62–67
51. Ducker TB, Salcman M, Perot PL Jr, Ballantine D (1978) Experimental spinal cord trauma, I: correlation of blood flow, tissue oxygen and neurologic status in dog. Surg Neurol 10:60–63
52. Ducker TB, Salcman M, Lucas JT, Garrison WB, Perot PL Jr (1978) Experimental spinal cord trauma, II: blood flow, tissue oxygen, evoked potentials in both paretic and plegic monkeys. Surg Neurol 10:64–70
53. Ducker TB, Salcman M, Daniell HB (1978) Experimental spinal cord trauma, III: therapeutic effect of immobilization and pharmacologic agents. Surg Neurol 10:71–76
54. Oishi M, Niimi T, Takagi S, Takeoka T, Seki T, Toyoda MN, Gotoh F (1978) Chemical control of cerebral circulation. Modification by a new vasodilator (YC-93). J Neurol Sci 36:403–410
55. Kistler JP, Lees RS, Candia G, Zervas NT, Crowell RM, Ojeman RG (1979) Intravenous nitroglycerin in experimental cerebral vasospasm: a preliminary report. Stroke 10:26–33
56. Bories J, Merland JJ, Thiebot J (1977) The intra-arterial injection of Iskedyl for hyperselective vascular exploration. Neuroradiology 14:33
57. Jeppsson PG, Olin T (1972) Lesions of the blood-brain barrier following selective injection of contrast media into the vertebral artery in rabbits. Acta Radiol [Diagn] (Stockh) 12:271–282
58. Epsen F (1966) Spinal cord lesion as a complication of abdominal aortography. Acta Radiol [Diagn] (Stockh) 4:47–61
59. di Chiro G (1974) Unintentional spinal cord arteriography: a warning. Radiology 112:231–233
60. Feigelson HH, Ravin HA (1965) Transverse myelitis following selective bronchial arteriography. Radiology 85:663–665
61. Kardjiev V, Semyonov A, Chankov T (1974) Etiology, pathogenesis and prevention of spinal cord lesions in selective angiography of the bronchial and intercostal arteries. Radiology 112:81–83
62. Henson RA, Parsons M (1967) Ischaemic lesions of the spinal cord: a illustrated review. Q J Med 36:205–222
63. Skalpe IO, Lundervold A, Tjorstad K (1980) Complications of cerebral angiography: comparing metrizamide (Amipaque) and meglumine metrizoate (Isopaque Cerebral). Neuroradiology 19:67–71
64. Salvesen S (1973) Local toxicity of metrizamide on intravascular injection. Effect on kidney, liver, and blood-brain barrier. Acta Radiol [Suppl] (Stockh) 335:166–174
65. Skalpe IO, Lundervold A, Tjorstad K (1977) Cerebral angiography with non-ionic (metrizamide) and ionic (meglumide metrizoate) water soluble contrast media. A comparative study with double-blind technique. Neuroradiology 14:15–19
66. Andrew E, Dahlstrom K, Sveen K, Renaa T (1981) Amipaque (Metrizamide) in vascular use and use in body cavities: a survey of the initial clinical trials. Invest Radiol 16:455–465

67. Grainger RG (1979) A clinical trial of a new low osmolality contrast medium. Sodium and meglumine ioxaglate (Hexabrix) compared with meglumine iothalamate (Conray) for carotid arteriography. Br J Radiol 52:781–786
68. Aulie A (1980) Effect of Iohexol, Metrizamide, and Ioxaglate on the blood-brain barrier. Acta Radiol [Suppl] (Stockh) 362:13–16
69. Siefert HM, Press WR, Speck U (1980) Tolerance to Iohexol after intracisternal, intracerebral and intraarterial injection in the rat. Acta Radiol [Suppl] (Stockh) 362:77–81
70. Skalpe IO (1981) The toxicity of the nonionic water soluble contrast media, Iohexol and Metrizamide (Amipaque), in selected vertebral angiography. Neuroradiology 20:237–239
71. Amundsen P, Dugstad G, Presthus J, Sveen K (1983) Randomized double-blind cross-over study of Iohexol and Amipaque in cerebral angiography. AJNR 4:342–343
72. Bryan RN, Miller SL, Roehm JOF Jr, Weatherall PT (1983) Neuroangiography with Iohexol. AJNR 4:344–346
73. Hindmarsh T, Bergstrand G, Ericson K, Olivecrona H (1983) Comparative double-blind investigation of meglumine metrizoate, metrizamide, and iohexol in carotid angiography. AJNR 4:347–349
74. Andrew E, Shaw D, Sveen K, Holager T, Dahlstrom K (1984) Adverse reactions with iohexol in the vascular field. Experiences from clinical trials. Invest Radiol 19:S143–S144
75. Ingstrup HM, Hauge P (1982) Clinical testing of Iohexol, Conray meglumine and Amipaque in cerebral angiography. Neuroradiology 23:75–79
76. Drayer B, Ross M, Allen S, France R, Bates M (1984) Iotrol myelography: initial clinical trial. Invest Radiol 19:S141
77. Alexander JC, Newman TJ, Sudilovsky A, Meyer JH (1984) Clinical experience with iopamidol in the United States. Invest Radiol 19:S146
78. Speck U, Siefert H-M, Klink G (1980) Contrast media and pain in peripheral arteriography. Invest Radiol 15:S335–S339
79. Bacarini L, de Nicola T, Gasparini D, Orlando P, Vassallo A (1982) Iopamidol (B 15,000), a nonionic water-soluble contrast medium for neuroradiology. Part II: results of a double-blind study of the lumbar epidural venous plexuses. Neuroradiology 23:147–152
80. Molyneux AJ, Sheldon PWE (1982) A randomized blind trial of Iopamidol and meglumine calcium metrizoate (Triosil 280, Isopaque Cerebral) in cerebral angiography. Br J Radiol 55:117–119
81. Muetzel W, Speck U (1983) Pharmacological profile of Iopromide. AJNR 4:350–352
82. Skalpe IO (1983) The toxicity of non-ionic water-soluble monomeric and dimeric contrast media in selective vertebral angiography. An experimental study in rabbits. Neuroradiology 24:219–223
83. Dandy WE (1919) Roentgenography of the brain after the injection of air into the spinal canal. Ann Surg 70:397
84. Dandy WE (1925) The diagnosis and localization of spinal cord tumors. Ann Surg 81:223
85. Jacobaeus HC (1921) On insufflation of air into the spinal canal for diagnostic purposes in cases of tumors in the spinal canal. Acta Med Scand 55:555
86. Petrovitch M (1981) Radiologic evaluation of the spinal cord. CRC, Boca Raton
87. Sackett JF, Strother CM (1979) New techniques in myelography. Harper and Row, Hagerstown
88. Shapiro R (1975) Myelography, 3rd edn. Year Book Medical Publishing, Chap. 14
89. Kido DK, Schoene W, Baker RA, Rumbaugh CL (1978) Metrizamide epidurography in dogs. Radiology 128:119
90. Bromagh PR, Bramwell RSB, Catchlove RFH et al. (1978) Peridurography with metrizamide: animal and human studies. Radiology 128:123
91. Hatten HP (1980) Metrizamide, lumbar epidurography with Seldinger technique through the sacral notch and selective nerve root injection. Neuroradiology 19:19

92. Capesius P, Babin AE (1978) Radiculosaccography with water soluble contrast media. Springer, Berlin Heidelberg New York
93. Collins HR (1975) An evaluation of cervical and lumbar discography. Clin Orthop 107:133
94. Haughton VM, Correa-Paz F (1977) Double contrast myelography. Invest Radiol 12:552
95. Servo A, Halonen V (1979) Double-contrast ventriculography with oxygen and water-soluble positive contrast medium, metrizamide (Amipaque). J Neurosurg 51:211
96. Drayer BP, Rosenbaum AF, Higman HB (1977) Cerebrospinal fluid imaging using serial metrizamide CT cisternography. Neuroradiology 13:7
97. Howland WJ, Curry JL, Butter AK (1963) Pantopaque arachnoiditis: experimental study of blood as a potentiating agent. Radiology 80:489
98. Young DA, Burney RE II (1971) Complication of myelography – transection and withdrawal of a nerve filament by the needle. N Engl J Med 285:156
99. Sinclair DJ, Ritchie GW (1972) Morbidity in post-myelogram patients. A survey of 100 patients. J Can Assoc Radiol 23:278
100. Tourtellotte WW, Haber AF, Heller GL, Somer JE (1964) Post-lumbar puncture headaches. Thomas, Springfield
101. Baker RA, Hillman BJ, McLennan JE, Strand RD, Kaufman SM (1978) Sequelae of metrizamide myelography in 200 examinations. Am J Radiol 130:499
102. Levine MC, White DW (1974) Chronic postmyelographic headache. A result of persistent epidural cerebrospinal fluid fistula. JAMA 229:684
103. Goff H, Goldstein AS, Ruskin R, Leopold HH (1971) Chronic post myelogram headache. Arch Neurol 25:169
104. Lieberman LM, Tourtellotte WW, Newkirk TA (1971) Prolonged post-lumbar puncture cerebrospinal fluid leakage from lumbar subarachnoid space demonstrated by radioisotope myelography. Neurology 21:925
105. Harris LM, Harmel MH (1953) The comparative incidence of post lumbar puncture headache following spinal anesthesia administered through 20 and 24 gauge needles. Anesthesiology 14:390
106. Hatfalvi BI (1977) The dynamics of post-spinal headache. Headache 17:64
107. Wiggli U, Oberson R (1975) Incidence of extra-arachnoid discharge following lumbar puncture. Schweiz Med Wochschr 105:235
108. Kieffer SA, Binet EF, Esquerra JV et al. (1978) Contrast agents for myelography: clinical and radiological evaluation of Amipaque and Pantopaque. Radiology 129:695
109. Strother CM (1979) Adverse reactions. In: Sackett JF, Strother CM (eds) New techniques in myelography. Harper and Row, Hagerstown, p 196
110. McLennan JE (1973) Prevention of post-myelographic and post-pneumoencephalographic headache by single dose intrathecal methyl-prednisolone acetate. Headache 13:39
111. Ahlgren P (1980) Early and late side-effects of water soluble contrast media for myelography and cisternography: a short review. Invest Radiol 15:264
112. Eldevik OP, Haughton VM, Ho KC, Williams AL, Unger GF, Larson SJ (1978) Ineffectiveness of prophylactic intrathecal methylprednisolone in myelography with aqueous media. Radiology 129:99
113. Dullerud R, Morland TJ (1976) Adhesive arachnoiditis after lumbar radiculography with Dimer-X and Depo-Medrol. Radiology 119:153
114. Hammer B, Lackner W (1980) Iopamidol, a new non-ionic hydrosoluble contrast medium for neuroradiology. Neuroradiology 19:119
115. Eldevik OP, Haughton VM, Sasse EA (1980) Elimination of aqueous myelographic contrast media from the subarachnoid space. Invest Radiol 15:260
116. Speck U, Schmidt R, Volkhardt V, Vogelsang H (1978) The effect of position on the passage of metrizamide (amipaque), meglumine iocarmate (Dimer X) and ioserinate (Myelographin) into the blood after lumbar myelography. Neuroradiology 14:251
117. Gutterman P, Bezier HS (1978) Prophylaxis of post-myelogram headaches. J Neurosurg 49:869

118. Zenglein JP, Baldauf E, Wasser P (1978) Effect of tiapride on the side effects of cerebrospinal fluid depletions in spinal puncture, pneumoencephalography and air myelography. Sem Hop Paris 54:413
119. Eldevik OP, Haughton VM, Sasse EA (1980) The effect of dehydration on the elimination of aqueous contrast media from the subarachnoid space. Invest Radiol 15:155
120. Eldevik OP, Nakken KO, Haughton VM (1978) The effect of dehydration on the side effects of metrizamide myelography. Radiology 129:715
121. Eldevik OP, Haughton VM (1978) The effect of hydration on the acute and chronic complications of aqueous myelography. An experimental study. Radiology 129:713
122. Lieberman P, Siegle RL, Kaplan RJ, Hashimoto K (1976) Chronic urticaria and intermittent anaphylaxis. Reactions to Iophendylate. JAMA 236:1495
123. Hurwitz SR, Suydam M, Steinberg A (1980) Aspiration of metrizamide following lumbar myelography. Radiology 136:789
124. Irstam L, Sellden U (1975) Side effects after lumbar myelography with dimeglumine iocarmate (Dimer-X). Further experiences. Acta Radiol [Diagn] (Stockh) 16:449
125. Grepe A, Widen L (1973) Neurotoxic effect of intracranial subarachnoid application of metrizamide and meglumine iocarmate. An experimental application in dogs in neuroleptic analgesia. Acta Radiol [Suppl] (Stockh) 335:102
126. Hindmarsh T, Grepe A, Widen L (1975) Metrizamide-phenothiazine interaction. Report of a case with seizures following myelography. Acta Radiol [Diagn] (Stockh) 16:129
127. Sovak M, Ranganathan R, Speck U (1982) Nonionic dimer: development and initial testing of an intrathecal contrast agent. Radiology 142:115
128. Sovak M, Ranganathan R (1982) Novel amino-dioxepane intermediates for the synthesis of new non-ionic contrast media. US patent no 4,341,756
129. Belloni G, Bonaldi G, Moschini L, Quilici N (1981) Cervical myelography with iopamidol. Neuroradiology 21:97
130. Belenger J, Simons M, Jean-Mart L, Davis A (1971) Evolution de la neuralographie. J Belge Radiol 54:347
131. Piper H (1929) Die Entwicklung der Myelographie. Roentgenpraxis 154:275
132. Sicard JA, Forestier A (1926) Roentgenologic explorations of the central nervous system with iodized oil (Lipiodol). Arch Neurol Psychiatr 16:420
133. Odine M, Runstrom G, Lindblom AF (1928) Iodized oils: an aid to the diagnosis of lesions of spinal cord and a contribution to the knowledge of adhesive circumscribed meningitis. Acta Radiol [Diagn] [Suppl] 7:1
134. Lindblom AF (1931) The effects of various iodized oils on the meninges. Acta Med Scand 76:395
135. Jaeger R (1950) Irritating effect of iodized vegetable oils on the brain and spinal cord when divided into small particles. Arch Neurol Psychol 64:715
137. Hughes R (1953) Chronic changes in the central nervous system following Thorotrast ventriculography. Proc R Soc Med 46:191
138. Nosik WA, Mortenson OA (1938) Myelography with Thorotrast and subsequent removal by forced drainage: an experimental study, preliminary report. Am J Roentgenol 39:727
139. Boyd JT, Langlands AO, Maccabe JJ (1968) Long-term hazards of Thorotrast. Br Med J 2:517
140. Arnell S, Lidström F (1931) Myelography with Skiodan (Abrodil). Acta Radiol 12:287
141. Lefft HH, Maclean JA Jr (1942) Visualization of the brain and spinal cord with diiodothyrosine-gelatin contrast medium, including observation on the fate of this material. Arch Neurol Psychiatry 48:343
142. Schober R (1964) Roentgen-Kontrastmittel und Liquor-Raum. Springer, Berlin Göttingen Heidelberg New York
143. Strain WH (1971) Radiocontrast agents for neuroradiology. In: Knoefel PK (ed) Encyclopedia of contrast media, vol II. Pergamon, Oxford, p 369
144. Kemp JD (1950) Contrast myelography: past and present. Radiology 54:477

145. Kieffer SA, Peterson HO, Gold LHA, Binet EF (1970) Evaluation of dilute pantopaque for large-volume myelography. Radiology 96:69
146. Greenberg MK, Vance SC (1980) Focal seizure disorder complicating iodophendylate myelography (letter). Lancet 1:312
147. Jones DF (1980) Postoperative convulsions due to iophendylate (Myodil). Report of a case and review of the causes of postoperative convulsions. Anaesthesia 35:50
148. Cristi G, Scialfa G, Di Pierro G, Tassoni A (1974) Visual loss: a rare complication following oil myelography. Case report and review of the literature. Neuroradiology 7:287
149. Occhiogrosso M, Troccoli V, Vailati G (1979) A rare complication following iodized myelography: late blindness. Case report. Acta Neurol (Napoli) 34:76
150. Perpetuo FO, Hurtado PS (1979) Diabetes insipidus after myelography. Report of a case. Arq Neuropsiquiatr 37:85
151. Lee SH (1976) Venous intravasation of pantopaque during myelography. Report of two cases and a review of the literature. J Can Assoc Radiol 27:111
152. Irstam L, Rosencrantz M (1973) Water-soluble contrast media and adhesive arachnoiditis. I. Reinvestigation of nonoperated cases. Acta Radiol [Diagn] (Stockh) 14:497
153. King AY, Khodadad G (1979) Intravasation of pantopaque during myelography. Surg Neurol 11:3
154. Jensen F, Reske-Nielsen E, Ratjen E (1979) Obstructive hydrocephalus following Pantopaque myelography. Neuroradiology 18:139
155. Kaufman P, Jeans WD (1976) Reactions to iophendylate in relation to multiple sclerosis. Lancet 2:1000
156. Luce JC, Leith W, Burrage WS (1951) Pantopaque meningitis due to hypersensitivity. Radiology 57:878
157. Burton CV (1978) Lumbosacral arachnoiditis. Spine 3:24
158. Barsoum AH, Cannillo KL (1980) Thoracic constrictive arachnoiditis after Pantopaque myelography: report of two cases. Neurosurgery 6:314
159. White AG (1972) Prolonged elevation of serum protein-bound iodine following myelography with Myodil. Br J Radiol 45:21
160. Ferry DJ Jr, Gooding R, Standefer JC, Wiese GM (1973) Effect of Pantopaque myelography on cerebrospinal fluid fractions. J Neurosurg 38:167
161. Rinaldi I, Gendron FG, Reach WF Jr, Harris WO Jr, Kopp JE, Reagan TF, Botton JE (1979) Contamination of Pantopaque by glass. Surg Neurol 11:295
162. Mindell HJ (1976) On the use of Pantopaque in renal cysts. Radiology 119:747
163. Raskin MM, Roen SA, Viamonte M Jr (1975) Effect of intracystic Pantopaque on renal cysts. J Urol 114:678
164. Vestby GW (1971) Percutaneous treatment of renal cysts. The triple contrast or Pantopaque method. Acta Radiol [Diagn] (Stockh) 11:529
165. Bergeron RT, Rumbaugh CL, Fang H, Cravioto H (1971) Experimental Pantopaque arachnoiditis in the monkey. Radiology 99:95
166. Klee JG, Praestholm J (1975) Comparison of iothalamate meglumine, metrizamide and iodophendylate in cerebral ventriculography. A clinical, radiological, and histopathological study in the rat. Invest Radiol 10:244
167. Gjerris A, Praestholm J, Klinken L (1978) Comparison of metrizamide and iodophendylate for cerebral ventriculography: a long-term ultrastructural study of the ventricular wall in the rat. Neuroradiology 15:79
168. Praestholm J, Klee JG, Klinken L (1976) Histological changes in the central nervous system following intraventricular administration of oil-soluble contrast media. An experimental study in the rat. Radiology 119:391
169. Yuen TG, Agnew WF, Rumbaugh CL (1976) Ultrastructural effects of Conray 60 and Pantopaque on ependyma and choroid plexus following intraventricular injections. Invest Radiol 11:112

170. Liu MS, Dobben GD, Szanto PB, Alrenga DP, Khin U, Arambulo AS, Forrest R (1976) Myelography with perfluoroctylbromide. Comparison with Pantopaque. Invest Radiol 11:319
171. Brahme F, Sovak M, Powell H, Long DM (1976) Perfluorocarbon bromides as contrast media in radiography of the central nervous system. Acta Radiol [Suppl] (Stockh) 347:347–459
172. Newton BN (1976) Iodine-containing organic carbonates as investigative radiopaque compounds. J Med Chem 19:1362
173. Newton BN (1978) Structure toxicity relationships of iodinated aromatic carbonates and related compounds. J Pharm Sci 67:1154
174. Ahlgren P, Praestholm J (1969) Complications of myelography with Methiodal. Nord Med 82:1600
175. Ahlgren P (1973) Long term side effects after myelography with water soluble contrast media: Conturex, Conray Meglumin 282 and Dimer-X. Neuroradiology 6:206
176. Skalpe IO (1976) Adhesive arachnoiditis following lumbar radiculography with water-soluble contrast agents. A clinical report with special reference to metrizamide. Radiology 121:647
177. Funkquist B, Obel N (1961) Effect on the spinal cord of subarachnoid injection of water-soluble contrast media. Acta Radiol 56:449
178. Betoulieres P, Temple JP, Janicot JY (1960) La radiculographie lombo-sacrée au Methiodal. J Radiol Electrol Med Nucl 41:447
179. Ferrand J, D'Eshouges JR, Barsotti J (1961) La radiculographie lombo-sacrée par substance iodée hydrosoluble et resorbable. Expansion scientifique française, Paris
180. Harvey JP, Freiberger RF, Werner G (1961) Clinical and experimental observations with methiodal, an absorbable myelographic contrast agent. Clin Pharmacol Ther 2:610
181. Ledoux-Lebard G, Heitz F, Laurent YM (1965) Incidents et accidents en myelographie. In: Fischgold H, Wackenheim A (eds) La radiographie des formations intrarachidiennes. Masson, Paris, p 203
182. Lindblom K (1947) Complications of myelography by Abrodil. Acta Radiol 28:69
183. Monroe D (1956) Lumbar and sacral compression radiculitis. N Engl J Med 254:243
184. Woringer E, Baumgartner J, Braun JP (1955) Le diagnostic de la hernie discale lombo-sacrée par la myelographie au mono-iodo-methane sulfonate de sodium. Nouv Presse Med 63:1584
185. Dietz H, Ulbricht W (1968) Zur Frage der Potenzstörungen nach lumbaler Myelographie mit positiven Kontrastmitteln. Acta Neurochir (Wien) 19:109
186. Praestholm J, Olgaard K (1972) Comparative histological investigation of the sequelae of experimental myelography using sodium methiodal and meglumine iothalamate. Neuroradiology 4:14
187. Albertson K, Doppman JL (1974) Meglumine diatrizoate v. iothalamate: comparison of seizure-inducing potential. Br J Radiol 47:265
188. Melartin E, Tuohimaa PJ, Dabb R (1970) Neurotoxicity of iothalamate and diatrizoates. I. Significance of concentration and cation. Invest Radiol 5:13
189. Boisen E, Lindholmer E (1971) Serious complications from myelography with meglumine iothalamate. An account of 324 lumbar myelographies together with a description of 2 cases of severe leg cramp. Nord Med 85:520
190. Campbell RC, Campbell JA, Heimburger RF et al. (1964) Ventriculography and myelography with absorbable radiopaque medium. Radiology 82:286
191. Heimburger RF, Kalsbeck JE, Campbell RL et al. (1966) Positive contrast cerebral ventriculography using water soluble media. J Neurol Neurosurg Psychiatry 29:281
192. Praestholm J, Lester J (1972) Complications of myelography with Conray meglumin. Acta Radiol [Diagn] (Stockh) 13:860
193. Oftedal SI, Sawhney BB (1970) Toxic effects of water-soluble contrast media for myelography. A polygraphic study in rabbits. Acta Neurol Scand [Suppl 43] 46:273
194. Weems TD, Cashion EL, Cunningham DL (1977) Microscopic effects of meglumine iothalamate. Ventriculography in canines. Neuroradiology 13:151

195. Slatis P, Autio E, Suolanen J, Norrback S (1974) Hyperosmolality of the cerebrospinal fluid as a cause of adhesive arachnoiditis in lumbar myelography. Acta Radiol [Diagn] (Stockh) 15:619
196. Irstam L, Sundstrom R, Sigstedt B (1974) Lumbar myelography and adhesive arachnoiditis. Acta Radiol [Diagn] (Stockh) 15:356
197. Skalpe IO (1976) Adhesive arachnoiditis following lumbar radiculography with water soluble contrast agents. Radiology 121:647
198. Shaw MM, Miller JD, Steven JL (1975) Effect of intracranial pressure of meglumine iothalamate ventriculography. J Neurol Neurosurg Psychiatry 38:1022
199. Skalpe IO (1973) Myelography with metrizamide, meglumine iothalamate, and meglumine iocarmate. Acta Radiol [Suppl] (Stockh) 335:57
200. Oftedal SI, Kayed K (1973) Epileptogenic effect of water soluble contrast media: an experimental investigation in rabbits. Acta Radiol [Suppl] (Stockh) 335:45
201. Hilal SK (1966) Hemodynamic responses in the cerebral vessels to angiography contrast media. Acta Radiol 5:211
202. Suzuki S, Kawaguchi S, Mita R, Iwabuchi T (1976) Ventriculography with methylglucamine iocarmate (Dimer-X). Experimental and clinical study. Acta Neurochir (Wien) 33:219
203. Suzuki S, Kawaguchi S, Mita R, Ito K, Iwabuchi T (1975) Ventriculography with methylglucamine iocarmate (Dimer-X). Experimental and clinical study. Neurol Surg (Tokyo) 3:849
204. Gonsette R (1971) An experimental and clinical assessment of water soluble contrast medium in neuroradiology: a new medium, Dimer-X. Clin Radiol 22:44
205. Ahlgren P (1972) Dimer-X. A new contrast medium for lumbar myelography without spinal anaesthesia. Acta Radiol [Diagn] (Stockh) 13.753
206. Hickel D, Reisner K, Dinkloh H (1979) A comparison of the side effects of watersoluble contrast media for lumbar myelography. ROEFO 130:470
207. Usbeck W, Assmann H (1977) Value of Dimer-X myelography in the diagnosis of lumbar intravertebral disk lesions. Zentralbl Neurochir 38:165
208. Nishikawa M, Yonekawa Y (1976) Dimer-X in the intracranial subarachnoid space – its toxicity. Neurol Surg (Tokyo) 4:543
209. Kun M, Alwasiak J, Gronska J (1978) Morphological changes in the CNS after Dimer X ventriculography. Neuroradiology 15:99
210. Haughton VM, Ho K-C (1980) Arachnoiditis from myelography with iopamidol, metrizamide and iocarmate compared in the animal model. Invest Radiol 15:267
211. Haughton VM, Ho K-C, Larson SJ, Unger GF, Correa-Paz F (1978) Comparison of arachnoiditis produced by meglumine iocarmate and metrizamide myelography in an animal model. A J Radiol 131:129
212. Autio E, Suolanen J, Nörrback S, Slätis P (1972) Adhesive arachnoiditis after lumbar myelography with meglumine iothalamate (Conray). Acta Radiol [Diagn] (Stockh) 12:17
213. Bidstrup P (1972) A case of chronic adhesive arachnoiditis after lumbar myelography with methiodal-natrium. Neuroradiology 3:157
214. Davies FM, Llewellyn RC, Kirgis HD (1968) Water-soluble contrast media myelography using meglumine iothalamate (Conray) with methylprednisolone acetate (Depo-Medrol). Radiology 90:708
215. Geller GE (1971) Komplikation bei der lumbalen Myelographie mit Conray 282 (Contrix 28). ROEFO 114:568
216. Weill F, Steinle R, Jacquet G, Bonneville JR, Prévetat N (1971) Incident sérieux aprés radiculographie au Contrix. J Radiol Electrol Med Nucl 52:535
217. deVelliers PD (1977) Myelography with a water-soluble contrast medium: a revision of technique and a review of results. S Afr Med J 52:751
218. Perrigot M, Pierrot-Deseilligny E, Bussel B, Held JP (1976) Paralysis following Dimer X radiculography. Nouv Presse Med 5:1120
219. Kuhner A, Hagenlocher HU, Ciba K, Krastel A (1977) Lesions of the cauda equina after dimer-X myelography. Neurochirurgia (Stuttg) 20:216

220. Walker N, Egli M, Wellauer J (1976) Side reaction after lumbar myelography with dimer-X. Z Orthop 114:793
221. Metrizamide, nonionic water soluble contrast medium (1973). Acta Radiol [Suppl] (Stockh) 335
222. Hol L, Kelly M, Salvesen S (1977) Metrizamide in biochemical properties of drug substances. In: Goldberg ME (ed) Academy Pharm, vol I. Sciences, Washington DC
223. Metrizamide (1977) Lindgren E (ed) Acta Radiol [Suppl] (Stockh) 355
224. Björk L, Ericksson U, Ingelman B (1969) Clinical experiences with a new type of contrast medium in peripheral arteriography. Am J Roentgen 106:418
225. Björk L, Erikson U, Ingelman B, Lindblad G (1976) Experiments with a new contrast medium in myelography. Acta Radiol [Diagn] (Stockh) 17:136
226. Klieger E, Schroeder E (1975) Synthesis of N-(3-acylamino-5-alkyl carbomoyl-2,4,6-triiodobenzoyl)amino acids as X-ray contrast agents. Eur J Med Chem 10:84
227. Hammer B (1978) Results of a double-blind study of 3 contrast media and technique for lumbo-sacral radiculography. Neuroradiology 17:45
228. Hammer B (1977) Meningeale Spätveränderungen durch wasserlösliche Myelographiekontrastmittel. ROEFO 126:145
229. Hammer B, Vogelsang H (1976) Erfahrung mit einem neuen wäßrigen Kontrastmittel für die lumbale Myelographie. Radiologe 16:412
230. Vogelsang H, Speck U, Becker P, Blumenbach L, Busse O (1976) Experience with a new water soluble contrast medium for lumbar myelography. Roentgenblaetter 29:201
231. Almen T (1969) Contrast agent design. Some aspects on the synthesis of water soluble contrast agents of low osmolality. J Theor Biol 24:216
232. Sovak M, Ranganathan R (1980) Stability of nonionic water-soluble contrast media: implications for their design. Invest Radiol 15:323
233. Salvesen S (1973) Acute toxicity tests of metrizamide. Acta Radiol [Suppl] (Stockh) 335:5
234. Gonsette RE (1973) Biologic tolerance of the CNS to metrizamide. Acta Radiol [Suppl] (Stockh) 335:25
235. Salvesen S (1973) Suboccipital injection of metrizamide into anesthetized and unanesthetized rabbits. Acta Radiol [Suppl] (Stockh) 335:93
236. Sawhney BB, Oftedahl SI (1973) Reactions of suboccipital injection of water-soluble contrast media in rabbits. Acta Radiol [Suppl] (Stockh) 335:67
237. Oftedahl SI (1973) Toxicity of water-soluble contrast media injected suboccipitally in cats. Acta Radiol [Suppl] (Stockh) 335:84
238. Oftedahl SI (1973) Intraventricular application of water-soluble contrast media in cats. Acta Radiol [Suppl] (Stockh) 335:125
239. Oftedahl SI, Sawhney BB (1973) Effect of water-soluble contrast media on cortically evoked potentials in the cat. Acta Radiol [Suppl] (Stockh) 335:133
240. Hilal SK, Douth GW, Burger L, Gilman F (1977) Effects of isotonic contrast agents on spinal reflexes in the cat. Radiology 122:149
241. Almen T, Golman R (1979) Pharmacology and toxicology of some intrathecal contrast media. In: Sackett JF, Strother CM (eds) New techniques in myelography. Harper and Row, New York, p 8
242. Drobeck HP, Duprey LP (1975) Acute intracisternal toxicity of Metriz. (300 mg I/ml) in newborn and young adult rabbits, internal report. Sterling-Winthrop Research Institute, Rennsalear, New York
243. Piwonka RW, Healey JF, Rosenberg FJ (1976) Intrathecal tolerance of metrizamide in chloralose-anesthetized cats. Invest Radiol 11:182
244. Wylie IG, Afshar F, Koeze TH (1975) Results of the use of a new water-soluble contrast medium, metrizamide, in the posterior fossa of the baboon. Br J Radiol 48:1007
245. Gonsette RE, Brucher JM (1977) Potentiation of Amipaque: epileptogenic activity by neuroleptics. Neuroradiology 14:27
246. Praestholm J (1977) Experimental evaluation of water-soluble contrast media for myelography. Neuroradiology 13:25

247. Skalpe IO, Torvik A (1975) Toxicity of metrizamide and meglumine iocarmate in the spinal subarachnoid space. Invest Radiol 10:154
248. Oftedahl SI (1973) Meningeal reactions to the water-soluble contrast media in cats. Acta Radiol [Suppl] (Stockh) 335:153
249. Suzuki S, Ito K, Iwabuchi T (1977) Ventriculography with nonionic water-soluble contrast medium, Amipaque (metrizamide): comparative experimental and clinical studies. J Neurosurg 47:79
250. Treten L, Salveson S (1973) Histology of the central nervous system of the rabbit after suboccipital injection of metrizamide. Acta Radiol [Suppl] (Stockh) 335:161
251. Haughton VM, Ho KC, Larson S et al. (1978) Arachnoiditis produced by metrizamide and meglumine iocarmate myelography compared in an animal model. Am J Roentgenol 131:120
252. Haughton VM, Ho KC, Larson S et al. (1978) Severity of arachnoiditis and the concentration of meglumine iocarmate. Am J Roentgenol 130:313
253. Haughton VM, Ho KC, Larson S et al. (1977) Arachnoiditis following intrathecal injection of blood and aqueous contrast media. Acta Radiol [Suppl] (Stockh) 355:373
254. Haughton VM, Ho KC, Unger GF (1977) Arachnoiditis following myelography with water-soluble agents: the role of contrast medium osmolality. Radiology 125:731
255. Haughton VM, Eldevik POP (1979) Complications form aqueous myelographic media: experimental studies. In: Sackett JF, Strother CM (eds) New techniques in myelography. Harper and Row, New York, p 184
256. Bartels JE, Bround KG (1980) Experimental arachnoiditis fibrosis produced by metrizamide in the dog. Radiology 21:78
257. Lee BCP, Gomez DG, Potts DG, Pavese AM (1981) Subacute reactions to intrathecal amipaque, metrizamide, Conray, and Dimer-X: a structural and ultrastructural study. Neuroradiology 20:229
275a. Sage M (1983) Kinetics of ureter-soluble contrast media in the central nervous system. AJNR 4:897–906
258. McChesney EW (1971) Routes and rates of excretion of radio-contrast agents. In: Knoefel PK (ed) Radiocontrast agents. Pergamon, London, p 335
259. McChesney EW, Hoppe JO (1957) Studies of the tissue distribution and excretion of sodium diatrizoate in laboratory animals. Am J Roent 78:137
260. Golman K (1976) Metrizamide in experimental urography. Invest Radiol 11:187
261. Golman K (1973) Excretion of metrizamide. Acta Radiol [Suppl] (Stockh) 335:253
262. Golman K, Dahl SG (1973) Absorption of metrizamide, diatrizoate, insulin and water from cerebrospinal fluid to blood. Acta Radiol [Suppl] (Stockh) 335:276
263. Amundsen P, Weber H, Hoel L, Golman K (1979) Excretion of metrizamide (Amipaque) in humans following lumbar subarachnoid injection. Acta Radiol [Diagn] (Stockh) 20:401
264. Lee BCP, Gomez GD, Potts DG, Pavese AM (1979) Passage of Amipaque (metrizamide) through the arachnoid granulations. Neuroradiology 17:185
265. Hindmarsh T (1975) Elimination of water-soluble contrast media from a subarachnoidal space: investigation with computer tomography. Acta Radiol [Suppl] (Stockh) 346:45
266. Fenstermacher JD, Bradbury MWB, Boulay GDU, Kendall BE, Radu EW (1980) The distribution of ^{125}I metrizamide and ^{125}I diatrizoate between blood, brain, and cerebrospinal fluid in rabbit. Neuroradiology 19:171
267. Golman K, Wiik I, Salveson S (1979) Absorption of a nonionic contrast agent from cerebrospinal fluid to blood. Neuroradiology 18:227
268. Arimitsu T, Di Chiro G, Brooks RA (1977) White-gray matter differentiation in computed tomography. JCAT 1:437–442
269. Kelley RE, Daroff RB, Sheremata WA (1980) Unusual effects of metrizamide lumbar myelography. Arch Neurol 37:588–589
270. Hindmarsh T (1977) Computer cisternography for evaluation of cerebrospinal fluid flow dynamics: future experiences. Acta Radiol [Suppl] (Stockh) 355:269
271. Skalpe IO (1977) Adverse effects of water soluble contrast media in myelography, cisternography, and ventriculography. Acta Radiol [Suppl] (Stockh) 355:280–293

272. Irstam L (1978) Lumbar myelography with amipaque. Spine 3:70
273. Drayer BP, Rosenbaum AE (1977) Metrizamide brain penetration. Acta Radiol [Suppl] (Stockh) 355:280–293
274. Hindmarsh T (1977) Metrizamide in selected cervical myelography. Acta Radiol [Suppl] (Stockh) 355:127
275. Dugstad G, Eldevik P (1977) Lumbar myelography. Acta Radiol [Suppl] (Stockh) 355:17
276. Nickel AR, Salem JJ (1977) Clinical experience in North America with metrizamide. Acta Radiol [Suppl] (Stockh) 355:409–416
277. Gulati AN, Guadagnoli DA, Quigley JM (1981) Relationship of side effects to patient position during and after metrizamide lumbar myelography. Radiology 141:113–116
278. Sykes RHD, Wasenaar W, Clark P (1981) Incidence of adverse effects following metrizamide myelography in nonambulatory and ambulatory patients. Radiology 138:625–627
279. Hauge O, Falkenberg H (1982) Neuropsychologic rcactions and other side effects after metrizamide myelography. AJR 139:357–360
280. Hekster REM, Prins HJ, Pennings-Braun AGM (1977) Lumbar myelography with metrizamide. Acta Radiol [Suppl] (Stockh) 355:38–40
281. Drayer BP, Rosenbaum AE (1977) Metrizamide brain penetrance. Acta Radiol [Suppl] (Stockh) 335:280
282. Drayer BP, Vassallo C, Sudilovsky A (1983) A double-blind clinical trial of iopamidol versus metrizamide for lumbosacral myelography. J Neurosurg 58:531–537
283. Caille JM, Guibert-Tranier F, Howa JM (1980) Cerebral penetration following metrizamide myelography. J Neuroradiol 7:3–12
284. Fenstermacher JD, Tatlack CS, Blasberg RD (1974) Transport of material between brain extracellular fluid, brain cells, and blood. Fed Proc 33:2070–2074
285. Winkler SS, Sackett JF (1980) Explanation of metrizamide brain penetration: a review. J Comput Assist Tomogr 4:191
286. Kerber CW, Sovak M, Ranganathan RS, Heilman CB (1983) Iotrol, a new myelographic agent: 1. radiography, CT, CSF clearance, and brain penetration. AJNR 4:317–318
287. Skalpe IO, Torbergsen T, Amundsen P, Presthus J (1973) Lumbar myelography with metrizamide. Acta Radiol [Suppl] (Stockh) 335:369
288. Irstam L (1978) Lumbar myelography with Amipaque. Spine 3:70
289. Hansen EB, Praestholm H, Fahrenkrug A, Bjerrum J (1976) A clinical trial of amipaque in lumbar myelography. Br J Radiol 49:34
290. Sackett JF, Strother CM, Quaglieri CE, Javid MJ, Levin AB, Duff TA (1977) Metrizamide – CSF contrast medium. Analysis of clinical application in 215 patients. Radiology 123:779
291. Sartor K (1979) Ascending and descending myelography with water-soluble contrast medium. A report on thoracic and cervical metrizamide myelography in 200 patients. Roentgenblaetter 32:251
292. Kaada B (1973) Transient EEG abnormalities following lumbar myelography with metrizamide. Acta Radiol [Suppl] (Stockh) 335:380
293. Hammer B, Lackner W (1980) Iopamidol, a new non-ionic hydrosoluble contrast medium for neuroradiology. Neuroradiology 19:119
294. Gelmers HJ (1979) Adverse side effects of metrizamide in myelography. Neuroradiology 18:119
295. Skalpe IO, Amundsen P (1975) Lumbar radiculography with metrizamide. A nonionic water-soluble contrast medium. Radiology 115:91
296. Richert S, Sartor K, Holl B (1979) Subclinical organic psychosyndromes on intrathecal injection of metrizamide for lumbar myelography. Neuroradiology 18:177
297. Picard L, Vespignani H, Vieux-Rochat P, Moret C, L'esperance G, Montaut J, Weber M, Roland J (1979) Serious neurological complications of metrizamide myelography. J Neuroradiol 6:3
298. Bastow M, Godwin-Austen RB (1979) Cervical myelopathy after metrizamide myelography. Br Med J 2:1262

299. Weber RJ, Weingarden SI (1979) Electromyographic abnormalities following myelography. Arch Neurol 36:588
300. Vogelsang H, Schmidt RE (1979) Spinal irritation after myelography with amipaque in patients with kyphoscoliosis. ROEFO 131:90
301. Rubin B, Horowitz G, Katz RI (1980) Asterixis following metrizamide myelography. Arch Neurol 37:522
302. Kelley RE, Daroff RB, Sheremata WA, McCormick JR (1980) Unusual effects of metrizamide lumbar myelography. Constellation of aseptic meningitis, arachnoiditis, communicating hydrocephalus, and Guillaine-Barre syndrome. Arch Neurol 37:588
303. Haughton VM, Ho KC (1979) The risk of arachnoiditis from experimental nonionic contrast media. S Afr Med J 56:631
304. Hansen EB, Fahrenkrug A, Praestholm J (1978) Late meningeal effects of myelographic contrast media with special reference to metrizamide. Br J Radiol 51:321
305. Ahlgren T (1978) Amipaque myelography with late adhesive arachnoidal changes. Neuroradiology 14:231
306. Amundsen P, Skalpe IO, Presthus J, Torbergsen T, Kaada B (1976) Metrizamide, the new water-soluble non-ionic contrast media for myelography. Clinical experience. Acta Radiol [Suppl] (Stockh) 347:453
307. Sortland O (1977) Cervical myelography with metrizamide using lumbar injection. Acta Radiol [Suppl] (Stockh) 355:141
308. Bradac GN, Kaernbach A (1981) Selektive zervikale Myelographie mit Metrizamid (Amipaque). Bericht über 102 Fälle mit lateraler C1/C2-Kontrastmitteleingabe. Radiologe 21:199
309. Lundervold A, Sortland O (1977) EEG disturbances following myelography, cisternography, and ventriculography with metrizamide. Acta Radiol [Suppl] (Stockh) 355:379
310. Gonsette RE, Brucher JM (1981) Neurotoxicity of novel water-soluble contrast media for intrathecal application. Invest Radiol [Suppl] 15:S254
311. Sovak M, Ranganathan R (1980) Stability of nonionic contrast media: implications for their design. Invest Radiol 15:S323
312. Hoey GB, Hopkins RM, Smith KR et al. (1981) Synthesis and biological testing of nonionic iodinated X-ray contrast media. Invest Radiol [Suppl] 15:S289
313. Sovak M, Nahlovsky B, Lang H, Lasser EC (1975) Preliminary evaluation of diiodophenyltriglucoside: an approach to the design of nonionic water-soluble radiographic contrast media. Radiology 117:717
314. Sovak M, Ranganathan R, Weitl FL, Lang J, Lasser EC (1979) Benzyl and phenyl hexosyl ethers as non-ionic contrast media: toxicological significance of the methylene group. Eur J Med Chem 14:257
315. Sovak M, Ranganathan R (1981) US patent no 4,243,653
316. Ranganathan RS, Sovak M (1981) Syntheses of new nonionic radiographic contrast media: acylamino-triiodophenyl ethers of sugars. Invest Radiol [Suppl] 15:296
317. Holtermann H (1973) Metrizamide: introduction. Acta Radiol [Suppl] (Stockh) 335:2
318. Felder E, Pitre D (1977) US patent no 4,001,323
319. Felder E, Pitre D (1979) US patent no 4,139,605
320. Pitre D, Felder E (1981) Development, chemistry, and physical properties of iopamidol and its analogs. Invest Radiol [Suppl] 15:301
321. Bonati F, Felder E, Tirone P (1981) New preclinical and clinical data. Invest Radiol [Suppl] 15:310
322. Gonsette RE, Liesenborgh L (1981) New contrast media in cerebral angiography: animal experiments and preliminary clinical studies. Invest Radiol [Suppl] 15:270
323. Morris TW, Francis M, Fischer HW (1979) A comparison of the cardiovascular responses to carotid injection of ionic and nonionic contrast media. Invest Radiol 14:217
324. Belan A, Benda K, Fabian J, Blake J (1978) Advantages of a new nonionic contrast medium: results of animal experiments. Ann Radiol (Paris) 21:279
325. Sovak M, Johnson M, Ranganathan R (1980) Neurotoxicity of new contrast media: effects of cisternography on lapine EEG spectrum. Invest Radiol 15:452

326. Sovak M, Siefert HM, Ranganathan R (1981) Combined methods for assessment of neurotoxicity: testing of new nonionic radiographic media. Invest Radiol [Suppl] 15:248

327. Sovak M, Deutsch JA, Ranganathan R (1982) Evaluation of intrathecal contrast media by aversion conditioning in rats. Invest Radiol 17:101

328. Spencer LP, Crisman CL, Mayhew IG, Kaude JV (1980) Acute neurotoxicity of iopamidol following subarachnoid application. Invest Radiol 15:411

329. Yu C, Wang J (1980) Deiodination kinetics of water-soluble radiopaques. J Pharm Sci 69:671

330. Pitre D, Felder E, Tirone P (1980) Radiopaque contrast media – preliminary studies of the metabolism of iopamidol in the dog, rabbit, and man. Farmaco 35:826

331. Golman K, Olivecrona H, Gustafson C et al. (1980) Excitation and depression of non-anesthetized rabbits following injection of contrast medium into SAS. Acta Radiol [Suppl] (Stockh) 362:83

332. Scaglione P, Marinoni EC (1982) The lumbar myelography with non-ionic water-soluble contrast. In: Proceedings of the XVth international congress of radiology, Brussels, 1981. Interimages, Luxembourg

333. Bockenheimer SAM, Hillesheimer W (1983) Clinical experience with iopamidol for myelography. AJNR 4:314–316

334. Bannon KR, Braun KF, Pinto RS, Manuell M, Sudilovsky A, Kricheff II (1983) Comparison of radiographic quality and adverse reactions in myelography with iopamidol and metrizamide. AJNR 4:312–313

335. Turski PA, Sackett JF, Gentry LR, Strother CM, Matozzi F (1983) Clinical comparison of metrizamide and iopamidol for myelography. AJNR 4:309–311

336. Trevisan C, Malaguti C, Manfredini M, Tampieri D (1983) Iopamidol vs. metrizamide myelography: clinical comparison of side effects. AJNR 4:306–308

337. Jacobsen T (1984) The preclinical development of iohexol. Invest Radiol 19:S142–143

338. Haalveson J (1980) Iohexol – introduction. Acta Radiol [Suppl] (Stockh) 362:9

339. Aulie A (1980) Effect of iohexol, metrizamide, and ioxaglate on the BBB. Acta Radiol [Suppl] (Stockh) 362:13

340. Salvesen S (1980) Acute intravenous toxicity of iohexol in the mouse and in the rat. Acta Radiol [Suppl] (Stockh) 362:73

341. Siefert HM, Press WR, Speck U (1980) Tolerance of iohexol post intracisternal, intracerebral, and intraarterial injection in the rat. Acta Radiol [Suppl] (Stockh) 362:77

342. Mutzel W, Siefert HM, Speck U (1980) Biochemical pharmacologic properties of iohexol. Acta Radiol [Suppl] (Stockh) 362:111

343. Aspelin P, Liessen MS, Almen T (1980) Effect of iohexol on human erythrocytes. I. Changes of red cell morphology in vitro. Acta Radiol [Suppl] (Stockh) 362:117

344. Aspelin P, Bink A, Almen T, Kiesewetter H (1980) Effect of iohexol on human erythrocytes. II. Red cell aggregation in vitro. Acta radiol [Suppl] (Stockh) 362:123

345. Aspelin P, Titel P, Almen T (1980) Effect of iohexol on red cell deformability in vitro. Acta Radiol [Suppl] (Stockh) 362:127

346. Andrew E, Shaw D, Sveen K, Holager T, Dahlstrom K (1984) Adverse reactions with iohexol in the vascular field: experiences from clinical trials. Invest Radiol 19:S143–144

347. Shaw DD, Mayes BA, Barbolt TA, Donikian MR (1984) Responses in cerebrospinal fluid white cell counts and protein concentrations in cynomolgus monkeys after single and repeated intracisternal injection of Omnipaque™. Invest Radiol 19:S136

348. Adams MD, Dean RT, Godat JF, Hoey GB, Hopkins RM, Lin Y, Rizzolo RR, Robbins MS, Valenti AV (1984) Preclinical studies with MP-328: a potential nonionic myelographic and angiourographic contrast agent. Invest Radiol 19:S135–S136

349. Sovak M, Ranganathan R, Lang H, Lasser EC (1978) Concepts in design of improved intravascular contrast agents. Ann Radiol (Paris) 21:283

350. Pfeiffer H, Speck U (1980) US patent no 4,239,747

351. Speck U, Mutzel W, Mannesmann G et al. (1981) Pharmacology of nonionic dimers. Invest Radiol [Suppl] 15:317
352. Sovak M, Ranganathan R (1983) Intermediates and synthesis of 2-amino-2-deoxyte-tritols. US patent no 4,389,526
353. Sovak M, Ranganathan R, Hammer B (1984) Early experience with iotrol, a nonionic isotonic dimer for intrathecal space. Invest Radiol 19:S139–S140
354. Sovak M, Ranganathan R, Haghighi N (1981) New nonionic intravascular contrast media. Presented at AUR, New Orleans, April, 1981. Invest Radiol 16:421
355. Hershkowitz N, Bryan RS (1981) Extra-cellular effects of radiographic contrast agents on rat hippocampus. Invest Radiol 16:393
356. Bryan RN (1984) Neuronal effects of water-soluble contrast agents. Report to Berlex Company, Fort Wayne, NJ. J Neuroradiol
357. Almen T, Golman K, Jacobsen T, Maly P, Olivecrona H, Salvesen S (1984) Testing of new myelographic contrast media in the subarachnoid space of rabbits: effects on animal behavior. Invest Radiol 19:S134–S135
358. Muetzel W, Press W-R, Weinmann H-J (1984) Preclinical experience with iotrol. Invest Radiol 19:S140–S141
359. Sovak M, Kerber CW, Ranganathan R, Bickford RG, Alksne J (1983) Iotrol, a new myelographic agent: 2. Comparative electroencephalographic evaluation by spectrum analysis. AJNR 4:319–322
360. Drayer B, Ross M, Allen S, France R, Bates M (1984) Iotrol myelography: initial clinical trial. Invest Radiol 19:S141

CHAPTER 6

Basic Methods of Investigative Neuroradiology

M. Sovak

A. Introduction

Experimental neuroradiology, like any other investigative radiological field, relies on interdisciplinary improvisation. The purpose of this text is not to review the field, but rather to present a choice of references which can readily be retrieved and which contain applicable methodology to contrast media (CM) research.

Functions of the CNS, due to their extreme complexity, cannot be described in simple terms of mechanistic measurements. Unfortunately, such a lack of methodology is precisely what often causes an a priori acceptance of the idea that nondetectability means nonexistence. When first intrathecal neuroradiographic CM in animals elicited but moderate and controllable seizures and no permanent damage ensued, use of CM in humans was justified. Only then did CM toxicity become apparent, often with catastrophic sequelae. To be reasonably certain that a novel CM has acceptable toxicity, experimental models must be developed which are sensitive and sophisticated enough to resemble the clinical situation.

Unfortunately, most current methods are not sufficiently sensitive to predict with accuracy what the more subtle neurotoxicity symptoms, epileptogenicity, and inflammatory potential of a new drug will be, once injected into a patient. The decision to proceed with the pharmaceutical development of a new CM is still too often based only on determination of systemic toxicity by lethal dose, and organ toxicity by effective dose. On the basis of animal tests, extremely low neurotoxicity was expected for such nonionic agents as metrizamide and iopamidol. Clinical tests found that these media indeed constituted a major improvement over previous compounds since the most severe manifestations of neurotoxicity were absent. On the other hand, the entire spectrum of side effects, euphemistically called "discomfort to the patient" and varying from headache to mental disturbances, could not be predicted at all (these aspects are discussed in more detail in the preceding chapter). In order to develop a better detection and understanding of CM neurotoxicity, methods of advanced neurophysiology and psychophysiology need to be adopted.

B. Anesthesia

The Animal Welfare Act and its amendments in the United States (and corresponding legislation in other countries), as well as ethics and common sense, dictate to a responsible investigator that everything possible should be done to minimize needless pain and discomfort to an experimental animal. To achieve this, general anesthesia is the most readily available, but its use is often research-defeating. Every anesthetic affects some organ system and therefore will interfere with the experiments, especially those aimed at elucidation of a physiological phenomenon rather than those mimicking a clinical situation. There are numerous examples in the literature that amply illustrate the point. For instance, epileptogenicity of metrizamide was suspected from studies in dogs anesthetized with neuroleptic drugs. Yet, epileptogenicity in these experiments was found later to be due mainly to an unexpected synergism of the CM with the anesthetic agent.

Even though it primarily affects the central nervous system, general anesthesia in neurological research has no alternative at present. It is obvious that, more than in any other discipline, the use of chronically instrumented animal models and limited local anethesia should be always considered. When this is not possible, agents causing minimal interference with the experimental protocol should be chosen.

Basic principles of anesthesia are described in more detail elsewhere in this book. In the following, relevant aspects for neuroradiological CM research are considered. References recommended for additional reading are [1–8]. An eminently readable book containing a wealth of concisely presented physiological and pharmacological information was published recently [9]. Should general anesthesia be needed in exotic species, a special review is available [10].

I. Premedication

Major or minor tranquilizers (i.e., benzodiazepines or phenothiazines) generally have no place in neurophysiology. If tachycardia, invariably elicited by barbiturates in all cats, dogs, and swine, has to be counteracted, the premedication agent of choice is morphine, 1–2 mg/kg s.c. 15–30 min before the experiment. Guinea pigs and rats require 2–5 mg/kg [1] while rabbits need a higher dose, 5–10 mg/kg. (Morphine and most of its analogs are extremely potent neural depressants in rats and rabbits, where they probably should be avoided altogether.)

Morphine should be avoided in the entire cat family since it induces a manic excitatory state and sometimes convulsions. If absolutely necessary, the i.m./s.c. dose for felines should not exceed 0.1 mg/kg [8].

Atropine is still the most easily handled anticholinergic drug which can be used in every mammal, with substantial differences among species, however. For dosages, see Chapt. 14.

Diazepam (Valium) is useful for controlling CM-elicited convulsion. Cats, dogs, pigs, primates, and rabbits require 1 mg/kg i.m. or i.v. while rats and guinea pigs need at least 2 mg/kg.

II. Injectable Anesthetics

Ketamine is used for introduction of anesthesia, especially in primates. It is preferably administered with atropine in all species, where it produces a short anesthesia. For rapid introduction, ketamine should be given intramuscularly; the doses vary greatly with different species. In chronically instrumentalized animals, the relative advantage of ketamine is induction of a rapid and short anesthesia for restraint. Ketamine is rapidly catabolized and, in our experience, its effects on the EEG of rats, rabbits, or monkeys vanish 1 h after the injection. It is important to note, however, that ketamine used for long anesthesia in acute experiments may induce myospasms during the waking period. They could easily be mistaken for irritative effects of CM.

Intravenous dosage of ketamine (mg/kg):

Primates	15
Swine	15
Rabbits	40–50
Rats	40–50
Mice	–
Guinea pigs	30
Cats	30

Anesthesia with *barbiturates* is simple to induce and to maintain. Unfortunately, barbiturates have profound effects on cardiovascular parameters as well as electrical and synaptic activity of the central nervous system. Thus, barbiturates can modify or even abolish reflex responses mediated by spinal cord and/or the carotid or cardiac reflexes. Furthermore, these drugs have an atropine effect on the autonomic nervous system. Following i.v. injection in dogs they elicit extreme tachycardia which cannot be stopped once induced, except by pacing; it can be prevented by morphine premedication. That combination, unfortunately, has a depressant effect on the EEG.

Barbiturates change the spectrum of EEG energy and have an antiepileptic effect.

As an alternative, *α-chloralose, alone or in combination with urethane,* can be employed, but only in acute experiments. It induces hemolysis and, because of its low water solubility, large volumes of 1% solution are required. Such volumes may temporarily change the electrolytic balance. α-Chloralose, nevertheless, is a suitable agent in experiments studying effects of CM on the CNS. Chloralose enhances spinal, baro-, and chemoreceptor reflexes and will thus "tilt" the likelihood of detecting irritating effects against the drug tested.

Chloralhydrate, because of its pronounced depressive effect, is not a suitable anesthetic in the field.

Possible alternatives to barbiturates are steroid combinations which, when given i.v., produce short duration anesthesia in rats, cats, pigs, and primates; the effects of alphaxolone-alphadolone on the EEG cardiac rate and output are smaller compared with the barbiturates. This agent is contraindicated in dogs, where it cats as a potent releaser of histamine.

Dosage of alphaxolone-alphadolone acetates (mg/kg) (adapted from [9]):

	i.m.	i.v.
Primates	12–18	6–9
Cats	12	9
Pigs	5	2

Rabbits	6–9
Guinea pigs	10–20
Rats	10–20
Mice	10–20

III. Volatile Anesthetics

Ether. Diethyl ether is an easy compound to use for rapid induction of anesthesia in small rodents, especially rats. A closed jar with a cloth soaked in ether or an improvised "evaporizer" consisting of soaked cotton in a small beaker fitting over the rat's nose is sufficient. Ether is dangerous in rabbits, where an overdose will usually result in suppression of the respiratory center activity. In higher species, ether, as an explosive, is too risky and, in fact, obsolete in view of the availability of other inhalational anesthetics.

Diphenylether, fluoroxine, methoxyfluorane, and *cyclopropane* are all flammable and explosive, and they all affect the brain electrical activity. Methoxyfluorane has the advantage that it can be applied via a nose-fitting funnel or in a jar to small rodents and rabbits; other in this group require a precision vaporizer.

Halothane. Although requiring a precision vaporizer, halothane is not explosive and anesthesia can be rapidly induced. Although the effects of halothane on the EEG are profound, they tend to disappear rapidly.

Electroanesthesia affects CNS electrical activity even after its discontinuation, and thus cannot be recommended for electrophysiological studies of the CNS.

Muscle relaxants should not be used alone to restrain the animal if pain is inflicted during the experiment. None of the muscle relaxants or paralytic drugs have an analgesic effect. Both succinyl choline and gallamine induce changes in the EEG of rabbits and monkeys, but curare (*d*-tubocurarine) does not seem to affect lapine EEG appreciably. *d*-Tubocurarine, however, has an atropine-like effect.

C. Neurovascular Experimental Methods

Methods applicable to the vascular testing of CM neurotoxicity are partly described in other chapters (Chaps. 3, 4, 6, Sect. B). These texts deal with the registration of the cardiovascular parameter changes in the cardiovascular system and the cardiovascular instrumentation. Registration of the electrophysiological activity in conjunction with vascular testing will be described elsewhere. In the following, methods aplicable to studies of CM on blood, CNS circulation, and neural tissue will be considered.

Effects of CM on blood rheology are toxicologically important. The behavior of blood-containing CM can be examined in a microscope flow chamber with a counter-rotating cone and plate fitted to an inverted microscope, preferably in conjunction with interference contrast optics [11]. A method to quantify the red-cell aggregation uses transmission photometry of flowing and rapidly stopped blood in a microscope flow chamber to obtain a so-called syllectograme, based on V/T where V is light transmission and T is time [12]. In vitro measurements of erythrocyte passage through the capillaries can be taken using a transluminated bat wing or hamster pouch [13, 14].

Many CM effects on the vasculature can be studied by measurement of flow dynamics of the *microcirculation* [15]. Blood flow can be determined using on-line photometry, utilizing photomultipliers, phototransistors, and video tubes. Coupled to a televised microscope, these devices (Instruments for Physiology and Medicine, Inc., San Diego, CA) automatically measure the transit time of blood elements in vessels up to 100 μm in diameter. Special correlators permit analysis of the pulsatile blood flow components and determination of the volumatic flow [16]. Although these methods were originally developed to be applied to readily exteritorizable organs (rabbit omentum, hamster cheek pouch, etc.), they were found adaptable to the skin and could therefore conceivably find use in the study of surface circulation of the CNS and its envelopes.

Organ perfusion can also be studied videodensitometrically, using fluoroscopy; the sensitivity of the method is sufficient to depict pulsatile flow in lungs [17] and would be applicable to the evaluation of CNS circulation, especially if assisted by blood-pool CM.

Experiments to study the effects of CM in cerebral angiography must be designed to separate the dynamic from the morphological effects of these drugs. The dynamic effects involve activation of receptors and a follow-up of a cascade or chain reaction in cerebral as well as systemic hemodynamics. The morphological effects include the cerebral microvasculature and, if CM penetrate to the neurons, the infrastructure of the CNS as well. A chronological review of the vascular dynamic studies of CM shows that the list of structures suspected to contain activated receptors grew ever longer; also, the investigative protocols demonstrated the necessity of accounting for feedback systems and autoregulative mechanisms, of both the cerebral and systemic hemodynamics [15–17].

For the assessment of total cerebral hemodynamics, a number of methods are available. In principle, an indicator is injected into the circulation and sampled at the return point. Such a marker can be a dye, isotope, isotope-labeled erythrocyte, or CM delivered only into the cerebral circulation which do not damage the blood-brain barrier. The theoretical background and practical applications of these methods have been reviewed in detail elsewhere [18, 19].

Cerebral blood flow can also be measured using diffusable markers, usually inert gases. The method, based on the well-known Fick principle, originally employed nitrous oxide. Because of the difficulties in measuring nitrous oxide accurately and rapidly, diffusable gaseous isotope techniques were introduced. ^{133}Xe, ^{135}Xe, and even ^{13}N$_2$O have been used to determine regional blood flow. Using multiple detectors placed around the head, it is possible to detect relatively minor and fast changes in the cerebral blood flow. These methods are reviewed in detail in specialized monographs [20, 21].

A noninvasive method, based on cranial *impedance plethysmography*, does not measure the cerebral, but preponderantly the total cranial, circulation [22]. *Light plethysmography* of the supraorbital artery can give some information on the condition of the internal carotid flow with which it is connected via the ophthalmic artery [23, 24]. *Thermography* has been used to measure the temperature changes of the supraorbital cutaneous segment. Change in temperature is proportional to the blood flow but, due to the lag caused by the high skin heat capacitance, the method, although useful in diagnosis of cerebral vascular disease, is not sensitive enough to detect subtle physiological changes [25].

Ultrasonic techniques using the Doppler principle can, by measuring the shift of the echo, determine the velocity of blood flow. Unfortunately, only certain well-exposed vessels are amenable to this investigation [26]. If the average cross-sectional area of the vessel segment measured is determined, for example angiographically, flow can be calculated by multiplying the velocity by the area. An electromagnetic flowmeter using an intravascular transducer and an electromagnetic field generated outside the body has been developed [27].

Assessment of cerebral hemodynamics at microcirculation level requires specialized approaches. These methods should take into consideration certain peculiarities of the brain capillary network. For instance, regional differences in the capillary density are considerable, with the parietal cortex and the thalamic ganglia having over twice the capillary density of the cranial nerve tissue or the white matter. It has also been shown that, in general, the capillary density is proportional to the density of synapses [28]. The subject, together with appropriate methodology, has been comprehensively reviewed elsewhere [29].

The cerebral capillaries contain the blood-brain barrier (BBB), a structure of great interest to CM research. The barrier can be damaged both by chemotoxicity and by hyperosmolality, and in this way is a direct indicator of CM toxicity. Damage to the BBB can be grossly assessed by injecting into the cerebral circulation a suitable marker. Originally, a protein-binding dye, trypan blue, was utilized. It could be detected visually in the brain tissue sliced after the injection [30–39].

Although the trypan-blue method was useful for gross assessment of damage to the BBB, it did not lend itself to quantification or elucidation of the pharmacotoxicological mechanisms. Techniques using either an isotope-containing compound like $^{197}HgAc_2$, an isotope-labeled CM, or a fluorescent tracer, enable the investigator to make some quantification. A combination of ^{32}P autoradiography with fluorescent microscopy and silver staining have been applied to the assessment of the BBB [40].

It is important to ensure that the CM tested is injected into exactly the same anatomical structure and that the blood flow is the same for different injections. This is especially important in smaller species where most of the flow in the common carotid artery enters the external carotid artery branch; ligations and/or supraselective injections are thus necessary.

To study the mechanism of breakage of the BBB is not without problems since to this day it has not fully been elucidated where the site of the BBB actually is. Light microscopy originally gave credence to a widespread belief that the BBB is located in the tight junctions of the capillary endothelium, since dyes with protein-binding capacity, when injected intravascularly, were not seen to transgress into the neurons while polar nonionic compounds and ions of small molecular weight did. Later electron microscopy found that the perineuronal, extracellular space which light microscopy considered empty in fact contains glial structures. This finding forced a revision of the concept confining the BBB solely to the tight junctions. These considerations are very aptly reviewed in a specialized monograph [41].

An excellent method for studying the BBB in conjunction with electron microscopy utilizes a horseradish peroxidase marker. This enzyme with a molecular weight of 40,000, as a result of its enzymatic activity produces a compound which can be intensely stained by osmium tetraoxide [42]. Another suitable marker is colloidal iron which, injected into previously damaged brain capillaries, was found in the astrocytes and in the basement membrane [43]. Another useful tracer is lanthanum hydroxide.

Although electron microscopy has a potential for detecting intracellular iodine stemming from the CM, it is doubtful whether this method is applicable when the quantities of CM leaked from the cerebral circulation into the tissue are very small.

It has been suggested, but not fully substantiated, that the BBB could be damaged by CM via activation of the serum complement system [35].

Interactions of CM with the serum complement system are nevertheless an important segment of CM toxicity [44]. Such interactions can be studied by a variety of basic direct and indirect methods [45]. The basic methodology has been further modified for greater sensitivity [46].

With the decreasing toxicity brought about by new intravascular CM, the sensitivity of toxicological methods must improve. Ultimately, methods for the study of CNS functions will have to be refined and applied to CM research. In this conjunction, an extremely important development is measuring the brain's metabolic activity. Mapping the local cerebral metabolic rate can be achieved by a labeled derivative of glucose 2-[^{14}C]-deoxy-D-glucose (DG), developed by SOKOLOFF et al. [21]. DG competes with glucose for uptake; it is catabolized to DG-6-phosphate (DG-6-P) which remains in the neuron. ^{14}C cannot be detected in vivo, but the ^{18}F derivative of DG can be utilized in positron computed tomography (CT). The method has been successfully applied in humans. A ring of detectors in the coronar plane measures the radiation, and the tomographic image is reconstructed from spacial resolution of the ^{18}F radiation loci, akin to the principles of X-ray CT. Such minute metabolic changes as responses of the visual cortex to optical stimulation can thus be detected [47, 48]. It is entirely possible that with the improvement of detector techniques and of the markers, the method will develop into a far more sensitive way of assessing the functions of the brain than studies of the cerebral blood flow.

An ingenious development which has not been carried further due to technology limitations uses a strong source of magnetic energy applied to the arteries of the cerebral circulation and detectors at the venous side to detect changes in proton state, making it possible to calculate noninvasively cerebral blood flow with reasonable accuracy [49, 50]. The recent dramatic improvements in nuclear magnetic resonance (NMR) technology should justify revival of the method. NMR tomography is currently emerging as an extremely promising method for evaluation of CNS morphology. To derive other pathophysiological information, it may be necessary to introduce specialized CM to be able to visualize the vascular component and/or the metabolic processes. NMR tomograms of the living brain are especially successful because of the high CNS content of lipids known to affect the proton relaxation times considerably. It is possible that specialized NMR imaging techniques alone will be able to depict local changes in vascular perfusion, but an appropriate manipulation of the normal/abnormal tissue contrast by contrast-enhancing agents may also be useful. In this conjunction, NMR contrast-enhancing or contrast-suppressing media affecting the proton behavior in specific physiological compartments should be developed.

In recent years, interventional vascular neuroradiology made sufficient progress to be applied clinically to correct various vascular malformations. The philosophy of this approach, supported by recent advances in imaging, has not yet been fully exploited, and additional research in this area is certainly needed. Cerebral angiography using CM sufficiently nontoxic to permit selective or subselective repeated injections is indispensable for future development of this field.

To test the toxicity of such media even under the most adverse conditions, animal models are needed. An experimental fistula between the common carotid artery and a branch of the external jugular vein and its percutaneous obstruction with cyanoacrylate has been described [51]. A relatively simple surgical technique simulating the human berry aneurysms in the carotid artery was the subject of a separate study [52]. Production of model aneurysms is especially important in view of the known neurosurgical dilemma: unoperated such intracranial aneurysms have a tendency to rupture, while peroperative mortality of emergency craniotomy is high. A technique of artificial percutaneous thrombosis of such aneurysms by injection of an embolizing material has been developed. Originally a needle was stereotactically placed within the aneurysm and a 1-A direct current was applied [53]. The method was further improved upon by introducing surgical adhesives, alone or in combination with a carbonyl iron powder, guided and confined to the aneurysm by a strong external magnetic field [54].

The tissue adhesive (cyanoacrylates) are monomers which polymerize upon contact with the moist tissues. Extensive research of a homologous series of alkyl alphacyanoacrylates resulted in derivatives which present a reasonable compromise between adhesive capabilities and toxicity. The chemistry and use of the tissue adhesives have been extensively reviewed [55]. The subject of interventional techniques in neuroradiology is reviewed elsewhere [56].

In a natural state animal models of atherosclerotic vascular diseases are difficult to find. In most species, cerebral vascular disease is rare. A notable exception is older pigs (8–14 years of age), which develop some sclerosis of aorta; nonthrombotic cerebral infarctions have also been reported [57].

In pigs, natural atherosclerosis predominantly affects the internal carotid arteries and the origins of the middle and anterior cerebral arteries. Also affected are proximal portions of the middle cerebral arteries, the anterior communicating system, the origin of the anterior cerebral and epicallosal arteries, and the origin of the posterior cerebral and posterior communicating arteries. The system of the vertebral and basillary arteries is affected to a lesser degree. No gross atherosclerosis is found in the terminal branches of the cranial arterial beds [58], nor does it appear in the arteries caudal to the rostral border of the pons under natural conditions.

It can therefore be seen that in pigs the sites of predilection are similar to those in the human condition, except for the small cortical infarct typical for humans.

Not unlike humans, cerebral infarctions in pigs result from ischemia caused by atherosclerotic severance of the arterial lumen rather than by thrombosis. Thromboembolic occlusion of the porcine cerebral arteries is seen only rarely, mainly in bacterial endocarditis. Both white and gray matter can be affected.

Systemic atherosclerosis can be experimentally induced in several species by methods reviewed in Chap. 3. Atherosclerosis can be produced in the dog, but only when the thyroid function is suppressed; the cat is extremely resistant to atherosclerosis and the rabbit, where transient ischemia and cholesterol diet easily produced aortic atherosclerosis, does not show severe changes in the cerebral circulation. There are several avian atherosclerosis models. The most easily accessible models of mammalian atherosclerosis of the cerebral vasculature are those with the rabbit and pig, in which severe lesions can be induced by dietary manipulations.

Normotensive *Macaca fascicularis* on a high cholesterol diet does not develop cerebral atheroclerosis; changes are found only at the carotid bifurcation, in the coronary ateries, and the aorta. If hypertension is added to this model by surgically produced coarctation of the thoracic aorta, cerebral atherosclerosis develops rapidly [59].

Cerebral infarction can be produced experimentally in any animal using thin silastic catheters directed by flow (mentioned elsewhere in this chapter), and maneuvered into a terminal branch of the area of interest; one of the cyanoacrylate bond glues is injected and the catheter immediately withdrawn. The extent of infarction can be checked by angiography, or, in order to visualize the thrombus, a mixture of the surgical glue with Pantopaque as a source of radiopacity can be employed [60].

Selective temporary breakdown of the BBB without infarction can be achieved by supraselective catheterization and injection of hypertonic solution of glucose or mannose.

Ulcerations and thromboembolism can be induced by electrocoagulation of the arterial wall by a thin wire passed through a catheter, maneuvered to the chosen site, and by applying a faradic current. This method, originally developed for production of pulmonary emboli, is also applicable to the production of intracranial hemorrhage.

Experimental cerebral vasospasm can be produced with intravenous nitroglycerin [61]. The method of production of *experimental trauma to the spinal cord* was developed both in monkey [62] and dog [63–65].

Infections and tumors in the brain can be produced only by surgical implantation.

D. Experimental Methods for the Subarachnoid Space

1. Choice of Animal

The *choice of animal* for studies of the subarachnoid space (SAS) is dictated by its size. In rats, although it is possible to aspirate CSF from the cisterna magna, the procedure is potentially traumatic. Rats, however, are eminently suitable for inject-and-leave studies; their cisterna magna is easily accessible. Rats are also ideally suited for direct intraventricular injection via an implanted chronic cannula. On the other hand, the aqueducts of rats, hamsters, and guinea pigs are too small to allow free passage of highly viscous CM (over 15–20 cps). The SAS of the lumbar area of cats and rabbits is difficult to enter and chronic or acute catheterization may be necessary via laminectomy from a higher level. In dogs, the SAS can be assessed by a suboccipital or lumbar puncture, but since dogs' posterior lumbar SAS is extremely narrow, a subdural injection and/or damage to the spinal cord is likely. In contrast, the ventral part of the SAS is much wider. The pig has a large posterior lumbar SAS and is thus an excellent animal for lumbar myelography, mimicking the clinical procedure in humans. In small primates (*Macaca mulatta* and *M. fascicularis*), lumbar SAS is small, and chronic catheterization via T12–L1 laminectomy and/or cisternal puncture may be necessary. On the other hand, primates are the only animals whose cauda equina resembles that of the human.

2. Methods of Access to the Subarachnoid Space

Lumbar Puncture. A lumbar puncture at the L2–L4 level in dogs, especially in the smaller species, may result in subdural injection. A method for entering the ventral subarachnoid space at the L4–L6 level through the spinal cord has been reported [66].

In pigs, at the level of L6–S1, the posterior SAS is wide enough to allow injections simulating the procedure used in humans [67].

In small monkeys (3-kg *Macaca*), injection at the L5 level is generally possible, but repeated attempts often result in entering the subdural space. Especially bothersome is when the CM enters both spaces, which is often difficult to discern on the spinal films. When the dose is small, CM can be maneuvered into the head. With the animal inverted, failure of CM to spread beyond the tentorial level and/ or a "beak" sign at the posterior part of the sella (Fig. 1) are indicative of a subdural injection.

In larger *Macacas* or baboons, even repeated lumbar injections are easily carried out. Small species, rabbits, rats, cats, etc., do not lend themselves to the lumbar approach – for the risk of trauma is too high.

Suboccipital puncture can be performed in practically any species. The technique requires a relatively fine cannula to prevent a meningeal tear, and injection must be made strictly in the midline. In all animals, maximal head flexion with resulting stretching of the nucheal muscles facilitates precise entry into the cisterna magna; the rule is to advance the needle along the occipital bone until resistance is felt at the level of the foramen magnum. When the cannula is minimally advanced at this stage, gentle aspiration should verify the presence of the clear liquor. It is imperative, especially in smaller species, that the aspiration be extremely slow and preferably small (Hamilton) syringes be utilized to prevent sudden decompression of the cisterna magna and resulting damage to the spinal cord.

In nonanesthetized rabbits (over 3 kg, and preferably larger), which can be restrained in rabbit boxes, the cisterna magna can be punctured with the head in the normal "sitting" position.

Suboccipital puncture in every species carries the risk of meningeal tear or inadvertent entry into a venous plexus. If the objective is to study the effect of CM on the leptomeninges, animals which do not show clear liquor should not be in-

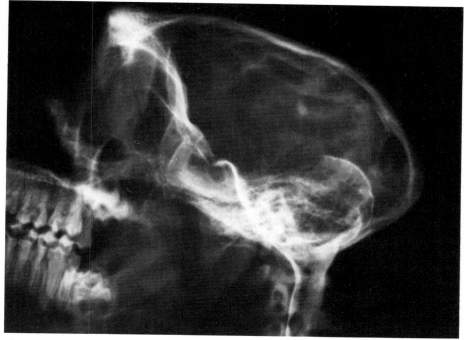

Fig. 1. Subdural injection of a contrast medium in a cynomolgus monkey

cluded in the protocol, since hemorrhage into the CSF is known to potentiate development of arachnoiditis.

Ventricular sampling can be accomplished following the usual clinical procedure (a burr hole in the parietal or frontal bone and a puncture of the lateral and/or the third ventricle). Another possibility is implantation of chronic cannulas. Rats are especially well suited for such chronic implantation. With stereotactic coordinates [68], a cannula is introduced into the lateral ventricle using a stereotactic holder. This is done by a midline incision over the sagittal suture, retraction of the scalp, and removal of the outer lamina of the parietal bone with a 0.5-mm dental drill. The inner lamina is perforated when the special cannula (Plastic Products, Inc.) is driven into the brain using stereotactic coordinates. Bleeding is stopped with wax and the implant is secured by cementing with an acrylic resin onto screws symmetrically inserted into both parietal bones. Since the cannula is supplied with an adapter, it is possible to attach a catheter and use this preparation in nonanesthetized rats for slow infusion; the animals heal in approximately 5 days.

A method of intraventricular CSF sampling in nonanesthetized monkey and dog was described recently [69]. A stereotactic atlas of monkey brain allowing adaptation of the stereotactic coordinates was developed [70]. In monkeys, chronic ventricular CSF sampling can also be accomplished by implanting a 2-mm outside diameter silicone catheter via the foramen magnum and through a dilated foramen of Magendi. The silicone catheter, whose tip is placed into the fourth ventricle, is connected to a subcutaneous Ommaya reservoir [71]. The ventricular landmarks for thalamic stereotaxy in *Macaca* have been reviewed [72]; however, the stereotactic coordinates were subsequently corrected using X-ray ventriculography [73].

A stereotactic method for injection of CM into cat ventricles has been described [74].

Pericerebral injection can be accomplished using a method well established in guinea pigs, which is also aplicable in rabbits and rats. The approach allows injection of CM to the close proximity of the brain cortex and the basal cisterns. A 1-mm opening is made with a dentist's drill off the center of the frontal bone at the level of the foramen supraorbitale. Care is taken not to perforate the dura mater. After stopping the bleeding with wax, a short beveled cannula is inserted into the anterior fossa of the skull base. Inadvertent entry into the venous sinus is a possibility, but the correct technique can be easily learned with the assistance of fluoroscopy. After the injection, the cannula can be retracted and the opening sealed with surgical bone wax [75]. This technique is not applicable in cats, dogs, or primates where the likelihood of entering the frontal venous sinus is high.

An *intrathalamic and/or pericerebral* injection in the rat can be made in lightly anesthetized animals. The technique is based on a peculiarity of the rat's anatomy which makes possible insertion of a small-gauge needle through a fissure in the area behind the zygomatic arch, delineated by the anterior part of the tympanic bulla and the posterior edge of the squamosal bone. The technique was originally described for manual injection [76]. Reproducible injections into the diencephalon can be made with a simple stereotactic apparatus capable of maintaining the given coordinates. Rat brain anatomy has been studied by microangiography and contact radiography [77–81].

Chronic Cannulation of the Spinal Subarachnoid Space. Although silastic catheters are not entirely innocuous and may, especially if rubbing against the leptomeninges, induce chronic inflammatory reaction, in general they tend to remain patent. They can be implanted not only into the cerebral ventricles, but also into the spinal SAS of a number of animals. Using a partial hemilaminectomy, the catheter can be inserted through a minimal incision of the dura and the arachnoid into the spinal SAS and advanced to a desired level, preferably in the ventral SAS. The dura and arachnoides are then sealed around the catheter using fine ophthalmic sutures and/or a tiny droplet of cyanoacrylate surgical glue. The catheter is then connected to a subcutaneously placed Ommaya resevoir [82]. In our experience, daily depression of the Ommaya resevoir to flush the catheter preserves its patency, and the animals can be used on a chronic basis for many months. This preparation, which also can be applied to cats, dogs, or pigs, has the advantage of providing safe access to the CSF (in nonanesthetized animals) without risk of infection or damage by puncture. The method is exceptionally relevant for studies of effects of intrathecal CM on the electrical activity of the brain.

The SAS is lined with sensitive membranes which are of great concern to CM toxicology. On the CNS side, the pia mater, a membrane composed of flat cells, adheres to the nervous tissue from which it is separated by a basement membrane and a layer of astrocytic processes. In the other direction, the subarachnoid space is delimited by the arachnoid membrane, which consists of two to three layers of the flat cells. These cells have a phagocytic capability and readily pick up particulate materials instilled into the CSF. In contradistinction to the pia, the arachnoid remains in close proximity to the dura mater throughout the SAS. There are also fibroblasts and collagen in the leptomeninges. The space between the arachnoid and pia is not hollow, but filled with numerous fine trabeculae which greatly increase the SAS surface area.

In contradistinction to the pia, the arachnoid contains a CSF barrier; therefore, a peroxidase tracer injected into the CSF does not penetrate through the arachnoid [83].

The subarachnoid space is completely filled with CSF formed predominantly in the choroid plexuses of the lateral third and fourth ventricles. The fluid is produced continuously, flowing from the fourth ventricle into the cisterna magna. The total volume of CSF varies from 10% of the brain weight in man and subhuman primates to 20% in lagomorphs and rodents. Especially in rats, the correlation can vary greatly and, therefore, experiments where the CSF volume is an important variable should be based on comparison of the same size rats and/or on an index of cranial cavity size, developed from frontal, posterior, or transverse dimensions.

The production rate of the CSF is 0.36% of the total volume per minute, while in most laboratory animals it varies from 0.4% to 0.6% of the total volume pr minute. The CSF is continuously absorbed by the arachnoid villi and granulations; only some 15% is absorbed by these structures in the spinal canal. With any experimentation with CSF it must be considered that the absorption of CSF is, to a great extent, dependent upon the pressure in the subarachnoid space which normally exceeds that in the veins by about 6 cmH$_2$O. Increase in the pressure can affect the velocity of CM absorption. The flow of CSF is unidirectional, made possible by valves in the villi. Large biomacromolecules can pass through easily. High viscosity, however, impedes the passage.

When jugular veins are compressed, the CSF in the spinal canal is absorbed faster relative to the cranial space due to the increase in driving pressure which increases the elimination of water-soluble CM from the SAS.

For the same reason, CM are also more rapidly eliminated in fully hydrated or overhydrated, rather than dehydrated, animals because dehydration reduces CSF production. It should be noted that hypothermia, alkalosis, acetazolamide, furosemide, oubain, spirolactone, amiloride, amphotericine, and vasopressin reduce the CSF formation substantially [84]. The relation of CSF dynamics and CM toxicity has been reviewed in detail elsewhere [85].

After injection, water-soluble CM show different ratios of blood : SCF, probably because of their different degrees of hydrophilicity 1 h after the injection. The ratio for metrizamide in rabbits is 0.04, while for iothalamate in dogs it is 0.05 [86].

Hydrophilicity does not seem to affect the rate of absorption of compounds from the CSF to the blood. Highly water-soluble CM, ionic or nonionic, have a similar biological half-life in CSF of about 4 h.

Studies involving effects of CM instilled into the SAS on CSF kinetics are best done with radioactively labeled compounds, preferably in nonanesthetized chronically instrumented animals. A rabbit model employing a cannula inserted into the cisterna magna by a suboccipital puncture (25-g Butterfly) was used for infusion of CM; the infusion pressure was controlled with a pressure transducer [87].

The extent to which CM affect the CSF kinetics can be studied by a number of CSF parameters. A multiregional model, helpful for understanding the CSF kinetics, has been developed [88]. It has been shown that not only positive CM but also air pneumoencephalography affects the CSF circulation [89]. The CSF can be sampled as previously mentioned from the cisterna magna of most species and from the lumbar subarachnoid space in dogs and pigs. For chronic sampling, an operatively placed catheter into the ventricle, cisterna magna, or the spinal SAS is necessary [90, 91].

Analysis of CSF for proteins can be a useful toxicological parameter, but increased leukocyte count (above 10 cells/mm^3) was found in rabbits after a simple cisternal puncture alone [92]. This finding may be relevant for studies of experimental arachnoiditis since the same author found that the incidence of histological changes was to some extent dependent upon the control CSF cell count. Increase in leukocyte count following a simple suboccipital puncture has also been reported for dogs [93] and cats [94].

Contrast media injected into CSF affect the blood pressure and heart rate; the CSF pressure is also affected. The CSF pressure can be measured using a venous pressure transducer, preferably of sufficient sensitivity to reflect the dynamic component. The standard water manometers used in clinical practice are not suitable for small animal experimentation. Intracranial CSF pressure can be measured with a microtransducer and a transmitter [95], and the CSF pulsations can also be studied by videodensitometry [96].

Inflammation of the envelopes of the CNS is a major concern when working with CM. In clinical practice, significant arachnoiditis usually develops only after a lag of many months. There is, however, a correlation between the degree of the early irritative effects and the occurrence of chronic late arachnoiditis. The subject has been discussed comprehensively [97]. Methods for arachnoiditis detection have been reviewed; they are based on abnormalities of the CSF and on the radiographic appearance of the envelopes [98]. For experimental arachnoiditis, rats, rabbits, dogs, and monkeys are suitable subjects. A good substrate for the study of arachnoiditis is the rat [99]. Large rats (male/female) of uniform weight (at least 400–500 g), stemming from a controlled pathogen-free source, are anesthetized with i.p. ketamine and their head fixed, half flexed, in a standard stereotactic holder. The neck is shaved and disinfected and through a 27-g cannula up to 100 μl of a CM at clinically useful concentration is injected over 1 min into the cisterna magna. The procedure is repeated for 4 weeks, once a week, prior to histological examination of the meninges away from the neck area. Special care has to be exercised before arachnoiditis in rabbits is attributed to myelography, however. The CNS of the rabbit apparently can harbor latent infections, resulting in leukocyte infiltration of the arachnoides. In fact, in rabbits, injection of almost any CM elicits some histologically detectable arachnoiditis.

In the dog, hyperosmolal solutions of metrizamide injected into the cisterna magna elicit arachnoiditis [100].

No matter which animal or which level of entry is chosen, design of the experiment should imitate the human condition. Thus, the animal should be kept in such a position as to retain the CM in the lumbosacral part of the spinal canal. This applies to dogs, pigs, and monkeys.

The only true models of human lumbar myelography are subhuman primates since they have cauda equina. Consequently, the CM can be injected into the lumbar SAS without risking a trauma. Moreover, the monkey's arachnoidea is a apparently very sensitive: the monomeric nonionic CM produce typical arachnoiditis changes on myelograms repeated 4 weeks after the first injection. In these studies, to determine the degree of chronic arachnoiditis, a repeat myelogram was also carried out at 12 weeks after the first injection of CM. By this method, the arachnoiditis scores were generated from the correlation of the myelographic findings and the histological examination [101, 102].

E. Toxicity Screening of Experimental Compounds

Screening of new compounds should be economical, rapid, and reliable. For evaluation of systemic toxicity, lethal dose determinations in cell cultures (organ or protozoan) and in small rodents are standard, widely accepted procedures which nevertheless do not necessarily reflect neurotoxicity. Different methods are employed by different laboratories. An example of a battery of tests was the subject of a review [103]. Such tests include computerized analysis of the EEG spectrum following cisternography and effective and lethal dose (ED_{50} and LD_{50}) determination by intra- and pericerebral injection in rats under short anesthesia; in nonanesthetized rats intraventricular injection in chronically cannulated animals makes ED_{50} and aversive conditioning, described in more detail below, possible. If the experimental compound passes these tests, experimentation in higher species, and finally in nonhuman primates, is justified [104].

1. Aversion Conditioning

Animal neurotoxicity of CM should be assessed by methods closely resembling clinical application. To this end, relevant methodology must be chosen to be able to predict clinical toxicity accurately. At present, an unequivocally qualified method, or animal model, does not exist. Instead, the decision to proceed with pharmaceutical development is often based only on systemic toxicity, ED_{50}, of neurofunctional deficits and electroneurophysiological and morphological data. Potential epileptogenicity of an intrathecally injected compound can be tested by animal EEG if precautions are taken to eliminate adverse effects of the CSF pressure disturbance. The inflammatory potential of a new compound can be determined by light and electron microscopy of the CNS envelopes. Intracerebral and intracisternal lethal and effective doses assess the "gross" neurotoxicity. Such tests, however, do not necessarily reveal subtle neurotoxicity manifestations encountered in clinical practice. For example, standard animal tests indicated extremely low clinical neurotoxicity of metrizamide, but results of clinical myelo- and cisternography did not confirm this expectation. Metrizamide was found to produce a high incidence of acute side effects, varying from nausea and headache to mental disturbances, including confusional states, amnesia, hallucinations, anxiety, nightmares, etc., described in more detail in Chap. 5. Similarly, animal tests indicated toxicological superiority of metrizamide to iopamidol, but clinical myelography with iopamidol demonstrated adverse effects similar in kind and frequency to those with metrizamide [105]. It is thus apparent that the tests utilized for evaluation of neurotoxicity should be chosen not because of their availability, but rather on the bais of their clinical relevance. The problem is that available electrophysiological and biochemical methodology is not suited for the detection of neurotoxicity manifestations more subtle than, for example, epileptogenicity.

Certain methods of behavioral research present a viable alternative: aversion conditioning has been applied in various species, but it is most conveniently conducted in rats. Rats have the unusual characteristic of avoiding any substance which has elicited malaise during previous exposure. The unusually good survival record of rats is often ascribed to this capability [106–108].

Aversion conditioning is a psychophysiological method previously used to evaluate a variety of pharmacological agents administered orally or intraperitoneally [106, 109–111]. Conditioning can be achieved with degustatory or olfactory stimulus to which the rat is exposed simultaneously with the test substance. The method was successfully applied to the evaluation of intrathecal CM [112]. Briefly, these rats were made thirsty and then offered water mixed with flavors which previously the animals were found to prefer. The rats were then subsequently injected with increasing doses. Later, the rats were offered water flavored with the prepared fragrance and the intake was quantified. From the ratio of the pre- to postinjection intake, a percentage avoidance/preference core was calculated as a measure of conditioning.

Like most psychophysiological methods, aversion conditioning data show extensive variability; consequently, to obtain statistically significant results animal groups of reasonable size must be employed. On the other hand, no other more accurate method is presently available which would be more sensitive. The doses employed are typically eight to ten times lower; thus, neural deficits are typically tested with 300 mg I/kg, while aversion was conditioned with as little as a single dose of 22.5 mg I/kg [112].

2. Electrophysiological Methods

Electrical activity of the brain, which can be recorded either by electroencephalogram (EEG) or electrocorticogram (ECoG), stems preponderantly from the outer layers of the cortex. The recorded potentials are caused by changes in the current flowing between the bodies of the neurons and the dendrites. Such changes are extremely rapid, based on the activity of both excitatory and inhibitory endings on the dendrites. Furthermore, current can flow from one dendrite to another, and the resulting EEG recording thus reflects a tremendously complex summation of hypo- and hyperpolarization within the neural tissue. The physiological basis of EEG is still largely unknown and thus a source of considerable speculation. Although a rather sensitive method for evaluation of neurotoxicity of CM, the EEG only reflects a disturbance without giving a clue to its origin. A number of references are available on the fundamentals of EEG [113–116].

Electrophysiology of the CNS can be studied directly either by recording the electrical activity of the neural tissue or by measuring its reactivity of stimulation. The secondary effects of CNS electrical activity can be measured by registration of electrical muscle activity using standard electromyographic techniques. For this purpose, any good amplifier with two electrodes adapted to cannulas which can be placed intramuscularly will suffice. More sophisticated techniques utilizing fine electrodes to measure firing of single muscle units are also available [117].

A direct measurement of CNS activity involves registration of the electrical activity of single or multiple neurons by the EEG. It has to be recognized that any anesthesia alters normal nervous functions of profoundly that data derived from anesthetized animals must be considered inferior to those obtained from awake animals. The only way to obtain an unadulterated EEG is to implant the electrodes into the skull, preferably without excision of the dura.

To record signals from a single neuron, special microelectrodes which contain a shock-absorber between the electrode and the connector can be utilized. Using micromanipulators, such electrodes can be placed in to the extracellular space to touch a neuron. A neuronal discharge in the cortex is registered by such electrodes in a field up to 100 µm in diameter. To minimize the cortical damage and meningeal reaction, microelectrodes should be sharp and have a gradual taper. The electrodes can be either connected to wires or to a subcutaneously implanted microtransmitter. The development in this area is so rapid that consultation of the latest publications on neurophysiology techniques is recommended.

To record gross neural potentials, electrodes must be placed as close to the cortex as possible. Scalp elektrodes are not suitable for long-term studies in unrestrained animals, mainly because of their vulnerability and the high impedance of the scalp. To implant an EEG electrode, the scalp of anesthetized experimental animals should be retracted off the skull and both laminas of the skull bone carefully perforated with a dental drill. At this point, an electrode consisting of either a silver ball connected to a wire can be placed on the dura, or a stainless, small screw can be set into the bone hole and advanced until it gently touches the dura. Cementing with an acrylic resin is a necessity. A number of specially designed electrodes are available for cerebral stimulation and/or recording from the depths.

The brains of both humans and lower animals generate continuous electric activity. When a large number of neurons fire in unison, regular patterns of frequencies result. Such patterns are remarkably similar in a variety of mammals [108].

A predominant rhythm occurs at frequencies of 8–12 Hz (alpha) as well as extremely slow waves of 2–4 Hz (delta). Like alpha, a fast rhythm of 18–30 Hz (beta) is occasionally recorded from the frontal lobes. It is uncertain whether beta is a harmonic of the alpha rhythm. The hippocampus is a source of a slow rhythm of 4–8 Hz (theta), which normally occurs in mammals.

As mentioned above, the rhythmic patterns result from synchronous firing of certain neurons. Arousal or irritation manifests itself by desynchronization of such patterns. In an experimental EEG, the effect of a drug-eliciting desynchronization cannot therefore be interpreted unequivocally.

Of experimental animals, monkeys have an EEG most similar to the human primate; normal encephalograms of cats, dogs, and pigs, and remarkably, guinea pigs have predictable, steady patterns of neuron firing. In contrast rabbit EEG contains spontaneous bursts of high-voltage fast activity, the so-called spindles which have to be taken into account in analysis of a response to CM. One possibility is to obtain long recordings for a computerized analysis to achieve averaging of the spindles [109, 110].

Desynchronization of the EEG rhythms originates from levels under the midbrain. Under normal circumstances, desynchronization is produced by the sensory input and also by the spontaneous activity of the reticular formation.

On the other hand, excessive *synchronization* can originate either from the cortex, in which case its lateralization can be demonstrated, or from a subcortical pacemaker. A variety of conditions can induce excessive synchronization, which manifests itself by large slow waves. Aneurysms, hypertension, vascular insufficiency, arteriovenous anomalies, and brain tumors all affect the metabolism of the CNS, thus eliciting slow wave activity which is not based on the usual impulse conduction. The exact mechanism of widespread synchronicity elicited by CM is not known, but it can be assumed that it is not related to charge on the molecule since certain nonionic compounds can also induce synchronization. More likely, the chemotoxicity of CM and possibly the hyperosmolality of solutions is responsible for the synchronized patterns. In evaluating the EEG obtained after experimental injection of CM into the SAS, it should be recognized that the potential of the EEG in assessing mental and emotional states has been greatly exaggerated and in applied pharmacology can serve only as a detector of gross disturbances. No correlation between temporary slow-wave activity and postmyelogram headache has been found [111].

An extremely important factor in CM neurotoxicity which can be examined by EEG is epileptogenicity, i.e., uncontrolled bursts of multiple neuronal firing. It is not quite certain what produces the massive neuronal discharge leading to convulsions. It can be assumed, however, that a drug changing the electrical environment of the neuron induces a massive depolarization of the neuron membrane potentials which then in turn can activate, by spreading, groups of cells at a fair distance from the original epileptic stimulus. Recognizing that most neurons apparently have the inherent capacity to discharge in a disorderly fashion, epileptogenicity of a CM can be understood as lowering the discharge threshold of the neurons. When certain CM and some other drugs are brought in contact with the brain tissue, they may elicit repetitive EEG spikes representing rapid high-voltage discharge. Such activity does not necessarily have to produce systemic convulsions.

The EEG picture of a seizure proceeds along fairly typical lines. Depending upon the compound and dose, low-voltage fast activity first, followed by an amplitude increase and generalized high-voltage spikes; due to the myoclonic activity at this point, the myogenic artifacts in EEG prevail. As the seizure progresses, the frequency of spikes usually decreases and high-voltage slow waves appear. Typically, after the seizure the overall electrical activity amplitude diminishes or almost disappears while only extremely slow frequencies prevail.

As mentioned above, registration of a meaningful encephalogram for studying CM effects should be done only with nonanesthetized experimental animals. Every anesthesia has profound effects on the EEG; even small doses of barbiturates affect the EEG profoundly. Amobarbital, pentobarbital, secobarbital, and thiopental all increase the beta rhythm, while phenobarbital depresses the alpha rhythm. Morphine and its synthetic analogs have a general effect of increasing the synchronization. Interestingly, chloralhydrate does not seems to alter the EEG pattern of normal sleep [118]. Phenothiazine derivatives in dog, man, and guinea pig have been shown to lower the threshold of epileptic firing for metrizamide (see Chap. 5).

A number of methods utilize unanesthetized animals. For example, in guinea pigs, a small opening is made in the frontal bone; CM is injected into the anterior fossa of the skull base; and the EEG is recorded from the frontal, parietal, and parietal/occipital scalp regions bilaterally [76]. In rabbits, it is possible to establish the instrumentation by administering a short-acting barbiturate followed by *d*-tubocurarine and assisted respiration and to record the EEG only after the effects of the anesthetic have disappeared. In this model, taking advantage of the anesthesia, at least three electrodes can be placed bilaterally into the outer lamina of the parietal and/or occipital bones [103]. Studies of short-acting myorelaxants were found to affect the EEG while *d*-tubocurarine produced appreciable changes.

Although it is possible to inject CM into the cisterna magna of nonanesthetized, restrained rabbits [88], a recording of scalp EEG is, in our experience, extremely difficult due to the myogenic artifacts. Gross epileptogenicity of CM was nevertheless assessed in anesthetized rabbits [119]. Cats are extremely useful for EEG recording in long-term experiments with implanted electrodes, but they do not tolerate restraint, inducing both myogenic and arousal artifacts in their EEGs.

Dogs have an unstable EEG which tends to oscillate rapidly between arousal and suppression; the best experimental animal is the monkey, especially if chronically instrumentalized as described elsewhere in this chapter. Awake monkeys can be trained to accept a temporary restraint either on a cradle or in a primate chair. Following shaving and skin disinfection, scalp intradermal electrodes can be used and up to eight channels recorded from each hemisphere. Unfortunately, while frowning during the procedure, the potently developed frontal muscles of the monkeys induce strong myogenic artifacts which often make use of frontal EEG channels impossible for analysis. We have found that limited infiltration of the scalp with procaine chloride (maximally 1 ml/kg 1% solution) tends to remove the frowning and improve the tracing quality. Xylocaine is not suitable in *Macaca* (both *M. mulatta* and *M. fascicularis*) due to the depressant effect on the CNS activity, specifically on the breathing center. In anesthetized animals, the effect of xylocaine can be potentiated by ketamine.

Although it is relatively easy to distinguish between normal EEG patterns and such dramatic changes as epileptic seizures and/or major frequency shifts, minor changes are more difficult to quantitate by visual estimation. There are essentially two aspects of EEG changes which are experimentally relevant: the average amplitude and the frequency spectrum. Average amplitude can be obtained using a simple electronic circuit integrating the area under the EEG curve [120]. With the advance of electronics, EEG spectrum analysis has become available also [121–123].

Spectrum analysis is a more sensitive method of evaluating the EEG, with frequency shifts brought in corelation with a drug dose. For this, complicated computers and programs have to be utilized. Usually, the spectrum for 0–20 Hz is arbitrarily divided into a number of bins which then store the EEG power, in arbitrary power units. This is accomplished by computerized Fourier analysis. The data can be treated by smoothing and hidden line suppression and displayed by various graphic forms. Methods of quantification of the power spectrum of the EEG useful in the evaluation of CM toxicity are available [103, 104]. Effects of CM on neural tissue can be assessed by changes of CNS responsiveness to electrical stimulation. Stimulation means inducing action potentials in neurons by applying external electrical current. The method has been well established in the peripheral nerves, where it is understood that an action potential fires when the transmembrane potential is decreased, i.e., when the cell is depolarized. Passive depolarization can result from resistive or capacitive current passing through the cell membrane. In the peripheral nerve, nerve fibers can be isolated and electrodes placed underneath. In the brain, because of the high current density, it is impossible to stimulate single neurons but it is possible to stimulate certain areas.

The effect of peripheral sensory stimuli on the cerebral electroactivity are too minute to be readily detectable by EEG tracing. Special averagers or digital computers can be used to store the responses, sum, and then average them up at the end of a series of stimuli. Because each stimulus also activates the computer, a summation finally eliminates the noise of the other EEG activity. For a review of this approach, see ref. [124]. Because the pattern of a normal evoked response is remarkably stable and reproducible, it is a valuable method for assessing neurotoxicity. The essence of this approach is to determine effects of the drug on the normal conduction of neural impulses, both in the afferent neuronal pathways and on the synaptic relays. Thus, prolonged *latency* of the response represents a slowed-down conduction of the impulse; while a *decreased amplitude* of the response signals a reduction of the afferent volley arriving to the cortex.

Visual, audio, and somatosensory potentials can be used to that end. A method for registration of somatosensory evoked potentials after instillation of CM into the dural sac to evaluate CM neurotoxicity in cats is available [125]. In essence, a peripheral nerve was stimulated, and the EEG was registered and processed using an averager.

The altered conductivity can be also studied by a reversed technique. Thus, a method of evoking corticospinal responses for evaluation of CM in cats is available. The cerebral cortex over the cruciate sulcus was unilaterally stimulated with rectangular waves of 10 mA at a frequency of 1 Hz. The evoked response was recorded from the opposite sciatic nerve, and the threshold level and amplitude changes were recorded [126]. This study suggested depression due to hypertonicity and excitation due to chemotoxicity.

Another approach to studying the effects of CM on the neural conductivity is examination of differences in the H-reflex. The H-reflex measures the excitability of the motor neurons of the anterior horns of the spinal cord. Two stimulating needle electrodes are placed 1–1 ½ cm apart adjacent to a peripheral nerve, and the stimulation current is adjusted to a level at which the H-reflex can be recorded from the ipsilateral muscle distal to the stimulating electrode with a different recording electrode placed into the periphery of the same extremity. To obtain statistically significant data, a number of responses are averaged using one of the standard computerized averagers available in every neurophysiology laboratory (averagers of cerebral evoked potentials are also applicable). The method was applied in cats to evaluate CM; toxicity was explained by adverse effects on the function of the large (group I) root fibers [127].

A variation of this technique, aimed at investigating the effect of CM on the monosynaptic reflex, measured the response amplitude and action potentials in the intradural nerve roots [128].

The physiological stimulators used in these studies are pulse generators which allow accurate determination of the output and frequency. They should be equipped with a stimulus isolation unit to eliminate shock artifacts when early responses are recorded. Either isolation transformers or the so-called RF isolators (Schmitt isolators) can be used.

The stimulus parameters can be expressed as strength of the stimulating current or as the time elapsed on a strength-duration curve. Thus, the smallest current evoking the response is rheobase, while twice rheobase on the strength-duration curve is known as chronaxie. The shorter the pulse, the more current is needed to evoke a response. It is important to realize that the intensity of stimulating current varies from one tissue to the other, mainly because of shorting. As a stimulus, a sinusoidal current at frequencies of 50–200 Hz with threshold responses occurring at 0.1 mA can be used, but rectangular pulses are also adequate.

References

1. Barnes CD, Etherington LG (1973) Drug dosage in laboratory animals, a handbook. University of California Press, Berkeley
2. Goodman LS, Gilman A (1980) Pharmacological basis of therapeutics. MacMillan, New York
3. Committee for the preparation of a technical guide for comparative anesthesia in laboratory animals (1969) Comparative anesthesia in laboratory animals. Fed Proc 28:1369–1586
4. Lumb WV, Jones EW (1973) Veterinary anesthesia. Lea and Febiger, Philadelphia
5. Melby EC, Altman NH (eds) (1974) Handbook laboratory animal science. CRC Press, Cleveland
6. Russell RJ, David TD (1977) A guide to the type and amount of tranquilizers, anesthetics, analgesics, and euthanasia agents for laboratory animals. Naval Medical Research Institute, Bethesda, p 36
7. Soma LR (ed) (1971) Textbook of veterinary anesthesia. Williams and Wilkins, Baltimore
8. Jones LM, Booth NH, McDonald LE (eds) (1977) Veterinary pharmacology and therapeutics, 4th edn. Iowa State Univ Press, Ames, Iowa
9. Green CJ (1979) Animal anesthesia. Laboratory animals, London
10. Stunkard JA, Miller JC (1974) An outline guide to general anesthesia in exotic species. Vet Med/Small Anim Clin 69:1181–1186
11. Schmid-Schöenbein H, Gosen J, Heinich L, Klose HJ, Volger E (1972) A counter-rotating "rheoscope chamber" for the study of the microrheology of blood-cell aggregation by microscopic observation and microphotometry. Microvasc Res 6:366–376

12. Aspelin P, Schmid-Schönbein H (1978) Effect of ionic and non-ionic contrast media on red cell aggregation in vitro. Acta Radiol [Diagn] (Suppl) 19:766–784
13. Almen T, Wiedemann MP (1968) Application of CM to the external surface of the vasculature. Invest Radiol 3:151–158
14. Wiedemann MP (1963) Passage of the arteriovenous pathways. In: Hamiton FW, Dow P (eds) Am Physiol Soc, pp 891–933 (Handbook of physiology, sect 2, vol 2)
15. Endrich B, Ring J, Intaglietta M (1979) Effects of radiopaque contrast media on the microcirculation of the rabbit omentum. Radiology 132:331–339
16. Intaglietta M (1977) Measurement of flow dynamics in the microcirculation. Med Instrum 11:149–152
17. Silverman NR, Intaglietta M, Simon AL, Tompkins WR (1972) Determination of pulmonary pulsatile perfusion by fluoroscopic videa densitometry. J Appl Physiol 33:147
18. Hilal SK (1974) Cerebral hemodynamics assessed by angiography. In Newton TH, Potts DG (eds) Radiology of the skull and brain, vol 2, angiography. Mosby, St Louis, p 1049
19. Fischer HW (1974) Contrast media. In: Newton TH, Potts DG (eds) Radiology of the skull and brain, vol 2, angiography. Mosby, St Louis, p 893
20. Ingvar DHI, Lassen NA (eds) (1977) Cerebral function, metabolism and circulation. Munksgaard, Copenhagen
21. Sokoloff L (1961) Local cerebral circulation at rest and during altered cerebral activity induced by anesthesia or visual stimulation. In: Kety SS, Elkes J (eds) Regional neurochemistry; the regional chemistry, physiology and pharmacology of the nervous system. Pergamon, New York, pp 107–117
22. Seipel JH (1967) The biophysical basis and clinical applications of rheoencephalography. Neurology 17:443–451
23. Fuster B (1977) Carotid cutaneous photoplethysmography test: a method to explore the carotid and vertebral basilar systems. Clin Electroencephalogr 8:6–26
24. Barns RW, Clayton JM, Bone GE, Slaymaker EE, Reinerton J (1977) Supraorbital photoplethysmography, simple accurate screening of carotid occlusive disease. J Surg Res 22:319–327
25. Wood EH (1965) Thermography in the diagnosis of cerebravascular disease. Radiology 85:270–283
26. Brisman R, Hilal SK, Tenner M (1972) Doppler ultrasound measurements of superior sagittal sinus blood velocity. J Neurosurg 37:312–315
27. Consigny PM, Baltaxe HA (1980) Measurements of blood vessel diameter and blood flow with an intravascular electromagnetic flow meter. Invest Radiol 15:396
28. Wolff HG (1938) The cerebral blood vessels – anatomical principles. Res Publ Assoc Res Nerv Ment Dis 18:29–68
29. Purves MJ (1972) The physiology of the cerebral circulation. Cambridge University Press, Cambridge
30. Broman T, Olsson O (1948) The tolerance of cerebral blood-vessels to a contrast medium of the diodrast group. Acta Radiol 30:326–342
31. Broman T, Olsson O (1956) Technique for pharmacodynamic investigation of contrast media for cerebral angiography. Effect on blood-brain barrier in animal experiments. Acta Radiol 45:96–100
32. Steinwall O (1958) An improved technique for testing the effect of contrast media and other substances on the blood-brain barrier. Acta Radiol 49:281–284
33. Fischer HW, Eckstein JW (1961) Comparison of cerebral angiographic media by their circulatory effects; an experimental study. Am J Roentgenol 86:166–177
34. Lundervold A, Engeset A (1966) Polygraphic recordings during cerebral angiography. Acta Radiol [Diagn] (Stockh) 5:368–380
35. Gonsette RE (1978) Animal experiments and clinical experiences in cerebral angiography with a new contrast agent (ioxaglic acid) with a low hyperosmolality. Ann Radiol (Paris) 21:271–273
36. Olin T, Redman H (1967) Experimental evaluation of contrast media in the vertebral circulation. Acta Radiol [Suppl] (Stockh) 270:216–227

37. Tornell G (1968) Bradycardial reactions in cerebral angiography induced by sodium and methyl-glucamine iothalamate (Conray). Acta Radiol [Diagn] (Stockh) 7:489–501
38. Jeppsson PG, Olin T (1970) Neurotoxicity of roentgen contrast media. Study of the blood-brain barrier in the rabbit following selective injection of contrast media into the internal carotid artery. Acta Radiol [Diagn] (Stockh) 10:17–34
39. Gonsette RE (1973) Biologic tolerance of the central nervous system to metrizamide. Acta Radiol [Suppl] (Stockh) 335:25–44
40. Gonsette RE, Liesenborgh L (1980) New contrast media in cerebral angiography: animal experiments and preliminary clinical studies. Invest Radiol 15:S270–S274
41. Bradbury M (1979) The concept of a blood-brain barrier. Wiley, Chichester
42. Graham RC, Karnovsky MJ (1966) The early stages of absorption of injected horseradish peroxidase in the proximal tubules of mouse kidney: ultrastructural chemistry by a new technique. J Histochem Cytochem 14:291–302
43. Clawson CC, Hartman JF, Vernier RL (1966) Electron microscopy of the effect of gram-negative endotoxin on the blood-brain barrier. J Comp Neurol 127:183–198
44. Lasser EC, Kolb WP, Lang JH (1974) Contrast media activation of serum complement system. (Letter) Invest Radiol 9:4A–6AS
45. Mayer MM (1971) Complement and complement fixation. In: Kabat EA, Mayer MM (eds) Experimental immunochemistry, 2nd edn. Thomas, Springfield, pp 133–240
46. Lasser EC, Lang JH, Sovak M, Kolb W, Lyon S, Hamblin AE (1977) Steroids: theoretical and experimental basis for utilization in prevention of contrast media reactions. Radiology 125:1–9
47. Phelps ME, Hoffman EJ, Huang SC, Kuhl DE (1978) ECAT: a new computerized tomographic imaging system for positron-emitting radiopharmaceuticals. J Nucl Med 19:635–647
48. Phelps ME, Kuhl DE, Mazziotta JC (1981) Metabolic mapping of the brain's response to visual stimulation: studies in humans. Science 211:1445–1558
49. Singer JR (1959) Blood flow rates by nuclear magnetic resonance measurements. Science 130:1652–1653
50. Singer JR (1960) Flow rates using nuclear or electron paramagnetic resonance techniques with applications to biological and chemical processes. J Appl Physics 31:125–127
51. Kerber CW (1975) Experimental arteriovenous fistula. Creation and percutaneous catheter obstruction with cyanoacrylate. Invest Radiol 10:10–17
52. Kerber CW, Buschman RW (1977) Experimental carotid aneurysms: simple surgical production and radiographic evaluation. Invest Radiol 12:154–157
53. Sawyer PN (1964) Bioelectric phenomena and intravascular thrombosis: the first 12 years. Surgery 56:1020–1026
54. Alksne JF, Smith RW (1977) Iron-acrylic compound for stereotaxic aneurysm thrombosis. J Neurosurg 47:137–141
55. Matsumoto R (1972) Tissue adhesives in surgery. Medical Examination Publishing Company, Flushing
56. Dubois PJ, Kerber CW, Heinz ER (1979) Interventional techniques in neuroradiology. Radiol Clin North Am 17:515–542
57. Luginbuhl H (1966) Comparative aspects of cerebral vascular anatomy and pathology in different species. In: Cerebral vascular diseases. Transactions of the conference on cerebral vascular diseases (5th). Grune & Stratton, New York
58. Luginbuhl H, Detweiler DK (1968) Animal models for the study of cerebrovascular disease. In: Proceedings of 1st symposium on animal models for biomedical research. Natl Acad Sciences, Washington DC, pp 35–41
59. Ferris EJ, Prusty S, Hollander W (1978) Radiologic evaluation of cerebrovascular disease in experimental atherosclerosis in a subhuman primate model. Invest Radiol 13:430
60. Cromwell LD, Harris AB (1980) Treatment of cerebral arteriovenous malformations: a combined neurosurgical and neuroradiological approach. J Neurosurg 52:705–708

61. Kistler JP, Lees RS, Candia G, Zervas NT, Crowell RM, Ojemann RG (1979) Intravenous nitroglycerin in experimental cerebral vasospasm. A preliminary report. Stroke 10:26–29
62. Bingham WG, Goldman H, Friedman SJ, Murphy S, Yashon D, Hunt WE (1975) Blood flow in normal and injured monkey spinal cord. J Neurosurg 43:162–171
63. Ducker TB, Salcman M, Perot PL Jr, Ballantine D (1978) Experimental spinal cord trauma. I: Correlation of blood flow, tissue oxygen and neurologic status in the dog. Surg Neurol 10:60–63
64. Ducker TB, Salcman M, Lucas JT, Garrison WB, Perot PL Jr (1976) Experimental spinal cord trauma. II: Blood flow, tissue oxygen, evoked potentials in both paretic and plegic monkeys. Surg Neurol 10:64–70
65. Ducker TB, Salcman M, Daniell HB (1978) Experimental spinal cord trauma. III. therapeutic effect of immobilization and pharmacologic agents. Surg Neurol 10:71–76
66. Funkquist B (1960) Lumbar subarachnoid puncture and injection in the dog. Nord Vet Med 12:805–812
67. Punto L, Suolanen J (1976) Testing of myelographic CM using the pig as an experimental animal. Invest Radiol 11:331–334
68. Konig JRF, Klippel RA (1967) The rat brain: a stereotaxic atlas of the forebrain and lower parts of the brainstem. Kreiger, Huntington
69. Smith AR, Freund H, Rossi-Fanelli F, Berlatzky Y, Fischer JE (1979) Long-term sampling of intraventricular CSF in the non-anesthetized monkey and dog. J Surg Res 26:69–73
70. Snider RS, Lee JC (1961) A stereotaxic atlas of the monkey brain. University of Chicago Press, Chicago
71. Wood JG, Poplack DG, Flor WJ, Gunby EN, Ommaya AK (1977) Chronic ventricular cerebrospinal fluid sampling, drug injections, and pressure monitoring using subcutaneous reservoirs in monkeys. Neurosurgery 1:132–135
72. Percheron G (1975) Ventricular landmarks for thalamic stereotaxy in *Macaca*. J Med Primatol 4:217–244
73. Féger J, Ohye C, Gallouin F, Albe-Fessard D (1975) Stereotaxic technique for stimulation and recording in non-anesthetized monkeys: application to the determination of connections between caudate nucleus and substantia nigra. Adv Neurol 10:35–45
74. Kun M, Alwasiak J, Gronska J (1978) Morphological changes on the CNS after Dimer X ventriculography. Neuroradiology 15:99–106
75. Gonsette RE, Brucher JM (1981) Neurotoxicity of novel water soluble CM for intrathecal application. Invest Radiol [Suppl] 15:S255–S259
76. Valzelli L (1964) A simple method to inject drugs intracerebrally. Med Exp 11:23–26
77. Schumacher M, Doller P, Voigt K (1979) Neuroradiologie der normalen und pathologischen Anatomie des Rattenhirnes. Fortschr Röntgenstr 131:293–299
78. Dor P, Salomon G (1970) The arterioles and capillaries of the brainstem and cerebellum: a microangiographic study. Neuroradiology 1:27–29
79. Levinger IM (1971) The cerebral ventricles of the rat. J Anat 108:447–451
80. Ikada K (1978) Cerebral angiography of the rat: technical note. J Neurosurg 49:319–321
81. Hebel R, Stromberg MW (1977) Anatomy of the laboratory rat. Williams and Wilkins, Baltimore
82. Hilal SK, Dauth GW, Hess KH, Hilman S (1978) Development and evaluation of a new water-soluble iodinated myelographic contrast medium with markedly reduced convulsive effects. Radiology 126:417–422
83. Nabeshima S, Reese TS (1972) Barrier to proteins within the spinal meninges. J Neuropath 31:176–177
84. Plum F, Siesjo BK (1975) Recent advances in CSF physiology. Anesthesiology 42:708–730
85. Potts DG, Gomez DG, Abbott GF (1977) Possible causes of complications of myelography with water-soluble contrast medium. Acta Radiol [Suppl] 355:390–402

86. Golman K, Dahl SG (1973) Absorption of labelled metrizamide, diatrizoate, inulin and water from cerebrospinal fluid to blood. Acta Radiol 335:276–285
87. Golman K, Olivecrona H, Gustafson C, Salvesen S, Almen T, Maly P (1980) Excitation and depression of non-anesthetized rabbits following injection of contrast media into the SAS. Acta Radiol 362:83
88. Partain CL, Wu HP, Staab EV, Johnston RE (1978) A multiregional kinetics model for cerebrospinal fluid. Radiology 127:705–711
89. Kinney AB, Blount M, Donohoe KM (1974) Cerebrospinal fluid circulation and encephalography. Nurs Clin North Am 9:611–621
90. Smith AR, Freund H, Rossi-Fanelli F, Berlatzky Y, Fischer JE (1979) Long-term sampling of intraventricular CSF in the unanesthetized monkey and dog. J Surg Res 26:69–73
91. Schmidt RC (1980) Mental disorders after myelography with metrizamide and other water-soluble contrast media. Neuroradiology 19:153–157
92. Praestholm J (1977) Experimental evaluation of water soluble contrast media for myelography. Neuroradiology 13:25–35
93. Melartin E (1970) Intracisternal toxicity of angiographic contrast media. Thesis, Turku, Finland
94. Oftedal SI (1973) Meningal reactions to water-soluble contrast media in cats. Acta Radiol [Suppl] (Stockh) 335:153–160
95. Lanner G (1977) New methods and findings in the measurement of intracranial pressure. Fortschr Med 95:2565–2569
96. Lane B, Kricheff II (1974) Cerebrospinal fluid pulsations at myelography: a video-densitometric study. Radiology 110:579–587
97. Burton CV (1978) Lumbrosacral arachnoiditis. Spine 3:24–30
98. Summer K, Traugott U (1975) Eosinophil leucocytes in the CSF after myelography. J Neurol 210:127–134
99. Skalpe IO, Torvik A (1975) Toxicity of metrizamide and meglumine iocarmate in the spinal subarachnoid space: an experimental study in rats with special reference to long-term effects. Invest Radiol 10:154–159
100. Bartels JE, Braund KG (1980) Experimental arachnoid fibrosis produced by metrizamide in the dog. Vet Radiol 21:78–81
101. Haughton VM, Ho KC (1981) Arachnoiditis from myelography with iopamidol, metrizamide and iocarmate compared in the animal model. Invest Radiol 15:S267–S274
102. Haughton VM, Ho KC, Larsen SJ, Unger GF, Correa-Paz F (1977) Experimental production of arachnoiditis with water-soluble myelographic media. Radiology 123:681–685
103. Sovak M, Ranganathan R, Johnson M (1980) Spectral analysis of lapine EEG: neurotoxicologic evaluation of new nonionic contrast media. Invest Radiol 15:452–456
104. Sovak M, Kerber CW, Ranganathan R, Bickford RG, Alksne JF (1983) Iotrol, a new myelographic agent: 2. comparative electroencephalographic evaluation by spectrum analysis. AJNR 4:319–322
105. Hammer B, Lackner W (1980) Iopamidol, a new non-ionic hydrosoluble contrast medium for neuroradiology. Neuroradiology 19:119–121
106. Garcia J, Hankins WG, Rusiniak KW (1974) Behavioral regulation of the milieu interne in man and rat. Science 185:824–831
107. Deutsch JA, Davis JK, Cap M (1976) Conditioned taste aversion: oral and postingestinal factors. Behav Biol 18:545–560
108. Revusky SH (1968) Aversion to sucrose produced by contingent X-irradiation; temporal and dosage parameters. J Comp Physiol Psychol 65:17–22
109. Deutsch JA, Hardy WT (1977) Cholecystokinin produces bait shyness in rats. Nature 266:196
110. Nachman M (1970) Learned taste and temperature aversions due to lithium chloride sickness after temporal delays. J Comp Physiol Psychol 73:22–30

111. Dragoin W, McCleary GE, McCleary P (1971) A comparison of two methods of measuring conditioned taste aversions. Behav Res Methods Instr 3:309–310
112. Sovak M, Deutsch JA, Ranganathan R (1982) Evaluation of intrathecal contrast media by aversion conditioning in rats. Invest Radiol 17:101–106
113. Kooi KA, Tucker RP, Marshall RE (1978) Fundamentals of EEG, 2nd edn. Harper and Row, New York
114. Scott E (ed) (1976) Understanding EEG. Druckworth, London
115. Low M (1973) The EEG handbook. Beckman Instruments, Schiller Park
116. Venables PH, Martin I (eds) (1967) Manual of psychophysiological methods. Elsevier/North Holland, Amsterdam
117. Basmajian JV, Kukulka CG, Narayan MG, Takebe K (1975) Biofeedback treatment of footdrop after stroke compared with standard rehabilitation technique: effects on voluntary control and strength. Arch Phys Med Rehab 56:231–236
118. Ellingson RJ, Houfek EE (1952) Seconal and chloralhydrate as sedatives in clinical electroencephalography. Electroencephalogr Clin Neurophysiol 4:93–96
119. Oftedal SI, Kayed K (1976) Epileptogenic effect of water-soluble contrast media; an experimental investigation in rabbits. Acta Radiol [Suppl] (Stockh) 335:45–56
120. Emde JW, Shipton HW (1974) A dual digital integrator for EEG studies. Electroencephalogr Clin Neurophysiol 37:185–187
121. Kellaway PE, Petersen E (eds) (1973) Automation of clinical electroencephalography. Raven Press, New York
122. Rémond AJG (ed) (1972) Handbook of electroencephalography in clinical neurophysiology, vol 4, part B. Elsevier, Amsterdam
123. Bickford RG (1979) Newer methods of recording and analyzing EEG. In: Klass DW, Daly DD (eds) Current practice of clinical electroencephalography. Raven, New York
124. Regan D (1972) Evoked potentials in psychology, sensory physiology and clinical medicine. Chapman and Hall, London
125. Oftedal SI, Sawhney BB (1973) Effects of water soluble contrast media on cortically evoked potentials in the cat. Acta Radiol [Suppl] (Stockh) 335:133–145
126. Hilal SK, Dauth GW, Burger LC, Gilman S (1977) Effect of isotonic contrast agents on spinal reflexes in the cat. Radiology 122:149–155
127. Allen WE, Van-Gilder JC, Collins WF III (1976) Evaluation of the neurotoxicity of water-soluble myelographic contrast agents by electrophysiological monitors. Radiology 118:89–95
128. Harvey JP, Freiberger RH (1965) Myelography with an absorbable agent. J Bone Joint Surg [Am] 47A:397–416

CHAPTER 7

Hepatic Disposition and Elimination of Biliary Contrast Media

J. L. Barnhart

A. Introduction

A variety of iodinated organic compounds are used clinically for oral cholecystography and for intravenous cholangiography. The specific physiologic and biochemical factors responsible for establishing the preference of these contrast media (CM) for hepatic elimination are not well established. Much of the early information concerning these organic compounds used as CM has been published [1]. In addition several more recent review articles have appeared [2–6]. However, during the past few years, a significant amount of new information has been reported about the mechanism of hepatic transport of many of these biliary CM. In addition, strides have been made in our understanding of hepatic and biliary physiology. The purpose of this chapter is to provide a general discussion of hepatic and biliary physiology and to summarize the more recent information concerning the pharmacology and hepatic disposition of biliary CM.

B. Anatomic Considerations

I. Liver Anatomy [7–10]

The liver is the largest of all the organs in the body and has both endocrine and exocrine functions. As an endocrine gland, the liver releases lipids, glucose, proteins, glycoproteins, and lipoproteins into the bloodstream. As a exocrine gland, the liver forms and secretes bile. Bile contains water, electrolytes, bile salts, cholesterol, phospholipids, bilirubin, and a number of drugs and hormones which have been biotransformed by the liver into inactive and, in some cases, active or toxic metabolites. Once formed, bile is delivered into a system of ducts that convey their contents to the small intestine. Before reaching the intestine, bile may be stored and concentrated by the gallbladder.

II. Liver Blood Flow

Special characteristics of the liver vasculature allow the liver access to a wide variety of substances [11]. First, blood is supplied to the liver by both arterial blood and portal venous blood. Most of the blood comes from the portal vein, which drains the digestive tract, pancreas, gallbladder, and spleen; the remaining blood is supplied via the hepatic artery. This dual blood supply provides the liver with two sources of nutrients. The portal vein transports nutrients absorbed in the digestive tract, hormones from the pancreas, and breakdown products of red blood cells from the spleen. On the other hand, the arterial source supplies the liver with oxygenated blood containing hormones from other parts of the body. This dual supply of blood to the liver has a special effect on compounds absorbed from the intestine. For instance, oral CM absorbed from the intestine are delivered to the liver through the portal blood and are exposed to hepatic extraction and elimination before entering the systemic circulation.

Blood flow through the liver is often regional. At any given time blood may be briskly percolating through liver tissue in one region while flow in the adjacent areas is stagnant. Such regional distribution of blood creates regions in which cells differ in their functional state. The sinusoidal capillaries that supply liver cells have an unusually porous lining, which allows blood-borne substances to diffuse readily through the capillaries to the liver-cell surface.

III. Classic Liver Lobule [10–13]

The first impression of the liver is that it is an enormous mass of cells permeated by numerous blood vessels and bile ducts. The liver's organization and function are best understood by dividing it into small repeating units referred to as liver lobules (Fig. 1). The classic liver lobule is polyhedral in shape and consists of interconnecting plates of hepatocytes that radiate toward a central vein located in the middle of the lobule. The classic lobule is bound on the periphery by groups of ducts and vessels, the most prominent of which is the conducting portal vein. Conducting portal veins branch at right angles to form distributing portal veins, which appear to delineate the periphery of the classic liver lobule and follow a path adjacent to that of larger portal vessels. Together, the portal venous blood and the arterial blood supply each lobule and mix upon entering a network of small sinusoidal capillaries within the lobule. Mixed blood, traveling via sinusoids, flows between intersecting plates of liver cells toward the middle of the lobule, where it empties into the central vein. From the central vein, blood flows into tributaries of the hepatic veins, which finally exit the liver to join the inferior vena cava.

IV. Hepatic Cellular Anatomy

Figure 2 shows the overall organization of liver tissue. Liver cells, or hepatocytes, are organized into intersecting plates, usually one cell thick. The intersecting plates are collectively called muralium [8], and the tunnel-like spaces penetrating the muralium are called lacunae. Liver capillaries, known as sinusoids, travel within the lacunae and thus supply surrounding hepatocytes with blood. Figure 3 shows how liver cells fit together to form interconnecting plates. The small bile canaliculi are extracellular channels formed by adjoining hepatocytes; they accumulate the bile secreted into them by the liver cells. The configuration of hepatocytes at any one moment depends largely upon regional blood flow and can be divided into four major shapes: A, octadedron; B, pentahedron; C, decadedron; and D, dodecahedron. The shape of a hepatocyte is determined by its location within the muralium of liver plates [8].

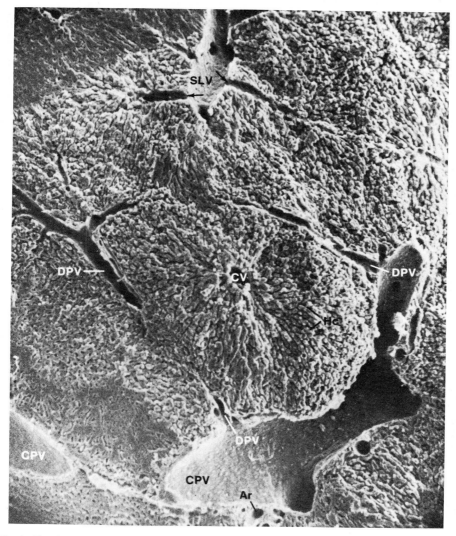

Fig. 1. Classic liver lobule. *Hc*, hepatocytes; *CV*, central vein; *CPV*, conducting portal vein; *DPV*, distributing portal vein; *Ar*, artery; *SLV*, sublobular vein. [7] × 130

The manner in which hepatocytes fit together to form bile canaliculi is shown in Fig. 4 [15, 16]. The bile canaliculi are extracellular channels which are formed between apposing hepatocytes. They are sealed off from the remainder of the extracellular space by tight junctions and are stabilized by desmosomes. Microvilli extend into the lumen of the canaliculus. The morphology of the bile canaliculus is altered during cholestasis and choleresis [16, 17]. A small extracellular space, termed the space of Disse, is present between the hepatocyte surface and the endothelial lining of the sinusoid. Exchange between the hepatocyte surface and

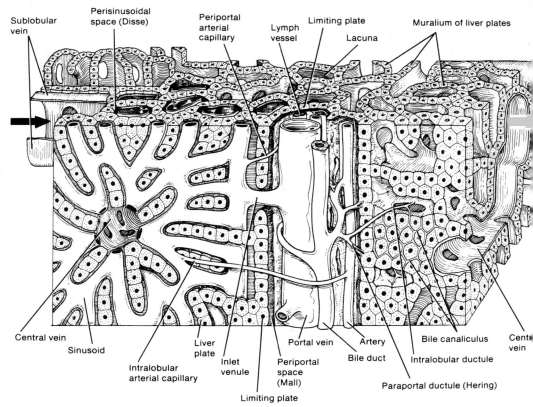

Fig. 2. Overall organization of liver tissue. (Redrawn from ELIAS and SHERRICK [8] by KESSEL and KARDON [7])

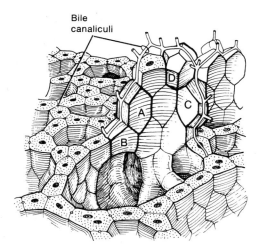

Fig. 3. Hepatocytes fitting together to form interconnecting plates. (Redrawn from ELIAS [14] by KESSEL and KARDON [7])

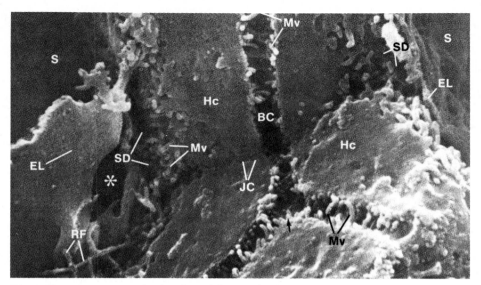

Fig. 4. Hepatocytes organized to form bile canaliculi. *Hc,* hepatocyte; *BC,* bile canaliculi; *JC,* junctional complexes; *Mv,* microvilli; *SD,* space of Disse; *EL,* endothelial lining; *RF,* reticular fibers; *, pore of endothelial lining. [7] × 14,170

blood occurs through the pores via the space of Disse. Under physiologic conditions, the space of Disse is quite small, almost nonexistent [18].

The transmission electron micrograph shown in Fig. 5 reveals some of the morphologic details of a liver parenchymal cell [19–24]. The nucleus (*N*) and the mitochondria (*M*) can be identified bvy their size and general shape. The Golgi complex (*G*) is likewise recognized by a characteristic form. It appears as a compact system of small membraneous sacs and associated small vesicles. This cell component plays an important role in the secretion of materials synthesized by the cell. The basophilic substance of the hepatic cell consists of clusters or stacks of thin membrane-limited vesicles (endoplasmic reticulum, *ER*) with numerous small particles, ribosomes, attached to their surfaces. Ribosomes are made up of RNA and protein and are responsible for the affinity for basic dyes. The ER extends throughout the cytoplasm and is referred to as the rough form of the ER when associated with ribosomes. The microbody (*Mb*) is another cytoplasmic component of the liver cell which is spherical in form and is about 0.5 μm in diameter. Lysomes (*Ly*) are dense bodies which are high in hydrolytic enzymes. The liver cell is also an important storage depot for metabolitites and glycogen. Glycogen deposits (*Gl*) are represented by groups of star-shaped granules. Lipid droplets are also seen occasionally.

The surface of the typical parenchymal cell is exposed to the space of Disse (*) beneath the endothelium (*En*) of the sinusoid (*Sn*) and is covered by numerous microvilli (*Mv*). These microvilli increase the surface area bathed by the fluid content of the sinusoid, which freely passes through the fenestrae in the endothelium. No basement membrane intervenes between the hepatic cell and the sinusoid endothelium, but a few connective tissue fibrils are occacionally found. The facing

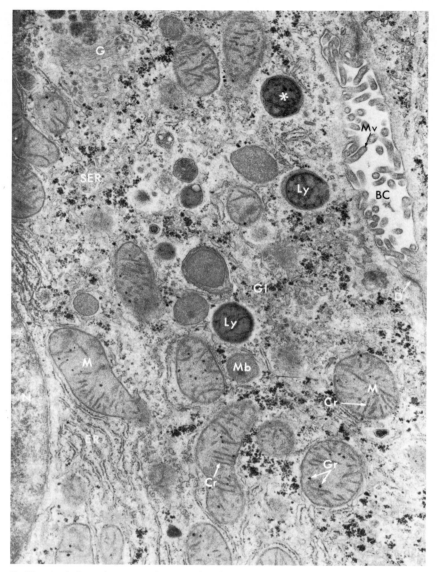

Fig. 5. Transmission electron micrograph of hepatic parenchymal cell. *N*, nucleus; *M*, mitochondria; *G*, Golgi complex; *ER*, endoplasmic reticulum; *SER*, smooth endoplasmic reticulum; *Mb*, microbody; *Ly*, lysosomes; *Gl*, glycogen deposits; ∗, space of Disse; *En*, endothelium; *Mv*, microvilli; *BC*, bile canaliculus; *Gr*, dense granule; *Cr*, cristae. [19] × 30,000

surfaces of adjacent hepatic cells are limited by smooth plasma membranes. These lie close to each other except in the region of the bile canaliculus (*BC*).

The fine structure of a cell or tissue is frequently clarified by the construction of a diagram of the whole or its parts. Such a diagram is given in Fig. 6 and represents a single parenchymal cell of the rat liver [18]. It is surrounded by and is

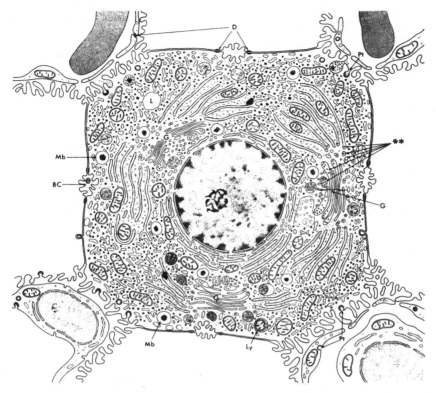

Fig. 6. Hepatocyte. *Mb*, microbodies; *BC*, bile canaliculus; *Ly*, lysosomes; *Pt*, pits or spherical depressions; *G*, Golgi complex; *D*, desmosomes; *L*, lipid granule; ∗∗, small granules showing the mechanisms of protein transport from the endoplasmic reticulum to the Golgi complex. [19]

closely contiguous with four other hepatic cells and four sinusoids or capillaries of the blood supply. The sinusoids are limited by thin endothelial cells with openings as illustrated. Kupffer cells also form part of the sinusoidal lining but are not represented in the diagram. Red blood cells are represented at the *top right* and *left corners* of the diagram; a white cell is on the *lower right*. It should be remembered, however, that diagrams are seldom absolutely correct in all they showm but are valuable primarily as an aid to our conceptual understanding of hepatic structure and how it relates to hepatic function.

V. Gallbladder Anatomy [7, 25]

The gallbladder is a pear-shaped sac located on the inferior surface of the liver. Bile produced by the liver may be shunted to the gallbladder, where it can be stored and concentrated before it is emptied into the duodenal portion of the small intestine. The gallbladder mucosa is folded and consists of a sheet of columnar epithelial cells anchored by a basement membrane to an underlying connec-

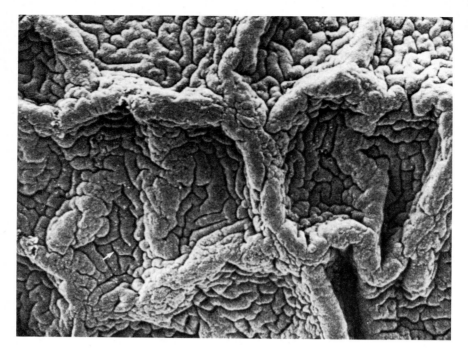

Fig. 7. Topography of the luminal surface of the rabbit gallbladder. [7] × 145

tive tissue layer (Fig. 7) [7]. The connective tissue beneath the epithelium is richly vascularized, because it is here that exchange of materials takes place (Fig. 8). The epithelial cells can transport material from the bile across their surface to underlying blood vessels. Beneath the folded mucosa of the gallbladder lie interlacing sheets of smooth muscle. When stimulated, the muscle sheets within the gallbladder wall contract, emptying bile into a duct system leading to the small intestine.

C. Biliary Physiology

I. Composition of Bile

Bile is a complex aqueous solution which is produced continuously by the liver and which consists of organic and inorganic solutes and water [26]. This body fluid has important digestive functions and also serves as a route for the excretion of a wide variety of endogenous and exogenous compounds. The tonicity of bile remains approximately equal to plasma although the rate of flow, composition, and total solid content vary widely at different times or under different, conditions of collection. There are also species differences in the composition of bile [27–34]. In general, the distribution of cations in bile is roughly similar to that in plasma in that the dominant cation is sodium. The biliary distribution of anions, on the other hand, is often very different from the anion distribution in plasma.

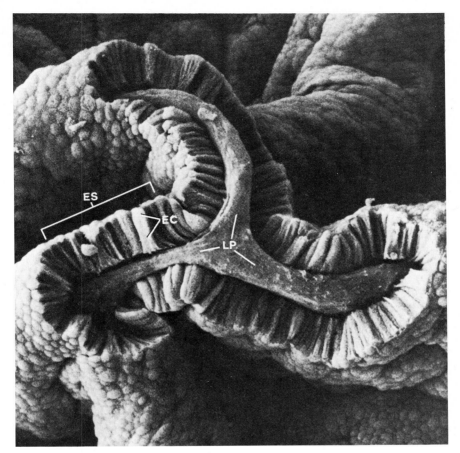

Fig. 8. Relationship of the epithelial sheet in the gallbladder to underlying tissue components. *LP*, lamina propria; *ES*, epithelial sheet; *EC*, epithelial cell. [7] × 695

Chloride concentrations ranging from 30 to 120 mEq/liter and bicarbonate concentrations from 11 to 120 mEq/liter have been reported in hepatic bile. In all mammalian species the naturally occurring bile acids are conjugated with glycine or taurine and have pK values appreciably lower than the lowest physiologic pH [26]. Consequently, these compounds appear in the bile as monovalent anions and usually constitute an appreciable, if not the dominant, fraction of the anions, making up most of the deficit between inorganic cations and anions. The pH of bile may vary from 5.9 to 7.8. Data available on bicarbonate concentration and pH appear to support the view that biliary P_{CO_2} is roughly comparable to plasma P_{CO_2}. The sum of all ions including bile salts is often much higher than total ionic concentration of plasma, despite the fact that bile is virtually an isotonic solution. The apparent discrepancy between ionic concentration and osmotic activity is attributable to the fact that the conjugated bile salt anions form large aggregates or micelles whose osmotic activity is very low [35].

II. Bile Formation

Bile flow can be divided into two types according to the probable anatomic site of entry of water into the biliary tree; that is, the bile canaliculi and the bile ductules [36]. Most of the water and important organic constituents are of canalicular origin arising from the parenchymal cells of the liver and excreted into the bile canaliculi (canalicular bile flow). The bile ducts and dictules add water and inorganic ions (ductular bile flow). Thus, when analyzing bile formation, it is necessary to consider both the canalicular and the ductular contributions to the total flow.

1. Canalicular Bile Flow

When bile salts such as taurocholate are administered intravenously, the rate of bile flow increases in direct linear relation to the amount of taurocholate excreted in bile (Fig. 9). This is a consistent finding in all species in which it has been tested [38]. The mechanism for this bile-salt-associated choleresis is believed to be the osmotic effect of the bile salt [5, 39]. Bile salts are actively transported across the canalicular membrane, a process that is accompanied by the appropriate counter ion to maintain electroneutrality and water flow to maintain bile osmolarity near that of plasma. The choleretic effect of an anion excreted in bile depends on the inherent choleretic properties of the compound and on the tendency of the compound and associated electrolytes to form micelles. Micelles have a negative effect on choleresis, since their formation effectively reduces the number of osmotically active particles in the bile. Thus, micelle-forming compounds are less choleretic than non-micelle-forming ones.

The reason that the choleretic reponses of compounds vary depending on the animal species and the chemical structure of the compound is unknown. The differences, however, are marked. A particularly potent choleretic compound, SC

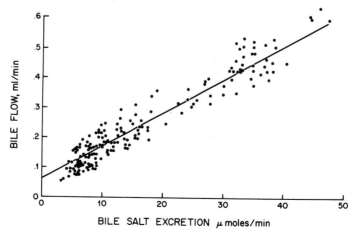

Fig. 9. Effect of bile salt excretion on the rate of bile flow in dogs infused with sodium taurocholate. $y = 0.0112x + 0.06$ ($r = 0.95$, $n = 169$). [37]

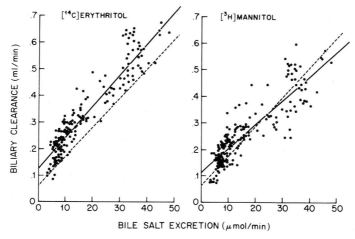

Fig. 10. Relationship between the biliary clearance of [^{14}C]erythritol and [^{3}H]mannitol and bile salt excretion during infusion of sodium taurocholate. *Broken lines* represent the regression line from Fig. 9 which describes the relationship between bile flow and bile salt excretion. *Left*, [^{14}C]erythritol clearance. $y = 0.0118x + 0.126$ ($r = 0.93$, $n = 169$). *Right*, [^{3}H]mannitol clearance. $y = 0.0092x + 0.111$ ($r = 0.88$, $n = 169$). [37]

2644 (beta-(2,4-diamethoxy-5-cyclohexylbenzoyl) propionic acid) is a highly effective choleretic in the dog [40] but does not cause choleresis in rats or guinea pigs [40]. Species differences in the magnitude of basal bile flow and in the choleretic response of bile salts have also been identified [41]. Basal rates of bile flow are variable between species, ranging from a low of 1.2 µl/min per kg for the caiman to a high of 160 µl/min per kg for the guinea pig [42]. Man has a relatively slow rate of 3.6 µl/min per kg [42].

Since canalicular bile is subject to modifications as it flows through the bile ductules and ducts, the rate at which bile emerges from the biliary tree is not necessarily a reliable measure of blow at the canalicular level. Experimentally, canalicular blow can be measured by using small neutral solutes such as erythritol and mannitol. These are low molecular weight compounds containing four and six carbon atoms, respectively, which equilibrate rapidly between plasma and liver-cell water and quickly penetrate the canalicular membrane. Both compounds are thought to be cleared into bile at a rate proportional to the rate of fluid production (Fig. 10). As can be seen, the regression coefficient for mannitol clearance is less than that for erythritol clearance (0.88 and 0.93, respectively). This is probably due to the larger molecular radius of mannitol, which results, at least in the dog, in partial restriction of its entry into bile.

When erythritol or mannitol clearances are used as a measure of canalicular flow and are plotted against bile salt excretion as shown in Fig. 10, extrapolation of this relationship to zero taurocholate excretion suggests that a fraction of canalicular flow occurs in the absence of bile salt excretion. This fraction of canalicular flow is designated the "bile salt-independent fraction" and represents a significant portion of canalicular flow in man [43], rat [32, 44], rabbit [45], hamster [46], as well as dog [47, 48]. A word of caution should be given about the method used to quantitate this fraction of bile flow, however. Recent evidence has raised some question about the generation of this fraction of bile. Data obtained from rats and monkeys indicate that the relationship between bile flow and bile salt excretion is curvilinear [49, 50] and is, therefore, an expression of many different regression lines rather than a single one. This suggests that bile salt-independent bile flow may not be real or that it may be somewhat variable. More information is needed before this can be determined.

The mechanism for the formation of bile salt-independent canalicular bile is believed to be the osmotic effect associated with active electrolyte transport. This is evidenced by several studies which have implicated a major role for sodium transport, as regulated by the enzyme Na^+,K^+-ATPase, in the basic mechanism underlying bile secretion by the hepatocyte. The data suggest that the mechanism for bile formation may be similar to the elaboration of electrolyte and water identified in many secretory epithelia [51–53]. Na^+,K^+-ATPase is found on the cell membrane and is responsible for maintaining low Na and high K concentrations inside the cell. Although the details are not understood completely, the enzyme translocates three sodium ions from the inside to the outside and two potassium ions from the outside to the inside of the cell [53]. The energy for this process is derived from hydrolysis of high-energy ATP molecules. Bile salt-independent canalicular bile flow has been correlated with Na^+,K^+-ATPase activity in membrane fractions isolated from hepatocytes under several experimental conditions [54, 55]. However, it was recently shown that bile salt-independent canalicular bile flow was induced by treatment with spironolactone [56]. In addition, this treatment caused an inhibition of Na^+,K^+-ATPase activity. These findings challenge this putative relationship between bile flow and solute transport by this enzyme.

Another phenomenon concerning the rate of canalicular bile flow is evident from the data shown in Fig. 10. The difference in the rate of bile flow between canalicular bile flow in the dog as determined by erythritol clearance (*solid line*) and the measured bile flow (*dashed line*) represents net ductular reabsorption of canalicular bile. The net reabsorption remains constant over a wide range of bile salt excretion. The magnitude of ductular reabsorption or secretion in species other than the dog is not well documented.

Thus, canalicular bile formation is composed of two portions; namely, a fraction associated with bile salt excretion (regression coefficient) and a fraction independent of bile salt excretion (*y*-axis intercept) (Fig. 10). This canalicular bile flow is modified further by net movements of water and electrolytes during passage through the biliary tree.

2. Ductular Bile Flow

Administration of the intestinal hormone, secretin, elicits a choleretic response in several animal species. This choleresis, however, is quite distinct from canalicular bile flow, because the bile produced is hyperosmotic and has a high concentration of bicarbonate [47, 57]. Clearance of mannitol and erythritol [48, 58] and other evidence [59] suggest that the bile generated by secretin originates in the bile ductules (ductular bile flow).

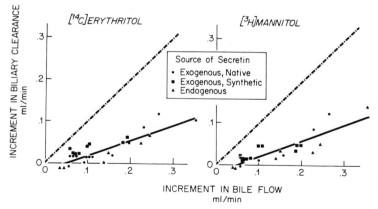

Fig. 11. Relationship between increments in biliary clearances of [^{14}C]erythritol and [^{3}H]mannitol and increment in bile flow induced by secretin. *Broken line* represents a slope of 1. *Left,* increment in [^{14}C]erythritol clearance. $y = 0.37x - 0.014$ ($r = 0.87$). *Right,* increment in [^{3}H]mannitol clearance. $y = 0.405x - 0.018$ ($r = 0.90$). [47]

Clearance studies indicate there is no increase in erythritol clearance into bile during secretin-induced choleresis [48–58]. It is reasoned that failure of erythritol to penetrate the ductular epithelium accounts for the lack of an increase in clearance during secretin-induced choleresis. This concept is not strictly correct, at least in the dog, as is shown in Fig. 11. These data indicate that both erythritol and mannitol do enter bile during secretin choleresis to a limited extent. This observation, originally noted in 1978 [47], has been substantiated by a recent report [60]. Although the inert marker is not completely excluded from bile during secretin choleresis as was previously believed, the concept that secretin acts primarily on the bile ducts remains a valid concept. However, it should be kept in mind that erythritol clearance may underestimate or overestimate canalicular bile flow, depending upon the extent of ductular flow [47]. Despite this limitation, the biliary clearance of erythritol and mannitol continues to be an important tool in differentiating canalicular flow from total bile flow, in much the same way that inulin clearance is used to distinguish glomerular filtration from the final urine flow.

III. Hepatocyte Cytoskeleton and Bile Flow

A possible role of microfilaments and microtubules has been postulated in bile secretion [61]. The role of microfilaments has been studied using cytochalasin, which blocks polymerization of monomeric actin [62], and phalloidin, which induces irreversible polymerization of monomeric actin into microfilaments [63]. Electron microscopy and morphometric analysis showed that phalloidin induced a marked increase in the thickness of the pericanalicular microfilament network with a parallel decrease in bile flow [64]. Phalloidin also decreased bile acid secretion into bile [64].

The role of microtubules in bile formation has been studied with colchicine and vinblastine which interfere with the structure of these organelles. Conflicting evidence has appeared on whether colchicine affects bile flow [65, 66]. However, recent data have indicated that colchicine had no effect on basal bile flow, but bile flow and bile salt excretion induced by a taurocholate load were decreased markedly [64]. Although these studies suggest a possible role of cytoskeletal and contractile proteins in the secretion of bile, these agents (cytochalasin B, colchicine, and phalloidin) may also have effects on the plasma membrane and, therefore, these results should be interpreted with care.

D. Pharmacokinetic Principles

In evaluating the potential of a drug to be used as an oral or intravenous contrast medium, several factors that normally influence drug disposition must be understood. In addition, it is necessary to determine how these factors affect the pharmacokinetic parameters that describe the time course of drug concentration in the body. For CM eliminated by the liver, the factors involved are (a) the rate of liver blood flow, (b) the activity of hepatic removal and excretion (or intrinsic clearance), (c) binding of the CM, and (d) the anatomy of the portal circulation. Quantification of hepatic elimination characteristics in vivo between different animal species or between different compounds has usually been limited to measurement of a plasma elimination half-life or its associated rate constant.

Half-life analysis has the advantages that it is easy to perform, does not require absolute blood concentrations, providing differences between levels at different time point can be measured accurately, and for most drugs is reproducible within the same subject on repeated measurement. The major disadvantage on the two physiologic variables: the volume of distribution (V_d) and clearance (Cl) according to

$$t_{1/2} = V_d \times \frac{0.693}{Cl}. \tag{1}$$

Thus a change in half-life might reflect a change in either parameter. A further consequence of the relationship of half-life and clearance is that a change in hepatic function will result in a reciprocal change in half-life. Thus, by definition, the changes in half-life are nonlinear with respect to function.

Volume of distribution (V_d) is a difficult parameter to deal with because the body seldom conforms to a single homogeneous compartment. In most cases, however, making this assumption does not lead to significant errors. Physiologically, V_d depends on a balance between drug binding in the blood compartment and the rest of the tissues in the body. If plasma binding is reduced, more drug distributes into the tissues and V_d increases.

In recent years, the clearance concept has been developed as an approach to describing hepatic disposition of compounds in terms of the basic drug elimination if the delivery of the compound is not rate limiting [67–69]. Hepatic clearance (Cl_h) is defined as the volume of blood cleared by the liver in unit time and is determined by liver blood flow (Q) and the extraction ratio (E) or efficiency of the liver such that

$$Cl_h = Q \times E. \tag{2}$$

Thus, hepatic clearance is a function of liver blood flow and the ability of the organ to extract the drug as it perfuses through the hepatic capillaries. The latter must be a reflection of the overall rate-limiting processes involved in elimination. In order to overcome the modifying effect of flow upon the removal process, the term total intrinsic clearance (Cl_i) is used to indicate the maximal ability of the liver to remove drug irreversibly by all pathways in the absence of any flow limitations.

Extraction ratio is determined by intrinsic clearance:

$$E = \frac{Cl_i}{Q + Cl_i}.$$

(3)

If the intrinsic clearance is low, then the rate of drug delivery by the liver blood flow is adequate to maintain actual or hepatic clearance at the same level as intrinsic clearance. Therefore, the hepatic clearance of compounds with low intrinsic clearance is independent of the rate of blood flow. This is illustrated in Figs. 12 and 13. However, if the intrinsic clearance is high, liver blood flow becomes rate limiting. For really high intrinsic clearance, E approaches 100% and hepatic clearance becomes equal to and limited by liver blood flow. Thus, the hepatic clearance of compounds with high intrinsic clearance is dependent on the rate of blood flow (Fig. 12, 13). For intermediate conditions, Cl_h is related quantitatively to both intrinsic clearance and liver blood flow.

The preceding relationships have been concerned with total drug concentrations in the blood. However, it is well recognized that many drugs are bound to blood proteins and, therefore, circulate as free and bound moieties. It is often assumed that only the unbound drug is available for extraction, but many examples exist in which the avidity of the hepatic extraction process is sufficiently high

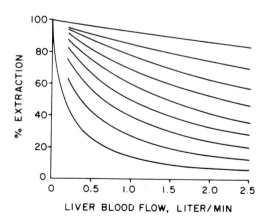

Fig. 12. The relationship between liver blood flow and hepatic extraction for drugs with varying extraction ratios. The individual curves reflect a 10% stepwise change in extraction at a normal flow of 1.5 liters/min, and therefore each is complementary to the equivalent curve in Fig. 13. [67]

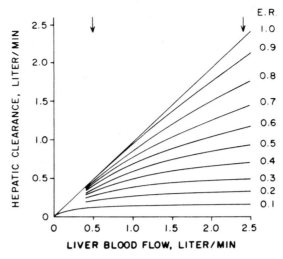

Fig. 13. The relationship between liver blood flow and total hepatic clearance for drugs with varying extraction rato is (*ER*). The *arrows* indicate the normal physiologic range of liver blood flow and the extraction values refer to a normal flow of 1.5 liters/min. [67]

that the drug may be removed from its binding sites during passage through the liver. Modification of Eq. (2) to take the blood binding into account indicates that

$$E = \frac{f_B \times Cl_i}{Q + f_B \times Cl_i}. \tag{4}$$

Two different types of extraction may, therefore, be invoked. Restricted extraction occurs when only the circulating free drug is removed, and nonrestrictive extraction occurs when both free and bound drug can be functionally removed by the liver, i.e., the removal of free drug leads to a dissociation of bound drug during passage through the liver, and some fraction of this released drug is extracted.

The effects of altered binding on the hepatic extraction of drugs with various values of intrinsic free clearance are illustrated in Fig. 14. When Cl_i is very high and Cl_h is dependent on liver blood flow, changes in f_B tend not to influence the hepatic clearance of a compound as the affinity of the compound for the liver far exceeds that for the plasma. This is called nonrestrictive elimination. Conversely, when Cl_i is very low, E is inefficient, and Cl_h is essentially equal to Cl_i and independent of Q. Under these circumstances, binding in blood tends to hinder elimination and Cl_h is proportional to f_B. This situation is called restrictive elimination. Between these extremes, both Q and Cl_i can influence Cl_h.

A brief comment about the oral route of drug administration seems appropriate. When given orally a series of barriers must be overcome in order for the drug to enter the systemic circulation. These include unfavorable gastrointestinal pH and metabolism by gut flora and intestinal mucosa. Even if a drug is fully absorbed into the portal blood, it may be eliminated by the liver before reaching the systemic circuit because of the anatomic arrangement of the portal circulation.

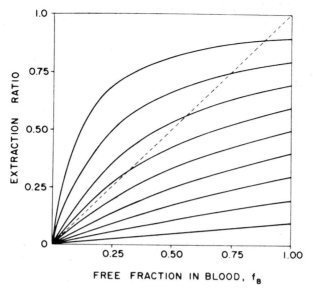

Fig. 14. The relationship according to Eq. (4) between the hepatic extraction ratio and the unbound fraction of drug in the circulating blood (f_B). The *dashed line* indicates when $E = f_B$; below this line extraction is limited to the unbound moiety whereas above the line non-restrictive extraction occurs. The individual curves represent different values of Cl_i/Q corresponding to 10% stepwise changes in extraction when $f_B = 1$. [67]

A compound with a high intrinsic clearance is absorbed from the gut and passes directly to the liver where a high proportion of the drug is extracted. Thus, only a small fraction of the compound administered reaches the systemic circulation and systemic availability is low. This is known as the "first-pass effect."

E. Cholecystographic and Cholangiographic Contrast Media

Successful radiographic visualization of the biliary tree is achieved by taking advantage of the liver's capacity to excrete certain organic compounds into the bile [2, 4]. When such organic compounds are made radiopaque by iodination, they are suitable for use as contrast media for opacification of the biliary tree. HOPPE and ARCHER developed such an organic compound for cholecystography in 1951 by testing a series of aromatic triiodoalkanoic acid derivatives [70]. Their compound (iopanoic acid, Telepaque) had greater efficiency and was far safer than the agents used previously. It has been estimated that more than 40 million doses of iopanoic acid have been administered since 1951 [2]. The basic structure of this molecule has been altered only slightly to produce other compounds which are now also commerically available as cholecystopaques. The primary goal of oral cholecystography is opacification of the gallbladder, which requires not only hepatic excretion, but also concentration of the CM by the gallbladder. In addition, an oral cholecystographic agent must have physicochemical properties that allow adequate absorption from the intestinal tract as well as preferential excretion by the liver into bile.

Compounds used for oral cholecystography are at present of limited value in visualization of the bile ducts. However, in 1953, sodium iodipamide (Biligrafin), a dimer of triiodobenzoic acid, was introduced, which can be administered intravenously and produces radiographic visualization of the common bile duct [71]. In 1955, sodium iodipamide was replaced by the methylglucamine salt (Cholegrafin). Subsequent compounds developed for intravenous cholangiography differ only slightly from iodipamide. These intravenous cholangiographic CM are currently utilized to obtain radiographic opacification of the common bile duct and to determine patency of the cystic duct [6]. Therefore, an intravenous CM must have physicochemical properties that allow intravenous administration and hepatic excretion of the compound in sufficient quantity and concentration to permit direct radiographic visualization of the bile ducts.

Currently, two major classes of compounds are being used as biliary CM: the triiodophenyl alkanoates for oral cholecystography (Table 1, Fig. 15) and the dimers of triiodobenzoic acid for intravenous cholangiography (Table 2, Fig. 16). The CM in both groups are organic anions and were specifically chosen for their high affinity for hepatic clearance. These anions are similar to compounds such as bilirubin, sulfobromophthalein (BSP), indocyanine green (ICG), and rose bengal, which have been used to test hepatic function and to study hepatic physiology. All of these compounds are organic anions that exhibit a high affinity for biliary excretion [72]. Despite the similarities between the CM and these organic anions, little basic biochemical or pharmacologic research was performed using the CM until recently.

I. Physicochemical Properties

There are several fundamental similarities in the chemical structure of the oral cholecystographic agents and the intravenous cholangiographic agents. Both types are aromatic triiodoalkanoic acid derivatives (Figs. 15, 16). The oral cholecystographic agents consist of a singly triiodinated benzene ring with a prosthetic group at the number one position and an amino group on the number three position. The intravenous CM are all dimers of triiodobenzoic acid and differ only in the length and composition of the polymethylene chain that connects the two iodinated benzene rings. The oral and intravenous biliary CM do not contain a prosthetic group on the number five position of the benzene ring. This appears to be an important structural feature that permits predominantly biliary, rather than renal, excretion of the compounds [73].

The oral cholecystographic agents differ from each other in the prosthetic group attached to the benzene ring and/or substitution on the amino group [1]. They are all polar lipids with a balance between hydrophilic and lipophilic groups that allows dissolution in the intestinal lumen, absorption, and hepatic excretion. There are marked differences in the water solubility of the oral cholecystographic agents, which is determined by variations in these two substituted groups [4]. Iopanoic acid is the least water soluble of the available oral cholecystographic agents. Subsequently, sodium tyropanoate (Bilopaque), the sodium and calcium

ble 1. Oral cholecystographic contrast media

mmon name	proprietary name	Manufacturer	Molecular weight (m.w.)		Iodine (%/m.w.)
			Acid form	Salt form	
anoic acid	Telepaque	Winthrop	571		66.7
date, calcium	Oragrafin, calcium	Squibb	598	1,234	63.7
date, sodium	Oragrafin, sodium	Squibb	598	620	63.7
ropanoate, sodium	Bilopaque	Winthrop	641	663	59.4
etamic acid	Cholebrine	Mallinckrodt	614		62.0
ronic acid	Oravue	Squibb	673		56.6
umetic acid		Schering	628		60.6

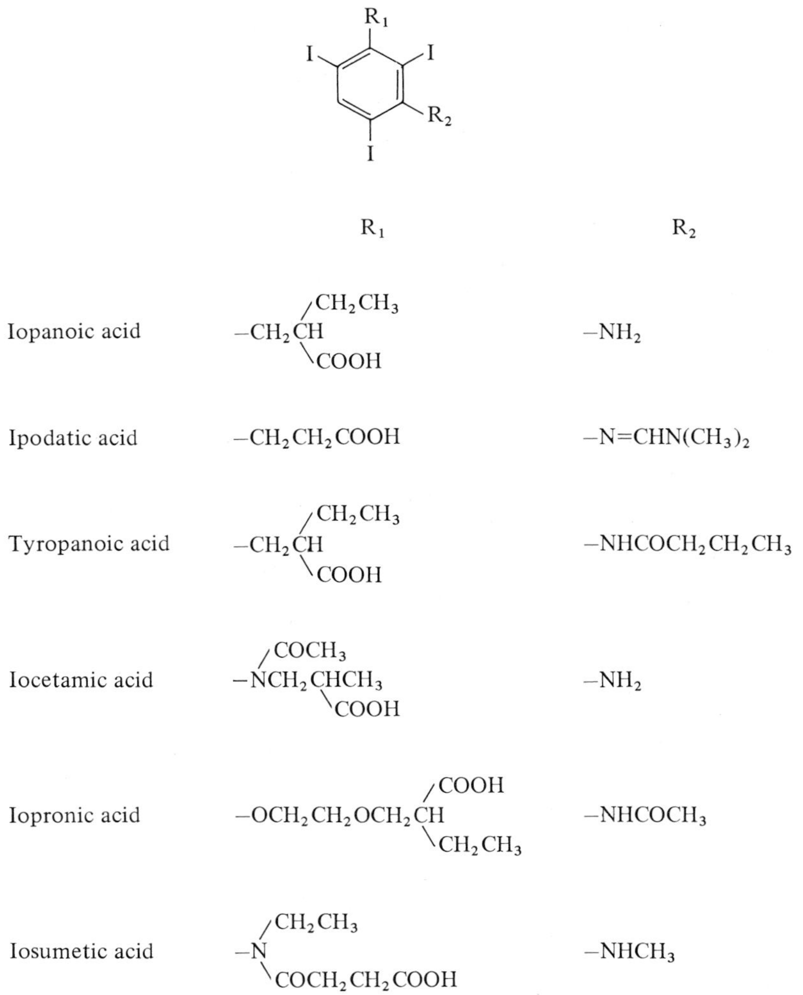

Fig. 15. Chemical formulas of oral cholecystographic contrast media

Table 2. Intravenous cholangiographic media

N-Methylglucamine salt of contrast media	Proprietary name	Manufacturer	Molecular weight(m.w.)		Iodine (%/m
			Acid form	Salt form	
Iodipamide	Cholografin	Squibb	1,140	1,530	66.8
Ioglycamide	Biligram	Schering	1,128	1,518	67.5
Iodoxamate	Cholevue	Winthrop	1,288	1,678	59.1
Iotroxamide		Schering	1,316	1,706	57.9
Iosulamide		Winthrop	1,376	1,764	55.3

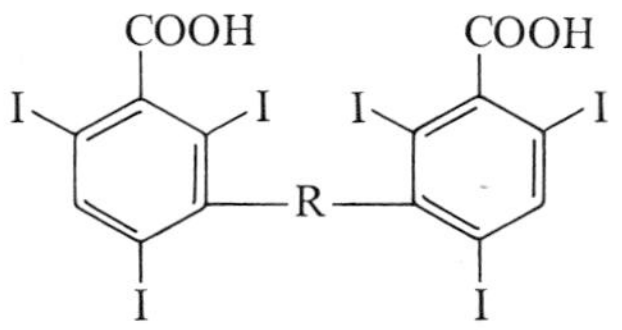

R

Iodipamide $-NHCO(CH_2)_4CONH-$

Ioglycamide $-NHCOCH_2-O-CH_2CONH-$

Iodoxamate $-NHCO(CH_2CH_2O)_4CH_2CH_2CONH-$

Iotroxamide $-NHCO(CH_2OCH_2)_3CONH-$

Iosulamide* $-NHCOCH_2CH_2SO_2CH_2CH_2CONH-$

$$* -N \begin{array}{l} COCH_3 \\ \\ CH_2CH_3 \end{array} \quad \text{at position 5}$$

Fig. 16. Chemical formulas of intravenous cholangiographic contrast media

salts of ipodate (Oragrafin), and iocetamic acid (Cholebrine) have been introduced for clinical use. These compounds are more soluble in water, but less lipid soluble than iopanoic acid [74].

The maximum solubility of several cholecystopaques in 0.15 M phosphate buffer at pH 7.4 and a temperature of 37 °C and their relative polarity between 0.15 M phosphate buffer and benzene was recently reported (Table 3) [74]. Values for relative polarities of these compounds varied in an apparent inverse manner with respect to maximum aqueous solubilities. Iopanoic acid is conjugated with

Table 3. Maximum aqueous solubility and partition ratio for seven cholecystopaques [74, 75]

Cholecystopaque	Maximum aqueous solubility (mM)	Partition ratio (benzene/buffer)
Iopanoic acid	0.61	31.96
Ipodate, calcium	1.87	4.93
Ipodate, sodium	3.75	8.23
Iocetamic acid	8.61	0.14
Iopanoate glucuronide	26.17	
Tyropanoate	26.48	0.49
Iopronic acid	29.84	0.07

Maximum solubility in 0.15 M phosphate buffer at 37 °C and partition ratios between benzene and 0.15 M phosphate buffer at 37 °C

glucuronic acid by the liver to form iopanoate glucuronide. That the conjugated form is more polar than the parent compound is evident by the much higher aqueous solubility of the conjugate (26.2 mM [75] compared with 0.61 mM for iopanoic acid) and by its lower partitioning into organic solvents such as ether, octanol, amyl alcohol, and heptane [76].

II. Intestinal Absorption

Oral cholecystographic CM are absorbed by passive diffusion across the gastrointestinal mucosa [77, 78]. However, in order for intestinal absorption of an oral cholecystographic agent to occur, the CM must first dissolve in the bulk water phase of the gastrointestinal lumen and diffuse across the poorly mixed layer of water (unstirred water layer) between the bulk water phase and the intestinal mucosa [77–79]. Therefore, ultimate absorption requires dissolution of the CM in both water and lipid [79].

Solubility of oral cholecystographic agents in the intestinal lumen is affected by the physical form of the CM, the pH of the intestinal fluid, and the presence of biologic detergents and bile salts [2, 77, 78]. The hydrogen ion concentration of the gastrointestinal lumen profoundly influences the ionization and the solubility of the oral cholecystographic agents [80–82]. These compounds are all weak acids with relatively wide ranges of aqueous solubility at the pH of the proximal small intestine (pH 6.5) [83]. At the pH of the proximal small intestine, iopanoic acid is poorly soluble in aqueous solutions. At pH 7.4, the solubility of tyropanoate is 50-fold greater than that of iopanoic acid. Ipodate and iocetamic acid are also more water soluble than iopanoic acid. Thus, under these limited conditions one might anticipate that the most widely used agent, iopanoic acid, would be so insoluble in the intestine that absorption might not occur.

Fortunately, the aqueous solubility of these polar lipids is also affected by the presence of bile salts in the intestinal lumen (Fig. 17) [80]. Bile salts are excreted by the liver, stored in the gallbladder, and emptied into the intestine in response to the hormone cholecystokinin (stimulated by fat and peptides in the intestinal

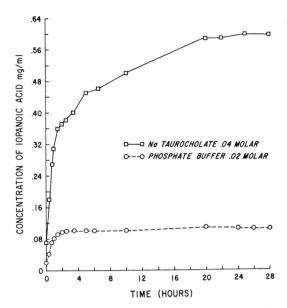

Fig. 17. Results of in vitro experiments comparing the rate of solution of dried iopanoic acid in 0.02 *M* phosphate buffer and in 0.04 *M* sodium taurocholate, pH 6.5. The rate of solution is much greater in the presence of bile salts, and the solubility is significantly higher. [80]

lumen) [83–86]. Bile salts increase the aqueous solubility of compounds like iopanoic acid by forming micelles [84]. Therefore, it appears likely that if bile salts are sequestered in the gallbladder, the aqueous solubility of a compound such as iopanoic acid would be severely limited, absorption would be incomplete, and ultimate radiographic opacification of the gallbladder might be impaired. The results of clinical studies support the thesis that impaired visualization of the gallbladder in normal patients after the first-dose cholecystogram is due at least in part to poor intestinal absorption of iopanoic acid [87].

The rate of permeation across the lipid barrier of the intestinal mucosa also influences the ultimate rate of disappearance of the oral cholecystographic compounds from the intestinal lumen [77–79, 84]. The permeation of a compound across a lipid membrane depends on the relative solubility of the compound in the lipid membrane and in the aqueous milieu in the intestinal lumen, i.e., the degree of partitioning between lipid and aqueous media.

Recent studies have been undertaken to define the specific characteristics of the intestinal mucosa and the properties of the various CM which determine their rates of intestinal absorption. The permeability coefficients varied inversely with the polarity of the compounds (Table 4, Fig. 18 a). However, the incremental changes in the coefficients were considerably less than the corresponding changes observed in the partition ratios. The rates of absorption of the more polar CM (tyropanoate, iopronic acid, and iocetamic acid) were greater than the less polar compounds (iopanoic acid, sodium ipodate, and calcium ipodate) under the con-

Table 4. Maximum rates of intestinal absorption of seven cholecystopaques [74, 75]

Cholecystopaque	Maximum aqueous solubility (mM)	Apparent passive permeability coefficient (μmol/min/loop/mM)	Calculated maximum rate of absorption at maximum aqueous solubility (μmol/min/loop)
Tyropanoate	26.48	0.143	3.79
Iopanoate glucuronide	26.17	0.076	1.98
Iopronic acid	29.84	0.060	1.79
Iocetamic acid	8.61	0.133	1.15
Ipodate, sodium	3.75	0.225	0.84
Ipodate, calcium	1.87	0.115	0.22
Iopanoic acid	0.61	0.264	0.16

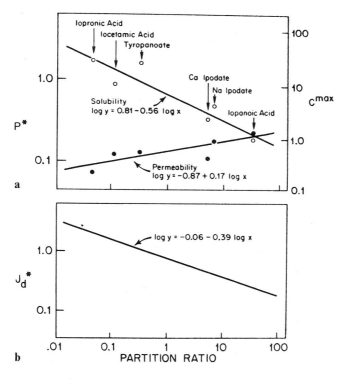

Fig. 18a, b. The effect of the relative polarity of a cholecystopaque on its maximum solubility, its apparent passive permeability coefficient, and its maximum rate of absorption from the gastrointestinal tract. In this diagram, the logarithm of the partition ratio of each cholecystopaque is plotted on the horizontal axis and represents a measure of the relative polarity of that compound. In **a**, the logarithms of the apparent passive permeability coefficients (P^*) and maximal solubility in phosphate buffer (C^{max}) are shown on the *vertical axis*. In **b**, the maximum rate of intestinal absorption (J_d^*) is shown: The values in **b** represent the product obtained when the two curves shown in **a** are multiplied together. [74]

ditions where bile acid micelles are not present and in which the resistance of the unstirred water layer is not rate limiting (Fig. 18 b). This latter condition is necessary because in reality the barrier to intestinal absorption is made up of two separate components, the lipid membranes of the mucosa and the unstirred water layers adjacent to the microvillus border [88–91].

From these data it can be postulated that iopanoic acid is absorbed at approximately one-fourth the rate of tyropanoate during oral cholecystography in fasted patients (large amounts of bile salts sequestered in the gallbladder). Less rapid absorption of iopanoic acid compared with iopronic acid, iocetamic acid, and ipodate can also be predicted in the clinical setting in fasted patients. The difference in the rate of absorption between iopanoic acid and tyropanoate may in part explain failure of the gallbladder to opacify when iopanoic acid was given to fasted normal human volunteers compared with the satisfactory gallbladder visualization obtained when tyropanoate was used [92].

Polar conjugates of compounds which have been excreted into bile are often poorly absorbed from the intestine, and recirculation, if it occurs, involves hydrolysis of the conjugate with subsequent absorption of the aglycone. However, some data suggest that iopanoate glucuronide may undergo enterohepatic recirculation [93, 94]. When iopanoate glucuronide was administered into the duodenum, a significant biliary excretion was found which reached a peak after 4 h [94]. Recent unpublished data confirm the finding of a significant enterohepatic circulation of iopanoate in dogs when administered as iopanoic acid or as iopanoate glucuronide [95]. Additional data have suggested that this recirculation occurred after the glucuronide moiety was hydrolyzed by beta-glucuronidase (produced by intestinal bacteria) in the intestine [94]. This conclusion was based on data showing a four- to fivefold decrease in biliary excretion of iopanoate in dogs whose gut flora was suppressed by antibiotics, neomycin and vancomycin.

However, recent data indicate that iopanoate glucuronide is absorbed more effectively than the parent compound in an isolated perfused intestinal loop of dogs [75]. The maximum aqueous solubility if iopanoate glucuronide is approximately 25 times greater than that of iopanoic acid while the permeability coefficient of iopanoic acid is increased by only a factor of three. This finding of a higher rate of absorption of the conjugated compound is consistent with the finding that the rates of absorption of more polar CM are greater than the less polar compounds [74].

An alternative explanation of the effect of antibiotics on enterohepatic recirculation is that histopathologic changes in the intestine induced by the antibiotic treatment result in decreased absorption [96, 97]. This malabsorption has been observed for a number of compounds after neomycin treatment [98]. In addition, fasting has been found to depress significantly the absorption of polar (salicylate) and nonpolar (antipyrene) drugs [99] and could also affect enterohepatic circulation of CM. The finding of a significant enterohepatic circulation of iopanoic acid [93, 94] and the realization that the intestinal mucosal membrane is more polar than had been assumed originally [90] suggest the need for additional studies into how this phenomenon of recirculation of CM affects opacification of the gallbladder and biliary tree in clinical practice.

III. Transport in Blood

After ingestion, the oral cholecystographic agents diffuse across the intestinal mucosa and enter the portal blood circulation. Studies in animals in which the lymphatic and portal venous concentrations of iopanoic acid were measured after oral administration of the compound reveal that the vast majority of iopanoate is present in the portal blood [2]. The amount of iopanoic acid removed in its first pass through the liver is not known.

Both the oral and the intravenous cholecystographic CM are transported in blood extensively bound to albumin by hydrophobic bonds [73, 100–103]. Iopanoic acid, which contains only one hydrophilic group and is the most hydrophobic of the biliary CM currently being used, is strongly bound to albumin. Albumin binding, therefore, appears to be important in increasing the solubility in plasma of the poorly water-soluble oral cholecystographic compounds.

Iopanoic acid and iophenoxic acid are both triiodophenyl alkanoates which have similar chemical structures. Nevertheless, the biologic half-life of iopanoate is only a few weeks compared with more than 2 years for iophenoxic acid [104]. It has been suggested that this difference in the rate of biliary elimination could be related to a difference in protein binding [105, 106]. However, another investigation indicated that iopanoic acid is more tightly bound than iophenoxic acid [103]. Although relatively few studies have been carried out to characterize these binding phenomena, it is evident that binding significantly influences hepatic events and dynamics [107]. Consequently, more research attention is needed in the area of drug-protein binding. These studies should include the calculation of binding parameters such as tissue binding, the extent of complexation of CM by red cells and blood vessels, the effect of binding on pharmacokinetic models and parameters, identification of protein active sites, and other molecular events associated with binding phenomena.

IV. First-Pass Effect

The liver has the ability to clear substances in one pass through the liver. This phenomenon has been termed the "first-pass effect" or presystemic hepatic elimination. The liver is in a very advantageous position for removing compounds from the blood after absorption by the gastrointestinal tract since this blood passes through the liver before it reaches the general systemic circulation. Thus, the liver presents a substantial fraction of the dose for hepatic elimination and gallbladder sequestration while preventing a sufficient amount of the CM from reaching the systemic circulation.

Clearance from the blood of compounds that have a significant first-pass effect is highly dependent on the liver blood flow [67–69]. Thus, compounds that are highly extracted from the plasma on the first pass through the liver are highly dependent on blood flow. These compounds reach a much lower concentration in the central blood compartment when they are administered orally or in the portal vein than if administered by other routes. No clear studies of the extent of the first-pass effect of oral CM have been published. However, it is evident that substantial blood concentrations of these oral compounds are found in man [108] and in dog [109] after oral administration. It would seem that although the first-pass hepatic clearance of these CM exist to some degree [1–5], it is not as extensive as for other compounds such as propranolol, which is not detectable in blood after administration into the portal vein [110].

V. Hepatic Uptake

Once the oral and intravenous CM enter the portal or central blood circulation, they pass through the hepatic sinusoids, enter the space of Disse, and are taken up by the hepatocytes across the sinusoidal hepatic-cell membrane [2, 6]. The factors that determine the selective hepatic uptake and the biliary excretion of these organic compounds have not been precisely delineated. Binding of the CM to plasma albumin partially limits their distribution to the vascular compartment and probably plays a role in reducing renal excretion by limiting glomerular filtration or tubular secretion. However, the degree of binding to plasma albumin of an organic compound is not necessarily related to the ultimate appearance of that compound in bile [1]. Indeed studies with the intravenous CM iodipamide [111], BSP [112], and bilirubin [113] indicate that albumin binding impedes the hepatic uptake. Studies in patients with hypoalbuminemia secondary to the nephrotic syndrome reveal that BSP clearance is decreased after albumin is administered intravenously [112].

Receptors on the sinusoidal liver-cell membrane or in the cytoplasma may be the factors that determine the preferential hepatic excretion of the biliary CM. Isolated liver-cell membranes have been shown to contain saturable binding sites for a number of other organic anions that are excreted into bile [114]. Unfortunately, with this experimental preparation, it is not possible to separate receptors on the sinusoidal membrane from those on the canalicular membrane. However, recent technical advances have now made it possible to isolate enriched subfractions of the live plasma membrane [115–117].

Pharmacokinetic data obtained with other organic compounds indicate that hepatic uptake is mediated by a rate-limiting active transport process [116–118]. Competition for hepatic uptake may explain the transient hyperbilirubinemia and BSP retention that have been demonstrated in some patients after the administration of iopanoic acid [121]. It may also explain the diminished biliary excretion of iodipamide found in dogs when iopanoic acid and iodipamide are administered together [122].

In general, however, very little is known about the mechanism by which most organic compounds cross the sinusoidal membrane of the hepatocyte. The recent introduction of an improved technique for isolating hepatocytes [123] has provided a valuable model for studying the uptake kinetics of a variety of compounds essentially free of the biliary excretion process. This technique has been used to characterize the hepatic uptake process of bile salts [124–126], BSP [127–129], ouabain [130], steroid hormones [131, 132], and amino acids [133]. Similar experiments have been performed using primary monolayer cultures of isolated rat hepatocytes [134–137]. These studies provide evidence that these compounds cross the hepatic plasma membrane by a carrier-mediated transport process.

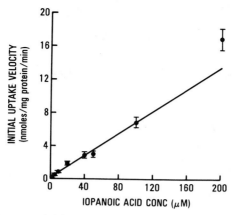

Fig. 19. Relationship between initial uptake velocity and substrate concentration of io-panoate. The initial uptake velocity is directly proportional to iopanoic acid concentrations and is nonsaturable up to 100 μM. The *slope of the line* represents an uptake rate constant of 0.067 nmol/(mg protein·min·μM) (r=0.995). Data obtained at 200 μM were not in-cluded in the calculated slope. [138]

Uptake of iopanoic acid was studied in 3-day primary cultures of rat hepato-cytes isolated by the collagenase perfusion method [123]. The inital uptake veloc-ity was directly proportional to iopanoic acid concentration and was nonsatur-able up to 100 μM (Fig. 19). Uptake was only slightly reduced when the incuba-tion was performed at 4 °C. In addition uptake was independent of sodium con-centration and was not inhibited by taurocholate. The data indicate that hepatic uptake of iopanoic acid occurs by passive diffusion. Bilirubin was also found to enter the isolated hepatocyte by passive diffusion [139]. Recently, however, data from isolate rat liver perfusion suggested that hepatic uptake of BSP and bilirubin is mediated by a liver-cell receptor for albumin [140, 141]. This conflicts with re-sults of previous studies [112, 113, 139]. It is apparent that more data are needed before any general concept of hepatic uptake can be formulated.

VI. Biotransformation

Oral contrast media, which are less soluble in water than the intravenous com-pounds, appear to be converted to more water-soluble conjugates prior to excre-tion in bile [139, 140]. Intravenous CM, however, do not appear to be metabolized [1]. Experimental data from rats, dogs, cats, and humans indicate that iopanoic acid is conjugated with glucuronic acid in the liver [142–144]. Other oral cholecys-topaques such as tyropanoate, ipodate, and iocetamic acid are also thought to be excreted as the glucuronide conjugate [1]. The hepatic intracellular site of glu-curonidation of these compounds has not been identified.

The hepatic biotransformation of the oral CM is thought to be similar to that of the endogenous organic anion, bilirubin, except that bilirubin is excreted pre-dominately as a diglucuronide rather than as a monoglucuronide like iopanoic acid [142, 143]. In addition, it is generally accepted that iopanoic acid, like bilirubin, is conjugated by the action of the microsomal enzyme glucuronyl transferase, which catalyzes the transfer of glucuronic acid. However, based on results from Gunn rats, it is now evident that this assumption was not correct. Gunn rats are a mutant strain of Wistar rat which has a hereditary defect in the enzyme uridine dephosphate (UDP)-glucuronyl transferase, which catalyzes the rate of glucuronidation of bilirubin and other substrates [147, 148]. Bilirubin excretion in the Gunn rat is greatly depressed due to a lack of conjugation of bilirubin to the glucuronide. Unpublished observations indicate that Gunn rats can excrete into bile iopanoic acid which was administered intravenously [149]. The CM in bile of the Gunn rat was identified as the glucuronide conjugate of iopanoic acid.

Recent studies have identified the presence of at least two forms of UDP-glucuronyltransferase in rat liver [150, 151]. One form is inducible by 3-methylcholanthrene and the other by phenobarbital. Indirect evidence indicates that bilirubin [152] and steroid hormones [153] may be glucuronidated by still other froms of the enzyme. Regardless, it is apparent that CM and bilirubin are conjugated by different forms of the UDP-glucuronyltransferase enzyme system.

Biotransformation by the liver of various biliary CM occurs. Using high-performance liquid chromatography (HPLC) and thin-layer chromatography (TLC), the bile of dogs infused with iopanoic acid, iocetamic acid, iopronic acid, and iosumetic acid was analyzed [154]. Only a single compound is detected in bile when iopanoic acid is administered (identified as the glucuronide conjugate). However, the parent compound and two metabolites were found in bile when either iocetamic acid or iopronic acid was infused [154]. Four metabolites and the parent compound were found with iosumetic infusion. In each case the uronic acid concentration present in bile suggests that the major metabolite for each compound is the respective glucuronide conjugate. These data indicate that the triiodophenyl alkanoates are extensively metabolized by the liver. However, the identity of most of the metabolites remains to be determined and, more important, the toxic potential of the metabolites remains to be established.

If the oral cholecystographic compounds are completely conjugated prior to excretion in bile, conjugation may be an important structural requirement for active transport from the liver into bile. This is not the case for BSP, which is excreted in bile in part without prior conjugation with glutathione [152]. Conjugation may be the rate-limiting step in the hepatic excretion of the oral CM, since the glucuronide of iopanoate established a higher maximum rate of biliary excretion than when iopanoic acid is administered [156].

VII. Biliary Excretion

Considerable data have accumulated indicating that excretion in bile of both the oral and intravenous CM is mediated by a carrier-mediated process involving carrier proteins in the liver-cell membrane that become saturated, thereby limiting the maximum rate of excretion of the CM [101, 157–164]. Figure 20 shows such a saturation curve for the biliary excretion of iopanoic acid. The site of the overall rate-limiting transport process for organic compounds has not been delineated, although it is generally believed to be located at the canalicular membrane.

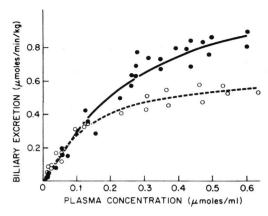

Fig. 20. The relation between the biliary excretion of iopanoic acid and plasma concentration in dogs. A continuous infusion of sodium taurocholate at a rate of 0.5 μmol/min per kilogram (*open circles, dashed line*) and 2.0 μmol/min per kilogram (*closed circles, solid line*). [165]

Among the biliary CM studied, iopanoic acid is unique in that the rate of excretion of bile salts in bile has a profound influence on the rate of biliary excretion of iopanoate [101, 160, 166, 167]. The results of several studies reveal a linear relation between the rate of iopanoate excretion in bile and the rate of bile flow produced by the infusion of the bile salt, taurocholate [166–168]. The calculated enhancement of maximum biliary excretion (*Em*) of iopanoate was 0.89 μmol/μmol bile salt excreted [169]. This calculated increase in the *Em* was 29 times greater than that measured for bilirubin [170] and eight times greater than that measured for BSP [155]. Enhancement by taurocholate has been observed in the biliary excretion of three other oral cholecystographic agents: iopronic acid, iocetamic acid, and iosumetic acid (0.3 μmol CM/μmol taurocholate excreted) [154]. It was reported that the maximum biliary excretion rate of ipodate and tyropanoate is not affected by bile salt excretion [162]. This is surprising since the chemical structures of ipodate and tyropanoate are similar to those of iopanoic acid. However, using a wider range of taurocholate infusion rates, it is now evident that the biliary excretion of these two oral CM is also enhanced by bile salt excretion [171].

Taurocholate infusion has no influence on the maximum rate of biliary excretion of several CM used for intravenous cholangiography, including iodipamide, ioglycamide, iodoxamate, iosulamide, and iotroxamide [158, 159, 162–164].

Taurocholate infusion results in an increase in bile flow by stimulating water movement across the bile canaliculi [172]. However, choleresis per se, whether produced by secretin, which stimulates water excretion across the bile ducts [172], or by SC 2644, which stimulates the bile salt-independent canalicular bile flow [40], does not affect the excretion rate of iopanoate [166, 173]. Therefore, it is clear that bile salts per se, independent of their choleretic effect, are the important determinants of iopanoate excretion.

The mechanism by which bile salts enhance the maximum biliary excretion of iopanoate and other oral CM has not been determined. Physicochemical inter-

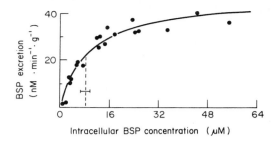

Fig. 21. Kinetics of canalicular BSP transport. BSP excretion rate versus the intracellular concentration of unbound BSP. (Drawn from data from FORKER [181] by SCHARSCHMIDT [182])

actions between bile salts and the organic anion in bile could play a role in preventing back diffusion of iopanoate across the canalicular membrane. The coupling ration of 0.89 during maximum excretion of iopanoate is consistent with molecular ratios found between certain lipids and bile salts in mixed micelles [174]. Because iopanoate is not choleretic [165, 169], it is possible that iopanoate is rendered osmotically inactive in bile by entry into bile salt micelles [165, 175]. The possible physiologic implications of aggregate formation or micelle formation by organic anions and bile salts remain speculative, and certain experimental findings appear inconsistent with a physiologically important interaction between mixed micelles and some organic anions [176–179].

Interaction at the level of the active transport process itself between the carrier for bile salts and the carrier for other anions remains an attractive explanation. This was postulated as the mechanism by which bile salts enhance the biliary excretion of BSP [180]. A plot of intracellular concentration against the steady-state biliary excretion of BSP was curvilinear (Fig. 21). Infusing taurocholate at a higher rate resulted in a higher curvilinear fit, suggesting that higher rates of BSP excretion are achieved at the same intracellular concentration when accompanied with a higher rate of bile salt excretion. The same conclusion was drawn for iopanoate excretion [183]. The hepatic cytosolic concentration of iopanoate was the same in rats infused with zero or 2 µmol/min per kg taurocholate. However, the rate of excretion was significantly higher during taurocholate infusion (Table 5).

Another possible mechanism by which bile salts could facilitate the biliary excretion of iopanoate is by recruitment of the centrilobular portions of the bile canaliculi increasing the capacity of the liver to transport [170]. Based on pharmacokinetic considerations, it has also been suggested that the enhancing effect of taurocholate was probably located at a step prior to canalicular transport, either hepatic uptake or conjugation [184].

Our findings in cultured hepatocytes show that the presence of 1.0 µM taurocholate in the incubation medium does not change the uptake of iopronic acid [185]. It is possible that taurocholate competes with iopanoic acid for binding to albumin in the medium, so that the unbound concentration of iopanoic acid is greater and that this results in a higher uptake velocity. However, taurocholate had no effect on the uptake of iopanoic acid in the presence of albumin. It seems

Table 5. Effect of presence or absence of taurocholate on biliary excretion of iopanoate in rats injected with iopanoic acid (IOP) or iopanoate glucuronide (IOP-G) [37]

Compound infused	IOP	IOP-G	IOP	IOP-G
Taurocholate (μmol/min/g liver)	0	0	2	2
Bile flow (μl/min/g liver)	1.80	1.81	2.48[a]	2.60[b]
Bile salt excretion (nmol/min/g liver)	48.5	58.6	97.9[a]	111.1[b]
Biliary excretion (nmol/min/g liver)	27.4	39.2[a]	47.0[a]	81.7[a,b]
Biliary concentration (μmol/ml)	15.2	21.0[a]	20.0[a]	39.8[b,c]

[a] Significantly different from value in column 1
[b] Significantly different from value in column 2
[c] Significantly different from value in column 3, P, 0.001

unlikely that the enhancement of iopanoate Em by taurocholate can be attributed to an effect on the uptake step.

Although oral CM have similar chemical structures, their maximum rates of biliary excretion are different (Table 6). In addition, when the oral agents are infused intravenously, the effect of taurocholate administration on Em was also variable. Differences in the transport maximums of the intravenous agents are also obvious (Table 6). These differences occur despite the similarity in their chemical structures and despite the lack of an effect of bile salts on their maximum rate of biliary excretion.

Generally, compounds excreted into bile have a strong polar group. Most compounds excreted into bile appear as more polar derivatives of the parent com-

Table 6. Maximum biliary excretion rates (E_m) of biliary contrast media in dogs

Taurocholate infusion (μmol/min/kg)	0.5	2.0
Triiodophenyl alkanoates		
Iopanoic acid	0.68	1.36
Ipodate	1.47	1.42
Tyropanoate	0.96	1.12
Iocetamic acid	1.07	1.24
Iopronic acid	0.85	1.22
Iosumetic acid	0.97	1.38
Triiodobenzyl dimers		
Iodipamide	1.20	1.15
Iodoxamate	1.60	
Ioglycamide	0.98	
Iotroxamide	1.63	1.66
Iosulamide	0.35	0.32

pound, having undergone hepatic biotransformation of a glucuronide, glutathione, glycine, or other conjugated moiety. Direct evidence for a higher affinity for the biliary transport for the more polar metabolite has been found for the glutathione conjugate of BSP. Both the parent compound and the glutathione conjugate of BSP are excreted into bile. The maximum rate of dye excretion into bile was greater when the performed glutathione conjugate of BSP (BSP-GSH) rather than BSP was administered intravenously to the dog [155], rat [186], and guinea pig [186]. The hepatic concentration of conjugated dye was similar regardless of whether BSP or BSP-GSH was infused, suggesting that conversion of BSP ot BSP-GSH did not limit dye transport when BSP was infused. Suppression of the formation of the more polar metabolite of bilirubin by methylating the carboxyl groups which normally form the glucuronide metabolite also reduces its bilirubin excretion [187]. In a study of various derivatives of sulfathiazole, a higher percentage of the dose of the more polar derivatives was excreted into bile. In addition, compounds which have two or three polar carboxyl or sulfonic acid groups in their structure (amaranth, phenolphthalein disulfate, iodocyanine green) are excreted into bile unchanged [187]. Despite these general findings relating biliary excretion and polarity of the compound, there is no definite study which has shown a direct relationship between degree of polarity and affinity for biliary excretion. Indeed from the available information it is not possible to determine whether the relative polarity of the test compound is related to biliary excretion or to a prior step in the overall elimination process, such as uptake, metabolism, or protein binding.

Another factor proposed to have a significant bearing on the extent to which a compound is excreted into bile is molecular weight. Generally, compounds with a molecular weight greater than a threshold value of 300–500 are excreted into bile to some degree [187–190]. Although the concept seems firm, it is not clear what effect molecular weight per se has on biliary excretion of compounds weighing more than the threshold value. There appears to be wide variation in the extent of biliary excretion between compounds of similar molecular weight [190].

The obvious explanation for the wide fluctuation in the extent of biliary excretion of compounds of similar molecular weight is that it is due to structural features of the organic compounds. It has been shown that shifting a single sulfonic acid group from one location to another in a number of dyes resulted in a four- to eightfold change in the extent of biliary excretion [191, 192]. Absence of a hydroxyl group [187], structural isomers [193], degree of saturation of aromatic ring [188], and homologous series differing in the number of methylene groups in the side chain [187] all seem to affect the extent of biliary elimination. However, the nature of the influence imparted by the chemical structure of the compound for biliary excretion remains unclear.

F. Concentration of Contrast Media

I. Choleresis

Contrast media are excreted into bile and induce an increase in bile flow in much the same way as taurocholate. For instance, bile flow increases by 21 µl for each

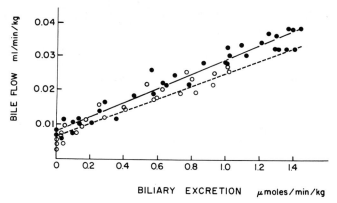

Fig. 22. Relationship between the rate of bile flow and biliary excretion of iodoxamate (*closed circles, solid line*) and iodipamide (*open circles, dashed line*). Iodoxamate: $y = 0.0219x + 0.0084$ ($r = 0.98$); iodipamide: $y = 0.0212x + 0.0068$ ($r = 0.96$). [158]

micromole of iodipamide or iodoxamate excreted into bile (Fig. 22). Although CM in general cause an increase in bile flow, the magnitude of the choleretic increments are variable as shown in Table 7. The increase in bile flow associated with the biliary excretion of the compounds varies from none with iopanoic acid excretion to 44 µl/µmol with RCK-136 [194].

RCK-136, an experimental CM, is a zwitterion with a basic ring structure similar to that of the other oral biliary CM in the chemical class of triiodophenyl alkanoates. The striking difference in the magnitude of the increment in bile flow elicited by the other alkanoates compared with RCK-136 emphasizes the fact that compounds of similar molecular structure induce a wide range of choleretic re-

Table 7. Choleretic increments induced by various contrast media in dogs

Compound	Choleretic increment (µl/µmol)
Oral compounds	
Iopanoic acid	0
Ipodate	8
Iosumetic acid	9
Iocetamic acid	10
Tyropanoic acid	10
Iopronic acid	17
RCK-136 (rat)	44
Intravenous compounds	
Iodipamide	21
Ioglycamide	22
Iodoxamate	22
Iotroxamide	23
Iosulamide	22

Table 8. Erythritol and mannitol clearances into bile during taurocholate- and iodoxamate-induced choleresis in dogs. [37]

	Taurocholate	Iodoxamate
$\dfrac{\text{Erythritol clearance}}{\text{Bile flow}}$	1.00	0.95
$\dfrac{\text{Mannitol clearance}}{\text{Bile flow}}$	0.71	0.74
$\dfrac{\text{Mannitol clearance}}{\text{Erythritol clearance}}$	0.69	0.67

sponses. In distinction, the intravenous CM are consistent in their degree of choleretic activity (21–23 µl/µmol) (Table 7).

In order to determine whether the increase in bile flow induced by iodoxamate, one of the intravenous CM, is canalicular or ductular in origin, biliary clearances of erythritol and mannitol were determined in dogs given iodoxamate and taurocholate (Table 8). The ratios of erythritol clearance and bile flow, mannitol clearance and bile flow, and mannitol and erythritol clearance are similar during choleresis induced by these two compounds. Erythritol enters bile to the same extent as the increase in bile flow with both iodoxamate and taurocholate, while mannitol entry is partially restricted with both compounds. Therefore, it appears that choleresis associated with iodoxamate transport into bile originates in the canaliculi.

II. Biliary Concentration

The concentration of CM in bile is one of the major determinants of the degree of radiographic visualization of the biliary tree. Figure 23 shows the relationship between the bile and plasma concentration in the dog of two intravenous agents, iodoxamate and iodipamide. The maximum biliary concentration that can be achieved with these agents is approximately 35 µmol/ml, a concentration which is approached in bile when plasma concentration is low. Higher plasma concentrations with concomitant greater rates of biliary excretion do not substantially increase the concentration of the CM in bile, because of the choleresis induced by the biliary transport of these compounds. Thus, there is an obligatory coupling between the CM and water which establishes a concentration maximum.

The rate of basal bile flow also influences the concentration of the CM. Basal bile flow consists of a bile salt-associated fraction, a bile salt-independent fraction, and the ductular bile flow. The influence of the basal bile flow on the biliary concentration of CM in the dog is illustrated in Fig. 24. In the theoretical condition, in which there is total absence of basal bile flow, the volume of bile would be determined solely by the choleresis associated with the excretion of the CM. The maximum concentration of iodoxamate and iodipamide would be 46 µmol/ml (reciprocal of the regression coefficient between biliary excretion and bile flow,

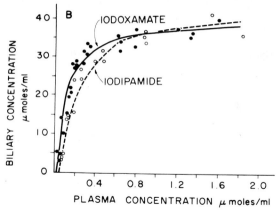

Fig. 23. Relationship in the dog between biliary concentrations of iodoxamate (*closed circles, solid line*), iodipamide (*open circles, dashed line*), and plasma concentration. The maximum biliary concentration for iodoxamate (39.3 µmol/ml) and iodipamide (42.5 µmol/ml) was estimated using a computer program for least-squares estimation of nonlinear equations. [158]

Fig. 22). The actual biliary concentration of the two compounds is less than the theoretical maximum value because of dilution by the basal bile flow.

The extent that the basal flow reduces the biliary concentration of CM varies with the rate of the basal flow. In the dog an increase of basal flow from 0.01 to 0.02 ml/min per kilogram reduces the maximum biliary concentration from 39 to 34 µmol/ml (Fig. 24). Since a biliary concentration of approximately 15 µmol/ml

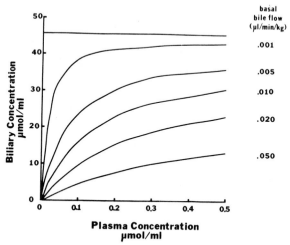

Fig. 24. Schematic representation of the effect of basal bile flow on biliary concentration of iodoxamate. The derived curves represent the relationship between biliary and plasma concentration of iodoxamate when basal bile flow is changed from zero (*horizontal line*) to 0.050 µl/min per kilogram. The calculated maximum biliary concentrations decreased (45.6, 44.8, 42.2, 39.2, 33.7, and 25.9 µmol/ml) when basal bile flow was increased (zero, 0.001, 0.005, 0.010, 0.020, and 0.050 µl/min per kilogram, respectively). [158]

iodoxamate is considered adequate to visualize the biliary tree [157, 195], the influence of basal bile flow appears to be insignificant. However, the plasma concentration of iodoxamate necessary to obtain a concentration of 15 µmol/ml in bile doubles (0.09 to 0.19 µmol/ml) when the basal bile flow is increased from 0.01 to 0.02 ml/min per kilogram. Thus, since the relationship between plasma concentration and rate of intravenous infusion of the CM appears to be linear [158, 159, 162, 163], the dose of CM required for minimum visualization of the biliary tree would double. Doubling the dose could be highly undesirable because of the toxicity of the agent.

III. Electrolyte Composition

The electrolyte composition of bile induced by taurocholate and iodoxamate is compared in Table 9. Despite the fact that clearance data suggest a similar site of origin for the choleretic increments induced by these two compounds, the composition of the bile created is different (Table 9). The sodium concentration in bile generated by taurocholate-induced choleresis appears to be higher than in bile formed during iodoxamate choleresis. However, in distinction to iodoxamate, bile salts entering micelles mask their full potential osmotic activity. Since sodium serves as the counter ion for both the osmotically active and inactive bile salts, the sodium concentration is higher in bile associated with taurocholate than in that associated with iodoxamate.

An important difference in electrolyte composition is the high concentration of bicarbonate in the bile increment associated with iodoxamate excretion (52.3 µEq/ml) (Table 9). SC 2644 is the only other compound which induces a bicarbonate-rich bile excreted at the canaliculus [40]. However, this compound is not transported into bile in sufficient quantities to function osmotically and is thought to act by activating electrolyte transport. These are the first data showing transport of bicarbonate in association with canalicular bile flow. Previously, bicarbonate-rich bile was believed to be associated solely with ductular bile flow.

It has not been determined whether the changes in bile composition associated with the biliary excretion of organic compounds such as the CM have clinical significance. It is clear, however, that the potent choleretic effect of cholangiographic CM imposes an obligatory restriction on the maximal concentration of

Table 9. Comparison of bile associated with taurocholate- and iodoxamate-induced increments in bile of dogs [37]

	Taurocholate	Iodoxamate
Sodium (µEq/ml)	179	147
Potassium (µEq/ml)	6.3	6.3
Chloride (µEq/ml)	63.0	59.2
Bicarbonate (µEq/ml)	24.3	52.3
Bile salt (µmol/ml	97.8	
Iodoxamate (µmol/ml)		39.6
Osmolality (mOsm/kg)	310	297

the agents in bile. It is hoped that a greater understanding of the mechanisms of choleresis will lead to the development of improved CM with more favorable excretion characteristics.

G. Gallbladder Function

Biliary excretion is the principal excretory route for biliary CM and their metabolites. Bile containing these compounds is influenced by the gallbladder in two ways: (a) by the concentration of bile by the absorption of water and electrolytes from bile in the gallbladder lumen, and (b) by the delivery of bile into the duodenum when the gallbladder contracts. These two physiologic functions act together to provide a concentrated solution of bile salts in the intestine at the proper time to aid in the digestion of fat.

The concentration of bile in the gallbladder has been the subject of intensive investigation in vitro. Since the gallbladder mucosa consists essentially of a single layer of epithelial cells, it provides an ideal model for in vitro investigation of transport mechanisms across epithelial membranes. These studies show that the gallbladder transports an isotonic solution whose principle solutes are sodium, potassium, chloride, and bicarbonate [196, 197]. DIAMOND [198], WHEELER [199], and DIETSCHY [200] have showed that both sodium and chloride are actively absorbed across the mucosa in the absence of a significant transepithelial electrical potential difference. It has also been demonstrated that chloride absorption is coupled in an electrically neutral fashion to sodium transport [201]. The energy for intracellular accumulation and transepithelial transport appears to be derived from the interaction between sodium and chloride entry into the cell and the electrochemical potential difference for sodium across the apical membrane [202]. Potassium moves across the gallbladder epithelium by passive diffusion [203]. Water transport, however, is secondary to active solute transport. Water absorption ceases when the concentration of chloride in the lumen is sufficiently low that cotransport of sodium and chloride stops. Water transport results from local osmotic forces created by the active transport of the solute into the lateral intercellular spaces in the epithelial membrane [204, 205].

Bile in the gallbladder is concentrated by water transport and is delivered to the intestine when the smooth muscle in the gallbladder wall contracts. Bile first enters the common bile duct where, after relaxation of the sphincter of Oddi, it flows into the duodenum. The major determinant of gallbladder motor activity is the hormone cholecystokinin (CCK). CCK stimulates contraction of the gallbladder [206] and relaxation of the sphincter of Oddi [207]. Its mechanism of action is independent of the autonomic nervous system and involves a direct effect on the muscle of the gallbladder wall [208, 209].

When the cystic duct is patent, CM enters the gallbladder. Once in the gallbladder, the CM is concentrated by the resorption of water by the gallbladder mucosa. A concentration of 0.25–1.0% iodine is required in the gallbladder for radiographic visualization [195, 210]. When the CM enters the gallbladder, it is diluted by the bile already present. Over a period of many hours, the gallbladder becomes radiopaque as it fills with CM that is gradually concentrated.

Since the first cholecystogram was reported by Graham and Cole in 1924, failure of the gallbladder to reabsorb water and to concentrate the CM has been assumed to be the major cause of nonvisualization of the gallbladder when cystic duct obstruction or extrabiliary problems are eliminated [2]. Later studies were initiated investigating the extent of in vitro water reabsorption in human gallbladders with cholecystitis and cholelithiasis immediately after cholecystectomy [211]. From these studies, it was apparent that some gallbladders that fail to visualize on cholecystography have the ability to transport water normally in vitro. Therefore, in some cases, nonvisualization cannot be attributed to failure of the gallbladder to reabsorb water and to concentrate the CM. In his classic review of gallbladder physiology, IVY suggested that reabsorption of CM by the gallbladder mucosa could also contribute to nonvisualization [212]. Indeed, it has been shown that conjugated iopanoate is readily absorbed from the inflamed gallbladder [213]. Thus, nonvisualization of the gallbladder may result from inadequate concentration of CM in the gallbladder due to failure to reabsorb water and/or reabsorption of the CM from the gallbladder.

In general, it is widely believed that a major portion of bile excreted by the liver is sequestered in the gallbladder [71]. However, data supporting this belief are sparse. Studies in baboons showing that during fasting hepatic bile partially bypasses the gallbladder to enter the duodenum so that a significant enterohepatic circulation continues even 48 h after fasting have been reported [214]. In addition, a recent report indicates that more than half of the bile secreted by night bypasses the gallbladder both in control subjects and in patients with cholelithiasis [215]. Much more information is needed about the sequestering function of the gallbladder to provide a basis for improving entry of CM into the gallbladder which would result in more efficient and safer cholecystography.

H. Enterohepatic Circulation

After being secreted into bile and deposited in the small intestine, CM may remain in the intestinal contents and be eliminated from the body via the feces. However, reabsorption from the intestine and re-entrance into the blood stream are also possible. This process is called enterohepatic circulation. The presence of an enterohepatic circulation could markedly prolong the plasma disappearance of a compound, especially if it went through a large number of cycles. The classic example of compounds which undergo this process is bile salts. Bile salts are normally excreted into bile and enter the duodenum. When the bile salts reach the ileum, they are actively reabsorbed. The return to the plasma leads to liver clearance and reexcretion into the bile. This enterohepatic circulation of bile salts serves as a mechanism for the reutilization of these physiologically important compounds.

Although many compounds can also undergo an enterohepatic circulation [216, 217], few are actively reabsorbed from the intestine. For those compounds secreted into bile in a lipid-soluble form, they can be reabsorbed through the intestinal mucosa by passive diffusion. More commonly, compounds are biotransformed or conjugated to a more polar form before their excretion into bile. This significantly changes their potential for passive reabsorption. Many compounds are excreted into the bile conjugated with glucuronic acid, but these polar conjugates may be hydrolyzed to more lypophilic forms by the bacterial enzyme beta-glucuronidase which is present in anerobic intestinal flora [218] and absorbed into the portal circulation [216]. Thus a decrease in the bacterial flora of the gastrointestinal tract will probably result in a decrease in the enterohepatic circulation of the polar conjugates excreted into bile [219].

The extent of enterohepatic circulation of oral CM is not accurately known [4]. Recently it was shown in dogs that about 30% of iopanoate glucuronide placed in the duodenum was recovered in bile [93] and that antibiotic treatment to reduce the bacterial flora resulted in a four- to fivefold decrease in the recovered CM [94]. In addition, iopanoate has been found in the stool of humans 5 days after administration of an oral dose [220]. During this period about 65% of the administered dose was recovered in the stool. These studies do not distinguish whether conjugated iopanoate is reabsorbed, intact, or after hydrolyzed. As pointed out earlier, the rates of absorption of polar CM are greater than had been originally thought [74, 75] and the possibility that the polar conjugates are partially absorbed intact remains a possible explanation for enterohepatic circulation for CM.

The fraction of the intravenous CM that enters the biliary tree would most likely be primarily excreted in the stool, since these are very highly water-soluble compounds.

J. Renal Excretion

Renal excretion is the other major route of elimination of the biliary CM. Data currently available suggest that only the water-soluble conjugated forms of the oral agents appear in urine [142, 143]. The water-soluble intravenous CM are excreted directly by the kidneys without chemical modification by the liver. Above a minimal plasma concentration, the renal excretion of both the intravenous CM and the oral agents are linearly related to the plasma concentration of the compound [157, 159, 162–164]. Therefore, unlike excretion of bile, the urinary excretion of the biliary CM appears to be a passive process across the glomerulus or renal tubule.

When the oral CM, iopanoic acid, ipodate, or tyropanoate are infused intravenously in dogs, no more than 5% of the infused dose is excreted into the urine [162, 166]. However, in studies in human subjects, 15%–35% of an orally administered dose of iopanoate is excreted in the urine [143, 221].

With the intravenous biliary CM, the urinary excretion rate is also linearly related to the plasma concentration or infusion rate of the compound. Studies in dogs have demonstrated that at high infusion rates, more than 20% of the infused dose is excreted in the urine. With slow infusion rates, less than 5% of the infused dose is excreted in urine. As the maximum capacity of the liver for excretion is approached with faster rates of infusion of the CM, the biliary excretion rate of the compound is increased by progressively smaller increments, and greater proportions of the infused dose appear in the urine [157]. In human studies, between 15% and 20% of the administered dose of iodipamide is eliminated in urine [157, 222, 223]. Studies in dogs with experimentally produced liver injury or partial biliary obstruction reveal that biliary excretion of iodipamide is reduced and renal excretion is increased [224, 225].

An important urinary factor which could have a major effect on the extent of urinary clearance of CM is urinary pH. The pronounced effect of urine pH on the renal clearance of salicylate and other drugs is well known [226, 227]. Generally, urinary excretion of compounds depends on the pH of urine if the pKa of the compound differs from the urine pH by about two units. Since the pH of urine ranges from approximately 4.5 to 8.0, the urinary excretion of these CM may be urinary pH dependent. In general, a substantial change in urinary excretion would be expected if the compound has a pKa of between 3.0 and 7.5. Triiodophenyl alkanoates are weak acids with pKa values within this range. an increase in urinary pH would increase the percentage of the compound in an ionized form and probably reduce the amount reabsorbed from the renal tubule and lead to an increase in the rate of urinary clearance. Urinary clearance of CM, however, plays only a minor role as a determinant for obtaining successful gallbladder visualization.

K. Toxicity

Serious reactions with the intravenous CM are much more common than with the oral CM. In a survey by ANSELL, iodipamide was associated with a higher incidence of toxicity than the renal CM [227]. In his series, there was one death per 5,000 examinations with iodipamide, compared with one death per 40,000 with intravenous pyelograms. The primary reactions associated with iodipamide are skin rash, cardiovascular collapse, and renal dysfunction [228, 229]. The mechanisms involved in the production of adverse reactions have not been clearly defined, but probably involve hypersensitivity reactions, direct cellular toxicity, critical enzyme inhibition, or vasoactive alterations in hemodynamics [1, 100]. It generally is assumed that the incidence of adverse reactions is related to the dose and rate of administration of the CM.

With oral cholecystographic CM, poor intestinal absorption may be a major factor in preventing serious toxic reactions when large and/or multiple doses are given. Minor side effects including nausea, vomiting, and diarrhea occur in nearly 50% of materials [230–239]. These problems appear to be dose related and may be due to a direct effect on the intestinal mucosa.

Impairment of renal function can occur after both oral and intravenous contrast studies and is the most serious toxic reaction [240–251]. Current data do not provide information to help distinguish the mechanism by which the CM produce nephrotoxicity [252]. Renal injury may result from systematic hypotension produced by a CM [85, 86, 252].

Although the nephrotoxicity of CM has been the subject of considerable research effort, careful studies evaluating the hepatotoxic potential of these agents have been lacking. In recent years, reports have appeared linking iodipamide administration to asymptomatic transaminase elevations [253] as well as to clinically apparent liver injury [254, 255]. One group has suggested that the agent is a direct hepatotoxin in humans [255]. A study was undertaken to determine the hepatotoxic potential of iodipamide in rats and to identify factors affecting it [256].

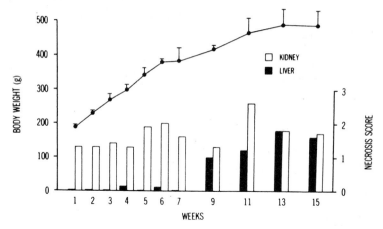

Fig. 25. Iodipamide liver and kidney necrosis related to age and growth. All animals were from the same shipment group and were started on the experiment at 190 g body wt. Time of the experiment is indicated on the *abscissa*. Four rats were injected with 2 mmol iodipamide/kg at each *time point* indicated and, 24 h later, they were killed and liver and kidney necrosis were graded histologically. The values shown are means. The weight of the rats studied at each time point is shown by the *closed circles* connected by *lines*. The *halfbrackets* indicate 1 SD. Necrosis is indicated by the *bars*. [256]

Iodipamide administered intraperitoneally or intravenously caused a characteristic type of necrosis which began in the midzonal area and spread to the centrilobular region. Only rats weighing 400 g or more developed necrosis when the dose administered was 2 mmol/kg. Rats weighing 200 g failed to develop liver necrosis even when given 3 mmol/kg (Fig. 25). Phenobarbital pretreatment provided little or no protection. Kidney tubular necrosis was also observed but occurred in young rats and in selenium-deficient rats which developed no liver necrosis. These results indicate that iodipamide is a hepatoxin in rats. There are a number of factors, age being the most striking, that modify its hepatotoxicity.

Further studies with older rats indicated that the biliary excretion of iodipamide and iopanoate was significantly reduced [257]. It appeared that the diminished excretion of iodipamide associated with aging may be responsible for the increased hepatotoxicity of iodipamide noted in older rats [256]. If the ability of the liver to excrete iodipamide and other CM is also reduced in older humans, older patients undergoing intravenous cholangiography with iodipamide may have a greater risk of receiving liver damage.

L. Future for Biliary Contrast Media

It seems likely that contrast media will continue to be used in the future for assessing liver function and gallbladder opacification. In addition, contrast media in conjunction with computed tomography could potentially be a very useful technique for future clinical investigations [258–267].

Acknowledgments. This study was supported in part by grant AM 21620 from the National Institutes of Health. The author was the recipient of Research Career Development Award AM 00680 from the United States Health Service.

References

1. Knoefel PK (1971) Radiocontrast agents, vols 1 and 2. International encyclopedia of pharmacology and therapeutics. Pergamon, New York
2. Berk RN, Loeb PM, Goldberger LE (1974) Oral cholecystography with iopanoic acid. N Engl J Med 290:204–210
3. Berk RN, Loeb PM (1976) Pharmacology and physiology of the biliary radiographic contrast materials. Sem Roentgenol 11:147–157
4. Loeb PM, Berk RN (1977) Biliary contrast materials. In: Berk RN, Clemett AR (eds) Radiology of the gallbladder and bile ducts. Saunders, Philadelphia, pp 71–100
5. Berk RN, Loeb PM (1977) Contrast materials for oral cholecystography. In: Miller RE, Skucas J (eds) Radiographic contrast agents. University Park Press, Baltimore, pp 195–222
6. Berk RN, Loeb PM, Ellzey BA (1977) Contrast materials for intravenous cholangiography. In: Miller RE, Skucas J (eds) Radiographic contrast agents. University Park Press, Baltimore, pp 223–250
7. Kessel RG, Kardon RH (1979) Tissue and organs: a text-atlas of scanning electron microscopy. Freeman, San Francisco
8. Elias H, Sherrick JC (1969) Morphology of the liver. Academic, New York
9. Miyai K, Abraham J, Linthicum SM, Wagner R (1976) Scanning electron microscopy of hepatic ultrastructure. Lab Invest 35:369–376
10. Rappaport AM (1958) The structural and functional unit in the human liver (liver acinus). Anat Rec 130:673–690
11. Rappaport AM (1963) Acinar units and the pathophysiology of the liver. In: Rouiller (ed) The liver: morphology, biochemistry, physiology, vol 1. Academic, New York, pp 265–328
12. Rappaport AM, Borowy ZJ, Lougheed WM, Lotto WN (1954) Subdivision of hexagonal liver lobules into a structural and functional unit. Anat Rec 119:11–34
13. Mall FP (1906) A study of the structural unit of the liver. Am J Anat 5:227–308
14. Elias H (1952) The geometry of the cell shape and the adaptive evolution of the liver. J Morphology 91:377–405
15. Motta P, Fumagalli G (1975) Structure of rat bile canaliculi as revealed by scanning electron microscopy. Anat Rec 182:499–513
16. Numchausky VA, Layden TJ, Boyer JL (1977) Effects of chronic choleretic infusions of bile acids on the membrane of the bile canaliculus. Lab Invest 36:259–267
17. Katsumi M, Richardson A, Mayr W, Javitt N (1977) Subcellular pathology of rat liver in cholestasis and choleresis induced by bile salts. Lab Invest 36:249–258
18. Grisham JW, Nopanitaya W, Compango J, Nagel AEH (1975) Scanning electron microscopy of normal rat liver: surface structure of its cell and tissue components. Am J Anat 144:295–322
19. Porter KR, Bonneville MA (1964) An introduction to the fine structure of cells and tissues. Lea and Febiger, Philadelphia
20. Palade GE (1953) An electron microscope study of the mitochondrial structure. J Histochem Cytochem 1:188–211
21. Palade GE, Siekevitz P (1956) Liver microsomes; an integrated morphological and biochemical study. J Biophys Biochem Cytol 2:171–200
22. Fawcett DW (1955) Observations on the cytology and electron microscopy of hepatic cells. J Natl Cancer Inst 15:1475–1503
23. Novikoff AB, Essner E (1960) The liver cell. Am J Med 29:102–131
24. Ashford TP, Porter KR (1962) Cytoplasmic components in hepatic cell lysosomes. J Cell Biol 12:198–200

25. Mueller JC, Jones AL, Long JA (1972) Topographic and subcellular anatomy of the guinea pig gallbladder. Gastroenterology 63:856–868
26. Wheeler HO (1968) Water and electrolytes in bile. In: Code CF (ed) Handbook of physiology, sect 6, alimentary canal. Am Physiology Soc, Washington, D.C., pp 2409–2431
27. Barnhart JL, Combes B (1975) Characteristics common to choleretic increments of bile induced by theophylline, glucagon and SQ 20009 in the dog. Proc Soc Exp Biol Med 150:591–596
28. Cook DL, Lawler CA, Calvin LD, Green DM (1952) Mechanism of bile formation. Am J Physiol 171:62–74
29. Rheinhold JG, Wilson DW (1934) The acid-base composition of hepatic bile. Am J Physiol 107:378–387
30. Scratcherd T (1965) Electrolyte composition and control of biliary secretion in the cat and rabbit. In: Taylor W (ed) The biliary system. Blackwell, Oxford, pp 515–529
31. Thureborn E (1962) Human hepatic bile. Composition changes due to altered entero-hepatic circulation. Acta Chir Scand [Suppl] 303:1–63
32. Klaassen CD (1971) Does bile acid secretion determine canalicular bile production in rats? Am J Physiol 220:667–673
33. Wheeler HO, Ramos OL (1960) Determinants of the flow and composition of bile in the unanesthetized dog during constant infusions of sodium taurocholate. J Clin Invest 39:161–170
34. Harrison FA (1962) Bile secretion in the sheep. J Physiol 162:212–224
35. Preisig R, Cooper HC, Wheeler HO (1962) The relationship between taurocholate secretion rate and bile production in the unanesthetized dog during cholenergic blockade and during secretin administration. J Clin Invest 41:1152–1162
36. Forker EL (1977) Mechanisms of hepatic bile formation. Ann Rev Physiol 39:323–347
37. Barnhart JL, Berk RN, Combes B (1980) Changes in bile flow and composition induced by radiographic contrast materials. Invest Radiol 15:5116–5121
38. Erlinger S, Dhumeaux D (1974) Mechanisms and control of bile water and electrolytes. Gastroenterology 66:281–304
39. Berk RN, Loeb PM, Cobo-Frenkel A, Barnhart JL (1976) Saturation kinetics and choleretic effects of iodoxamate and iodipamide. An Experimental study in dogs. Radiology 119:529–535
40. Barnhart JL, Combes B (1978) Characterization of SC 2644-induced choleresis in the dog. Evidence for canalicular bicarbonate secretion. J Pharmacol Exp Ther 206:190–197
41. Klaassen CD (1972) Species differences in the choleretic response to bile salts. J Physiol 224:259–269
42. Cornelius CE (1976) Rates of choleresis in various species. Digestive Dis 21:426–428
43. Boyer JL, Bloomer JR (1974) Canalicular bile secretion in man. Studies utilizing the biliary clearance of (14-C) mannitol. J Clin Invest 54:773–781
44. Boyer JL (1971) Canalicular bile formation in the isolated perfused rat liver. Am J Physiol 221:1156–1163
45. Erlinger S, Dhumeaux D, Berthelot P, Durmot M (1970) Effect of inhibitors of sodium transport on bile formation in the rabbit. Am J Physiol 219:416–422
46. King JE, Schoenfield LG (1971) Choleresis induced by sodium taurocholate in isolated hamster liver. J Clin Invest 50:2305–2312
47. Barnhart JL, Combes B (1978) Erythritol and mannitol clearance with taurocholate and secretin-induced cholereses. Am J Physiol 234:E146–E156
48. Wheeler HO, Ross ED, Bradley SE (1968) Canalicular bile production in dogs. Am J Physiol 214:866–874
49. Balabaud CP, Kron KA, Gumucio JJ (1977) The assessment of the bile salt nondependent fraction of canalicular bile water in the rat. J Lab Clin Med 89:393–399
50. Baker AL, Word RAB, Moosa AR, Boyer JL (1979) Sodium taurocholate modifies the bile acid independent fraction of canalicular flow in the rhesus monkey. J Clin Invest 64:312–320

51. Frizzell R, Field M, Schultz S (1979) Sodium-coupled chloride transport by epithelial tissues. Am J Physiol 236:F1–F8
52. Diamond JM (1971) Standing-gradient model of fluid transport in epithelia. Fed Proc 30:6–13
53. Sweadner K, Goldin S (1980) Active transport of sodium and potassium ions: mechanism, function, and regulation. N Engl J Med 302:777–783
54. Layden TM, Boyer JL (1976) The effect of thyroid hormone on bile salt-independent bile flow and Na^+,K^+-ATPase activity in liver plasma membranes enriched in bile canaliculi. J Clin Invest 57:1009–1018
55. Reichen J, Paumgartner G (1977) Relationship between bile flow and Na^+,K^+-adenosine-triphosphotase in liver plasma membranes enriched in bile canaliculi. J Clin Invest 60:429–434
56. Sneller M, Crawford S, Miner PB Jr (1980) Dissociation of bile salt independent bile flow (BSIBF) and hepatic (Na^+-K^+)ATPase activity induced by spironolactone and canrenone. Gastroenterology 79:1055
57. Preisig R, Cooper HL, Wheeler HO (1962) The relationship between taurocholate secretion rate and bile production in the unanesthetized dog during cholinergic blockage and during secretin administration. J Clin Invest 41:1152–1162
58. Forker EL (1967) Two sites of bile formation as determined by mannitol and erythritol clearance in the guinea pig. J Clin Invest 46:1189–1195
59. Wheeler HO, Mancusi-Ungaro PL (1967) Role of bile ducts during secretin choleresis in dogs. Am J Physiol 210:1153–1159
60. Nicholls RJ (1979) Biliary mannitol clearance and bile salt output before and during secretin choleresis in the dog. Gastroenterology 76:983–987
61. Fisher MM, Phillips MJ (1979) Cytoskeleton of the hepatocyte. In: Popper H, Schaffner F (eds) Progress in liver diseases, vol VI. Grune and Stratton, New York, pp 105–121
62. Brenner SL, Korn ED (1979) Substoichiometric concentrations of cytochalasin D inhibit actin polymerization. Additional evidence for an F-actin trendmill. J Biol Chem 254:9982–9985
63. Dubin M, Maurice M, Feldmann G, Erlinger S (1978) Phalloidin-induced cholestasis in the rat: relation to changes in microfilaments. Gastroenterology 75:450–455
64. Erlinger S (1980) Microfilaments, microtubules, and their role in the pathophysiology of cholestasis. The American Association for the Study of Liver Disease. Postgraduate course "Cholestasis. Update on pathophysiology, diagnosis and management," 1980
65. Stein O, Sanger L, Stein Y (1974) Colchicine-induced inhibition of lipoprotein and protein secretion into the serum and lack of interference with secretion of biliary phospholipids and cholesterol by the rat liver in vivo. J Cell Biol 62:90–103
66. Gregory DH, Vlahcevic ZR, Prugh MF, Swell L (1978) Mechanism of secretion of biliary lipids: role of microtubular system in hepatocellular transport of biliary lipids in the rat. Gastroenterology 74:93–100
67. Wilkinson GR, Shand DG (1975) A physiological approach to hepatic drug clearance. Clin Pharmacol Therap 18:377–390
68. Keiding S, Andreasen PB (1979) Hepatic clearance measurements and pharmacokinetics. Pharmacology 19:105–110
69. Rane A, Wilkinson GR, Shand DG (1977) Prediction of hepatic extraction ratio from in vitro measurement of intrinsic clearance. J Pharmacol Exp Ther 200:420–424
70. Hoppe JO, Archer S (1951) Aryl triiodo alkanoic acid derivatives as cholecystographic media. Fed Proc 10:310
71. Wise RE (1962) Intravenous cholangiography. Thomas, Springfield
72. Levine WG (1978) Biliary excretion of drugs and other xenobiotics. Ann Rev Pharmacol Toxicol 18:81–96
73. Lasser EC (1966) Pharmacodynamics of biliary contrast media. Radiol Clin North Am 4:511–519
74. Janes JO, Dietschy JM, Berk RN, Loeb PM, Barnhart JL (1979) Determination of the rate of intestinal absorption of oral cholecystographic agents in the dog jejunum. Gastroenterology 76:970–977

75. Janes JO, Berk RN, Barnhart JL (1980) Observations on the intestinal absorption of intact Telepaque glucuronide. Gastroint Radiol 5:83–84
76. Cooke WJ, Cooke L (1977) Biliary excretion of iopanoate glucuronide by the rat. Drug Metab Dispos 5:368–376
77. Hogben CAM, Tocco DJ, Brodie BB, Schanker LS (1959) On the mechanism of the intestinal absorption of drugs. J Pharmacol Exp Ther 125:275–282
78. Jollow DJ, Brodie BB (1972) Mechanisms of drug absorption and of drug solution. Pharmacology 8:21–32
79. Wilson FA, Dietschy JM (1972) Characterization of bile acid absorption across the unstirred water layer and brush border of the rat jejunum. J Clin Invest 51:3015–3025
80. Goldberger LE, Berk RN, Lang JH, Loeb PM (1974) Biopharmaceutical factors influencing intestinal absorption of iopanoic acid. Invest Radiol 9:16–23
81. Taketa RM, Berk RN, Lang JH, Lasser EC, Dunn CR (1972) The effect of pH on the intestinal absorption of Telepaque. Am J Roentgenol 114:767–722
82. Nelson JA, Moss AA, Golbert HI, Benet LZ, Amberg J (1973) Gastrointestinal absorption of iopanoic acid. Invest Radiol 8:1–8
83. Fordtran JA, Locklear TW (1966) Ionic content of small bowel fluid. Am J Dig Dis 11:503–521
84. Carey MC, Small DM (1972) Micelle formation by bile salts: physical, chemical and thermodynamic considerations. Arch Intern Med 130:506–525
85. Go VA, Hofmann AF, Summerskil WH (1970) Pancreozymin bioassay in man based on pancreatic enzyme secretion: potency of specific amino acids and other digestive products. J Clin Invest 49:1558–1564
86. Ertran A, Brooks FP, Ostrow JD, Arvan DA, Williams CN, Cerda JJ (1971) Effect of jejunal amino acid perfusion of exogenous cholecystokinin on the exocrine pancreatic and biliary secretions in man. Gastroenterology 61:686–692
87. Evens G, Schroer C, Koehler PR (1971) Importance of contrast absorption in evaluation of nonvisualized gallbladder. Radiology 98:365–372
88. Westergaard H, Dietschy JM (1974) Delineation of the dimensions and permeability characteristics of the two major diffusion barriers to passive mucosal uptake in the rabbit intestine. J Clin Invest 54:718–732
89. Wilson FA, Dietschy JM (1974) The intestinal unstirred layer: its surface area and effect on active transport kinetics. Biochim Biophys Acta 363:112–126
90. Dietschy JM, Westergaard H (1975) The effect of unstirred water layers on various transport processes in the intestine. In: Csaky TZ (ed) Intestinal absorption and malabsorption. Raven, New York, p 197
91. Dietschy JM, Sallee VL, Wilson FA (1971) Unstirred water layers and absorption across the intestinal mucosa. Gastroenterology 61:932–934
92. Loeb PM, Berk RN, Janes JO, Perkin L (1978) The effect of fasting on gallbladder opacification during oral cholecystography. A controlled study in normal volunteers. Radiology 126:395–401
93. Goldberg HI, Lin SK, Thoeni R, Moss AA, Brito AC (1977) Recirculation of iopanoic acid after conjugation in the liver. Invest Radiol 12:537–541
94. Thoeni RF, Goldberg HI, Moss AA, Lin SK, Brito AC (1978) Observation of the metabolism of iopanoyl (Telepaque) glucuronide in dogs treated with antibiotics. Invest Radiol 13:241–246
95. Cox SR, Barnhart JL (1978) Unpublished observations
96. Jacobson ED, Prior JT, Faloon WW (1960) Malabsorptive syndrome induced by neomycin: morphologic alterations in the jejunal mucosa. J Lab Clin Med 56:245–250
97. Dobbins WO, Merrero BA, Manabach CM (1968) Morphologic alterations associated with neomycin induced malabsorption. Am J Med Sci 255:63–75
98. Jacobson ED, Faloon WW (1961) Malabsorptive effects of neomycin in commonly used doses. JAMA 175:187–196
99. Orr JM, Benet LZ (1975) The effect of fasting on the role of intestinal absorption in rats: preliminary studies. Dig Dis Sci 20:858–865
100. Lang JH, Lasser EC (1967) Binding of roentgenographic contrast media to serum albumin. Invest Radiol 2:396–400

101. Cooke WJ, Mudge GH (1975) Biliary and urinary excretion of iopanoic acid in the dog. Invest Radiol 10:25–34
102. Lin SK, Moss AA, Riegelman S (1977) Iodipamide kinetics: capacity-limited biliary excretion with simultaneous pseudo-first-order renal excretion. J Pharm Sci 66:1670–1673
103. Fehske KJ, Miller WE (1978) The interaction of iopanoic and iophenoxic acids with human serum albumin. Res Comm Chem Path Pharmacol 19:119–127
104. Mudge GH, Strewler GS, Desbiens N, Berndt WO, Wade DN (1971) Excretion and distribution of iophenoxic acid. J Pharmacol Exp Ther 178:159–172
105. Berndt WO, Mudge GH, Wade DH (1971) Hepatic slice accumulation of iopanoic and iophenoxic acids. J Pharmacol Exp Ther 179:85–90
106. Sudlow G, Birkett DH, Wade DN (1973) Spectroscopic techniques in the study of protein binding: the use of 1-anilino-8-naphthalene-sulfonate as a fluorescent probe for the study of the interactions of iophenoxic and iopanoic acids to human serum albumin. Mol Pharmacol 9:649–657
107. Vallner JJ (1977) Binding of drugs by albumin and plasma protein. J Pharm Sci 66:447–465
108. Loeb PM, Berk RN, Janes JO, Perkin L, Moore J (1978) The effect of fasting on gallbladder opacification shunting oral cholecystography: a control study in normal volunteers. Radiology 126:395–401
109. Hunter TB, Fon GT, Berk RN, Capp MP (1981) Concentration and excretion of contrast agents during oral cholecystography as measured by computer tomography in dogs. Invest Radiol Gastrointestinal Radiol 6:349–352
110. Shand DG, Rangno RE, Evans GH (1972) The disposition of propranolol. II. Hepatic elimination in the rat. Pharmacology 8:344–352
111. Song CS, Beranbaum ER, Rothschild MA (1976) The role of serum albumin in the hepatic excretion of iodipamide. Invest Radiol 11:39–44
112. Grauz H, Schmid R (1971) Reciprocal relation between plasma albumin level and hepatic sulfobromophthalein removal. N Engl J Med 284:1403–1406
113. Barnhart JL, Clarenburg R (1973) Factors determining clearance of bilirubin in perfused rat liver. Am J Physiol 225:497–507
114. Cornelius C, Ben-Ezzer J, Arias IM (1967) Binding of sulfobromophthalein sodium (BSP) and other organic anions by isolated hepatic cell plasma membranes in vitro. Proc Soc Exp Biol Med 124:665–667
115. Song CS (1969) Plasma membrane of rat liver. Isolation and enzymatic characterization of a fraction rich in bile canaliculi. J Cell Biol 41:124–132
116. Boyer JL, Reno D (1975) Properties of $(Na^+ + K^+)$-activated ATPase in rat liver plasma membranes enriched with bile canaliculi. Biochim Biophys Acta 401:59–72
117. Wisher MH, Evans WH (1975) Functional polarity of the rat hepatocyte surface membrane. Isolation and characterization of plasma-membrane subfractions from the blood-sinusoidal, bile-canalicular and contiguous surfaces of the hepatocyte. Biochem J 146:375–388
118. Goresky CA (1965) The hepatic uptake and excretion of sulfobromophthalein and bilirubin. Can Med Assoc J 92:851–857
119. Scharschmidt BF, Waggoner JG, Berk PD (1975) Hepatic organic anion uptake in the rat. J Clin Invest 56:1280–1292
120. Vonk RJ (1978) Transport of drugs in isolated hepatocytes. The influence of bile salts. Biochem Pharmacol 27:397
121. Bolt RJ, Dillon R, Pollard HM (1961) Interference with bilirubin excretion by a gallbladder dye: report of a case. N Engl J Med 265:1043–1044
122. Goergen T, Goldberger LE, Berk RN (1974) The combined use of oral cholecystopaque media and iodipamide. Radiology 111:543–548
123. Berry MN, Friend DS (1969) High-yield preparation of isolated rat liver parenchymal cells. A biochemical and fine structural study. J Cell Biol 43:506–520
124. Schwarz LR, Burr R, Schwenk M, Pfaff E, Greim H (1975) Uptake of taurocholic acid into isolated rat-liver cells. Eur J Biochem 55:617–623

125. Anwer MS, Korker R, Hegner D (1975) Bile acids secretion and synthesis by isolated rat hepatocytes. Biochem Biophys Res Commun 64:603–609
126. Anwer MS, Dorker R, Hegner D (1976) Cholic acid uptake into isolated hepatocytes. Hoppe-Seylers Z Physiol Chem 375:1477–1486
127. Schwenk M, Burr R, Schwarz L, Pfaff E (1976) Uptake of bromosulphthalein by isolated liver cells. Eur J Biochem 64:189–197
128. van Bezooijen CFA, Grell T, Knook DL (1976) Bromosulfophthalein uptake by isolated liver parenchymal cells. Biochem Biophys Res Commun 69:354–361
129. Stege TE, Loose LD, DiLuzio NR (1975) Comparative uptake of sulphobromophthalein by isolated Kupffer and parenchymal cells. Proc Soc Exp Biol Med 149:455–461
130. Eaton DL, Klaasen CD (1978) Carrier-mediated transport of oubain in isolated hepatocytes. J Pharmacol Exp Ther 205:480–488
131. Breuer H, Rao ML, Rao GS (1974) Uptake of steroid hormones by isolated rat liver cells. J Steroid Biochem 5:359
132. Rao ML, Rao GS, Holler M, Goreuer H, Schattenberg PJ, Stein WD (1976) A phenomenon indicative of carrier-mediation and simple diffusion. Hoppe-Seylers Z Physiol Chem 367:573–584
133. LeCam A, Freychet P (1977) Neutral amino acid transport. Characterization of the A and L systems in isolated rat hepatocytes. J Biol Chem 252:148–156
134. Bissell DM, Hammaker L, Meyer UA (1973) Parenchymal cells from adult rat liver in nonproliferating monolayer culture. J Cell Biol 59:722–734
135. Guzelian PS, Bissell DM, Meyer UA (1977) Drug metabolism in adult rat hepatocytes in primary monolayer culture. Gastroenterology 72:1232–1239
136. Kletizien RF, Pariza MW, Becker JE, Potter VR, Butcher FR (1976) Induction of amino-acid transport in primary cultures of adult rat liver parenchymal cells by insulin. J Biol Chem 251:3014–3020
137. Hatoff DE, Hardison WG (1979) Induced synthesis of alakaline phosphatase by bile salts in rat liver cell culture. Gastroenterology 77:1062–1067
138. Barnhart JL, Hardison WG, Witt BL, Berk RN (1983) Uptake of iopanoic acid by isolated rat hepatocytes in primary culture. Am J Physiol 244:G630–G636
139. Iga T, Eaton PA, Klaassen CD (1979) Uptake of unconjugated bilirubin by isolated rat hepatocytes. Am J Physiol 236:C9–C14
140. Ockner R, Weisiger R, LysenkO N (1980) Specific and saturable binding of ^{125}I-albumin to rat hepatocytes: further evidence for a surface membrane albumin receptor. Gastroenterology 79:1041
141. Weisiger R, Jollan J, Ackner R (1980) An albumin receptor on the liver cell may mediate hepatic uptake of sulfobromophthalein and bilirubin: bound ligandin, not free, is the major uptake determinant. Gastroenterology 79:1065
142. McChesney EW, Hoppe JO (1956) Observations on the absorption and excretion of the glucuronide of iopanoic acid by the cat. Arch Int Pharmacodyn Ther 105:306–312
143. McChesney EW, Banks WF (1965) Urinary excretion of three oral cholecystographic agents in man. Proc Soc Exp Biol Med 119:1027–1030
144. McChesney EW, Hoppe JO (1954) Observations of the metabolism of iopanoic acid by the cat. Arch Int Pharmacodyn Ther 99:127–140
145. Gartner LM, Arias IM (1969) Formation, transport, metabolism and excretion of bilirubin. N Engl J Med 280:1339–1345
146. Schmid R (1973) Bilirubin metabolism in man. N Engl J Med 287:703–709
147. Carbone JV, Grodsky GM (1957) Constitutional nonhemolytic hyperbilirubinemia in the rat: defect of bilirubin conjugation. Proc Soc Exp Biol Med 94:461–463
148. Arias IM (1959) A defect in microsomal function in nonhemolytic acholuric jaundice. J Histochem Cytochem 7:250–252
149. Barnhart JL, Witt BL (1978) Unpublished data
150. Bock KW, Josting D, Lilienblum W, Pfeil H (1979) Purification of rat-liver microsomal UDP + glucuronyltransferase. Separation of two enzyme forms inducible by 3-methylcholanthrene or phenobarbital. Eur J Biochem 98:19–26

151. Matsui M, Nagai F, Aoyagi S (1979) Strain differences in rat liver UDP-glucuronyl-transferase activity towards androsterone. Biochem J 179:483–487
152. Bock K W, V Clausbruch UC, Ottenswalder H (1978) UDP-glucuronyl transferase in perfused rat liver and in microsomes: V. Studies with Gunn rats. Biochem Pharmacol 27:369–371
153. Lucier GW, McDaniel OS, Hook GER (1975) Nature of the enhancement of hepatic uridine diphosphate glucuronyltransferase activity by 2,3,7,8-tetracholodibenzo-p-dioxine in rats. Biochem Pharmacol 24:325–334
154. Barnhart JL, Berk RN, Czuleger PC (1979) Biliary excretion of three cholecysto-graphic contrast agents in dogs: iocetamic acid, iopronic acid, and iosumetic acid. Invest Radiol 14:79–87
155. Barnhart JL, Combes B (1976) Biliary excretion of dye in dogs infused with BSP or its glutathione conjugate. Am J Physiol 231:399–407
156. Barnhart JL, Parkhill BJ, Cobo-Frenkel A, Berk RN, Loeb PM (1978) Iopanoate glucuronide: procedure for its isolation and purification and pharmacokinetics of its biliary excretion. Invest Radiol 13:347–355
157. Loeb PM, Berk RN, Feld GK, Wheeler HO (1975) Biliary excretion of iodipamide. Gastroenterology 68:554–562
158. Berk RN, Loeb PM, Cobo-Frenkel A, Barnhart JL (1976) Saturation kinetics and choleretic effects of iodoxamate and iodipamide – an experimental study in dogs. Radiology 119:529–535
159. Loeb PM, Barnhart JL, Berk RN (1979) Iotroxamide – a new intravenous cholangio-graphic agent. Comparison with iodipamide and the effect of bile salts. Radiology 125:323–329
160. Nelson JA, Staubus AE, Riegelman S (1975) Saturation kinetics of iopanoate in the dog. Invest Radiol 10:371–377
161. Rosati G, Schiantaretti P (1970) Biliary excretion of contrast media. Invest Radiol 5:232–243
162. Berk RN, Loeb PM, Cobo-Frenkel A, Barnhart JL (1977) The biliary and urinary ex-cretion of sodium tyropanoate and sodium ipodate in dogs. Invest Radiol 12:85–95
163. Loeb PM, Berk RN, Cobo-Frenkel A, Barnhart JL (1976) The biliary and urinary ex-cretion of ioglycamide in dogs. Invest Radiol 11:449–458
164. Berk RN, Barnhart JL, Nazareno G, Witt BL (1981) The potential of iosulamide meglumine as a contrast material for intravenous cholangiography. Invest Radiol 16:240–244
165. Berk RN, Loeb PM, Cobo-Frenkel A, Barnhart JL (1976) The biliary and urinary ex-cretion of iopanoic acid. Pharmaco-kinetics, influence of bile salts and choleretic ef-fect. Radiology 120:41–48
166. Berk RN, Goldberger LE, Loeb PM (1974) The role of bile salts in the hepatic excre-tion of iopanoic acid. Invest Radiol 9:7–15
167. Moss AA, Amberg JR, Jones PS (1972) Relationship of bile salts and bile flow to bili-ary excretion of iopanoic acid. Invest Radiol 7:11–15
168. Dunn CR, Berk RN (1972) The pharmacokinetics of Telepaque metabolism: the rela-tion of blood concentration and bile flow to the rate of hepatic excretion. AJR 114:758–766
169. Loeb PM, Barnhart JL, Berk RN (1978) The dependence of the biliary excretion of iopanoic acid on bile salts. Gastroenterology 74:174–181
170. Goresky CA, Haddad HH, Kluger WS, Nadeau BE, Bach GG (1974) The enhance-ment of maximal bilirubin excretion with taurocholate-induced increments in bile flow. An J Physiol Pharmacol 52:389–403
171. Barnhart JL, Berk RN (1979) Unpublished observations
172. Forker EL (1977) Mechanisms of hepatic bile formation. Annual Rev Physiol 39:323–347
173. Berk RN, Dunn CR (1972) The effects of secretion on the hepatic excretion of Tele-paque. Radiology 103:585–587
174. Carey MC, Small DM (1972) Micelle formation by bile salts. Physical-chemical and thermodynamic considerations. Arch Intern Med 30:506–527

175. Feld GK, Loeb PM, Berk RN (1975) The choleretic effects of iodipamide. J Clin Invest 55:528–535
176. Benet S, Delage Y, Erlinger S (1979) Influence of taurocholate, taurochenodeoxycholate, and taurodehydrocholate on sulfobromophthalein transport in bile. Am J Physiol 236:E10–E14
177. Delage Y, Dumont M, Erlinger S (1976) Effect of glycodihydrofusate on sulfobromophthalein transport maximum in the hamster. Am J Physiol 231:1875–1878
178. Scharschmidt BF, Schmid R (1978) The micellar sink. A quantitative assessment of the association of organic anions with mixed micelles and other macromolecular aggregates in rat bile. J Clin Invest 62:1122–1131
179. Vonk RJ, Jekel P, Meijer DKF (1975) Choleresis and hepatic transport mechanisms. II. Influence of bile salt choleresis and biliary micelle binding on biliary excretion of various organic anions. Naunyn Schmiedebergs Arch Pharmacol 290:375–387
180. Gibson GE, Forker EL (1974) Canalicular bile flow and bromosulfophthalein transport maximum: the effect of a bile salt independent choleretic, SC 2644. Gastroenterology 66:1046–1053
181. Forker EL (1977) Canalicular anion transport. In: Berk PD, Berlin NI (eds) Chemistry and physiology of bile pigments. DHEW Publication Number 77-1100. US Government Printing Office, Washington, pp 383–389
182. Scharschmidt BF (1980) Secretion of organic anions and bile acids: possible role of macromolecular aggregates in bile (the micellular sink). From postgraduate course. The American Association for the Study of Liver Disease, Chicago
183. Barnhart JL, Berk RN, Janes JO, Witt BL (1980) Isolation, hepatic distribution and intestinal absorption of the glucuronide metabolite of iopanoic acid. Invest Radiol 15:5109–5115
184. Staubus AE, Berk RN, Loeb PM, Barnhart JL (1978) Saturation kinetics of iocetamic acid: evaluation of indirect pharmacokinetic techniques and comparison with iopanoic acid. Invest Radiol 13:85–92
185. Barnhart JL, Hardison WG, Witt BL, Berk RN (1983) Uptake of iopanoic acid by isolated rat hepatocytes in primary culture. Am J Physiol 244:G630–G636
186. Whelan G, Combes B (1971) Competition by unconjugated and conjugated sulfobromophthalein sodium (BSP) for transport into bile. Evidence for a single excretory system. J Lab Clin Med 78:230–244
187. Smith RL (1973) The excretory function of bile. Wiley, New York
188. Hirom PC, Millburn P, Smith RL, Williams RT (1972) Molecular weight and chemical structures as factors in the biliary excretion of sulphonamides in the rat. Xenobiotica 2:205–214
189. Hirom PC, Millburn P, Smith RC (1976) Bile and urine as complementary pathways for the excretion of foreign organic compounds. Xenobiotica 6:55–64
190. Hirom PC, Millburn P, Smith RL, Williams RT (1972) Species variations in the threshold molecular-weight factor for the biliary excretion of organic anions. Biochem J 129:1071–1077
191. Iga T, Awazu S, Nogami H (1971) Pharmacokinetic study of biliary excretion. III. Comparison of excretion behavior in xanthene dyes, fluorescein and bromsulphthalein. Chem Pharm Bull (Tokyo) 19:297–303
192. Iga T, Awazu S, Hanano M, Nogami H (1970) Pharmacokinetic studies of biliary excretion. I. Comparison of excretion behavior in azo dyes and indigo carmine. Chem Pharm Bull (Tokyo) 18:2431–2437
193. Ryan AJ, Wright SE (1960) The excretion of some azo dyes in rat bile. J Pharm Pharmacol 13:492–495
194. Sovak M, Barnhart JL, Ranganathan R, Schulze PE, Siefert HM, Speck U (1981) Development and preliminary pharmacological evaluation of a zwitterionic oral cholecystographic agent. Invest Radiol 16:513–516
195. Edholm P, Jacobson B (1959) Quantitative determination of iodine in vivo. Acta Radiol 52:337–346

196. Ravin IS, Johnson CG, Riegel C (1932) Studies of gallbladder function. VII. The anion-cation content of hepatic and gallbladder bile. Am J Physiol 100:317–327
197. Grim E, Smith GA (1957) Water flux rates across dog gallbladder wall. Am J Physiol 191:555–560
198. Diamond JM (1962) The mechanism of solute transport by the gallbladder. J Physiol 161:474–502
199. Wheeler HO (1963) Transport of electrolytes and water across the wall of rabbit gallbladder. Am J Physiol 205:427–438
200. Dietschy JM (1964) Water and solute movement across the wall of the everted rabbit gallbladder. Gastroenterology 47:395–408
201. Frizzell RA, Feld M, Schultz SG (1979) Sodium-coupled chloride transport by epithelial tissues. Am J Physiol 236:F1–F8
202. Frizzell RA, Duffey ME (1980) Chloride activities in epithelia. Fed Proc 39:2860–2864
203. Dietschy JM, Moore EW (1964) Diffusion potentials and potassium distribution across the gallbladder wall. J Clin Invest 43:1551–1560
204. Diamond JM (1971) Standing-gradient model of fluid transport in epithelia. Fed Proc 30:6–13
205. Tormey J McD, Diamond JM (1967) The ultrastructural route of fluid transport in the rabbit gallbladder. J Gen Physiol 50:2031–2060
206. Ivy AC, Oldberg E (1928) Hormone mechanism for gallbladder concentration and evacuation. Am J Physiol 86:599–613
207. Sandblom P, Boegtlin WL, Ivy AC (1935) The effect of cholecystokinin on the choledochoduodenal mechanism. Am J Physiol 113:175–180
208. Yau WM, Makhlouf GM, Edwards LE (1973) Mode of action of cholecystokinin and related peptides on gallbladder muscle. Gastroenterology 65:451–456
209. Amer MS (1972) Studies with cholecystokinin in vitro. III. Mechanism of the effect on the isolated rabbit gallbladder strips. J Pharmacol Exp Ther 183:527–534
210. Jaffee H, Wachowski TJ (1942) Relation of density of cholecystographic shadows on the gallbladder to the iodine content. Radiology 38:43–51
211. Berk RN, Wheeler HO (1972) The role of water reabsorption by the gallbladder in the mechanism of nonvisualization at cholecystography. Radiology 103:37–40
212. Ivy AC (1934) The physiology of the gallbladder. Physiol Rev 14:1–102
213. Berk RN, Lasser EC (1964) Altered concepts of the mechanism of nonvisualization of the gallbladder. Radiology 82:296–302
214. Small DM, Beaudoin M, Shaffer E, O'Brian J, Williams L (1975) The gallbladder and the enterohepatic circulation. In: Advanced bile acid research. Stuttgart, Schattauer
215. Van Berge-Henegouwen GP, Hoffmann AF (1978) Nocturnal gallbladder storage and emptying in gallstone patients and healthy subjects. Gastroenterology 75:879–885
216. Smith RL (1966) The biliary excretion and enterohepatic circulation of drugs and other organic compounds. Prog Drug Res 9:299–360
217. Plaa GL (1975) The enterohepatic circulation. In: Gillette JR, Mitchell JR (eds) Concepts in biochemical pharmacology 3. Berlin, Springer, p 130 (Handbook of experimental pharmacology, vol 28 pt 3)
218. Kent TH, Fischer LJ, Marr R (1972) Glucuronidose activity in the intestinal contents of rat and man and relationship to bacterial flora. Proc Soc Exp Biol Med 140:590–594
219. Bokenbaum HG, Bekersky I, Jack MC, Kaplan SA (1979) Influence of gut microflora on bioavailability. Drug Metab Rev 9:259–279
220. Schroder JS, Rooney D (1953) Excretion of 3(3-amino-2,4,6-triodophenyl)-2-ethyl-propanoic acid (Telepaque) by man. Proc Soc Exp Biol Med 83:544–546
221. Schroder JS, Rooney D (1953) Excretion of 3-(3-amino-2,4,6-triiodophenyl)-2-ethyl-propanoic acid (Telepaque) by man. Proc Soc Exp Biol Med 83:544–546
222. Fischer HW (1966) Physiologic and pharmacologic aspects of cholangiography. Radiol Clin North AM 4:625–632

223. Shames DM, Moss AA (1974) Iodipamide kinetics in the dog. A multicompartmental analysis. Invest Radiol 9:141–148
224. Burgener FA, Fischer HW (1975) Intravenous cholangiography in normal subsequently liver-damaged dogs. Radiology 114:519–524
225. Burgener FA, Fischer HW, Adams JT (1975) Intravenous cholangiography in different degrees of common bile duct obstruction. Invest Radiol 10:342–350
226. Smith PK, Gleason HL, Stoll CG, Ogorzalek S (1946) Studies on the pharmacology of salicylates. J Pharmacol Exp Ther 87:237–255
227. Levy G, Tsuchiya T, Amsel LP (1972) Limited capacity for salicyl phenolic glucuronide formation and its effect on the kinetics of salicylate elimination in man. Clin Pharm Therap 13:258–268
228. Ansell G (1970) Adverse reactions to contrast agents. Invest Radiol 5:374–384
229. Lindgren P, Saltzman GF (1974) Increase of subcapsular renal pressure after intravenous iodipamide and other parenteral contrast media. Acta Radiol (Diagn) 15:273–280
230. Benisek GJ, Gunn JA (1962) A preliminary clinical evaluation of a new cholecystographic medim. Bilopaque. AJR 88:792–796
231. Burhenne HJ (1963) Bilopaque: a new cholecystographic medium. Radiology 81:629–631
232. Han SY, Witten DM (1974) Clinical trial of Bilopaque oral cholecystography. Evaluation of time of optimal and peak opacification of the gallbladder. Radiology 112:529–532
233. Moskowitz H, Milidow E, Osmun GP (1973) Sodium Tyropanoate evaluation of new oral cholecystographic agent. NY State J Med 73:271–277
234. Parks RE (1974) Double blind study of four oral cholecystographic preparations. Radiology 112:525–528
235. White WW, Fischer HW (1962) A double blind study of Oragrafin and Telepaque. AJR 87:745–748
236. Juhl JH, Cooperman LR, Crummy AB (1963) Oragrafin, a new cholecystographic medium. Radiology 80:87–91
237. Hekster REM (1968) Results of comparative radiographic, clinical and clinical-chemical studies in iocetamic acid and iopanoic acid. Radiol Clin Biol 37:338–352
238. Tishler JM, Gold R (1969) A clinical trial of oral cholecystographic agents: Telepaque, sodium Oragrafin and calcium Oragrafin. J Can Assoc Radiol 20:102–105
239. Russell JG, Frederick PR (1974) Clinical comparison of tyropanoate sodium, ipodate sodium and iopanoic acid. Radiology 112:519–523
240. Berndt WO, Mudge GH (1968) Renal excretion of iodipamide. Invest Radiol 3:414–426
241. Lindgren P, Nordenstam H, Slatzman GF (1966) Effects of iodipamide on the kidneys. Acta Radiol (Diagn) 4:129–138
242. Peters GA, Hodgson JR, Donovan RJ (1966) The effect of premedication with chlorpheniramine on reactions to methylglucamine iodipamide. J Allergy 38:74–83
243. Craft IL, Swales JD (1967) Renal failure after cholangiography. Br Med J 2:736–738
244. Rene RM, Mellinkoff SM (1959) Renal insufficiency after oral administration of a double dose of cholecystographic medium; report of 2 cases. N Engl J Med 261:589–592
245. Fink HE, Roenick WJ, Wilson CP (1964) An experimental investigation of the nephrotoxic effects of oral cholecystographic agents. Am J Med Sci 247:201–216
246. Teplick JG, Myerson RM, Sanen FJ (1965) Acute renal failure following oral cholecystography. Acta Radiol (Diagn) 3:353–368
247. Harrow BR, Winslow OP (1966) Renal toxicity following oral cholecystography with Oragrafin. Radiology 87:721–728
248. Canalis CO, Smith GH, Robinson JC (1969) Acute renal failure after the administration of iopanoic acid as a cholecystographic agent. N Engl J Med 281:89–91
249. Meway J, McGeown MG, Kumar R (1970) Renal failure after radiological contrast material. Br J Med 4:717–721

250. Schiro JC, Ricci JA, Tristan TA, Levin DM (1974) Transient renal insufficiency secondary to iopanoic acid. P Med 74:57–58
251. Burgener FA, Fischer HW (1978) Nephrotoxicity of sodium iopanoate in hydrated and dehydrated dogs. Invest Radiol 13:247–254
252. Mudge GH (1970) Some questions of nephrotoxicity. Invest Radiol 5:407–421
253. Scholz RJ, Johnson DO, Wise RE (1975) Intravenous cholangiography: optimum dosage and methodology. Radiology 114:513–518
254. Stillman AE (1974) Hepatotoxic reaction to iodipamide meglumine injection. JAMA 228:1420–1421
255. Sutherland LR, Edwards LA, Medline A, Wilkinson RW, Connon JJ (1977) Meglumine iodipamide (Cholografin) hepatotoxicity. Ann Intern Med 86:437–439
256. Burk RF, Barnhart JL (1979) Iodipamide hepatotoxicity in the rat. Gastroenterology 76:1363–1367
257. Barnhart JL, Berk RN (1979) Reduction in biliary transport of bile salts, iodipamide and iopanoic acid in aging rats. Gastroenterology 77:A4
258. Stanley RJ, Sagel SS, Levite RG (1977) Computed tomography of the liver. Radiol Clin North Am 15:331–348
259. Gold JA, Zeman RK, Schwartz A (1979) Computed tomographic cholangiography in a canine model of biliary obstruction. Invest Radiol 14:498–501
260. Dean PB, Kivisaari L, Kormano M (1978) The diagnostic potential of contrast enhancement pharmacokinetics. Invest Radiol 13:533–540
261. Moss AA, Schrumpf J, Schnyder P (1979) Computed tomography of focal hepatic lesions: a blind clinical evaluation of the effect of contrast enhancement. Radiology 131:427–430
262. Prando A, Wallace S, Bernardino ME (1979) Computed tomographic arteriography of the liver. Radiology 130:697–701
263. Stephens DH, Sheedy II PF, Hattern RR (1977) Computed tomography of the liver. Am J Roentgenol 128:579–590
264. Violante MR, Dean PB (1980) Improved detectability of VX2 carcinoma in the rabbit liver with contrast enhancement in CT scanning. Radiology 134:237–239
265. Dean PB, Biolante MR, Mahoney JA (1980) Hepatic CT contrast enhancement: effect of dose, duration of infusion, and time elapsed following infusion. Invest Radiol 15:158–161
266. Fon GT, Hunter TB, Berk RN, Capp MP (1980) The effect of diet and fasting on gallbladder opacification during oral cholecystography in dogs as measured by computed tomography. Radiology 136:585–593
267. Harson A, Davis MA, Seltzer SE, Paskins-Hurlburt AJ, Hessel SJ (1980) Heavy metal particulate contrast materials for computed tomography of the liver. J Comp Assisted Tomog 4:642–648

CHAPTER 8

Laboratory Techniques for Studying Biliary Contrast Media

J. L. BARNHART

A. Introduction

Little training is provided for researchers in the proper care and handling of laboratory animals, selecting the best species for use in research projects, selecting the proper experimental technique to obtain the data which will provide them with the information needed to answer the questions being asked, or preparing for the technical problems which need to be avoided or anticipated and handled so that the desired project will not be a waste of time, resources, and energy. Sometimes a poor experiment carried out carefully and meticulously will be of some scientific value despite shortcomings in the original experimental design. However, a well-conceived study, regardless of its intellectual clarity and brilliance, will be of little or no value when pursued without the necessary laboratory background or experience, without the proper techniques, and without proper awareness of the possible technical difficulties. Assumptions drawn from data which are obtained using techniques not clearly understood, obtained using improper techniques, and obtained from ignorance of potential difficulties of techniques can lead the researcher to reach mistaken conclusions about the questions being asked.

Each researcher must determine for himself whether the procedural aspects of his research projects are correct and proper. The ultimate responsibility for the outcome of the project must still rest upon the researcher and not on those assigned to do the actual data collection. For this reason it is important that the techniques used in the laboratory are familiar to the investigator at least in principle, if not by actual experience.

The purpose of this chapter is to provide a preliminary guide for those who are not familiar with routine laboratory equipment or with in vivo and in vitro techniques used in studying biliary contrast media (CM) and for those who are not comfortable in handling laboratory animals which are to be used in their research projects. The chapter will cover some basic information concerning the variety of laboratory animals which are readily available for laboratory studies; the proper care, handling, and restraint of these animals in the laboratory; the proper technique for obtaining samples of blood and bile; a variety of in vivo and in vitro animal preparations available for studying biliary CM in animals; some basic information concerning a few laboratory instruments; and some routine assays often utilized by researchers when studying biliary CM.

The limitation of most research projects is that imposed on it by the techniques available. The information provided in this chapter reflects my personal bias and opinion on some established research techniques and procedures. It is provided with the understanding that it serve as a guide to those who have not had the opportunity to spend the necessary time in the laboratory to become familiar and comfortable with preparing animals for experimental studies or with laboratory equipment and techniques.

B. Choice of Animal Species

An increasingly more important role is being placed each year on the use of animal models to gain an understanding of the pathophysiologic mechanism in humans and an understanding for the prevention and control of disease processes in humans. Considerable resources are being expended to support research using experimental animals. At present an enormous amount of information can be found in the literature which is concerned with the use of animals in medical research [1–3]. More complete and detailed information can be obtained from a variety of other sources [4, 5].

Proper care and management of experimental animals during a study are important to the outcome of the study. In addition, there is considerable concern both inside and outside the research community that animals used in research laboratories are not abused or treated in a cruel manner. It is imperative that every research laboratory adopt a code for their laboratory personnel to follow in handling laboratory animals. An excellent code to adhere to is provided by the following principles developed by the American Association of Laboratory Animal Science, the National Academy of Sciences, and the National Society for Medical Research for the care of laboratory animals [6].

1. Animals used for experimental purposes must be lawfully acquired. Standards for their care shall be in strict compliance with federal, state, and local laws, and with pertinent government and institutional regulations.

2. Scientific institutions shall maintain a standing committee, or other appropriate administration body, to set policies and guidelines for the use and care of animals in experiments conducted under their auspices. These policies and guidelines shall be in accordance with the recommendations of the Institute for Laboratory Animal Resources.

3. Experiments involving live animals must be performed by, or under the immediate supervision of, a qualified biological scientist.

4. The housing, care, and feeding of all experimental animals shall be supervised by a properly qualified veterinarian or other biological scientist competent in such matters.

5. All laboratory animals must receive every consideration for their comfort; they must be kindly treated, properly fed, and their surrounds kept in a sanitary condition.

6. In any operation likely to cause greater discomfort than that attending anesthetization, the animal shall first be incapable of perceiving pain and be maintained in that condition until the operation is ended, except that whenever anesthetization would defeat the purpose of the experiment, the experiment must be specifically approved and supervised by the principal investigator in accordance with procedures established by the institutional committee.

a) If an acute study does not require survival, the animal must be killed in a humane manner at the conclusion of the experiment by a procedure that ensures immediate death, in accordance with practices established by the institutional committee. The animal is not to be discarded until its death is certain.
b) If the nature of the study is such as to require survival of the animals, acceptable techniques established by the institutional committee must be followed.
c) The postoperative care of animals must be such as to minimize discomfort during convalescence, in accordance with acceptable practices in veterinary medicine.

These principles must be followed and applied before any animal can be used for research purposes.

A compendium of normal values of several species of experimental animals is valuable since biological investigations must be related to normal and disease states in the human. The ranges of normal values for laboratory animals can provide criteria for the selection of the appropriate laboratory animal for use in the research project. Data in Table 1 are provided as a guide to normal values of various parameters in a number of animal species used in research laboratories. Many factors such as age, sex, nutritional status, and environmental factors affect these average values.

Table 1. Biological data of experimental animals and humans [5]

Species	Average life span (years)	Average age at puberty	Average gestation period (days)	Litter size	Body temperature (°C)	Blood volume (ml/kg body wt.)
Mouse (*Mus musculus*)	4	35 days	4	1–12	36.5	74.5
Rat (*Rattus norvegicus*)	5	50 days	21	1–9	37.3	58.0
Hamster (*Mesocricetus auratus*)	1.9	45 days	18	2–12	36.0	72.0
Guinea pig (*Cavia porcellus*)	6	62 days	68	1–8	37.9	74.0
Rabbit (*Oryctolagus cuniculus*)	13	7 months	30	1–12	38.8	69.4
Dog (*Canis familiaris*)	22	7 months	61	1–12	38.9	92.6
Pig (*Sus scrofa*)	27	7 months	114	4–6	39.3	69.4
Sheep (*Ovis aries*)	20	7.5 months	150	1–4	38.8	58.0
Monkey (rhesus) (*Macaca mulatta*)	29	2.5 years	168	1	38.8	75.0
Man (*Homo sapiens*)	73	13.5 years	278	1	36.9	77.8

Table 2. Constituents present in serum of mouse, rat, hamster, guinea pig, rabbit, dog, pig, sheep, rhesus monkey, and human

Constituents	Mouse mean (range)	Rat mean (range)	Hamster mean (range)	Guinea pig mean (range)
Total protein (g/dl)	6.18 (4.00–8.62)	7.56 (4.70–8.15)	5.20 (5.00–6.80)	5.35 (5.00–6.80)
Albumin (g/dl)	3.03 (2.52–4.84)	3.68 (2.70–5.10)	2.58 (2.10–3.90)	2.58 (2.10–3.90)
Alkaline phosphatase (IU/liter)	19.2 (10.5–27.6)	87.6 (56.8–128)	70.0 (54.8–108)	70.0 (54.8–108)
Alanine transaminase (SGPT) (IU/liter)	13.0 (2.10–23.8)	23.8 (17.5–30.2)	41.7 (24.8–58.6)	41.7 (24.8–58.6)
Aspartate transaminase (SGOT) (IU/liter)	35.8 (23.2–48.4)	63.2 (45.7–80.0)	46.8 (26.5–67.5)	46.8 (26.5–67.5)
Lactic dehydrogenase (LDH) (IU/liter)	134 (75.0–185)	91.2 (61.0–121)	49.5 (24.9–74.5)	49.5 (24.9–74.5)
Bilirubin (mg/dl)	0.72 (0.10–0.90)	0.30 (0.00–0.55)	0.31 (0.00–0.90)	0.31 (0.00–0.90)
Cholesterol (mg/dl)	64.4 (26.0–82.4)	26.5 (10.0–54.0)	29.4 (16.0–43.0)	29.4 (16.0–43.0)
Creatinine (mg/dl)	0.76 (0.30–1.00)	0.48 (0.20–0.80)	1.39 (0.62–2.18)	1.39 (0.62–2.18)
Glucose (mg/dl)	88.6 (62.8–176)	74.5 (50.0–135)	92.2 (82.0–107)	92.2 (82.0–107)
Urea nitrogen (mg/dl)	19.4 (13.9–28.3)	14.6 (5.0–29.0)	23.4 (9.00–31.5)	23.4 (9.00–31.5)
Sodium (mEq/liter)	136 (128–145)	146 (143–156)	124 (120–146)	124 (120–146)
Potassium (mEq/liter)	5.32 (4.85–5.85)	6.26 (5.40–7.00)	4.96 (3.80–7.95)	4.96 (3.80–7.95)
Chloride (mEq/liter)	108 (105–110)	102 (100–110)	94.4 (90.0–115)	94.4 (90.0–115)
Bicarbonate (mEq/liter)	25.5 (20.0–31.5)	22.4 (12.6–32.0)	21.4 (12.8–30.0)	21.4 (12.8–30.0)

Values are means for the male and female of each species and were calculated from data accumulated by MITRUKA and RAWNSLEY [5]

It is important that the animal species be carefully chosen for any experiment in order to prevent the waste of animal lives and the waste of time, effort, and money of the researcher. Many experimental animals have been studied in great detail and much is known about their anatomy, physiology, and biochemistry [1–3, 5, 6]. Modern experimental medicine employs a wide variety of animals and searches continuously for additional animals that may be a better choice in the study of a particular disease. At present, animals that are commonly employed to study biliary physiology and pharmacology fall into the following groups: (a) rodents and rabbits; (b) carnivores such as dogs and cats; (c) ungulates or hoofed animals such as horses, sheep, and goats; and (d) primates.

Rabbit mean (range)	Dog mean (range)	Pig mean (range)	Sheep mean (range)	Rhesus Monkey mean (range)	Man mean (range)
6.80 (6.00–8.30)	6.70 (4.90–9.60)	8.68 (4.80–10.30)	7.00 (5.70–9.10)	7.03 (5.90–8.70)	6.71 (6.60–8.30)
3.22 (2.42–4.05)	3.39 (2.12–4.00)	3.89 (1.80–5.60)	3.76 (2.70–4.55)	3.52 (1.80–4.60)	4.19 (3.50–4.70)
10.2 (4.10–16.2)	17.1 (7.90–26.3)	63.5 (35.0–110)	96.6 (69.5–125)	9.15 (3.00–29.0)	25.0 (19.0–69.0)
64.1 (48.5–78.9)	42.3 (24.5–60.0)	28.0 (10.5–45.0)	42.0 (25.0–70.0)	24.0 (3.50–45.0)	9.71 (6.00–40.0)
70.2 (42.5–98.0)	57.0 (36.0–77.5)	35.8 (30.0–61.0)	81.6 (40.0–123)	28.3 (12.5–44.2)	13.4 (80.0–55.0)
81.4 (33.5–129)	71.8 (30.0–112)	63.5 (32.0–100)	77.5 (44.0–112)	178 (30.0–320)	198 (85.0–283)
0.31 (0.00–0.74)	0.23 (0.00–0.50)	0.18 (0.00–0.60)	0.22 (0.00–0.60)	0.48 (0.50–1.32)	0.74 (0.90–1.10)
25.6 (10.0–80.0)	180 (137–275)	152 (76.0–174)	100 (50.0–140)	140 (100–220)	192 (170–328)
1.63 (0.50–2.65)	1.22 (0.80–2.05)	1.78 (1.00–2.60)	1.88 (0.70–3.00)	1.39 (1.00–2.00)	1.10 (0.80–1.50)
132 (78.0–155)	121 (80.0–165)	87.5 (60.0–136)	88.4 (55.0–131)	82.8 (43.0–148)	97.5 (80.0–120)
18.4 (13.1–29.5)	14.4 (5.00–23.9)	15.2 (8.00–24.0)	26.0 (15.0–36.0)	11.4 (7.00–23.0)	14.0 (8.00–26.0)
144 (138–155)	146 (139–153)	146 (135–152)	152 (140–164)	154 (143–164)	142 (135–155)
6.08 (3.70–6.80)	4.48 (3.60–5.20)	5.90 (4.90–7.10)	5.05 (4.40–6.70)	5.10 (3.79–6.67)	4.25 (3.60–5.50)
103 (92.0–112)	112 (103–121)	102 (94.0–106)	118 (115–121)	113 (103–118)	103 (98.0–109)
23.5 (16.2–31.8)	22.0 (14.6–29.4)	30.2 (24.5–35.0)	26.6 (21.2–32.1)	30.1 (21.5–38.6)	27.5 (22.0–33.0)

Although the principal physiologic and biochemical mechanisms in animals and in humans are similar, considerable variation exists in the normal concentration of the many constituents present in blood. Even within each species a considerable range of values can be found. This is due to differences in age, sex, breed, environment, time of day, and a variety of other factors. Some basic data are provided in Table 2, which shows the normal mean value and normal range of total protein, albumin, some representative enzyme activities, and some of the chemicals found in the serum of the mouse, rat, hamster, guinea pig, rabbit, dog, pig, sheep, monkey, and human.

Of particular interest for studies concerning biliary CM is the rate of bile formation. There is a remarkable variation in the rates of endogenous bile formation

Table 3. Endogenous rates of bile flow in laboratory animals [7]

Species	Bile flow rate (µl/min/kg body wt.)	Ratio of flow rates (animal/man)
Man	3.6	1.0
Dog	5.6	1.5
Cat	13	3.6
Pony	19	5.3
Monkey	20	5.5
Chicken	22	6.1
Sheep	43	11.0
Rat	65	18.0
Mouse	69	19.2
Rabbit	85	23.6
Guinea pig	160	44.4

between laboratory animals (Table 3) [7]. In general, herbivores have higher bile flow rates than other species. A variety of physiologic factors influence the magnitude of these values. However, much of the variation between these endogenous rates of bile production must be attributed to inherent species characteristics. It should also be noted that the rat and pony do not have gallbladders.

C. Anesthesia

Four stages or divisions have been arbitrarily set to describe the depth of consciousness in general anesthesia. These criteria were established by Guedel in 1920 using ether as an anesthetizing agent. This agent does not cause respiratory depression and is unusual in this characteristic [8]. However, the general description of anesthesia using ether as model agent provides a good basis upon which to administer anesthesia to laboratory animals. The stages of general anesthesia are as follows [8]. I. Stage of analgesia – lasts until the animal has lost consciousness. II. Stage of delirium – extends from the loss of consciousness to the beginning of surgical anesthesia. Excitement and involuntary activity may be present to a varying degree. This stage should be reduced to a minimum because of the possible harm from the thrashing of the animal that can be self-inflicted and that can be inflicted on the person administering the anesthetic. III. Stage of surgical anesthesia – this stage extends from the end of stage II until cessation of spontaneous respiration. The transition to stage III can be recognized by: (a) disappearance of the respiratory irregularity of stage II due to the loss of psychic influences and interruption of voluntary pathways; (b) absence of the eyelid and conjunctival reflexes and the fact that the eyelids no longer blink when the lashes are touched; and (c) the loss of pedel reflex when the toes of the hind limb are vigourously sqeezed. Stage III is further divided into four planes, numbered 1 to 4, in order of increasing depth of anesthesia. The major differences in physical signs in the various planes relate to the character of the respiration, the character of the eyeball movements, the presence or absence of certain reflexes, and the size of the pupils [9]. The cessation of all respiratory effort makes the passage from plane 4 to stage IV. IV. Stage of respiratory paralysis – this stage is characterized primarily by respiratory arrest. It is characterized by purely abdominal respiration, dilating pupils with loss of a light reflex, falling blood pressure, and the disappearance of the pink or rosy color of the mucous membranes.

Diethyl ether and barbiturate compounds are widely used as general anesthetics for laboratory animals.

Diethyl Ether. Diethyl ether is a volatile general anesthetic which can be used as the sole anesthetizing agent or as a preanesthetic medication. It is a potent agent which can be used to bring the animal through all planes of surgical anesthesia to respiratory arrest. It has good analgesia so that the animal is not aware of surgical operation. However, it is irritating to the respiratory tract and can cause flow of saliva when under light anesthesia. Ether is absorbed and eliminated from the pulmonary epithelium. This versatile anesthetic can be used safely and effectively. Its effects on a variety of normal body functions must be considered by the researcher, but these effects are in general minor.

Barbiturates. Perhaps the most widely used intravenous general anesthetic agent in experimental animals is the barbiturate class of compounds. Intravenous anesthetics differ from inhalational agents such as diethyl ether in a very practical way. Once injected, there is practically nothing that can be done to facilitate the removal of the injected drug. The temporal course of anesthetic effects from induction and rapidly deepening narcosis to gradual emergence from the anesthetic effect depends almost entirely upon the progressive redistribution of the drug within the body. Usually metabolic degradation and excretion of the anesthetic during the period of anesthetic administration is negligible [10]. The brain receives a large fraction of the initial dose because this tissue is well perfused with blood. As time passes the relatively poorly perfused areas of the body gradually come into equilibrium with the bloodstream content of barbiturate, with the result that the concentration of the anesthetic in the blood gradually declines.

Barbiturates are general depressants and capable of depressing, reversibly, a wide range of biological functions [8]. The central nervous system is quite sensitive to barbiturates and unconsciousness is caused primarily by blocking the central brain-stem core. Barbiturates are potent respiratory depressants, affecting both the drive of respiration and the mechanism responsible for the rhythmic character of respiratory movements [8]. However, when the drugs are given in additive or hypnotic doses, direct actions on peripheral structures are absent or negligible.

Other drugs are used in the laboratory for a variety of purposes. A few of these and some general comments about each are listed below.

Chlorpromazine. This compound gives good sedation and some analgesia when used as a preanesthetic. It reduces the amount of general anesthesia needed but is not always predictable. This drug can serve as an antiemetic and can produce behavioral changes in excited, fractious, unmanageable animals. It has adrenergic-blocking activity and may produce epinephrine reversal. Average dose in dogs is 0.23 mg/kg body wt. given intravenously.

Lidocaine. Lidocaine is a potent local anesthetic with a potency about twice that of an equal concentration of procaine. Systemic side reactions and local irritant effects are few. Some nausea, muscle twitching, and chills have been observed. This drug is used for infiltration anesthesia, for nerve block, and for saddle block anesthesia. Lidocaine is also used on mucous membranes as an aqueous solution or jelly and on minor burns and abrasions as an ointment. Because lidocaine is effective without a vasoconstrictor and is so dissimilar in structure to procaine, it is often the drug of choice where these conditions are indicated.

Morphine. As a preanesthetic, morphine gives good analgesia, good hypnosis, and usually produces emesis which may be indicated prior to surgery. Morphine may be used to control coughing and diarrhea and to alleviate pain. It is sometimes used to treat dyspnea. This drug, however, will develop tolerance and is highly addictive. The usual dose for dogs is 1–1.4 mg/kg body wt., subcutaneous.

Secobarbital Sodium. This drug is very similar to pentobarbital except that it is shorter acting. Its duration of action is approximately 45 min. The recommended dose for dogs os 1 ml/10 kg body wt.

Promazine Hydrochloride. Promazine has the ability of a tranquilizer in reducing excitement without causing depression of the central nervous system to the state of hypnosis. It is used in many experimental animals. It provides a drug for reducing struggle and for facilitating the handling of animals in the laboratory.

Thiopental Sodium. This drug is an ultra-short-acting barbiturate. It is recommended for basal anesthesia, short surgical procedures, physical exams, and radiography. Given at the recommended dosage, this compound has a wide safety margin. Dose depends on use.

Thimylal Sodium. This drug is an ultra-short-acting thiobarbiturate. Its short duration of action in comparison to pentobarbital is believed to be due to the rapidity with which it is absorbed by the fat depots of the body. This compound has few cumulative effects when administered on successive days. The recommended dosage is 3.6 mg/kg body wt.

D. Holding and Restraint

Rats. Holding and restraining rats while administering the anesthetic can cause anxiety. Care should always be practiced when handling rats or any other laboratory animal. Use of gloves is recommended for persons unfamilar in the proper technique of animal handling. Figures 1 and 2 show ways of restraining a rat for intraperitoneal administration of a compound. Notice that the rat is securely restrained without harming the animal. A rat can be transferred from one location to another by its tail. However, be sure to pick the rat up by the middle part of the tail since if picked up by the end the tail will sometimes break or the skin on the tail will come off.

Dogs. Proper restraint of larger experimental animals such as dogs while administering an intravenous anesthetic or collecting a sample of blood is very important. First the hair on the fore paw where the compound will be administered

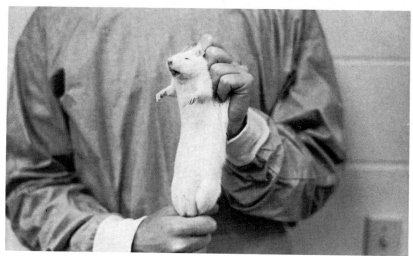

Fig. 1. Technique for holding a rat for intraperitoneal injection

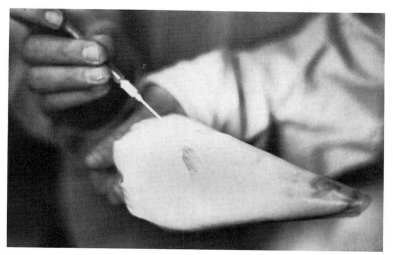

Fig. 2. Polyethylene cone used to restrain a rat

into the cephalic vein should be clipped to obtain an unrestricted view of the skin. The person restraining the dog should have one arm behind the dog's head while holding the dog's muzzle. Secure the leg receiving the injection with the other hand (Fig. 3). Blood flow through the vein should be occluded by the restrainer by placing one's thumb across the cephalic vein in the elbow joint and rolling the thumb outward. The vein should become apparent. If not, pump the dog's paw several times to move more blood into the vein.

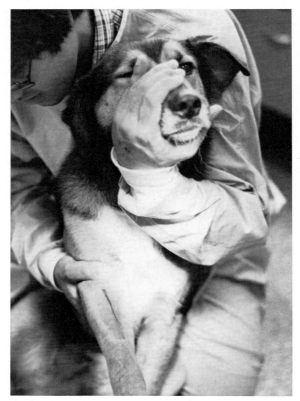

Fig. 3. Restraint of a dog for venipuncture of the cephalic vein

Restraint of dogs for venipuncture of the saphenous (Fig. 4) and the jugular veins (Fig. 5) provides additional techniques for administering compound and for collecting blood from dogs. Most dogs do not object to venipuncture when restrained as shown.

E. Administration of Anesthetic

Rats. Rats and other small laboratory animals can be anesthetized for general surgical procedures with the short-acting volatile liquid, diethyl ether. Place cotton or gauze soaked with ether in the bottom of a closed container made of glass or other transparent material (such as an aquarium) and cover tightly. Allow a few minutes for the ether vapors to saturate the air in the chamber. Rats are placed in the chamber and left until the animal has reached the proper level of anesthesia. The proper level of anesthesia is recognized when the rat lies limply on its side and does not retract its leg when its toe is pinched or blink its eye when the cornea is touched with the tips of a forceps.

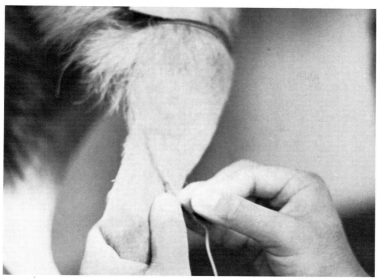

Fig. 4. Restraint of a dog for venipuncture of the saphenous vein

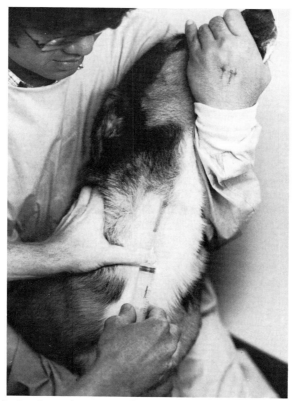

Fig. 5. Restraint of a dog for venipuncture of the jugular vein

After removing the rat from the anesthesia jar, anesthesia can be prolonged using ether by placing a piece of cotton or gauze which is saturated with ether in a small beaker or cone and placing it a few centimeters from the rat's nose so that the animal continually breathes a mixture of air and ether. The level of anesthesia is controlled by moving the ether closer or further from the rat's nose.

Sodium pentobarbital is administered to small laboratory animals such as rats by intraperitoneal injection, that is, into the abdominal body cavity. The anesthetic is absorbed by the intestines and transported to the brain by blood. The best site for injection is the midline of the abdomen and level with the anterior edge of the hind limbs. Feel the rat's abdominal wall for three different layers: (a) the skin, (b) the abdominal muscles, and (c) the intestines. The injection is made by stretching the abdominal wall and sharply inserting a fine-gauge needle (25 gauge) through the skin and muscle layers. Be sure the tip of the needle is through the muscles but free to move in the peritoneal cavity. Draw back on the plunger of the syringe to determine that the tip of the needle is not in a blood vessel and then administer the prescribed dose. Intraperitoneal doses of anesthetic are ofter larger than i.v. doses. Therefore, direct administration of an i.p. dose into a blood vessel will be too large and will probably kill the animal. The anesthetic takes about 15 min to have a maximum effect and should last 60–90 min. If the pentobarbital has not had an effect within 20 min, it is likely that the compound was injected into the intestine, into the urinary bladder, or under the skin. In any of these cases more anesthetic must be administered to obtain general anesthesia. However, the investigator must use his judgment as to how much additional drug to administer. It is best to give a series of small doses until the desired depth of anesthesia is obtained.

The recommended dose for rats is 6 mg/100 g body wt. [If the pentobarbital is in standard injectable form (65 mg/ml), the usual dose is 0.1 ml/100 g body wt.] This is a reasonable guide for determining the appropriate dose to administer to other small laboratory animals. The optimum dose for each species, however, will be slightly different.

Dogs. Administering an i.v. anesthetic to dogs can be relatively easy when the animal is properly restrained. Figures 3–5 illustrate the proper technique in restraining dogs for venipuncture. Clip the hair and clean and sterilize the skin with an alcohol wipe. Insert the needle (20- to 22-gauge) through the skin into the vein. Pull back on the plunger of the syringe to draw a small volume of blood into the syringe. This ensures that the end of the needle is in the vein and not in the surrounding tissue. The person holding the dog should release any pressure on the vein while still securing the leg while the anesthetic is administered in two stages. First, approximately one-half of the dose should be administered quickly. If the dog remains in a stage of delirium, more of the dose should be given. After a few minutes, the remainder of the dose is given in small increments. This is done so that the proper level of anesthesia can be obtained and not passed. If too much drug is administered, there is little that can be done to reverse the situation. However, if the last part of the dose is administered slowly to obtain the desired level of anesthesia, a high degree of success in properly anesthetizing the dog can be expected.

The proper depth of anesthesia for surgery is obtained when the animal's breathing is regular at approximately 10 breaths/min, its pupil reflex is present, and it responds only slightly to pressure placed on the hind paw. Make sure that the dog has not swallowed its tongue and that the airway is free of obstruction. Once anesthetized, the animal should not be left unattended.

The recommended i.v. dose of sodium pentobarbital for the dog is 50–65 mg/kg body wt.

F. Cannulation of Veins

In the rat there are four peripheral veins which are easy to trace and cannulate. These are the two jugular (external) veins in the neck and the two femoral veins in the hind limbs (Fig. 6). The jugular veins are close to both the trachea and carotid artery and are larger in diameter than the femoral veins. However, the jugular vein is short and has a tendency to collapse.

Prepare a length of tubing (PE 50) for cannulation by cutting a smooth tip at one end with a razor blade (scissors will leave a rough edge). Insert a blunt needle into the other end of the tubing. Select the needle size so that the shaft of the needle fits snugly inside the cannula. Saline (0.9% NaCl) containing 500 units heparin/ml should be available to fill the tubing to prevent blood from clotting in the end of the cannula.

Femoral Vein Cannulation. With the rat lying on its back, make a cut about 2 cm long with coarse scissors through the skin overlying the region where the hind limb joins the trunk of the body. This reveals two branches of the femoral vein, one draining the skin and the other the muscles of the hind limb. These two vessels join together and from this point about 1.5 cm of femoral vein can be traced before it enters the body cavity. Clear the connective tissue covering this part of the vein. The vein, artery, and nerve trunk are together in the connective sheath. The artery is smaller than the vein and is lighter in color. The nerve trunk is white. Carfully separate the vein from the nerve and artery by blunt dissection. Place two loose ligatures around the vein. Tighten the ligature on the distal end of the vessel as far away from the body wall as possible while holding back on the proximal ligature. With a pair of fine scissors, make an oblique cut into the vein approximately halfway through the vessel. While holding the free ends of the tightened ligature to provide some support, insert the tip of the cannula into the vein far enough so that the cannula can be secured by tying the other ligature.

Jugular Vein Cannulation. The technique employed in cannulating a jugular vein is exactly the same as those described for the femoral vein. Jugular veins are located superficially along the side of the lower end of the neck (Fig. 7). Although the jugular veins are usually larger in diameter than the femoral veins, they are less muscular and tend to collapse with manipulation. A jugular vein cannula in place in an anesthetized rat is shown in Fig. 8.

Cannulation of Veins in Dogs. Because the veins in dogs are much larger than in rats, the technique for cannulating blood vessels in dogs is easier. The procedure is basically the same as used in rats except that a larger diameter cannula tubing (PE 90 to 160) is used.

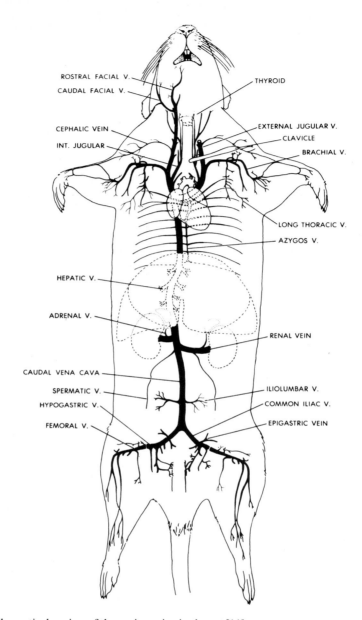

Fig. 6. Schematic drawing of the major veins in the rat [11]

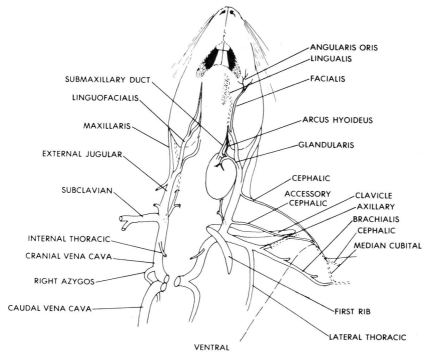

Fig. 7. Schematic drawing of ventral view of cranial veins in the rat [11]

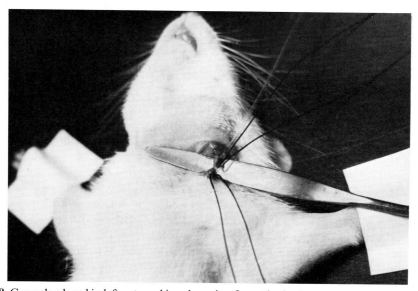

Fig. 8. Cannula placed in left external jugular vein of anesthetized rat

G. In Vivo Animal Preparation

In addition to the standard puncture, cannulation of the bile duct is required for
most studies of the biliary excretion of contrast media. There are anatomic differences in the biliary system between dogs and rats. Dogs have gallbladders while
rats do not, and therefore data in the rat cannot be influenced by this organ. The
steps required to cannulate the rat and dog common bile duct are described below.

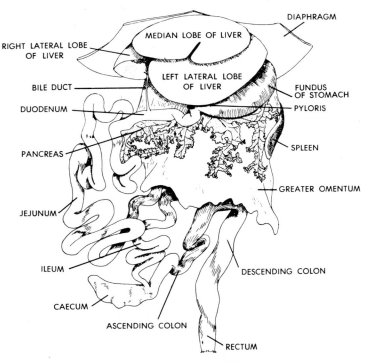

Fig. 9. Schematic drawing of abdominal viscera of rat [11]

Cannulation of Rat Bile Duct. The rat should be properly anesthetized (see
p. 428), placed on its back, and its legs secured to a board. Inasmuch as the rate
of bile flow decreases when body temperature falls [12, 13] it is important to maintain the rat's body temperature near normal using a lamp or a heating pad. Make
a midline incision in the abdominal area from the xiphoid process to the pubic
region. Figure 9 shows the abdominal viscera and the anatomic arrangement of
the bile duct, liver, and duodenum. Find the bile duct in the loop of duodenum that
is tucked under the right side of the intestine near the liver (Fig. 10). The duct appears as a thin, firm vessel. Place two ligatures around the duct approximately
one-half the distance between the liver and the duodenum. The pancreatic duct
joins the bile duct at the distal end and must be avoided in the cannulation. Carefully expose a short (1-cm) segment of the duct and place two loose ligatures

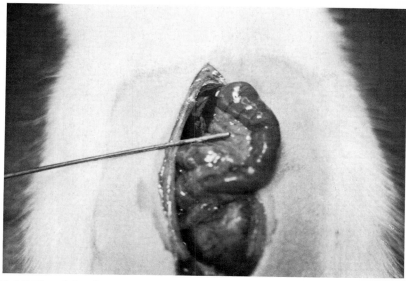

Fig. 10. Midline abdominal incision of a rat with the loop of intestine which contains the common bile duct exposed. The common bile duct is located at the end of the pointer

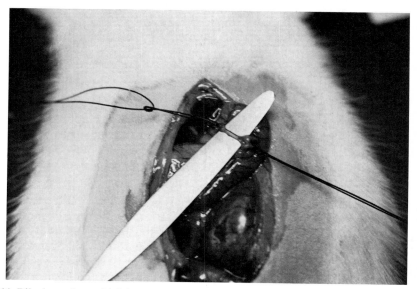

Fig. 11. Bile duct of rat which is exposed and ready for cannulation

around it approximately one-half the distance between the liver and the duo-denum. Support the bile duct from beneath with a spatula blade, tie the distal li-gature (Fig. 11), and make a small hole in the bile duct proximal to the ligature with a sharp needle or fine pair of scissors. Prepare a short piece of polyethylene

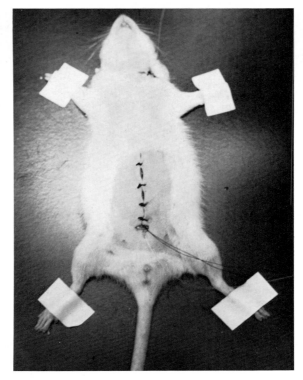

Fig. 12. Anesthetized rat with a cannula in its left external jugular vein and in its bile duct

tubing (PE 10, approximately 20 cm in length) by making a smooth point on one end with a razor blade. The cannula is inserted into the bile duct with a pair of small forceps. The ligature proximal to the point of cannulation is secured to hold the cannula in place. Verify that bile flows freely and close the abdominal incision (Fig. 12).

Cannulation of Dog Bile Duct. Most animal species have a gallbladder. In order to collect hepatic bile quantitatively, the cystic duct of the gallbladder must be ligated. To prepare an acute biliary fistula in a dog, the animal should be anesthetized with a general anesthetic such as sodium pentobarbital. Secure the dog on its back by tying its legs to the surgery table. Clip the hair in the abdominal area as close to the skin as possible. Place an appropriate-sized tracheal cannula in the dog's air passage to aid in the animal's unobstructed breathing. This is especially important if the animal is to be kept anesthetized for more than an hour. Mucus tends to accumulate with time in the trachea when the dog is on its back. This can lead to problems in maintaining an open passage for free and easy breathing.

A midline laparotomy is performed to expose the liver and gallbladder and bile duct. This is accomplished by cutting the skin from the xiphoid of the throxic area to the pubic region. To avoid excessive bleeding, carefully cut through the abdominal muscle layers along the linea alba. The linea alba appears as a whitish line along the abdominal midline and is avascular. If the incision is not made along the midline, muscle tissue will be cut and this will result in bleeding. The free flow of blood from severed vessels should be stopped by tying with suture thread or clamped with hemostats. Small vessels from which blood seems only to ooze slowly can be ignored. These vessels will stop bleeding due to the blood-clotting mechanism.

Once the midline abdominal incision has been completed, the next step is to ligate the cystic duct which leads from the gallbladder to the common bile duct. In the dog the gallbladder and the cystic duct are sometimes attached to the liver. Therefore, care should be exercised in the placement of the ligature around the cystic duct to avoid tearing the liver parenchyma, causing excessive bleeding and injury to the hepatic tissue. Next, locate the common duct and follow the duct from the cystic duct to the duodenum. Sometimes more than one bile duct can be found in the dog. Once the common bile duct is identified, place a ligature around it near the duodenum. Place a second ligature proximal to the first and free the tissue from around the duct between the two ligatures. Secure the distal ligature, cut a small opening in the duct between the two ligatures, insert a piece of tubing (PE 10) into the common duct, and secure the proximal ligature. Take care in the final positioning of the cannula in the common duct so that the end of the cannula is not in either the right or left hepatic ducts. These ducts are found proximal to the cystic duct and drain bile from the right and left lobes of the liver before joining to form the common bile duct. Once the position of the cannula is verified, secure the cannula in place by placing additional ligatures around the duct and cannula. Close the incision and collect bile from the cannula. Be sure to maintain the proper level of anesthesia throughout the surgery and throughout the study. Also, body temperature should be maintained near normal using a heating pad or lamp.

Chronic Preparations. Considerable data concerning biliary CM have been obtained from dogs fitted with a Thomas cannula [14–20]. One design of Thomas cannula used in dogs is illustrated in Fig. 13. This technique requires the removal of the gallbladder and the placement of the cannula through the abdominal wall and through one side of the duodenum across from the Papilla of Vater [21]. The common bile duct enters the duodenum through this papilla. If the Thomas cannula is placed correctly, removal of the cannula stopper exposes the duodenum and the papilla of Vater. The dog can be taught to lie on its side while a piece of tubing is passed through the opening in the Thomas cannula and inserted into the common duct through the papilla. Thus, the dog can be used in many studies provided sufficient time has lapsed between studies for the dog to recover from the previous study. These studies can be performed with the dog alert and awake or anesthetized. My personal bias is to perform the study with the dog awake to avoid any possible complication in interpreting the data caused by the anesthetic drug being used.

Placement of the bile duct cannula requires the dog to lie quietly on its left side with the Thomas cannula easily accesible. Remove the plug from the Thomas cannula and aspirate any intestinal contents present around the papilla. Some-

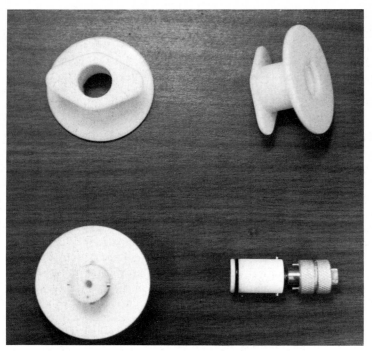

Fig. 13. Thomas cannula designed by Milton Bates and made of Teflon. The outside rim is 50 mm in diameter; the center hole is 16 mm in diameter; the distance between the outer and inner rims is 18 mm; the thickness of the rims is 4 mm

times it is difficult to find the papilla. The best way to avoid this difficulty is by having the Thomas cannula properly placed in the duodenum at the time of surgery. If the papilla is not in the field of vision when the plug of the cannula is removed, it is not possible to place a cannula into the bile duct. After locating the papilla, insert a surgical probe through the papilla into the common duct. The path through the papilla and into the duct is slightly upward and to the right. Therefore, the probe should have a slight curve at the end to facilitate its entry. The polyethylene tubing (PE 50) used to cannulate the bile duct is put through the middle of a cork stopper which fits into the hole of the Thomas cannula. Next insert the cannula into the bile duct about 6–8 cm. Slide the cork into the hole of the Thomas cannula to hold the bile duct cannula in place (Fig. 14). Stand the dog in position supported with a heavy canvas sling (Fig. 15). If bile does not flow readily, a little suction on the bile duct cannula is sometimes needed to get the flow of bile started.

Surgical Preparation of Thomas Cannula. The surgical preparation of Thomas-cannulated dogs should be performed by an accomplished surgeon. The following surgical procedure is used to fit a dog with a Thomas cannula. The dog is anesthetized and a laparotomy performed. The gallbladder is removed. The

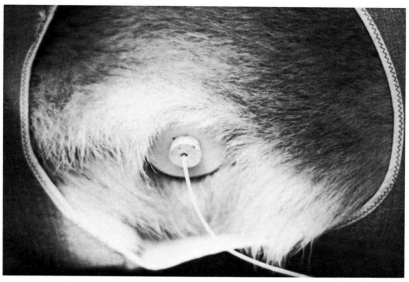

Fig. 14. Thomas cannula with a piece of tubing inserted into the common bile duct of a dog

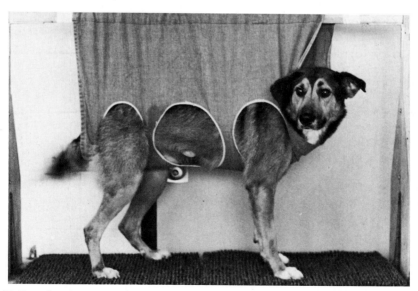

Fig. 15. Dog fitted with Thomas cannula is stationed with a canvas sling in an upright position

common bile duct is located and traced to its entry point into the duodenum. The wall of the duodenum directly across from the anticipated location of the papilla of Vater is cut to expose the intestinal mucosa. Locate the papilla and insert a small piece of tubing into the bile duct to verify its identity (Fig. 16).

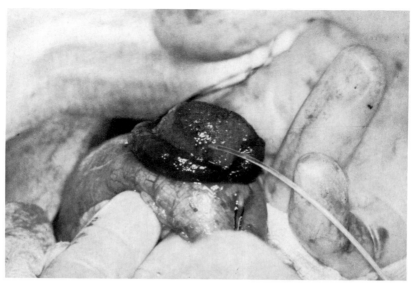

Fig. 16. Loop of dog intestine which has been cut to expose the papilla of Vater. A piece of tubing has been inserted through the papilla into the common bile duct

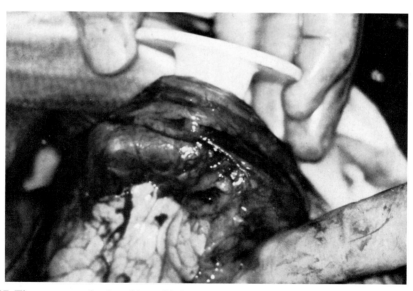

Fig. 17. Thomas cannula placed into the dog duodenum

The next step for placing the Thomas cannula in place is very critical. After positioning the cannula so that the hole in the cannula is directly over the papilla, the cannula is secured in place (Fig. 17). The outer rim of the cannula is exteriorized through an opening through the side of the right abdominal wall (Fig. 18).

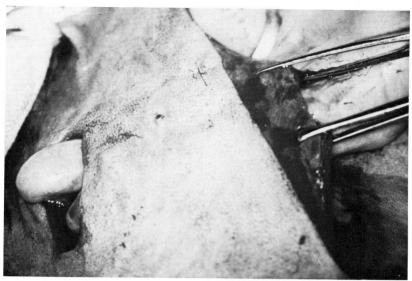

Fig. 18. Opening in the dog's right abdominal wall through which the outer rim of the Thomas cannula is exteriorized

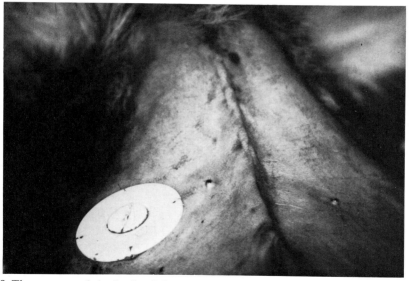

Fig. 19. Thomas cannula in the dog following its surgical placement

The incisions should be closed (Fig. 19) and the dog allowed 3–4 weeks to recover from the surgical procedure.

T-Tube Chronic Fistula. In many large animals it is not possible to use the Thomas cannula, for both practical and technical reasons. However, if a chronic biliary preparation is desired in these animals, a "T-tube" cannula can be used. Again it is important, as it was with the Thomas cannula preparation, that an accomplished surgeon be responsible for all the surgical steps involved in fitting the animal with a T-tube. The initial surgical procedure requires a laporotomy and the removal of the gallbladder. Next the short portion of the T-tube is inserted into the common bile duct through a slit cut parallel to the bile duct. In some species the common bile duct is only a few centimeters in length. Placement of the T-tube into the duct can be difficult. Suture the tube in place. The long end of the cannula is exteriorized through the right abdominal wall and plugged. The animal is allowed to recover from the surgery.

The cannula should be cleared of any material that may plug it by allowing the cannula to drain for a short period at least once a week. If the cannula becomes plugged, carefully pass sterile saline through the tube. It is often necessary to tape the exteriorized end of the cannula to the side of the animal so that the cannula will not be pulled out by the animal's scratching or chewing of the cannula. Data obtained from sheep and horses fitted with T-tube biliary cannulas have been published [22–25].

H. In Vitro Liver Preparations

Isolated Rat Liver Perfusion. An established technique for studying hepatic physiology, biochemistry, and pharmacology is perfusion of isolated rat liver. Hepatic metabolism and function are studied in an in vitro situation in which circulating medium is perfused through the liver. This system makes possible the regulation of liver perfusion parameters and provides a convenient means for analyzing hepatic metabolic function within the controllable conditions established by perfusion. However, today the investigator has several choices as to the type of perfusion system to use. The basic choices include whether to remove the liver from the rat or to perfuse the liver in situ and whether to use apparatus which provides for hydrostatic pressure or pump-driven flow of the perfusion medium.

Most of the techniques for isolated rat liver perfusion currently found in the literature are modifications of the procedure introduced by Miller et al. [26]. The modification by Hems et al. [27] of the Miller technique in which the liver is determined by hydrostatic pressure will be the basis for the following description for perfusing isolated rat livers.

Animals. Rats weighing 150–300 g serve as liver donors. Anesthesia is with pentobarbital sodium or with diethyl ether.

Perfusion Medium. Perfusion medium contains (a) physiologic saline prepared as follows: 100 vols 0.9% NaCl, 4 vols 1.15% KCl, 3 vols 1.22% $CaCl_2$, 1 vol 2.11% KH_2PO_4, 1 vol 3.8% $MgSO_4 \cdot 7H_2O$, and 21 vols 1.1% $NaHCO_3$; (b) bovine serum, fraction V (BSA); and (c) washed bovine blood cells. Freshly drawn bovine blood is centrifuged at 200 g for 10 min. The plasma and buffy layers are removed by suction. The cells are washed twice with 0.9% NaCl and once with physiologic saline. The washing solution is separated and removed from the cells by centrifugation at 2,000 g for 10 min.

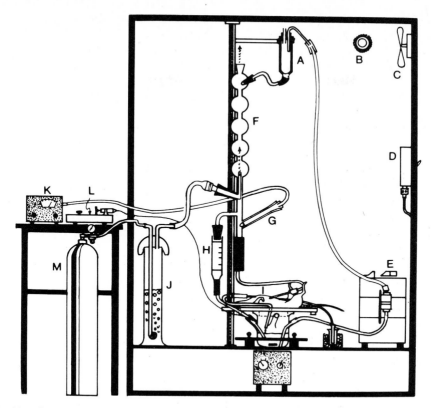

Fig. 20. Diagram of the apparatus used to perfuse isolated rat livers. The perfusion apparatus is housed in a thermostatically controlled environmental chamber which measures $76 \times 91 \times 117$ cm. *A*, filter strains medium before entering liver; *B*, cone coil heater heats chamber to specified temperature; *C*, fan moves air across heater to maintain uniform temperature throughout chamber; *D*, control panel; *E*, pulsatile pump moves perfusion medium from reservoir to filter; *F*, film oxygenator provides surface for oxygenating red blood cells; *G*, temperature probe monitors temperature of medium; *H*, perfusion flowmeter measures overflow rate to provide an indirect measure of perfusion flow; *I*, rat; *J*, oxygen scrubber humidifies gas to minimize evaporation of perfusion medium; *K*, thermostat controls the temperature of perfusion medium by regulating heater; *L*, infusion pump provides continuous infusion of test compounds; *M*, bottled gas, 95% oxygen/5% carbon dioxide

The volume of medium needed for each perfusion is 120 ml. Heparin (100 units) and antibiotic (0.1 ml Combiotic) are added to 100 ml physiologic saline. The desired amount of BSA (0–4 g/dl) is dissolved in this solution. Washed red blood cells from 60 ml bovine blood are combined with the physiologic saline-BSA solution. The pH of the medium is adjusted to 7.4 with 0.25 M NaOH or 0.25 M HCl. If the medium is not being used immediately, it should be covered and refrigerated at 4 °C. Every effort should be made to reduce bacterial contamination since the solution is a very good growth medium for microorganisms. Storage of medium for longer than 24 h is not recommended because no glucose has been added for red blood cell metabolism, and excess antibiotic needed to

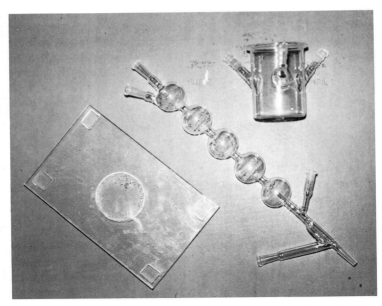

Fig. 21. Rat board, perfusion oxygenator, and perfusion medium reservoir used in isolated rat liver perfusion

control bacterial growth may affect perfusion results. Each investigator should establish a standard method for the collection, preparation, and use of red blood cells in the perfusion. Although bovine red blood cells are used in this method, other workers have used rat cells or human cells obtained from banked blood no longer suitable for transfusion. Use of fresh bovine erythrocytes greatly reduces hemolysis during perfusion (a problem when aged human cells are used). The inconvenience and expense of bleeding ten or more rats for each perfusion is also avoided.

Perfusion Apparatus. The basic perfusion apparatus used is as described by HEMS et al. [27]. It is housed in a thermostatically controlled environmental chamber. Figure 20 shows the complete perfusion apparatus.

The rat board is made of 1.3-cm Plexiglas (15×23 cm) (Fig. 21). A circular piece of Plexiglas attached to the center of the board provides the stability needed for placing the board on top of the medium reservoir. The reservoir consists of a 7.6×10.2-cm jar with three side arms equally spaced (Fig. 21). The reservoir is held in place by a Plexiglas square with a 7.6-cm hole raised above the platform directly beneath the reservoir. The total length of the oxygenator is 43 cm with the bulbs 4.4 cm in diameter (Fig. 21). The flowmeter is made from a 25-ml pipette. Flexible plastic tubing (Tygon: outer diameter, 0.5 cm) is used to connect the plastic tubing to the pump, filter, and flowmeter. Other connections to the oxygenator are made with ground glass fittings.

Preliminary Start-up Procedure. After the animal has been anesthesized, the apparatus must be made ready to receive the liver for perfusion immediately after surgery. This entails circulating the medium, bringing the chamber to the correct temperature, bubbling oxygen through the scrubber, and stirring the reservoir medium with the magnetic stirrer. The glassware and tubing are thoroughly rinsed with water before assembling. A screw clamp under the filter is adjusted to keep the filter from completely emptying during each cycle of the pump. This helps to prevent foaming of the medium in the oxygenator and fluctuations of the perfusion pressure. A screw clamp is also attached to the rubber tubing beneath to oxygenator to prevent the medium from foaming. Thus, connecting the cannulated animal into the perfusion circuit can be performed quickly and easily.

Surgical Procedures. The animal is taped to the board so that the hole in the board is between the worker and the right side of the animal on its back. This allows correct positioning for cannulation and subsequent tube placement.

The skin on the right hind leg is cut to expose the femoral vein. Heparin (100 units) is injected with a small needle and syringe. Heparin prevents the animal's blood from clotting in the liver during the surgical and hook-up procedures.

The abdominal cavity is opened with a midline incision from the pubic area to the xiphoid. The intestines are gently removed from the abdominal cavity and placed on the animal's left side. Laying the intestines on a 10×10-cm moist gauze sponge helps to prevent their drying during surgery. The hepatic portal vein, inferior vena cava, right kidney, and bile duct should be exposed. A loose ligature is placed around the vena cava just cranial to the right renal vein.

The bile duct is cannulated with a 20-cm length of polyethylene tubing (PE 10) beveled with a sharp razor blade to provide a smooth pointed end. The bile duct is isolated, supported on the underside with a pointed spatula blade (Fig. 11), and ligated at a point just distal to the exposed area. With the aid of a dissecting microscope, a fine-gauge needle (25 G) is used to open the bile duct. The cannula is inserted into the bile duct with a pair of small forceps. A ligature is tied proximal to the point of cannulation to hold the cannula in place. Verify that bile flows freely from the cannula and trim the ends of the ligatures. The cannula is taped to the left hind leg in order to keep it out of the way during the remainder of the surgical procedure.

The hepatic portal vein is prepared for cannulation by carefully isolating the vein and placing two loose ligatures around it. These ligatures should be approximately 1 cm apart and 3–5 cm distal to the point where the vein divides to enter separate lobes of the liver.

The remainder of the surgical procedure should be done quickly and smoothly. The blood flow to the liver is interrupted from this point in time until the liver is inserted into the perfusion circuit. The remaining steps include (a) portal vein cannulation, (b) vena cava cannulation, (c) ligation of the vena cava at the area of the right renal vein, and (d) insertion of cannulated liver preparation into the perfusion circuit. With practice, this time lapse can be held to around 1 min.

A small pair of hemostats is placed around the portal vein to stop blood flow and to provide support for the cannulation. The vein is held firmly with fine-tipped forceps while a small cut is placed in the vein between the forceps and hemostats using fine-pointed scissors. The cannula (PE 190) is inserted and firmly tied. The tip of the cannula should not be against the liver tissue. The thorax is immediately opened with scissors from the diaphragm to the neck region. The phrenic nerves are cut. A ligature is placed under the vena cava between the heart and diaphragm. The cannula (PE 240) is pushed through the right atrium into the vena cava until the tip of the cannula reaches the diaphragm. The cannula is secured with the ligature.

The loose ligature which was placed earlier around the vena cava in the abdominal cavity is secured. The animal is transferred to the perfusion apparatus where the liver is placed into the perfusion circuit.

Final Start-up Procedure. Figure 22 is a diagram of the perfusion apparatus after completion of the hook-up procedure. The portal cannula is connected to the tubing coming from the oxygenator and the vena cava is connected to a piece

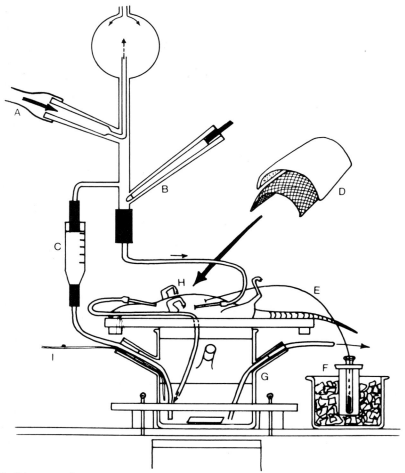

Fig. 22. Diagram of apparatus after starting perfusion of rat liver. *A*, gas inlet; *B*, temperature probe; *C*, overflow meter; *D*, wire cage and moist gauze sponge; *E*, bile duct cannula; *F*, bile collection tube and ice bath; *G*, medium reservoir; *H*, rat; *I*, tubing from infusion pump

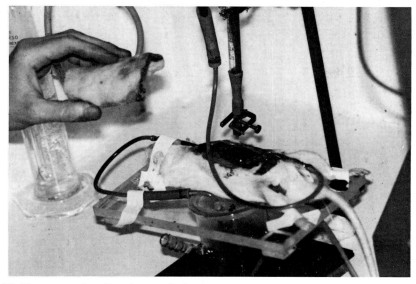

Fig. 23. Placement of rat liver into perfusion apparatus

of tubing which returns the perfused medium to the reservoir. Careful attention should be given to avoid twisting either cannula since this will restrict flow through the liver. Taping the cannula in place helps to avoid this problem. After establishing the proper alignment to allow free flow of bile, the cannula is taped to the animal. This step avoids unwanted movement of the cannula during the collection of bile.

The screw clamp previously placed on the inlet tubing is removed, placed under the overflow meter, and adjusted to keep the overflow tubing full, thus preventing the medium from foaming.

The intestines are removed. This eliminates any influence they might have on liver position and temperature. A moist sponge on a wire cage is placed over the liver (Fig. 23). The entire area is covered with a piece of thin plastic wrap in order to minimize moisture loss and to provide a humid environment for the liver. Thus, the liver is enclosed in a separate, well-defined chamber with a humid environment.

Perfusion Measurements and Sampling (Fig. 24). Bile is collected in pre-weighed tubes which are placed in an ice bath. Tubes are changed at periodic intervals. Samples of the circulating medium are taken with a syringe and needle from the rubber tubing under the oxygenator or from the rubber tubing in the exit flow before returning to the medium reservoir. Thus, samples can be taken before and/or after flow through the liver.

The rate of medium flow through the liver is determined by the pressure difference formed by the distance between the overflow outlet on the oxygenator and the portal cannula. It can be changed by moving the oxygenator in the appropri-

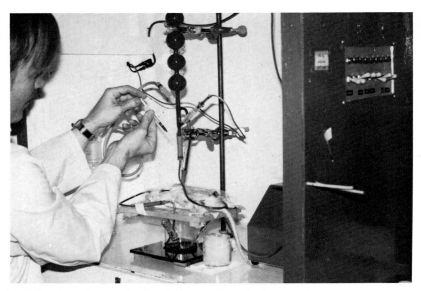

Fig. 24. Collection of a sample of perfusion medium during a study

ate direction. This flow rate is determined indirectly to avoid disrupting flow through the liver. Since the pump is working at a set rate, the overflow rate provides sufficient information to calculate the perfusion rate by difference.

Material can be added or removed from the reservoir through one of the side arms. Compounds are also continuously added to the medium by an infusion pump placed outside the chamber. Tubing from the pump is placed through a hole in the side of the chamber and into the medium.

At the completion of the experiment, the apparatus should be completely disassembled. The oxygenator and reservoir are washed with water and stored with cleaning solution (sodium dichromate and concentrated sulfuric acid). The filter is washed with water and stored in a graduated cylinder filled with a detergent or KOH solution. Some may want to discard the filter after each use. All tubing and cannulas are washed and stored in water or in dilute chemical disinfectant. The filter and tubing are periodically replaced. Proper cleanup helps to avoid technical problems which will arise in subsequent perfusions.

Isolated Hepatocytes. Increasingly, isolated hepatocytes are being utilized to study biological phenomena and have contributed to the understanding of cellular functions, transport, and metabolism. Isolated cell preparations provide the investigator with several advantages, such as: the functions of cells can be studied in the absence of other cells, the medium surrounding the cells can be controlled precisely, many samples can be taken from a single batch of cells, and several studies can be performed with a single batch of cells.

The preparation of isolated hepatocytes from liver requires a method that ruptures intracellular bonds and "tight junctions." A major advance in preparing isolated hepatocytes accompanied the introduction of a mixture of collagenase and hyaluronidase to digest these intracellular junctions without seriously affecting the structure of the plasma membrane. Subsequently, BERRY and FRIEND introduced a method of recirculating the enzyme solution through the liver, which made recoveries of hepatocytes from the liver of greater than 60% both possible and routine [28]. This technique has promise as a tool for better characterization of the hepatic transport mechanisms of radiographic agents.

These isolated cells are used in studies as obtained immediately after their preparation or after they form a monolayer of cells on a culture plate. Both techniques are utilized extensively. The basic difference in preparing cultured hepatocytes is that the cells are placed in culture plates for at least a day to allow the cells to stick or form a layer of cells which are attached to the bottom of the dish. There are numerous variations to the basic technique for isolating hepatocytes and for forming monolayer plates of hepatocytes. No single method has been accepted as the best or preferred technique. Therefore, the following description of the technique for isolating and plating rat hepatocytes is offered as an introduction to this very popular technique.

The technique to be described for preparing isolated cells is a modification of that used by BERRY and FRIEND [28] as reported by HATOFF and HARDISON [29]. Rats weighing from 150 to 250 g are anesthetized with ether, and a midline laparotomy is performed. The absominal area is sterilized with ethanol and shaved prior to surgery. The inferior vena cava is ligated just above the right renal vein and the portal vein cannulated with a 14 G catheter for inlet of buffer. Infusion of calcium-free Hank's balanced salt solution (HBSS) is begun immediately. The thorax is opened and the superior vena cava cannulated through the right atrium for drainage. Approximately 100 ml HBSS at 39 °C is perfused through the liver and discarded. Next, 50 ml 0.5% collagenase (with high clostripain activity in addition to the usual trypsin/protease activity) in HBSS containing 3 mM CaCl$_2$ (39 °C) is recirculated in situ for 20 min. The recirculating apparatus need not be as sophisticated as was described above in the discussion of the perfused liver technique. The liver is then removed, minced into 25 ml sterile collagenase solution, and shaken gently for 10 min at 37 °C. The supernatant fluid containing parenchymal and nonparenchymal hepatic cells was removed and placed into 10 ml culture medium. [Culture medium used in this preparation is Eagle's basal medium (BEM) containing heat-inactivated horse serum 16% (v/v), sodium bicarbonate 20 mM, 10 mM HEPES buffer, 250 U/liter insulin, 100,000 U/liter penicillin G, 100 mg/liter streptomycin, and 250 µg/liter amphotericin B.] The remaining undigested tissue is treated with additional collagenase and the process repeated. The supernatants are combined and placed in a refrigerated centrifuge at 4 °C. The centrifuge is stopped just as 500 g (1,500 rpm) centrifugation is reached. The supernatant, containing mostly nonparenchymal cells, is discarded and the pellet washed twice with 20 ml culture medium. This preparation is again centrifuged at 500 g and the supernatant removed. Cells are resuspended in about 20 ml culture medium.

The viability of the isolated cells is determined by staining with trypan blue. One hundred microliters of cell suspension is placed in 1 ml 0.9% NaCl solution with 2.5 mg/ml trypan blue. Cells are counted in a standard hemocytometer chamber. Those cells excluding trypan blue are considered viable with intact membranes. Those cells that take up trypan blue are considered to have leaky membranes and not viable. Yields should be around 100 million cells per gram liver with greater than 90% exclusion of trypan blue. These isolated cells can be used in studies for up to 2–3 h after their preparation or they can be used to make primary cultures.

To make culture plates, cell suspensions are made to contain 350,000 cells/ml and 1.5 ml is plated in plastic tissue culture dishes (26 × 33 mm well). These plates are maintained in a 37 °C incubator (5% CO_2, 95% air). Cells form a confluent monolayer in the bottom of the dish after 1 day.

From 1–3 days after plating the isolated cells, transport or metabolism studies can be performed. The plates are removed from the incubator and washed three times with 37 °C phosphate-buffered saline. One milliliter of Hanks-Hepes buffer is added to each plate, which is allowed to equilibrate in a 37 °C water bath for 10 min. At this time the test compound is added and incubated for the prescribed time interval. The reaction is stopped by washing the cells three times with cold saline, and the cells are removed from the plate with 1 ml 0.2 M NaOH.

Subcellular Fractionation of Liver [30]. The interest by the biochemist in the subcellular function of cells has brought forth a variety of techniques designed to study individual subfractions and components of the cell. This has resulted in studies concerning the hepatic metabolism, distribution, binding, and excretion of a large number of endogenous and exogenous compounds. The techniques require the preparation of subcellular fractions by homogenizing liver tissue and subsequently separating the various cellular components by differential centrifugation. This section will provide a general description of the technique for preparing a liver homogenate and for fractionating the homogenate into cellular mitochondrial, microsomal, and cytosolic fractions [30].

Preparation of Liver Homogenate. Rats are anesthetized with ether and their livers perfused in situ with approximately 20 ml ice-cold buffer A [50 mM Tris-HCl (pH 7.5), 25 mM KCl, 5 mM $MgCl_2$, 250 mM sucrose]. This can be done using a 20-ml syringe with a # 18 gauge needle and injecting the buffer through the portal vein after the vena cava or the femoral veins are cut. This allows an outflow for blood and for the injected buffer. Add 2–10 ml buffer A/g liver and disrupt the tissue using a Teflon pestle and glass homogenizer tube. The homogenizer tube is moved up and down relative to the stationary pestle through 8–12 excursions. The pestle rotates rapidly so that this process yields a homogenate consisting of dilute cell sap, nuclei, mitochondria, microsomes, and some unbroken cells. It is easier and faster to homogenize a number of small pieces of liver rather than a few large pieces. In addition, homogenization should be done in the cold and as quickly as possible.

Preparation of Subcellular Fractions. Preparation of the subcellular fractions is accomplished by differential centrifugation of the liver homogenate. All centrifugations are performed at 4 °C. First, the crude homogenate is filtered through two layers of nylon gauze. This will eliminate any large fragments not adequately homogenized. To obtain the cytosoli and microsomal fractions, centrifuge the homogenate at 18,000 g for 15 min. The pellet is discarded. The supernatant is centrifuged for 120 min at 100,000 g. The resulting supernatant is the cytosolic or soluble fraction of the liver. The pellet contains the microsomes. To remove adsorbed cytosolic proteins, the microsomal pellet is resuspended in buffer A containing 200 mM KCl but no sucrose and centrifuged at 100 g for 50 min. The resulting pellet is resuspended in buffer A and is the microsomal fraction.

Nuclear and mitochondrial fractions are obtained using a similar technique as described above. The liver is perfused free of blood using buffer B [20 mM Tris-HCl (pH 7.45), 3 mM MgCl$_2$, 320 mM sucrose] and is homogenized as described. The homogenate is centrifuged at 800 g for 10 min. This pellet is twice resuspended in buffer B and centrifuged at 800 g for 10 min. The pellet is the nuclear preparation. The supernatant from the first nuclear pellet contains the mitochondria. This solution is centrifuged at 7,000 g for 10 min. The pellet is resuspended in 0.25 M sucrose/1 mM MgCl$_2$ and centrifuged at 24,000 g for 10 min. This centrifugation is repeated. The pellet is resuspended in the sucrose/MgCl$_2$ solution and is the mitochondrial preparation.

J. Instrumental Methods of Analysis

I. Spectrophotometer [31]

Spectrophotometers are instruments designed for measuring absorption of radiant energy levels at specified wavelengths. A spectrophotometer capable of absorbing light in the ultraviolet (190–360 nm) and visible (340–700 nm) range of the spectrum is one of the most versatile instruments found in most experimental laboratories. These instruments have a stable light source (a tungsten lamp for the visible range and a deuterium source for the ultraviolet region) which is set to beam a light of a particular wavelength through a test solution. Light energy which passes through the solution is caught by a photoelectric cell and converted into an electrical signal that is projected upon a scale.

The intensity of the light passing through a solution depends on how thick a layer of material the light has to traverse and the concentration of the absorbing material in the solution. These two relationships are expressed in the Law of Lambert and Beer.

$$\text{Log}\, I_o/I = kCd$$

where I_o is the intensity of light entering the solution, I is the intensity of light emerging from the solution, C is the concentration of solution in grams per liter, d is the diameter of the cuvette or length of the light path through the solution, and k is a constant depending on the wavelength of light, temperature, and nature of solution.

Transmittance is the ability of a solution to transmit light and is equal to I/I_o. The term *absorbance* (A) or *optical density* (OD) is the negative logarithm of transmittance. Therefore, $A = kCd$, and a linear relationship exists between absorbance and the concentration of solute in solution. Cuvettes usually have the same path length (1 cm) and d becomes a constant which may be included in the value for k so that $A = aC$. The value for a (absorptivity or extinction coefficient) depends on the wavelength of light selected. However, at a given wavelength there is a lin-

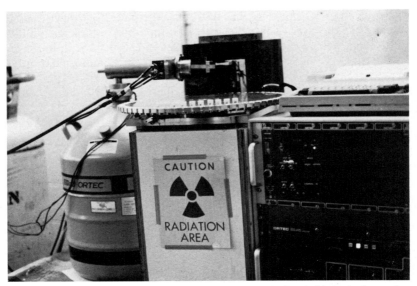

Fig. 25. Fluorescent excitation equipment used to analyze iodine in biological samples

ear relationship between the absorbance and concentration of solute in solution. Therefore, compounds which absorb light in the ultraviolet or visible spectrum can be quantitated.

II. Fluorescent Excitation Analysis [32]

Fluorescent excitation analysis (FEA) is used to measure the concentration of iodine in a variety of biological tissues such as blood, bile, and urine (Fig. 25). FEA is a form of X-ray energy spectrometry and is a technique for identification and quantification of elements. The basis of its function is the electronic makeup of atoms. The atom is a spherical shell which consists of negatively charged electrons bound to a positively charged nucleus by an electrostatic force in well-defined orbits, or shells. The binding energy of these electrons is the minimum energy required to lift an electron free of the nucleus. The energy of a given shell is related to the charge of the nucleus (atomic number). The removal of an electron out of its shell and from the atom constitutes an excitation of the atom, raising its energy from the stable state. Electrons from a higher shell will transfer to the vacant site to try to regain a stable energy configuration. This is accomplished by emission of electromagnetic radiation (photon) which carries an amount of energy equal to the energy difference between the two electron shells. In X-ray energy spectroscopy, this emission is detected and is a measure of the emitted energy.

Iodine is measured in biological fluids and tissues using the principles of X-ray energy spectrometry. Figure 26 shows the functional components of an FEA system designed to measure iodine. A radioactive source, ^{241}Am, excites the sample containing iodine. This results in the emission of characteristic fluorescent X-ray line spectra of iodine. The X-rays from the specimen are incident on a semicon-

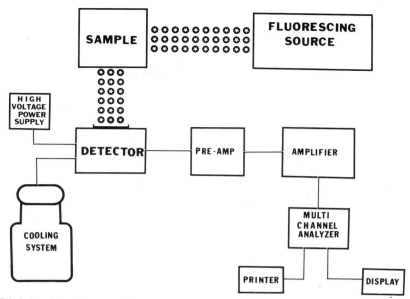

Fig. 26. Schematic diagram of components comprising the fluorescent excitation analysis apparatus

ductor detector (silicone/lithium) that gives a pulse directly proportional to the energy of the X-ray.

The selection of an excitation source is important for the element being assayed. The energy threshold for X-ray fluorescence of a particular element is defined as the absorption edge. Gamma photons or X-rays used to excite an element must have energies which exceed the K absorption edges of the element by only a few KeV. The ^{241}Am (gamma rays, 59.6 KeV) source can be used to measure elements other than iodine, such as barium and lithium. In addition, substituting ^{109}Cd for ^{241}Am as the exciter source provides the FEA system with the capacity to measure other elements such as bromine, manganese, and copper.

In order for the detector to be efficient, the general absorption properties of the conductor materials should be high. Thus, materials with a higher atomic number are selected. The crystal in the detector must be pure. Impure crystals trap the charges with loss of signal and possible polarization. For these reasons a silicone-lithium (Si/Li) detector is used. Lithium compensates for impurities and created a highly resilient and sensitive material when used with silicone. The detector is encapsuled in an evacuated area with a thin beryllium window. Because the mobility of lithium is very high at room temperature, it will diffuse and precipitate if not kept cooled to liquid nitrogen temperature (-196 °C).

It is possible to quantitate the amount of iodine present in solution since the detected count rate by the detector is proportional to the weight fraction of iodine. This technique also allows detection of iodine in samples of a variety of physical forms without altering the capability of the instrument to detect the weight fraction of iodine. This technique has several advantages for measurement in biological tissues.

1. FEA analysis of iodine is nondestructive to the sample.
2. Material analyzed may be in a variety of physical forms such as solid, liquid, powder, slurry, or gas.
3. Sample preparation is minimal.
4. FEA analysis is sensitive to low concentration ranges.
5. Elements in addition to iodine can be detected.

III. Chromatographic Analysis [31]

Chromatography is the selective removal of the components of a mobile phase while flowing past or through a stationary phase. The component which is held less strongly will move through the stationary phase at a higher rate than the more strongly held component. This results in a migration of the components into separate regions on the stationary phase. In order for separation of a mixture to occur by phase distribution, the components of the mixture must have different distribution coefficients. If the coefficients of the solutes are similar in the particular chromatographic mobile and stationary phases selected, the individual solutes will only be partially separated.

Thin-Layer Chromatography. Thin-layer chromatography (TLC) is a form of solid-liquid adsorption chromatography in which the stationary phase is a solid. The components of a liquid passing through it are separated by selective adsorption to the surface. A solid adsorbent is spread as a thin layer on a piece of glass or rigid plastic. The most popular solid support material is silica or alumina mixed with a small amount of binder. A small amount of sample is placed near one edge of the plate. The TLC plate is then placed in a chamber containing the mobile-phase solvent. The solvent is allowed to ascend from the bottom to the top of the plate. As the solvent migrates up the plate, the solutes in the sample migrate at different rates depending on their partition between the mobile and stationary phases. After the mobile phase has moved to near the top, the plate is removed from the solvent, dried, and analyzed. Several methods are available for the general detection of the separated solutes. If the solutes are colorless, but fluorescent, they can be irradiated with UV light to indicate their location. The plate can also be sprayed with various agents (sulfuric acid, potassium permanganate) which react chemically with solutes to form colored products. Another useful method for detecting solutes is placing the plate in a vessel with iodine vapor. Many organic compounds adsorb the iodine and form brownish products.

TLC is very useful in detecting small quantities (10^{-9} g) although sample sizes as large as 500 µg may be used. It is a relatively easy and rapid technique. Quantitative analysis of the separated solutes is sometimes possible by removing and analyzing each spot separately. TLC is used primarily for qualitative analysis of samples and for the initial separation of samples which are to be further separated by other techniques.

High-Performance Liquid Chromatography (Fig. 27) [33]. With the development of high-performance or high-pressure liquid chromatography (HPLC),

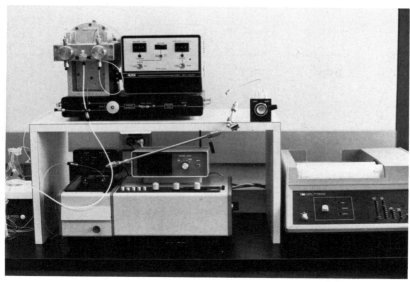

Fig. 27. High-performance liquid chromatography apparatus

complex mixtures can now be separated into individual components and these components analyzed qualitatively and quantitatively. This technique has gained wide acceptance and has seen rapid growth, due to the development of high-efficiency columns, sensitive and specific on-line detection systems, and microprocessors for data analysis. Perhaps the major reason for the important role of HPLC in biomedical research is the development of the reversed-phase technique (RPLC).

The column used in RPLC is made up of bonded phases made by reacting a long-chain hydrocarbon with a chloro-silane reactive group with a hydroxylated silica gel. The bonding reaction results in the hydrophilic surface of silica gel being converted to an essentially hydrophobic surface consisting of a hydrocarbonaceous layer.

Therefore, in reversed phase, the stationary phase (octadecyl-, octyl-, or phenyl-silica packings) is less polar than the mobile phase (typically water/methanol or water/acetonitrile mixtures). Substances thus elute in a general order of decreasing polarity. This is the reverse order of most chromatography and hence the name reversed phase. Thus, mobile-phase strength increases with decreasing polarity. In that sense, acetonitrile is a "stronger" solvent than water.

The basic components needed for an HPLC system are shown in Fig. 28. Those components include a solvent delivery system, an injection port, a column, a detector, and a device to record the data. Columns consist of stainless steel tubes of varying lengths (10–30 cm) with diameters of a few millimeters. These columns are available packed with a wide variety of stationary phases. The mobile phase is propelled at a uniform flow rate through the column using a pump designed to maintain a constant flow rate at elevated pressures. The pressure depends upon

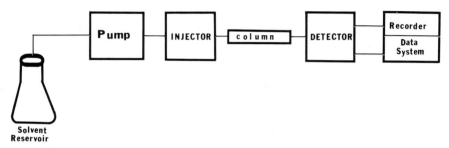

Fig. 28. Schematic diagram of components of a high-performance liquid chromatography apparatus

the characteristics of the column, the solvent, and the rate of solvent flow. A small volume (5–30 µl) of the sample is introduced at the head of the column. In the column, the solutes in the sample are partitioned between the liquid mobile phase and the solid stationary phase. Depending on the characteristics of the mobile and stationary phases employed, the solutes in the injected sample will be separated by pasage through the column. This separation is thought to be due to several properties such as polarity, viscosity, and molecular size. After leaving the column, the separated solutes pass through a detector with a flow-through cell. In this way the solutes are quantitated as they are eluted from the column. The most useful and popular detector is the ultraviolet-visible spectrophotometer. However, detection by refractive index, fluorescence, flame ionization, electrochemical measurements, infrared, and mass spectrometry has been used.

HPLC offers several advantages over other chromatographic techniques: (a) speed – in most instances analysis times are between 5 and 60 min; (b) high resolution and sensitivity; (c) reuseable columns – many samples can be analyzed with a single column, and the rate at which the column decays depends on the type of samples and solvents used and on the overall care of the column; (d) ability to separate ionic from nonionic compounds; (e) simplicity of operation; and (f) easy sample recovery.

K. Methods of Analysis

I. Bilirubin [34]

Background. Bilirubin is the major bile pigment and is formed primarily by the metabolism of hemoglobin. The liver removes bilirubin from blood, makes it water soluble by conjugating with glucuronic acid, and excretes the bilirubin glucuronide into bile. The traditional method for its analysis was introduced by Van den Bergh in the early 1900s. Bilirubin is coupled with diazotized sulfanilic acid (*p*-diazobenzenesulfonic acid) to form an azo dye. The color of the dye is pH dependent and is pink in acid conditions and blue in alkaline conditions. Two types of bilirubin products are thought to be determined by this reaction. The "direct" reacting products are diazotized in the absence of an accelerating agent. These products consist of the more polar conjugated water-soluble derivatives, i.e., glucuronides and sulfates. The "indirect" product reacts with the diazo reagent very slowly unless an accelerating agent (methyl alcohol) is added and is thought to be the unconjugated bilirubin. the sum of these two forms is termed "total" bilirubin.

Reagents
1. Bilirubin diluent: 5.2 g sodium carbonate; 5.2 g sodium chloride; dilute to 1 liter with water
2. Diazo stock: 1 g sulfanilic acid in 15 ml HCl (conc); dilute to 1 liter with water
3. Sodium nitrite: 0.5% solution
4. Diazo reagent: 0.3 ml $NaNO_2$; 10 ml diazo stock

Procedure
1. Blank: 2 ml diazo stock; add 100 μl sample and mix; add 2 ml methanol and mix
2. Sample: 2 ml diazo reagent; add 100 μl sample and mix; add 2 ml methanol and mix
3. Set samples in dark for 30 min to permit development of color
4. Read absorbance of each sample against its blank at 560 nm.

Notes. The time between the mixing or each sample with diazo reagent and determining its absorbance should be constant. Assay the samples in duplicate. A standard curve should be made with bilirubin concentrations between 1 and 30 mg/dl.

II. Iodine (Chemical) [35]

The following procedure includes modifications introduced by Drs. J. Lang and E. Lasser, University of California, at San Diego (personal communication).

Background. The iodine present in organic compounds can be determined by a wet chemical assay. The organically bound iodine (KI) is oxidized to iodate (IO^-) by digesting the samples with chloric acid. The iodate is then reduced to iodine (I_2) with an excess of an acidic solution of iodide. The iodine is then titrated with thiosulfate to a starch end point.

Reagents
1. Stock thiosulfate: 0.05 M; add 2.5 g $Na_2S_2O_3 \cdot 5H_2O$ to a total volume of 100 ml with freshly boiled water; store in amber-colored bottle
2. Working thiosulfate: 0.005 M or 0.001 M; dilute stock solution fresh 1:10 for 0.005 M $N_2S_2O^=$ or 1:50 for 0.001 M $S_2O_3^=$ in amounts needed
3. Stock iodate: 0.1 M; dry 1 g KIO_3 at 150 °C; weigh out 0.375 g and dilute to 100 ml with water; this is stable in refrigerator
4. Working iodate: 0.00909 M; dilute stock iodate 1:11 by adding 2 ml stock to 20 ml water; prepare fresh
5. Phosphoric acid: 85%
6. Phenophthalein: 0.1%
7. NaOH: 5 M
8. Starch-CdI_2 reagent: 0.06 M; dissolve 11 g CdI_2 in approximately 300 ml water and boil gently 15 min until colorless; filter and add water to approximately 800 ml and cool; add 2.5 g soluble starch; bring to a final volume of 1 liter; store in an amber dropper bottle

9. Chloric acid: 28%. Caution! Wear protective glasses and apron and work in a fume hood. Hot perchloric acid is explosive in the presence of organic materials. Use clean glassware and guard against contamination especially with organic solvents such as alcohols. Dissolve 500 g $KClO_3$ in 900 ml hot water in a large (3- to 4-liter) Erlenmeyer flask. (Complete solution is unnecessary.) Add perchloric acid (72%) (375 ml) very slowly, stirring in small portions at a time. Allow to cool and keep in freezer for at least 24 h. Filter with suction through a large Buchner funnel.

Sample Size. The optimal should contain 0.05 mg iodine. For plasma and bile use 0.1 ml. For samples expected to have low iodine concentration use 1–2 ml. Samples should be run in triplicate.

Digestion. Add 1 ml 28% chloric acid to the sample in a 25×100-mm test tube. Cap with a 25-mm funnel and place in a heating block at 90°–100 °C for 15–20 min until the yellow color disappears. The funnels prevent evaporation. Once the sample is clear, increase the temperature to 160 °C and remove the funnels. Continue heating until heavy white fumes are given off and the volume is reduced (0.05–0.1 ml). This digested material is stable for at least 2–3 days.

Titration. For a sensitive color reaction the volume should remain small. Dilute the residue with a few drops of water and one drop of phenolphthalein. Add 5 M NaOH dropwise until a pink color persists. Att two drops 85% H_3PO_4. Add two to three drops CaI_2 and titrate immediately with 0.005 M thiosulfate using a micrometer-driven syringe burette.

Standardization. Add two drops H_3PO_4 and three drops starch-CdI reagent to a 1 ml sample of working KIO_3. Do in triplicate. Titrate with 0.01 M $S_2O_3^=$. Since the weight of $Na_2S_2O_3$ is not easily calculated and it is not easily dried it is necessary to back titrate with KIO_3 to calculate the actual normality of $S_2O_3^=$ used in the assay.

III. Bile Salts [36]

Background. One of the methods available for quantitation of bile salts in biological fluids is an enzymatic assay using NAD^+-dependent 3α-hydroxysteroid dehydrogenase obtained from *Pseudomonas testosteroni*. This enzyme reacts with the 3α-hydroxyl groups of steroids, forming a keto group and NADH, which is measured spectrophotometrically.

Reagents
1. Hydrazine hydrate: 1 M (50 ml hydrazine hydrate in 1 liter distilled water)
2. Potassium phosphate: 0.1 M, pH 9.4
3. NAD 5 mM (33 mg/10 ml)
4. Enzyme (hydroxysteroid dehydrogenase)

Enzyme Solution
1. 0.5 g enzyme (crude hydroxysteroid dehydrogenase) + 50 ml ice-cold distilled water
2. Twenty minutes ultrasonication, probe intensity setting at 70

3. Centrifuge in refrigerated centrifuge at 18,000 rpm for 20 min (10 °C)
4. Freeze samples in 5.0-ml lots; store in freezer; the enzyme remains stable in freezer
5. To prepare for use add 10 ml cold water to each 5 ml enzyme solution

Method
1. Set up four standards in duplicate using 10, 20, 40, and 60 µl taurocholate standard (0.15 mM/10 ml in methanol). Use the same amount of reagents as samples.
2. Blank: 10 µl taurocholate standard + same amount of other reagents while substituting 0.25 ml water in place of NAD.
3. Samples: 5–10 µl bile + 2.0 ml phosphate buffer + 0.5 ml hydrazine hydrate + 0.25 ml NAD + 1.0 ml enzyme. Incubate the samples at 37 °C for 1 h. Cool and read at 340 nm on spectrophotometer.

IV. Protein [37]

The Lowry protein determination is widely used and is a simple assay to perform. There are two distinct steps leading to the final color with protein: (a) reaction with copper in alkali and (b) reduction of the phosphomolybdicphosphotungstic reagent by the copper-treated protein.

Reagents
1. Reagent A: 0.2 g $CuSO_4 \cdot 5H_2O$ + 0.6 g Tris (2-amino-2-hydroxymethyl-1,3 propanediol); bring to a volume of 100 ml with water
2. Reagent B: 10% Na_2CO_3 in 0.5 M NaOH
3. Phenol reagent: 10 ml phenol reagent (Folin and Cioalteu's phenol reagent, 2 M + 100 ml water

Procedure
1. Add 1.0 ml reagent mixture (10 ml reagent B + 1.0 ml reagent A) to 1 ml sample or protein standard
2. Incubate for 10 min at room temperature
3. Add 3.0 ml phenol reagent, mix, and place in water bath (50 °C) for 10 min
4. Remove from bath and cool. Read absorptivity at 670 nm.

Notes. The blank is made by adding 1 ml water rather than the sample. Make a standard curve for albumin up to 0.3 mg/ml. The slope of the line when plotting absorptivity at 670 nm versus albumin concentration is not linear at high concentrations (approximately 0.5 mg/ml and above).

Acknowledgments. The author wishes to express his sincere thanks and appreciation to Brenda Witt for her significant contribution and assistance in preparing this chapter. He was supported in part by grant Am 21620 from the National Institutes of Health.

References

1. Hafez ESE (1970) Reproduction and breeding techniques for laboratory animals. Lea and Febiger, Philadelphia
2. Mitruka BM, Rawnsley HM, Vadehra DV (1976) Animals for medical research. Models for the study of human disease. Wiley, New York

3. Universities Federation for Animal Welfare (1976) The UFAW handbook on the care and management of laboratory animals, 5th edn. Churchill Livingstone, New York
4. Federation of American Societies for Experimental Biology (1969) Comparative anesthesia in laboratory animals. Miller EV, Ben M, Cass JS (eds) Fed Proc 28:1373–1586
5. Mitruka BM, Rawnsley HM (1977) Clinical biochemical and hematological reference values in normal experimental animals. Masson, New York
6. Kaplan HM, Timmons EH (1979) The rabbit. A model for the principles of mammalian physiology and surgery. Academic, New York
7. Cornelius CE (1976) Rates of choleresis in various species. Digest Dis 21:426–428
8. Goodman LS, Gilman A (1975) The pharmacological basis of therapeutics, 5th edn. Macmillan, New York
9. Gillespie NA (1943) The signs of anesthesia. Curr Res Anesth Analg 22:275–282
10. Raventos J (1954) The distribution in the body and metabolic fate of barbiturates. J Pharm Pharmacol 6:217–235
11. Chiasson RB (1975) Laboratory anatomy of the white rat, 3rd edn. Brown, Dubuque
12. Vanlerenberghe J (1965) The effects of hypothermia on biliary function. In: Taylor W (ed) The biliary system, a symposium of the NATO Advanced Study Institute. Blackwell, Oxford, pp 263–276
13. Roberts RJ, Klaassen CD, Plaa GL (1967) Maximum biliary excretion of bilirubin and sulfobromophthalein during anesthesia-induced,alteration of rectal temperature. Proc Soc Exp Biol Med 125:313–316
14. Wheeler HO, Ramos OL (1960) Determinants of the flow and composition of bile in the unanesthetized dog during constant infusions of sodium taurocholate. J Clin Invest 39:161–170
15. Wheeler HO, Meltzer JI, Bradley SE (1960) Biliary transport and hepatic storage of sulfobromophthalein sodium in the unanesthetized dog, in normal man, and in patients with hepatic disease. J Clin Invest 39:1131–1144
16. Berk RN, Goldgerger LE, Loeb PM (1974) The role of bile salts in the hepatic excretion of iopanoic acid. Invest Radiol 9:7–15
17. Berk RN, Loeb PM, Cobo-Frenkel A, Barnhart JL (1976) Saturation kinetics of choleretic effects of iodoxamate and iodipamide. Radiology 119:529–535
18. Berk RN, Loeb PM, Cobo-Frenkel A, Barnhart JL (1977) The biliary and urinary excretion of sodium tyropanoate and sodium ipodate in dogs. Invest Radiol 12:85–95
19. Loeb PM, Barnhart JL, Berk RN (1978) The dependence of the biliary excretion of iopanoic acid on bile salts. Gastroenterology 74:174–181
20. Nelson JA, Staubus AE, Riegelman S (1975) Saturation kinetics of iopanoate in the dog. Invest Radiol 10:371–377
21. Thomas HE (1941) An improved cannula for gastric and intestinal fistulas. Proc Soc Exp Biol Med 46:260–265
22. Gronwall R, Cornelius CE (1970) Maximum biliary excretion of sulfobromophthalein sodium in sheep. Am J Dig Dis 15:37–48
23. Alpert S, Mosher M, Shanske A, Arias IM (1969) Multiplicity of hepatic excretory mechanisms for organic anions. J Gen Physiol 53:238–247
24. Gronwall RR, Engelking LR, Anwer MS, Erickson DF, Klentz RD (1975) Bile secretion in ponies with biliary fistulas. Am J Vet Res 36:653–654
25. Engelking LR, Gronwall R (1979) Effects of fasting on hepatic bile acid clearance. Proc Soc Exp Biol Med 161:123–127
26. Miller LL, Bly CG, Watson ML, Bale WF (1951) The dominant role of the liver in plasma synthesis. A direct study of the isolated perfused rat liver with the aid of lysine-ε-^{14}C. J Exp Med 94:431–453
27. Hems R, Ross BD, Berry MN, Krebs HA (1966) Gluconeogenesis in the perfused rat liver. Biochem J 101:284–292
28. Berry MN, Friend DS (1969) High-yield preparation of isolated rat liver parenchymal cells. J Cell Biol 43:506–520
29. Hatoff DE, Hardison WGM (1979) Induced synthesis of alkaline phosphatase by bile acids in rat liver cell culture. Gastroenterology 77:1062–1067

30. Strange RC, Chapman BT, Johnson JD, Nimmo IA, Percy-Robb IW (1979) Partitioning of bile acids into subcellular organelles and the in vivo distribution of bile acids in rat liver. Biochim Biophys Acta 573:535–545
31. Willard HH, Merritt LL Jr, Dean JA (1965) Instrumental methods of analysis, 4th edn. D Van Nostrand, Princeton
32. Woldseth R (1973) All you ever wanted to know about x-ray energy spectrometry. Kevex, Burlingame
33. Johnson EL, Stevenson R (1978) Basic liquid chromatography. Varian, Ralp Alto
34. Malloy HT, Evelyn KA (1937) The determination of bilirubin with the photoelectric colorimeter. J Biol Chem 119:481–484
35. Zak B, Boyle AJ (1952) A simple method for the determination of organic bound iodine. J Am Pharmacol Assoc 41:260–262
36. Turley SD, Dietschy JM (1978) Re-evaluation of the 3α-hydroxysteroid dehydrogenase assay for total bile acids in bile. J Lipid Res 19:924–928
37. Lowry OH, Rosebrough NJ, Farr AL, Randall RJ (1951) Protein measurement with the folin phenol reagent. J Biol Chem 193:265–275

CHAPTER 9

Contrast Media in Lymphography

M. Sovak

A. Introduction

The diagnostic potential of visualization of lymphatic vessels and lymph nodes was recognized soon after the discovery of X-rays. A variety of heavy metal salts, sodium or potassium iodides, and bromides were injected intralymphatically into cavities as well as into soft tissues. Lymphograms were produced but serious tissue damage resulted [1, 2]. In 1931, it was found that Thorotrast, a thorium-containing colloid, which at the time was believed to be a biologically inert substance, would, upon injection into the pleural space of animals, visualize the thoracic and diaphragmatic lymph vessels [3]. Also, the newly discovered iodized oil, Lipiodol, instilled into the maxillary sinus, successfully demonstrated lymphatic drainage of the maxillary area [4].

Although oils or Thorotrast produced a dense contrast in the lymphatic vessels draining the various cavities, these media failed to visualize the trunk nodes. Interstitial injection of either Lipiodol or Thorotrast did not produce useful lymphograms; the more distant structures were poorly visualized and most of the contrast medium tended to remain at the injection site, sometimes for a long period. In 1952, Kinmonth discovered that subcutaneous injections of a small amount of organic dye resulted in coloration of the lymphatic vessels adjacent to the injection site, thereby allowing their identification and direct cannulation [5]. This approach led to widespread clinical use of direct lymphography, mainly with iodized oils, but not without reservations concerning side effects.

Several studies have suggested that direct lymphography may expulse malignant cells from the lymph nodes and thus cause tumor dissemination [6–8]. Moore research remains to be done; however, there is no doubt that the method of direct access to the lymphatic system has many more applications than being purely a diagnostic radiographic procedure.

The intralymphatic route has been utilized for immunization, in conjunction with antineoplastic vaccine therapy [9]. The attractive possibility of injecting oil as a carrier of radioactive iodine, or of other cytostatic drugs, for therapeutic purposes into the lymphatic vessels has also been explored. These methods are reviewed elsewhere [10, 11].

Unsuccessful attempts have been made with a combination of chlorophyll and the contrast medium Lipiodol ultrafluid, in the hope that staining lymph nodes would make them easier to see during pelvic lymphadenectomy [12]. Chlorophyllated Lipiodol produced extensive aggregation of macrophages in the oil-filled spaces of the lymph nodes, and the lymphograms were found to contain artifacts simulating advanced metastatic disease [13].

B. Methods of Lymphography

For visual identification, lymphatics can be colored by intradermal or sub-cutaneous injection of trypen blue or Alphafurine 2G, preferably in a mixture with a local anesthetic [14]. Fluorescein-aided isolation of lymphatics has also been suggested. (The cannulation, dosage for injection, and radiographic techniques are described in detail in a standard monograph [15].) It appears that complications of lymphography are mostly caused by contrast media (CM), but the technique itself has some inherent risks, as well, i.e., infections at the cannulation site and lymphangiitis. Four classes of CM were radiologically explored for direct lymphography: isotopes, water-soluble materials (Urokon, Diodrast, Cholografin), iodized oils, and particulate CM (Thorotrast and stannic oxide).

Isotope scanning has been carried out using ^{131}I-labeled human serum albumin and radioactive colloidal ^{198}Au. The method found limited use in imaging but has been used extensively to study retention, distribution, and excretion patterns of CM in the lungs and other organs [16–19]. Experimental lymphography in animals was summarized at the time [20]. Particulate CM based on iodinated polymer polystyrene and on polymerized hydroxyethyl tetraiodophthalate, intended primarily for colloidal hepatosplenography, were developed but not pursued further [21].

Thorotrast was a successful CM thanks to its apparent inertness, but when the carcinogenic properties were recognized the CM was removed from human use. The choice of a CM for lymphography thus became narrowed to the iodized oils and the water-soluble CM.

Water-soluble materials could be injected rapidly (20–30 ml 76% Urografin injected from 1 to 5 min) but they did not visualize the lymph nodes beyond the inguinal or iliacal level. The water-soluble materials also caused burning pain in the extremities; they diffused rapidly out of the lymphatic system, and became considerably diluted intralymphatically by lymph influx from pelvic lymphatics [22]. Water-soluble CM were found to diffuse through both inflammatory and necrotic tissues and to conceal lymph node detail. In direct comparison with oils and particulate CM, water-soluble CM failed to depict experimental lymph node lesions produced in dogs [19].

By exclusion, these early observations established the iodized oils as the only viable CM in lymphography. Further research has concentrated on studying their pharmacokinetics and developing new formulations aimed at reduction of the toxicity.

Several attempts have been made to modify the viscosity of the oily CM. Addition of ether to Ethiodol, to decrease the viscosity, was explored both in dogs [23] and man [24]. Although the addition of ether substantially decreased the oil viscosity, reduced the injection pressure, achieved rapid filling, and produced no apparent adverse effects in dogs, a burning sensation in the legs was reported by the patients. Details of the pharmacology of iodized oils, their distribution, transformation, elimination, and toxicity have been summarized [25].

Chemically, the oil from which CM are derived is a mixture of glyceryl esters and linoleic, palmitic, oleic, and steric acids. In Ethiodol (Lipiodol Ultrafluide) upon iodination and transesterification, a mixture of mono and di-iodo ethyl stearates predominates as the major component of the oily CM. Compared with the aromatic carbon-iodine bond, the aliphatic carbon-iodine bond such as found in the stearates is weak. It is easily broken by oxidation, light, heat, or enzymatic processes in vivo. Following breakdown, inorganic iodides are formed which diffuse into most body compartments and are in part responsible for the adverse physiological effects observed with oily CM.

In spite of its high viscosity (25 cps at 37 °C), Ethiodol can be handled by a variety of commercial and improvized injectors to allow the injection rates requires for opacification. For different parts of the lymphatic system, the rates range from 0.1 to 0.5 ml/min [26]. During steady injection into the lymphatic vessels, the oil gradually fills the trunk and then the nodes. Depending upon the quantity injected, all lymphatics and nodes up to the junction of the thoracic duct with the subclavian vein can be filled. Vasomotility of lymphatics expels the oil from the trunk, but CM remains in the nodes for periods of time ranging from weeks to years. The mechanism of CM clearance from the nodes depends on mechanical washout, on macrophage activity, and very probably on concurrent deiodination [27]. An inflammation develops in the nodes resulting in a slight increase of the nodes following the procedure. A chronic foreign body reaction with pronounced fibrocytosis is, however, practically never encountered. As noted above, the rate of disappearance of CM from the nodes varies considerably. Some studies have reported more prolonged storage of CM in abnormal as compared with normal lymph nodes [28]. Another study found a longer retention of CM in females [29]. A study of 500 patients found no significant difference between retention of CM in males or females, but in those patients 20 years old or less, CM appeared to dissipate more rapidly [30].

Hypersensitivity reactions that can be ascribed to iodinated oil manifest themselves as urticaria, fever, allergic dermatitis, edema of the limbs, and, rarely, sialitis [31]. Cases of anaphylactic shock reported in the course of lymphography were attributable to the organic dyes, alphazurene 2G, or the patent blue violet [32]. Fever can be expected to occur in 5%–10% of cases. The overall incidence of hypersensitivity reaction to oil CM was reported as 1:800, based on 32,000 lymphograms.

Extravasation of the oil along the lymphatic vessels or nodes is attributable to excessive pressure. Three coincident cases of severe hypersensitivity dermatitis have been reported [33]. Rarely, CM can break through lymphovenous shunts, especially in cases where there is a malformation of the lymphatics. It has been reported that lymphangiography in a patient with Hodgkin's disease produced diffuse opacification of the kidneys [34].

The most frequently encountered serious adverse reaction to lymphography results from the rapid spilling of CM into the venous system via the emptying thoracic duct. Since pulmonary circulation acts as a fine filter, the *oil embolism* is most frequently found. Chest roentgenograms usually show fine nodularity and even arborization patterns in the lungs, especially in the upper lobes and the bases. The incidence of pulmonary infarcts was given as 1:400; for pulmonary edema, 1:3,200; and for pneumonia, 1:2,500 [8]. The incidence of the clinically nonmanifest pulmonary oil embolism was reported as 50% of the studies [35].

If the embolism is massive, immediate hypotension, cyanosis, and electrocardiographically demonstrable right ventricular strin pattern can be seen. The incidence of hypotensive crisis was found to be 1:5,000 [35]. The oil, once trapped in the pulmonary circulation, is subject to histochemical degradation, i.e., deiodination and β-oxidation. Small oil granulomatous changes were found by one study [36] but no chronic sequelae were reported. The fate of oil in the lungs and the pathophysiological mechanisms involved have been dealt with extensively [8].

More serious embolization complications are encountered when the pulmonary circulation filter fails and a large quantity of the CM is lodged in the terminal circulation of vital organs.

Cerebral disorders attributable to the embolization of the cerebral arteries occur with an incidence of 1:3,500; they are usually associated with the use of larger amounts of the oil, i.e., above 20 ml [34]. Other authors reported detecting emboli in the spleen sinuses and in the glomerular capillaries of the kidneys [6]. Experimental work carried out in rabbits found increased incidence of kidney and brain embolism in irradiated rabbits. The authors concluded that irradiation of the lung tissue hampers the filter ability of the pulmonary circulation [31].

From this account, it can be seen that the use of iodized oils is a compromise justified only by lack of viable alternatives. Considering that embolization constitutes the majority of adverse reactions, it would be of major importance if a nonembolizing material could be found.

The ideal CM for lymphography should be deliverable noninvasively, and be able to visualize the trunk and all lymphatic nodes while being locally and systemically inert, acutely as well as chronically. Present efforts to develop new CM have this goal.

C. Physiology and Pharmacology of Lymphokinetics

If lymphography is to be improved, a thorough knowledge and understanding of lymphatic physiology and of basic experimental methods is indispensable.

Anatomy of the lymphatic system has been reviewed in a number of monographs. General and special anatomy of the lymph system from the subcellular up to the organ level, including histology, is well described in the works of YOFFEY and COURTICE [37] and RUSZNYAK et al. [38, 39]. There are also a number of excellent textbooks and atlases of lymphography available [40].

Anatomical studies at the subcellular level have made important contributions to the current understanding of lymph production [41].

Lymph forms from the interstitial fluid, which in turn is a continuum of plasma. Therefore, it is useful to consider lymph an integral part of the body fluid's compartmentalized system, forming what may be called the body's "internal milieu." Composition of lymph has been studied thoroughly; its components, including electrolytes, glucose, nonprotein nitrogen, urea, amino acids, creatinine, uric acid, bilirubin, and enzymes have been extensively investigated [42, 43]. A related subject, tissue fluid pressure and composition, was reviewed in an excellent monograph, which also contains descriptions of useful experimental models [44].

If radiographic CM were to be delivered into the lymphatic vessels by means other than direct cannulation, it would have to enter lymph from the interstitial space rapidly and at a high concentration. The task of the lymphatic system is to remove not only the aqueous, but also large molecular weight and particulate materials which have found their way into the interstitial space. The mechanism and dynamics of lymph flow have been studied in man, cats, dogs, rabbits, goats, rats, sheep, cows, calves, as well as lambs in utero and lower vertebrates [45]. Lymphodynamics are known to be affected by the activity of the striated muscles, by breathing, by intestinal peristalsis, as well as by autorhythmicity of the lymphatic vessels [46]. Propulsion of lymph by autorhythmic contractions of the lymphatic vessels is apparently a highly individual phenomenon varying greatly according to species as well as among individuals of the same species [47].

Autorhythmicity of the lymphatics has been described in a variety of animals and in man [48]. These studies demonstrate that lymphatic vessels move in spontaneous rhythmic contraction with a frequency of 1–5 min and that the contraction wave progresses along the lymphatic segments in a cranial direction. The frequency apparently can be activated by stimulation of the sympathetic nerve fibers [49]. In the mesenterial lymphatics, innervation is accomplished via the splanchnic and vagal nerves, which contain vasoconstrictive autonomic fibers [50]. Factors stimulating the contraction of lymphatic vessels have been investigated by collecting lymph vessels of the intestinal mesentery of guinea pigs and rats. Intralymphatic pressure changes were found to coincide with opening and closing of the valves, with contraction frequency clearly dependent upon intralymphatic pressure. Contraction frequency also correlated with lymphatic wall tension, thus proving myogenic mechanism of the contraction. The highest frequency recorded in a single vessel was 18 min [51].

In mammals, lymph flow in different organs as well as the total lymph flow varies. The variations, among others, are caused by inflow-outflow differences. As a result, the amount of liquid entering the capillary bed is larger than its outflow; the excess liquid enters the interstitial space. Pressure within the interstitial space is nearly constant under normal circumstances and is regulated by increased or decreased lymphatic drainage. This mechanism is an important factor in homeostasis.

A number of drugs can influence lymph flow in three ways: by affecting the vasomotor activity of the lymph vessels, by affecting the rate of formation of the interstitial fluid, or by affecting the permeability of the collecting lymphatics.

In the interstitium, compounds which are water soluble exert osmotic pressure. Osmotic pressure has been found to regulate the exchange of materials across the capillary wall. This principle, called the Starling hypothesis, assumes that in a steady state the concentration of osmotically active large molecules in the tissue fluid is always adjusted so that the effective osmotic pressure exerted by the plasma balances the capillary pressure. This delicate balance is basically achieved between the hydrostatic blood pressure in the capillaries and the osmotic attraction of the blood for the surrounding fluid. A disturbed balance, such as is found in states of low plasma protein concentration, will result in edema formation.

When a water-soluble hyperosmolal CM is injected interstitially, plasma filtration is increased locally in order to restore osmotic balance. As a result, more interstitial fluid is formed and the lymphatic flow increases, thus diluting the CM. In addition, due to its hyperosmolality and relatively small molecular size, CM tends to escape readily from the lymphatic vessels.

Water and low molecular weight molecules dissolved in water move across the capillary wall by the diffusion process, which transports approximately 5,000 times more water per weight unit of tissue than filtration and absorption. Since the diffusion of hydrosoluble molecules is also determined by the size of the pores in the capillary endothelium, substances with a molecular weight of more than 60,000 rarely cross capillary walls. Lipid-soluble molecules diffuse by a different mechanism: they are able to pass through lipid membranes and can therefore have a very large molecular weight. Certain compounds or particles can be transported across the capillary wall by pinocytosis, which entails encapsulation of the foreign substance by the surface membrane of a cell and then the active transport of the vesicle to the opposite cellular wall.

It is important for the study and design of lymphographic CM to know how water-soluble compounds (proteins), lipids, and particles of large molecular weight enter the lymph.

Most *proteins* in lymph originate from plasma, from which the smaller protein molecules continually escape into the interstitial fluid. It is surmised that they enter the lymphatic vessels as a result of pressure in the interstitium. Compounds which create a hypoosmolar environment vis-à-vis the body milieu apparently enter the lymphatics readily. It is contended that proteins can be phagocytized by the lymphatic endothelium, but it is not certain whether this mechanism actively contributes to the transport of proteins from the interstitial tissue. The largest amount of proteins appears in the interstitial space of the liver and the intestines.

Fats can constitute a major lymph component because lymph is a major transport mechanism for nutritional fats. Those fatty acids which have more than 10–12 carbon atoms are esterified in the intestinal mucosa to triglycerides. Following formation of complexes with proteins, cholesterol, and some form of phospholipids, they enter the lymphatics as chylomicrons. Distinct from crystalloids, fats are absorbed from the interstitial space at an extremely slow rate. Thus, injection of ^{131}I-labelled triolein into the muscle showed that only 17% cleared in 24 h [52]. Since fat is not readily transported into the lymphatics from the interstitial space, oily CM must be delivered by direct cannulation.

How larger *particles* are transported into the lymph capillaries is not immediately clear. Lymph capillaries are closed at their ends, enabling particles to enter only by being phagocytized by the endothelial cells or by entering through the spaces between the endothelial cells. It has been suggested that increases of interstitial pressure distend the lymphatics, thus creating apertures among the endothelial cells allowing the larger particles to pass. It has been observed that particles up to 110 μm could be absorbed from the tissue into the lymphatic system. Unfortunately for radiology, the rate of absorption of particles from the interstitial space is extremely slow. Particulate CM thus do not produce usable lymphograms upon injection into the tissue.

From the serous cavities or organs, the lymphatics take up particles much faster. Injection of Thorotrast into the pleural space resulted in early opacification of the lymphatics and some efferent lymph nodes [3]. Another study showed that injection of a suspension of 2- to 3-μm particles of 2,3,5,6-tetra-iodoterephthalic acid into the canine tonsils, thyroid, testes, and mammary glands produced good early opacification of adjacent lymphatics and nodes as well [53].

Lymph formation and lymph propulsion in the lymphatic system can be influenced by a number of drugs. It is thus conceivable that pharmacological manipulations of lymphatic kinetics could prove useful in conjunction with lymphographic CM. A number of drugs have been shown to affect lymph formation by changing the permeability of the plasma lymph barrier, and by changing the lymphodynamics. General reviews of the subject are available [54, 55]. The literature on the subject is extremely voluminous; therefore the present survey will be confined to studies considered relevant to further developments of CM for lymphangiography.

A number of substances have been found to have a direct effect on the lymphatic vessels. For example, the enzyme hyaluronidase was shown to increase substantially the lymphatic transport of protein, and a dramatic increase in experimentally injected anthrax bacilli following hyaluronidase has also been described [56]. The authors concluded that the enzyme increased the permeability of the lymphatic vessels by enlarging the pores in the lymph capillary walls [57]. It has been suggested that hyaluronidase facilitates entrance of particles or larger molecules into the lymph vessels by loosening the structure of the connective tissue. Hyaluronidase was thus recommended for use with lymphangiography. Angiotensin, vasopressin, noradrenaline and adrenaline, serotonin, and histamine all increase thoracic duct lymph flow, while it is decreased by the hypotensive agents, hexamethonium chloride or trimethaphen camphosulfonate (Arfonade). Compounds known to enhance intestinal motility have been shown to increase thoracic duct lymph flow as well. This applies to choline, vasopressin, serotonin, and, to some extent, certain acetylcholine derivatives [37]. Hydergine, a dehydrogenated ergotoxine, has been proposed as a pharmacological agent for the enhancement of the lymph flow. In animals, Hydergine increases the capillary filtration area by decreasing the tone of precapillary sphincters without changing peripheral vascular resistance. A combination of 5,6-benzo-α-pyrone (coumarin) and a γ-pyrone (troxerutin) was shown to have positive ino-, dromo, rhythmotropic, and angiospasmolytic effects on lymphatics and was thus recommended for routine use in lymphangiography: it has been argued that by increasing the lymphatic flow the injection pressure can be decreased, thereby reducing the risk of oil embolism and metastatic dissemination of malignant cells [58]. Apparently, by their vasotropic and antiinflammatory qualities, benzopyrones have a protective effect against experimental lymphostatic edema [58] and experimental pancreatitis [59].

The effect of different pharmacological agents on isolated lymphatic vessel rhythmicity has been studied. It was found that L-arginine added into the perfusate increased the contraction frequency three times while also increasing the tone of the lymphatics. This effect could be counteracted with ornithine. Local application of adrenaline in the mesentery of rats produced doubling of the contraction frequency. Isolated lymphatics from the mesentery of guinea pigs confirmed the stimulating effect of adrenaline, which could be counteracted with ergotamine. Similar effects could be produced with histamine and counteracted with antistin. A negative chronotropic effect was produced by atropine and papaverine while caffeine and strychnine were positively chronotropic [60, 61].

A strong lymphokinetic effect of coumarin combined with rutine derivative has been demonstrated and introduced into clinical practice (Venalot) [61, 62]. A carefully conducted study in dogs and patients has shown that a mixture of Ethiodol with Venalot significantly accelerated the lymph flow, enabling the injection pressure to be lowered and the CM dose to be reduced from 8–10 to 5 ml for the same diagnostic yield. The same effect could be demonstrated with an intravenous but not an intramuscular injection of Venalot [63].

Lymphokinetic and lymphodilatory effects have also been observed with derivatives of pyridine-3-carboxylic acid (nicotinic acid) bound to a xanthine (theophylline) base. The drug was administered intralymphatically and resulted in a shortening of the time needed to take the lymphograph with Ethiodol [64, 65].

Since vasomotility of the lymphatics is under control of the autonomic nervous system, it is likely that lymphatic flow could be influenced by nerve stimulation. The literature in this area is scarce and contradictory. Application of faradic current to the peripheral fibers of the sciatic nerve or to the tissue immediately surrounding the lymphatic vessels resulted in acceleration of the lymph flow. Nevertheless, the authors concluded that the observed contraction of lymphatics was not neurally mediated [66]. An experimental study in dogs has shown that stimulation of the sciatic nerve or the sympathetic trunk by faradic current resulted in constriction of the lymphatics, which could be prevented by sympathectomy [67].

D. Animal Models in Investigative Lymphangiology

Within the mammal family, man has a unique lymphatic system, which, with the exception of certain large primates, can only be partly approximated in experimental animals. Most studies have been conducted with rabbits, cats, rats, and dogs, although these species have a significantly smaller number of lymphatic trunks and nodes than man. Dogs furthermore are known to be more resistant than man to substances eliciting sterile lymphadenitis and perilymphadenitis [68].

It should also be appreciated that there is a tremendous difference in the physiology of lymphatics not only among different species, but also among the lymphatic systems of organs or regions [37, 69]. Classical microcirculation models are applicable to lymphangiological investigations, such as the rabbit ear chamber [70], the hamster cheek pouch, and the wing of an immobilized nonanesthetized bat [71].

Techniques for collection of lymph from various organs usually require fine surgical methods and the use of specialized catheters, adjusted to a particular species. A technique for collection of intestinal lymph in the rat has been reported [72]. Efferent cardiac and pulmonary lymphatics have been studied in the dog [73], including a technique for long-term catheterization of the canine thoracic duct allowing daily lymph sampling for periods in excess of 12 days [74].

A canine model of regeneration of lymphatics appears in ref.[75]. Models of lymphogenous encephalopathy in dogs and rats were described elsewhere in the same publication [76].

Lymphaticovenous communications have received a great deal of attention and have been investigated in several species [77, 78]. In addition, models of lymphaticovenous communications have been reviewed [75].

In one study, experimental ascites was produced by constriction of the inferior caval vein in order to study abdominal paracentesis and its effects on thoracic duct lymph dynamics [79].

Models of obstructive lymphopathies are difficult to produce in animals because of the capacity of practically every species studied to develop alternative outflow pathways rapidly. Obstruction of the lymphatics in the dog's inguinal region produced transient swelling of the limbs; however, a sufficient collateral lymphatic outflow was established in 3 months.

The techniques of lymphostasis involve ligations of the thoracic ducts in dogs and rats, surgical obstruction of cisterna chyli in rats, and use of sclerosing agents injected directly into the main lymphatics, i.e., injection of silica powder suspended in a 2½% solution of quinine into the mesentery lymphatics. In one study, application of clips to occlude hilar and capsular lymphatics of dog kidneys was used [80]. Experimental lymphedema could also be produced in dogs by infecting them with Brugia [81]. A lymphedema and elephantiasis model has also previously been described [82]. In addition, models of filariasis developed in dogs, cats, and primates have been reviewed [85].

Lymphangiography has been carried out in a number of species, especially dogs and rabbits as the most easily accessible models for studies of the lymphatic system and organ lymphangiography [75, 19]. Lymphangiography of canine cardiac and pulmonary mediastinal lymphatics has also been described [84]. Experimental lymphangiography with description of the lymphatic anatomy is available for cats [85] and monkeys, i.e., drill, baboon, rhesus, vervet, patas, and owl monkeys [86]. The lymphatic system of the rhesus monkey was the subject of a separate study [87]. Lymphangiography in the rat following injections of CM into the testes and prostate is has been used [88].

E. Experimental Contrast Media for Lymphography

The major drawback of contemporary lymphangiography is the procedure's invasiveness and length as well as the toxicity of the iodized oil. The oils, by being immiscible with lymph, tend to globulize. Therefore, lymphatic structures smaller than the oil globules cannot be radiographically detected. Further, oil entering the pulmonary circulation can produce pulmonary infarcts by a mechanical obstruction. On the other hand, by being ecluded from the aqueous milieu of the organism, the interaction of the oil with the biomacromolecules is limited. This explains the relatively low acute chemotoxicity of the oily media.

There were several attempts to develop emulsions in the hope that such formulation could provide indirect lymphography and better visualization. None of these developments have yet reached a stage of general clinical acceptance [89–94].

At Guerbet Laboratories, a mixture of ethyl esters of iodinated fatty acids of poppyseed oil and nonionic surface-tension-reducing agent was tested, with ambiguous results. The intravenous LD_{50} in mice and rats of the new agent, AG-52-315, turned out to be three times higher than for Ethiodol (6.5 g/kg vs 1.8 g/kg). Encouraged by the low toxicity, presumably attributable to the reduction of embolism incidents, the authors obtained lymphograms in dogs and humans. The lymphograms were comparable to those obtained with Ethiodol, but an acute inflammatory reaction within the lymphatic system was found. The authors attributed the intralymphatic toxic effect to the emulsifying agent as well as to the toxicity of the oil itself, which, by emulsification, gained a large area of contact with the organism [94]. It was demonstrated that retrosternal indirect lymphography could be performed with an emulsion injected infradiaphragmatically in rabbits; however, a chronic inflammatory reaction developed in the peritoneum with lymphangiitis and perilymphadenitis [95].

The task of producing stable, nontoxic ethiodized oils led to a number of new preparations; however, the resulting emulsions were found suitable primarily for i.v. hepatosplenography, in conjunction with computed tomography [96]. (See also Chap. 13.)

A radical departure from emulsions was the synthesis of the bis-hydroxyethyl ester of 2,3,5,6-tetra-iodoterephthalic acid by Bracco Industries. The suspended particles had an average diameter of 2–3 μm and the iodine content of the suspension was 480 mg I/ml. The suspension is stable for about 1 year at 5 °C. Injections of this suspension into the tonsils, thyroid, mammary glands, and testes of dogs led to good visualization of the adjacent nodes and lymphatic trunks. A nonspecific inflammatory reaction, disappearing after 4 weeks, was noted [53].

An innovative approach using indirect lymphography was reported from Schering AG. The authors described a nonionic dimer with a high viscosity (32.9 cps at 37 °C of 300 mg I/ml, a molecular weight of 1,608 and iodine content of 47%).[1] This compound remains water soluble when in highly concentrated aqueous solution, but upon exposure to a large surface and some dilution it falls out of solution, forming an extremely fine emulsion. Furthermore, the compound has a low osmotic pressure so that at 300 mg I/ml it is hypoosmolar vis-à-vis the body milieu. Inasmuch as the precipitated microcrystals retain some water solubility, the new compound, Iotasul, does not embolize [97].

Iotasul was used to opacify, by intracutaneous slow infusion, the lymph drainage system of the eye, face, and neck regions of dogs [98, 99]. Further investigations revealed that such indirect lymphography can depict lymphatic structures which have previously not been amenable to visualization by the direct approach [100]. Interdigital intracutaneous infusion of Iotasul in pigs gave good visualization of the inguinal and para-aortic lymph nodes and vessels, with rates varying from 6.6 to 16.5 ml/h of 300 mg I/ml solutions [101].

Potential CM for lymphography emerged with the introduction of C_6 and C_8 perfluorocarbons. These liquids, known for their extreme chemical inertness, are also known to absorb large amounts of oxygen, which originally led to their experimental use as plasma expanders [102]. Bromine substitution for one of the fluorines resulted in stable compounds whose radiographic potential was recognized [103]. [The subject is also treated elsewhere in this book (Chaps. 1, 6). Fur-

---

[1] See Introduction, p. 11, Fig. 3a

ther investigations were made of two compounds, the perfluorooctyl and the perfluorohexyl bromides, both clear, volatile liquids with low surface tension. The specific density of $C_8F_{17}B_r$ is 1.092 and its surface tension is 18.2 dynes/cm^2; for $C_6F_{13}B_r$ specific density is 1.089 and surface tension is 16.4 dynes/cm^2.] Both compounds have a low viscosity and are insoluble in water. The perfluorooctyl bromide compound was also tested in comparison with Ethiodol for lymphography in dogs [104], cats, rabbits, and rats [105]. Due to its low viscosity, perfluorocarbon could be infused more rapidly than Ethiodol. Complete visualization of the lymphatic system from the point of infusion to the outlet of the thoracic duct was obtained in both cats and rabbits. The lymph nodes remained opacified even 8 months after lymphangiography; after 3 years there was still a considerable amount present in the lymph nodes of the subject dogs. It has been reported that lymph nodes exposed to perfluorocarbon contained no chronic inflammatory changes such as are known with Ethiodol. The LD_{50} in cats was estimated at about 1 ml/kg body wt.

Indirect lymphography of diagnostic value could not be achieved with either neat or emulsified perfluorocarbon. Excretion of perfluorocarbons from a mammalian organism is extremely slow, the main mechanism being removal by macrophage activity. Although perfluorocarbons, because of their extreme chemical inertness, were expected to be biologically inert, macrophage activation and development of nonspecific tumoricidal properties of peritoneal exudate cells following exposure to perfluorocarbon were reported [106].

References

1. Capua A (1934) Iniezioni di thorotrast colloidale nella cavita peritoneale per lo studio della diffusione del mezzo di contrasto per le vie linfatiche. Radiol Med (Torino) 21:289–294
2. Dotti E (1934) Erforschung der Funktion der Lymphgefäße und Lymphdrüsen mittels Röntgendarstellung nach subkutaner Injektion von Thoriumdioxyd (Tierexperimente). Fortschr Geb Roentgenstr 50:615–618
3. Menville LJ, Ané JN (1934) A roentgen study of the absorption by the lymphatics of the thorax and diaphragm of thorium dioxide injected intrapleurally into animals. AJR 31:166–172
4. Pfahler GE (1932) A demonstration of the lymphatic drainage from the maxillary sinuses. AJR 27:352–356
5. Kinmonth JB (1972) The lymphatics; diseases, lymphography and surgery. Arnold, London
6. Schaffer B, Koehler PR, Daniel CR, Wohl GT, Riveria E, Meyers WA et al. (1963) A critical evaluation of lymphangiography. Radiology 80:917–936
7. Desmons M, Ramioul H (1964) Essaimage néoplastique périlymphatique après lymphographie dans un cas de tumeur mélanique du pied. J Radiol Electrol 45:703–705
8. Koehler PR (1967) Lymphography. Complications and accidents. In: Ruttimann A (ed) Progress in lymphology. Thieme, Stuttgart, pp 306–307
9. Juillard GJF, Boyer PJJ (1977) Intralymphatic immunization: current status. Eur J Cancer 13:439–440
10. Edwards JM (1972) Endolymphatic radiotherapy. In: Kinmonth JB (ed) The lymphatics. Arnold, London, pp 364–389
11. Kiusk H (1971) Technique of lymphography and principles of interpretation. Green, St. Louis, pp 284–307
12. Averette HE, Viamonte MI, Fergusson JH (1963) Lymphangiodenography as a guide to lymphadenectomy. Obstet Gynecol 21:682–686

13. Jackson RJA (1970) Chlorophyllated lipiodol ultrafluid as a contrast medium: an explanation for the disadvantages attending its use. In: Viamonte M, Koehler PR, Witte M, Witte C (eds) Progress in lymphography. Thieme, Stuttgart, pp 179–183

14. Fischer HW (1977) Introduction to angiographic contrast agents. In: Miller RE, Skucas J (eds) Radiographic contrast agents. University Park Press, Baltimore, p 465

15. Doss LL, Alyea JL, Waggoner CM, Schroeder TT (1980) Fluorescein-aided isolation of lymphatic vessels for lymphangiography. AJR 134:603–604

16. Fischer HW (1962) Intralymphatic introduction of radioactive colloids into the lymph nodes. Radiology 79:297–301

17. Heinzel F, Rosler M (1966) Quantitative investigation of the dynamics of intralymphatically applied substances. In: Ruttimann A (ed) Progress in lymphology. Thieme, Stuttgart, pp 248–253

18. Heinzel F, Rösler H, Ruttimann A, Wirth W (1968) Kinetische Untersuchungen nach intralymphatischer Applikation radioaktiver Substanzen. Radiologe 8:154–158

19. Fischer HW (1959) Lymphangiography and lymphadenography with various contrast agents. Ann NY Acad Sci 78:799–808

20. Tjernberg B (1956) Lymphography as an aid to examination of lymph nodes; preliminary report. Acta Soc Med Ups 61:207–214

21. Thomas SF, Dummel RJ, Patterson JA, Madden JD, Dummel GM (1959) Uniform colloidal dispersion for hepatolienography. Ann NY Acad Sci 78:793–798

22. Fuchs WA (1965) Lymphographie und Tumordiagnostik. Springer, Berlin Heidelberg New York

23. Jonsson K, Anderson JH, Osborne B, Wallace S (1977) Ether-dissolved ethiodol for lymphangiography: an experimental study. AJR 129:1047–1050

24. Ronneburg HP (1976) The addition of ether to contrast medium lipiodol ultrafluid – a proven modification of lymphographic examinations. Radiol Diagn (Berl) 17:523–524

25. Svoboda M (1971) Radiocontrast agents for lymphography. In: Knoefel PK (ed) The international encyclopedia of pharmacology and therapeutics, sect 76, pt II. Pergamon, Oxford, pp 413–429

26. Kiusk H (1971) Technique of lymphography and principles of interpretation. Green, St. Louis

27. Wendth AF, Moriarty DF, Cross UF, Vitale P (1968) Urinary bladder opacification following lymphangiography. Radiology 91:762–763

28. Blaudow K, Banaschak A (1968) Die Bedeutung der Lymphographie für gynäkologische Karzinome. Radiol Diagn (Berl) 9:661–668

29. Gerteis W (1972) Darstellungsmethoden des Lymphgefäßsystems und praktische Lymphographie. In: Von Messen H (ed) Lymphgefäß-System – Lymph vessel system. Springer, Berlin Heidelberg New York, pp 595–636 (Handbuch der allgemeinen Pathologie, vol 3/6)

30. Teske H-J, Kalkowski B (1977) On the persistence of an oily contrast medium (lipiodol ultrafluid®) in normal and abnormal lymph nodes. In: Mayall RC, Witte MH (eds) Plenum, New York, pp 157–161

31. Davidson JW (1969) Lipid embolism to the brain following lymphography: case report and experimental study. AJR 105:763–771

32. Koehler PR (1968) Complications of lymphography. Lymphology 1:116–120

33. Redman HC (1966) Dermatitis as a complication of lymphangiography. Radiology 86:323–326

34. Kiusk H (1971) Technique of lymphography and principles of interpretation. Green, St. Louis, pp 43–51

35. Bron KM, Baum S, Abrams HL (1963) Oil embolism in lymphangiography: incidence, manifestations and mechanism. Radiology 80:194–202

36. Clouse ME, Hallgrimsson J, Wenlund DE (1966) Complications following lymphography with particular reference to pulmonary oil embolization. AJR 96:972–978

37. Yoffey JM, Courtice FC (1970) Lymphatics, lymph and the lymphomyeloid complex. Academic Press, New York

38. Rusznyák I, Földi M, Szabó G (1967) Lymphatics and lymph circulation; physiology and pathology. Pergamon, Oxford
39. Kampmeier OF (1969) Evolution and comparative morphology of the lymphatic system. Thomas, Springfield
40. Gooneratne BWM (1974) Lymphography, clinical and experimental. Butterworth, London
41. Kalima TV, Collan Y, Kalima SH (1977) Variations of lymphatic endothelial cell junctions in experimental conditions. In: Mayall RC, Whitte MH (eds) Progress in lymphology. Plenum, New York, pp 7–12
42. Yoffey JM, Courtice FC (1970) Lymphatics, lymph and the lymphomyeloid complex. Academic, New York, pp 236–246
43. Rusznyák I, Földi M, Szabó G (1967) Lymphatics and lymph circulation; physiology and pathology. Pergamon, Oxford, pp 566–592
44. Hargens AR (ed) (1981) Tissue fluid pressure and composition. Williams and Wilkins, Baltimore
45. Rusznyák I, Földi M, Szabó G (1967) Lymphatics and lymph circulation; physiology and pathology. Pergamon, Oxford, pp 511–565
46. Málek P (1967) Pathophysiological and radiological aspects of lymphovenous anastomosis. Experientia [Suppl] 14:197–203
47. Yoffey JM, Courtice FC (1970) Lymphatics, lymph and the lymphomyeloid complex. Academic, New York, pp 187–189, 220–222
48. Kinmonth JB, Taylor GW (1964) Chylous reflux. Br Med J 1:529–532
49. Gross F, Haefeli H (1952) Motion picture analysis of blood circulation stimulators on the blood vessels of the mesotestis of the rat. Physiol Pharmacol Acta 10:C4–6
50. Mislin H (1975) The functional organization of vasomotoric lymph drainage. In: Gregl A (ed) Lymphographie und Pharmakolymphographie. Fischer, Stuttgart, p 10
51. Hargens AR, Zweifach BW (1977) Contractile stimuli in collecting lymph vessels. Am J Physiol 233:H57–H65
52. Schaffer B, Koehler PR, Daniel CR, Wohl GT, Riveria E, Meyers WA, Skelley JF (1963) A critical evaluation of lymphangiography. Radiology 80:427
53. Chiappa S, Campani R, Felder E, Ferrari D, Tirone P (1979) Experimental lymphography by intratissue injection of a crystal suspension. In: Málek P, Bartoš V, Weissleder H, Witte MH (eds) Lymphology. Proc of the VI international congress, Prague, 1977. Thieme, Stuttgart, pp 359–362
54. Vogel G (1972) Pharmacology of the lymph and the lymphatic system. In: Von Messen H (ed) Lymphgefäß-System – Lymph vessel system. Springer, Berlin Heidelberg New York, pp 363–404 (Handbuch der allgemeinen Pathologie, vol 3/6)
55. Vogel G (1979) Pharmacology of the lymph and the lymphatic system. In: Malek P, Bartos V, Weissleder H, Witte MH (eds) Lymphology. Proc of the VI international congress, Prague, 1977. Thieme, Stuttgart, pp 205–210
56. Schaffer B, Koehler PR, Daniel CR, Wohl GT, Riveria E, Meyers WA, Skelley FJ (1963) A critical evaluation of lymphangiography. Radiology 80:917–930
57. Kinmonth JB (1952) Lymphangiography in man. Method of outlining lymphatic trunks in man. Clin Sci 11:13–20
58. Mayall RC, Mayall ACDG, Mehri ET, Ferretti UR, Villani MV (1977) Lymphokinetics-lymphangiographic demonstration of lymphokinetic effect of benzopyrone. In: Mayall RC, Witte MH (eds) Progress in lymphology. Plenum, New York, pp 179–196
59. Bartoš V, Kolc J, Málek P (1979) The effect of Venalot on experimental pancreatitis in dogs. In: Málek P, Bartoš V, Weissleder H, Witte MH (eds) Lymphology. Proc of the VI international congress, Prague, 1977. Thieme, Stuttgart, pp 231–233
60. Mislin H (1961) Experimenteller Nachweis der autochthonen Automatie der Lymphgefäße. Experientia 17:29–30
61. Mislin H (1971) Effect of coumarin from Melilotus officinalis on the function of lymphangion. Arzneim Forsch 21:852–853
62. Kinmonth JB, Taylor GW, Harper RAK (1955) Lymphangiography by radiological methods. J Fac Radiols (Lond) 6(4):217–223

63. Krajnovic P (1975) Application of Venalot in lymphography. In: Gregl A (ed) Lymphographie und Pharmakolymphographie. Fischer, Stuttgart
64. Benda K (1977) Pharmakolymphographie. Radiol Diagn (Berl) 18:289–300
65. Brůna J, Šůnová J (1979) Technique and possibilities of clinical pharmacolymphography. In: Málek P, Bartoš V, Weissleder H, Witte MH (eds) Lymphology. Proc of the VI international congress, Prague, 1977. Thieme, Stuttgart, pp 355–357
66. Rovière H, Valette G (1937) Physiologie du système lymphatique „Formation de la lymphe, circulation lymphatique normale et pathologique". Masson, Paris
67. Bellinazzo P, Monteverde G (1953) Effects of the sympathetic nervous system on the circulation of the lymph in the limbs, experimental research by means of Thorotrast lymphography. Minerva Chir 8:731–740
68. Guerbet M, Bismuth V, Desprez-Curely JP, Gluckman A, Bourdon R (1970) Lymphangiography with new oily contrast media. In: Viamonte M, Koehler RP, Witte M (eds) Progress in lymphology II. Thieme, Stuttgart, p 181
69. Vogel G, Ströcker H (1967) Original differences in capillary permeability – investigations of the penetration of polyvinyl pyrrolidone and endogenous proteins from plasma in the rabbit lymph. Pfluegers Arch Gesamte Physiol 294:119–126
70. Clark ER, Clark EL (1936) Observations on living mammalian lymphatic capillaries: their relation to the blood vessels. Am J Anat 60:253–298
71. Wiedemann MP (1963) Patterns of the arteriovenous pathways. In: Handbook of physiology, sect 2 – Circulation, vol 2. American Physiol Soc, Washington DC, pp 891–933
72. Dennhardt R, Gartemann H (1979) Technique for the collection of intestinal lymph with an extracorporeal intestinal lymphatic-vena cava shunt. In: Malek P, Bartos V, Weissleder H, Witte MH (eds) Lymphology. Proc of the IV international congress, Prague, 1977. Thieme, Stuttgart, pp 88–91
73. Leeds SE, Uhley HN, Meister RB (1977) The cardiac and pulmonary efferent lymphatics. Folia Angiol 25:65
74. Nelson AW, Swan H (1969) Long-term catheterization of the thoracic duct in the dog. Arch Surg 98:83–86
75. Danese CA (1968) Regeneration of lymphatic vessels. In: Mayerson HS (ed) Lymph and the lymphatic system. Springfield, Illinois, pp 53–73
76. Foldi M (1968) Lymphogenous encephalography. In: Mayerson H (ed) Lymph and the lymphatic system. Springfield, Illinois, p 169
77. Job TT (1918) Lymphatico-venous communications in the common rat and their significance. Am J Anat 24:467–491
78. Takashima T, Benninghoff DL (1966) Lymphatico-venous communications and lymph reflux after thoracic duct obstruction: an experimental study in the dog. Invest Radiol 1:188–197
79. Witte MH, Witte Cl, Kintner K, Thomas D (1979) Effect of abdominal paracentesis on thoracic duct lymph dynamics in experimental ascites. In: Malek P, Bartos V, Weissleder H, Witte MH (eds) Lymphology. Proc of the VI international congress, Prague, 1977. Thieme, Stuttgart, pp 138–141
80. Burn JI (1974) Obstructive lymphopathy. In: Gooneratne BWM (ed) Lymphography, clinical and experimental. Butterworth, London, pp 34–55
81. Schacher JF, Sulahian A, Edeson JFB (1969) Experimental lymphoedema in dogs infected with Brugia spp. Trans R Soc Trop Med Hyg 63:682–684
82. Drinker CK, Field ME, Homans J (1934) The experimental production of edema and elephantiasis as a result of lymphatic obstruction. Am J Physiol 108:509–520
83. Gooneratne BWM (1974) Lymphography in experimental filariasis. In: Gooneratne BWM (ed) Lymphography, clinical and experimental. Butterworth, London, pp 83–122
84. Leeds SE, Uhley HN, Meister RB (1979) Application of direct cannulation and injection lymphangiography to the study of the canine cardiac and pulmonary efferent mediastinal lymphatics. Invest Radiol 14:70–78
85. Gooneratne BWM (1972) The lymphatic system of cats outlined by lymphography. Acta Anat 81:36–41

86. Gooneratne BWM (1974) Simian lymphography. In: Gooneratne BWM (ed) Lymphography, clinical and experimental. Butterworth, London, pp 165–176

87. Gooneratne BWM (1972) Lymphatic system in rhesus monkeys (*Macaca mulatta*) outlined by lower limb lymphography. Acta Anat 81:602–608

88. McCullough DL (1975) Experimental lymphangiography: experience with direct medium injection into the parenchyma of the rat testes and prostate. Invest Urol 13:211–219

89. Johansson S, Sternby NH, Theander G, Wehlin L (1966) Iodinated oil emulsion for lymphography. Acta Radiol [Diagn] 4:690–704

90. Vialla M, Colin R (1964) Essai comparatif entre les methodes d'opacification lymphatique avec produits hydrosolubles et liposolubles. J Radiol Electrol 45:190–192

91. Fischer HW (1966) Experiences in seeking an Ethiodol emulsion for lymphography. Invest Radiol 1:29–36

92. Koehler PR (1965) Radiographic visualization of the substernal lymph nodes. Radiology 85:565–567

93. Penning L, Kerckhoffs HP (1967) Comparative experimental evaluation of several types of emulsified oily radiopaque materials in the cranial subarachnoid space. Radiology 88:730–735

94. Teplick JG, Haskin ME, Skelley J, Wohl GT, Sanen F (1964) Experimental studies with a new radiopaque emulsion. Radiology 82:478–485

95. Roth S, Hiort U, Joseph K, Jost F, Kalbfleisch H, Müller H, Vielhauer E (1979) Indirect lymphography and lymph scintigraphy of the retrosternal lymphatics with a new contrast emulsion and its isotope. In: Malek P, Bartos V, Weissleder H, Witte MH (eds) Lymphology. Proc of the VI international congress, Prague, 1977. Thieme, Stuttgart, pp 352–355

96. Grimes G, Vermess M, Gallelli JF, Girton M, Chatterji DC, et al. (1979) Formulation and evaluation of ethiodized oil emulsion for intravenous hepatography. J Pharm Sci 68:52–56

97. Siefert HM, Mützel W, Schöbel C, Weinmann H-J, Wenzel-Hora BI, Speck U (1980) Iotasul, a water-soluble contrast agent for direct and indirect lymphography. Results of preclinical investigations. Lymphology 13:150–157

98. Wenzel-Hora BI, Siefert HM, Grüntzig J (1982) Animal experimental studies of indirect lymphography of the eye, face and neck regions using Iotasul. Lymphology 15:32–35

99. Grüntzig VJ, Wenzel-Hora BI, Siefert HM (1982) Die indirekte Lymphographie am Auge und im Gesichts-Hals-Bereich mit Iotasul im Tierexperiment. Fortschr Röntgenstr 136:592–594

100. Wenzel-Hora BI, Kalbas B, Siefert HM, Arndt JO, Schlösser HW, Huth F (1981) Iotasul, a water-soluble (non-oily) contrast medium for direct and indirect lymphography. Lymphology 14:101–112

101. Apitzsch DE, Kroll H-U, Zühlke HV (1981) Indirect caudal lymphography using a new water-soluble contrast agent – animal experimental studies in pigs. Lymphology 14:95–100

102. Clark LC, Kaplan S, Becattini F (1970) The physiology of synthetic blood. J Thoracic Cardiovas Surg 60:757–773

103. Long DM, Liu MS, Szanto PS, Alrenga P (1972) Initial observations with a new X-ray contrast agent – radiopaque perfluorocarbon. Rev Surg 29:71–76

104. Liebner EJ (1977) Evaluation of perfluoroctylbromide for lymphography in the dog: comparison with Ethiodol. Invest Radiol 12:368–372

105. Long DM, Nielson MD, Multer FK, Lasser EC, Liu MS, Russell S (1979) Comparison of radiopaque perfluorocarbon and Ethiodol in lymphography. Radiology 133:71–76

106. Miller ML, Stinnett JD, Clark LC (1980) Ultrastructure of tumoricidal peritoneal exudate cells stimulated in vivo by perfluorochemical emulsions. J Reticuloendothel Soc 27:105–118

CHAPTER 10

Contrast Media in Computed Tomography

P. B. DEAN and D. B. PLEWES

A. Introduction

Computed tomography (CT) produces remarkably accurate cross-sectional images of the human body, which are based on small differences in the X-ray attenuation among the various body tissues. The anatomic location, shape and size, homogeneity, and attenuation characteristics of structures in the body are used by the radiologist to determine their identity in the CT images. Based on this information, the radiologist attempts to determine whether a sequence of CT images represents normal anatomy or whether a pathologic lesion is present. Contrast media are routinely given to the patient prior to and during CT scanning to increase the attenuation coefficients of at least some of the tissues and organs or of their lumens. This is done to render some pathologic lesions and some normal anatomic structures more readily detectable so as to help in their differential diagnosis. This chapter will review the nature of contrast enhancement (CE) and the various applications of both conventional and experimental contrast media (CM) to computed tomography.

B. Basic Aspects of Computed Tomography Relevant to Contrast Enhancement

Computed tomography images are two-dimensional representations of the X-ray properties of a transaxial "slice" of tissue of depth ranging from 1.5 to 13 mm, depending on the machine manufacturer. Images are obtained by a suitable reconstruction algorithm which combines data from projections taken from many angles throughout the slice. Since the CT number of any one pixel is the result of manipulations of data from all the measured projections, the imaging artifacts arising in CT are unlike those characteristic of conventional radiography.

The projection data used in CT imaging are gathered in a number of ways, depending on the "generation" of the CT apparatus used. Currently, most CT scanners are either third- or fourth-generation machines. Third-generation scanners use a multiple detector array mechanically linked to an X-ray source that rotates around the patient. A fourth-generation scanner uses a stationary detector array that encircles the patient. The detectors are sequentially irradiated by a scanning X-ray fan from a rotating tube.

The imaging properties of CT are unique in that it exhibits a relatively poor spacial resolution (0.5 up to 2.5 cy-mm) compared with conventional radiography (5–8 cy-mm). However, this reduced resolution is offset by several other key

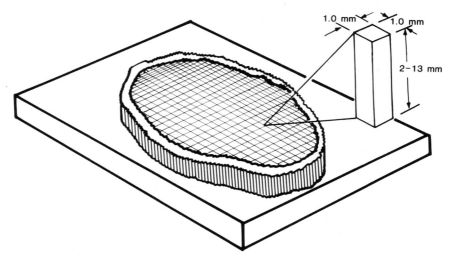

Fig. 1. Approximate size and shape of a CT "voxel." The exact dimensions will depend upon the scanner manufacture

factors which include improved scatter rejection, true tomographic imaging, and significantly improved contrast or density resolution. Under optimal conditions, it has been shown that with conventional radiographic techniques the minimum subject contrast perceptible above the film noise is about 2% [1]. However, CT images have a minimum perceptible subject contrast of about 0.2%–0.4%, [2], roughly a five- to tenfold increase in density resolution. This fine-density resolution allows in vivo monitoring of subtle CM uptake and washout in various tissues.

The density resolution of CT images is dependent upon several factors related to image noise, which include reconstruction algorithm, resolution, patient dose, detector geometry, and image structure. The relationship between the variance in the CT number of homogeneous object, patient dose, and imaging resolution has been the subject of several studies [3, 4] and it has been shown that:

$$\sigma^2 \propto \frac{1}{W^3 D \cdot h},$$

where σ^2 is the image variance, W is the image resolution, h is the slice thickness, and D is the peak surface dose. Thus, any attempt to improve resolution with a fixed image noise is done with substantial increase in patient dose. For example, for a fixed noise a twofold increase in resolution would require an eightfold increase in patient dose. CT images may exhibit many subtle artifacts that will cause the magnitude of the CT data to reflect inaccurately the attenuation properties of the tissues being scanned. It is not our purpose to outline these artifacts in any detail in this article as they have been reviewed elsewhere [5]. However, one of the many important artifacts which influence the CT image is the phenomenon of partial volume averaging. Figure 1 shows the shape of the volume elements over

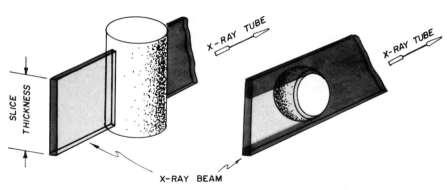

Fig. 2. Illustration of the partial volume artifact. A single attenuation measurement through a cylinder will show greater attenuation than the measurement through a sphere of the same diameter and material if the diameter is less than the scan beam width

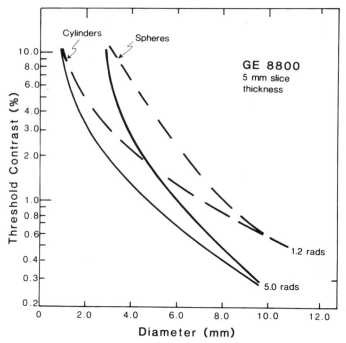

Fig. 3. Contrast detail curves for cylinders and spheres of the same material [7]

which the CT attenuation data are determined and can be seen as a rectangular parallelepiped of dimensions roughly $1 \times 1 \times 10$ mm, depending upon the scanner manufacturer. (A good review of many of the technical parameters of CT scanners is found in [6].) Thus, objects that partially protrude into the scanning beam may exhibit less attenuation than an object of identical physical makeup which totally covers the beam as shown in Fig. 2. This can result in a significant reduction in the measured CT attenuation for objects that partially fill the beam. Figure 3 illustrates this point by plotting the curve relating the minimum detectable subject contrast as a function of object diameter. For cylinders scanned with their long axis perpendicular to the scan plane we see that increasing the cylinder diameter reduces the necessary material contrast before it becomes imperceptible. This characteristic curve is generally referred to as a "contrast detail" [2] curve. When we scan objects that are spherical in shape so that partial volume averaging is significant, the contrast detail curves assume a new position [7, 8]. It is clear that objects of size approaching the X-ray beam width or smaller require greater intrinsic contrast to be resolved than that necessary for a cylinder of similar diameter and material having an axial orientation.

From the above discussion it is evident that in order for small objects to be detectable, their X-ray attenuation must differ substantially from that of the surrounding medium. One of the major reasons for using CM in CT is to render small lesions detectable by increasing the differences in their attenuation between these lesions and their surroundings [9]. The degree of enhancement as well as the pattern of enhancement may also provide information valuable in differential diagnosis.

C. Measurement of Contrast Enhancement with Computed Tomography

I. Contrast Enhancement from Iodine

The CT scanner offers the potential of accurately measuring the concentration distribution of iodine throughout the body. Study of the subtle variations in the distribution of CM in different tissues can be made with both a spatial and concentration resolution unequaled by any other clinical radiographic technique. The first step in quantitating the iodine uptake typical of clinical doses of CM is to establish the degree to which low iodine concentrations influence CT data. This will depend to some extent upon the scanner used, the tube filtration and kilovoltage, and the size, shape, and attenuation of the object being scanned.

To illustrate the effect of enhancement characteristic of iodine, a 25-cm circular lucite water phantom containing syringes of various known iodine concentrations was scanned on a GE 7800 scanner. The results of this experiment are shown in Fig. 4, where the response up to 10 mg I/ml is linear with a regression coefficient of 0.998 [10].

To characterize this response, we will define the "specific iodine" enhancement as the slope of the regression line at low iodine concentrations expressed in $\frac{HU \times ml}{mg\,I}$. The specific enhancement for the three scanning fields applicable to this phantom are shown in Table 1 and shows a small variation in response with the calibration files used for reconstruction [10]. We can obtain a first approximation of this parameter from measurements of the equivalent energy of the CT spectra (E_{eff}) [11] and the mass attenuation coefficients, μ, for iodine and water [12]. On

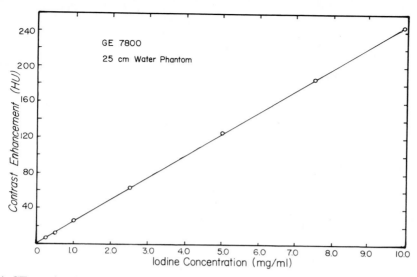

Fig. 4. CT number (HU) versus iodine concentration. Measured on a GE 7800 with a medium-body calibration file. [10]

Table 1. Specific iodine enhancement (GE 7800)

$\dfrac{\text{HU} \cdot \text{ml}}{\text{mg I}}$	Calibration file		
	Head	Medium body	Large body
	24.26	24.84	24.34

this basis the specific enhancement of iodine reduces to:

$$\text{specific enhancement} = \frac{\mu_{\text{iodine}}(E_{eff})}{\mu_{\text{water}}(E_{eff})}. \tag{1}$$

The results of this calculation are shown in the first row of Table 2 for various tube kilovoltages. The results of experimental measurements of specific enhancement from three literature sources are also included in Table 2. The general agreement between various scanners is reasonably consistent; however, there is some variation that indicates that for similar tube kilovoltages the specific enhancement may differ among scanners.

Measurements of optimum beam energies for imaging iodine have been made by KELLER [13] and have shown that on the basis of maximizing iodine enhancement with respect to image artifact an energy of 100 kVp appears to be optimal. However, these authors found that maximum enhancement with minimum patient dose was obtained at 80 kVp on an EMI CT 1010 using plastic bags filled with water.

Table 2. Specific iodine enhancement

Source	Machine	kVp				
		Phantom[b] thickness (cm)	80	100	120	140
Theory[a]	–	21.4/2.54	–	34.5	24.31	19.46
Table 1	GE-7800	24.0/1.2	–	–	25.34[c]	–
Ref. [19]	EMI	24.0/1.2	–	32.5	25.6	20.6
Ref. [31]	EMI	–	45.2	32.0	25.0	–
Ref. [32]	EMI	–	–	–	26.0	–

[a] Effective energy, water attenuation coefficient from Ref. [11]. Iodine attentuation coefficient from Ref. [12]
[b] Water thickness (cm)/lucite thickness (cm)
[c] Using large body calibration file

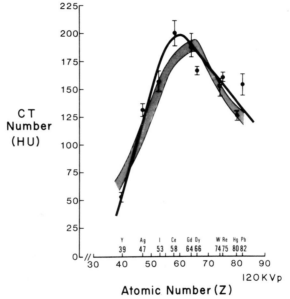

Fig. 5. Variation in enhancement with atomic number of 5 mg/ml concentration of absorber. The *shaded area* is the result of numeral calculation with data points resulting from phantom measurements. [14]

II. Contrast Enhancement from Other High Atomic Number Absorbers

It is well known that per gram of material iodine is slightly more attenuating than lead in the diagnostic energy range. However, this simple conclusion should not exclude the possibility of materials of atomic numbers between that of iodine and lead which may maximize the specific enhancement ratio for CT. The enhancement with materials of atomic numbers ranging from yttrium ($Z = 39$) to lead ($Z = 82$) has been calculated and measured at various tube potentials by SELTZER [14]. Figure 5 shows the measured and calculated enhancement as a function of

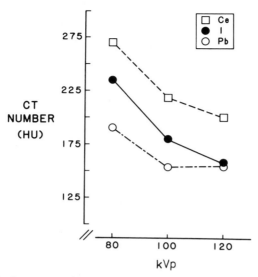

Fig. 6. Variation of enhancement for cerium (*squares*), iodine (*solid circles*), and lead (*open circles*) as a function of tube kilovoltage (4-mm aluminum total filtration) at concentrations of 5 mg/ml of absorber. [14]

atomic number for a 120-kVp beam. The results indicate that the specific enhancement reaches a maximum value around an atomic number of 58 (cerium). The shape of this curve can be explained by considering the position of the *K*-absorption edge of the element in the photon spectrum. At low atomic numbers the attenuation coefficient is relatively small; however, the bulk of the spectrum of photons have energy above the *K*-edge of the material. As the atomic number increases the attenuation coefficient increases and we would expect a net increase in attenuation; however, a larger portion of the spectrum will have photons of energy below the *K*-edge. At some atomic number the gain in attenuation by increasing the atomic number is exactly compensated by the loss in attenuation from low-energy photons interacting with *L* rather than *K* shell electrons. A further increase in atomic number causes a net reduction in absorption as the bulk of the spectrum interacts with the material below its *K*-edge.

The effect of beam energy is shown in Fig. 6 for tube kilovoltages of 80–120 kVp. However, an interesting point is that iodine shows a specific enhancement of 76% of that of cerium at 120 kVp. It is thus necessary to consider whether the relatively modest advantage in attenuation over iodine offered by materials of higher atomic number warrants the pharmacologic development necessary to make a clinically realistic alternative to currently existing iodinated CM from these elements of high atomic number. The behavior of these elements in biologic systems also needs to be tested, as many of them are highly toxic.

D. Image Manipulation

The detection of lesions that exhibit only a small differential attenuation change from normal parenchyma with CE can prove to be a difficult task when dealing with organs that are relatively inhomogeneous or when lesions are near organ boundaries. The presence of such a background may impair lesion detection in either the enhanced or nonenhanced scans. Attempts to minimize the perturbing effects of this structural background have involved imaging the iodine distribution itself. This has been done in two ways: viewing an image corresponding to the difference of the pre- and postcontrast-enhanced scans (subtraction) [15–17] or using the K-edge [18] or dual-energy [19] methods to construct images corresponding to the iodine distribution in tissues in the postcontrast-injected scan.

I. Subtraction

In this technique a precontrast injection scan is subtracted from the contrast-enhanced scan on a pixel by pixel basis. Ideally the final image corresponds to the iodine distribution and is free of any structure of the tissue itself. However, in practice this subtraction approach is far from ideal due to several scanning artifacts adding structural noise to images, tending to confound interpretation. Patient motion and differences in the beam-hardening patterns (due to the presence of iodine in the postcontrast injection scan) may introduce error in the iodine intensity in the subtracted image unless great care is taken to restrict patient motion and maintain low iodine concentrations in the tissue of interest. Nonlinear partial volume averaging may cause streaks across the image if iodine concentrations reach high levels [20]. However, in addition to these artifacts there will be an increase in imaging noise due to the image subtraction itself. This will, under ideal situations, be the limiting factor in the iodine image precision. It can be easily shown that the variance of the iodine density (g/cm^2) in the *projection data* is given by:

$$\sigma_i^2 = (\sigma_c^2 + \sigma_{nc}^2)/\mu_i^2 \, ,$$

where σ_{nc}^2 and σ_c^2 are the pre- and postcontrast-enhanced projection data variances and μ_i is the mass attenuation coefficient of iodine at the effective beam energy. For low iodine concentrations we can simplify this to:

$$\sigma_i = \sqrt{2}\sigma_c/\mu_i \, . \tag{2}$$

The minimum iodine precision in the *image* depends upon several scanner parameters including spatial resolution, choice of filter function, number of views, and projection data variance. The interrelationship between these parameters has been well documented [3,4]. Since the first three of these parameters will vary among scanners, we have chosen to deal only with the projection data variances in this and the following analysis to give a measure of the *relative* noise performance of the various image manipulation schemes.

II. Multiple Energy Methods

ZATZ [19] has shown the possibility of imaging iodine directly by subtracting images from scans made at 100 and 140 kVp as originally suggested by HOUNS-FIELD [21]. Results from this work indicate a specific iodine enhancement of approximately 12 HU ml/mg I after subtraction, a value about half that obtained with the pre- and postinjection subtraction method. This would indicate that the

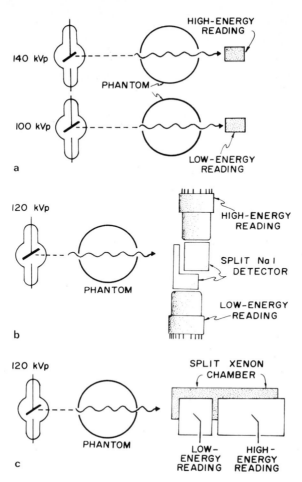

Fig. 7 a–c. Methods of dual-energy CT. The dual-scan method is shown in **a**, the "split" detectors using either a scintillator **b** or a xenon ionization chamber **c**. [10]

minimum concentration of iodine determinable with the dual-energy method shoud be about twice that of pre-post iodine subtraction. The fundamental approach to iodine determination by multiple energy methods has been well described by REIDERER [18], who concluded that iodine concentrations of 0.25 mg I/ml could be just resolved, at the expense, however, of considerable increase in scan time (several minutes) over that currently available due to reduced X-ray tube output required by K-edge filtration methods.

Figure 7 shows some of the alternatives for dual-energy scanning [10]. The dual kVp method (Fig. 7 a) uses high- and low-energy sets of projection data obtained by switching the tube potential. This has generally been accomplished by conducting two scans each with different tube potentials. Patient motion between scans can cause registration artifacts that limit the utility of this method. The "split detector" method [22–25] (Fig. 7 b, c) circumvents this problem by collecting the two sets of projection data simultaneously. One detector is used to filter the beam incident on a second detector. By this means the measured spectra of the two detectors shift to give a high- and low-energy pair of readings. This has been proposed for both scintillation and xenon detectors. Figure 8 shows the absorbed energy spectra for the high- and low-energy data for both the dual-kVp and a split-sodium iodine detector. It is clear that there is considerable spectral

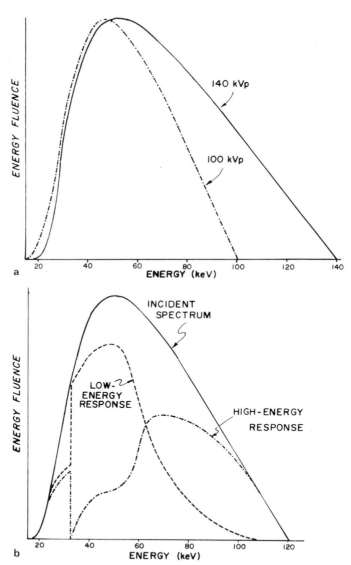

Fig. 8 a, b. Spectra of detected photons for the high- and low-energy reading. Dual-kVp scans shown in **a** with a NaI split detector shown in **b**

Table 3. Iodine precision simulation conditions

Tube-detector distance	100 cm
Total tube filtration	5.0 mm AL
Phantom	20 cm water
Detector area	1.0 cm^2
Tube mAs	kVp/120.0 (mAs)

overlap between the two sets of projection data, which is the primary cause of reduced imaging precision obtained with these methods.

If the attenuation data of the high-energy, A_h, and the low-energy, A_l, beams is due to tissue-like absorbers and iodine alone then:

$$A_h = \mu_{th}\varrho_t + \mu_{ih}\varrho_i \, ,$$
$$A_l = \mu_{tl}\varrho_t + \mu_{il}\varrho_i \, , \tag{3}$$

where μ_{th} and μ_{tl} are the *tissue* attenuation coefficients and μ_{ih} and μ_{il} are the iodine attenuations for the high- and low-energy beams. The parameters ϱ_t and ϱ_i are the projected tissue and iodine densities. We can rearrange Eq. (3) to yield the iodine density as:

$$\varrho_i = \frac{\mu_{tl}A_h - \mu_{th}A_l}{\mu_{ih}\mu_{tl} - \mu_{il}\mu_{th}}. \tag{4}$$

The variance in this measurement can be easily shown to be:

$$\sigma_i^2 = \{\mu_{tl}^2\sigma_h^2 + \mu_{th}^2\sigma_l^2\}/D^2 \, , \tag{5}$$

where

$$D = \mu_{ih}\mu m_{tl} - \mu m_{il}\mu_{th} \tag{6}$$

and σ_h^2 and σ_l^2 are the projection variances of the high- and low-energy measurements.

This result, which has been documented by several authors [18, 26], shows that the parameters "D," which we will call the "conditioning parameter," is central to the iodine noise determination and may be thought of as a measure of effective energy difference between the high- and low-energy projection data.

To estimate the relative precision of these two methods of direct iodine imaging Eq. (5) was evaluated using a continuous X-ray spectrum [10]. The conditions of the simulation are outlined in Table 3, which can be used to alter the following precision values for a more realistic scanner design.

The attenuation coefficients for the water and iodine measurements were evaluated using the expression [27]:

$$\mu = \int \mu(E)\,\phi(E)\,dE \, , \tag{7}$$

where $\mu(E)$ was obtained by log-log interpolation of iodine attenuation data [10] and $\phi(E)$ is the normalized detector energy spectra of the high- or low-energy

Table 4. Iodine noise (mg/cm^2)

	Dual kVp			Split	Pre-post subtraction
Beam kVps	100/140	80/140	80/120	120	120
mAs	1.2/.85	1.5/.85	1.5/1.0	1.0	2.0
Phantom surface [a] exposure (mR)	89	80	71	46.4	92
Iodine noise mg/cm^2 (SD)	0.82	0.52	0.68	0.78	0.32
SD × $\sqrt{mR}$ (mg/cm^2 mR$^{1/2}$)	7.72	4.66	5.77	5.31	3.07

[a] Calculated from ref. [28] assuming the phantom was centered between the source and detector. Single-phase X-ray source

beams. The data were calculated for a constant tube heat loading for each of the procedures.

Table 4 shows the iodine noise from Eq. (7) for the dual kVp combinations of 100/140, 80/140, and 80/120, a "split" sodium iodide detector, and the pre-post contrast subtraction method.

The exposure to the surface of the phantom (without backscatter) and standard deviation of the iodine projection measurement is shown for each technique [28]. We can directly compare the iodine noise for each of these techniques if tube loading is our only concern. However, if we wish to estimate the iodine noise on the basis of constant patient exposure, we can obtain an estimate of this by considering the parameter of the iodine noise time, the square root of exposure [2], which is shown in the last row. This indicates that the pre-post subtraction method offers minimum noise for a given patient exposure. The multiple energy methods exhibit some 1.5- to 2.5-fold greater noise for the same exposure. The result should not be unexpected as we may think of the pre-post subtraction method measuring the iodine attenuation over the entire spectrum of photons, but the dual-energy method measuring the iodine attenuation only over portions of the spectra that are *not* common to the high- and low-energy beams.

III. High Atomic Number Absorbers and Dual-Energy Computed Tomography

This section will extend the analysis of dual-energy CT for iodine detection to consider the influence of other high atomic number absorbers [10]. As was mentioned earlier the key to the noise properties of the dual-energy method involves the energy separation between the two sets of projection data as measured by the conditioning parameter, D of Eq. (6). Figure 9 shows a plot of the conditioning parameter for a 100/140-kVp dual-energy scan for water and an absorber of variable atomic number. This plot shows that the conditioning parameter appears to maximize at an atomic number of $Z = 58$. Figure 10 shows a plot of the standard

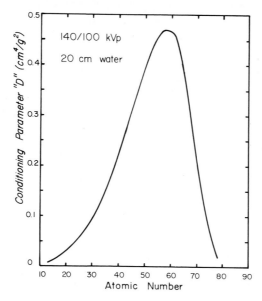

Fig. 9. Variation in dual-energy conditioning parameter D (see text) with atomic number. Dual-energy calculation made with beams of 100 and 140 kVp, 5-mm aluminum filtration, and 20-cm water path length. [10]

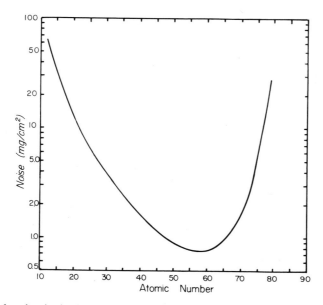

Fig. 10. Calculated noise in the projection data of the CM as a function of CM atomic number. Calculations made with 100/140 kVp. See Table 3 for more details on beam and detector parameters. [10]

Table 5. Effect on Z in dual-energy CT

Parameter	Dual-energy method			
	100/400	80/140	80/120	Split NaI
Z_{min}	57	58	58	53–58
D_x (cm⁴/g²)	0.493	0.960	0.764	0.631
Noise (mg/cm²)	0.753	0.505	0.678	0.78

deviation of the projected unknown element density versus the atomic number as evaluated from Eq. (5). Again, our conclusion is that the imaging noise reaches a broad minimum near the atomic number of 58.

To illustrate the effect of various dual-energy protocols on the noise, Table 5 summarizes the material atomic number (Z) for minimum imaging noise using the exposure parameters of Table 7. The overriding message from this analysis is that cerium ($Z = 58$) offers a noise advantage as a CM over iodine; although, as in the single-energy case, the improvements are modest. This points out that the choice of iodine as an absorber for diagnostic X-rays is close to optimal in the single- or dual-energy schemes that we have tested. This review of dual-energy techniques is by no means complete as several combinations of beam filtration and kilovoltage selection are conceivable. It is possible that the use of the K-edge filters with different tube kilovoltages may offer some sensitivity advantages for materials of high atomic number over iodine (S. Riederer, personal communication).

E. Dynamic Scanning

I. Conventional Computed Tomography Equipment

Reduction in scan time with the advent of third- and fourth-generation scanners has not only reduced patient motion artifacts but allows the possibility of observing the temporal response of various tissues to a bolus of CM. Early work on the dynamics of CM was conducted using the first-genertion EMI scanner with a scan time of approximately 5 min. Faster scan times with short time delays between scans offer more frequent sampling in dynamic studies. Further reductions in the effective scan time have been introduced by many manufacturers, with a technique which uses only a portion of the scan data normally analyzed in conventional reconstruction. Third- and fourth-generation scanners typically collect data from at least a 360° rotation; however, a "segmented reconstruction" can be obtained from data collected over an angle equal to 180° plus the fan angle as shown in Fig. 11. This approach uses only the data which represent unique angular views of the patient and for most scanners corresponds to about 210°. This zone of segmented reconstruction can be shifted throughout the scanner rotation to give serial images from scan motion. It is obvious that a good portion of the data between adjacent partial scans is redundant and as the time delay between images decreases the data redundancy increases. This has led most manufacturers to settle on three images per rotation. The times for full and partial scans are shown in Table 6 for some of the major scanner manufacturers, who are currently using dynamic routines. The number of partial reconstructions for each rotation is generally fixed at three to four with a few exceptions. Another important parameter that is central to the dynamic study issue is the number of dynamic scans that can be conducted without tube overload. This clearly depends upon the efficiency of photon utilization of the scanner, X-ray tube heat loading and dissipation characteristics, and the exposure techniques used during the individual scans. Table 6 indicates the tube heat-loading capacities for the various scanners in question.

II. Artifacts

The rapid changes in patient attenuation due to a circulating bolus of CM can produce scan artifacts in static CT. A study of this problem has shown that with cylindrical objects of time-varying attenuation, the images were artifact free within the cylinder, with a CT number corresponding to the time-averaged density over the duration of the scan [29]. The artifacts produced outside the cylindrical flow are similar in nature to motion artifacts, with the amplitude of the artifact decreasing with increasing distance from the cylinder, as shown in Fig. 12. The orientation of these streaks corresponds to the beginning and end of the bolus injection. The magnitude of these changes depends upon the nature of the bolus time-density profile but generally decreases as the temporal rate of change of bolus density decreases. In many practical cases the rate of change is sufficiently small to be of no consequence (Fig. 12).

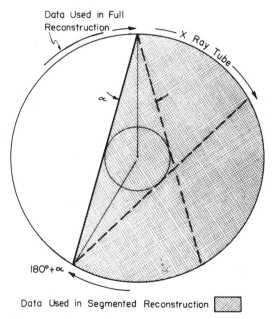

Fig. 11. Schematic of segmented, reconstruction principle. Conventional scans use data collected over 360° while segmented scans use data from a smaller region corresponding to 180° plus the fan angle α. [10]

Table 6. Survey of dynamic scanners

Scanner	Scan geometry "generation"	Shortest partial scan time (s)	Shortest full scan time (s)	Minimum interscan time (s)	Shortest full scan cycle (s)	Partial reconstruction time (s)	No. of partial reconstructions per 360° rotation	X-Ray tube heat capacity (heat units)
CGR 10,000	3rd	–	3.4	4	15.3	24	–	850,000
Elscint 2002FF	3rd	1.3	1.3	0.7	2	12	–	water cooled
GE 9800	3rd	1.3	2	2.3	4.3	18	3	700,000
Imatron C-100	4th	0.05	0.05	0.008	0.058	10	1	9,000,000
Philips T 350	3rd	3	4.8	3.2	8.0	10	3	1,350,000
Picker 1200 SX	4th	1.0	1.5	0.8	2.5	12	5	1,000,000
Siemens DR3	3rd	1.4	3.0	1.7	4.7	0	3	1,750,000
Technicare 2060	4th	–	2	4.8	6.8	10	–	1,500,000
Toshiba TCT-60A	3rd	2.7	4.0	2.0	6.0	15	3	1,500,000

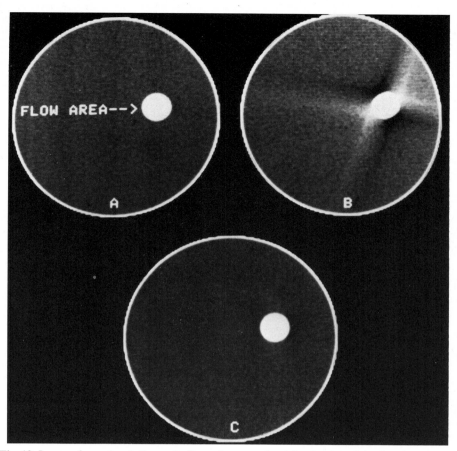

Fig. 12. Images from simulations of a flow phantom. In A the density of the flow is constant during the scan at 1.25 g/ml. In B the density of flow changes throughout the scan with a 1-s bolus during a 4.8-s scan. The bolus had a density of 1.25 g/ml with zero rise and fall time. In C the bolus increased linearly from 1 to 1.25 over 2 s and returned to 1.0 linearity over the next 2 s. Artifacts are visible outside the flow in B but not in C due to the long rise and fall times. The CT numbers in the flow area for all three conditions correspond to the time averaged CT density over the scan. [30]

These studies have been extended to the case of elliptical objects of varying eccentricity [30]. The CT density inside the ellipse was no longer equal to the time-averaged bolus CT density but was dependent upon several geometrical and temporal factors. Figure 13 shows the average CT density inside the ellipse relative to the true time average density of the bolus for a 1-s bolus injection passing through an ellipse of varying eccentricity with the initial X-ray beam inclined at angles of $0°$, $45°$, and $90°$ to the major axis. Note that the mean CT density relative to the time average bolus density is 1.0 at an eccentricity of 1.0 (circular), with the error increasing with increasing eccentricity. Figure 14 shows the effect of mean CT density on an ellipse of eccentricity of 2.0 for various times of bolus injection and initial projection angles. These curves suggest that as the bolus time approaches half the scan time, so that the bolus is present during transmission through both the major and minor axes, the error is reduced. In general the errors may be less than 10% when bolus lengths are greater than half the scan time.

III. Very High Speed Scanners

Principal limiting factors in the rapidity with which a CT scanner can operate are the beam current and heat capacity of the X-ray source. The time required for most single-tube scanners to expose one image is 1–5 s. Two approaches have been taken to allow scans to be made at times of approximately 50 ms.

The first approach uses a semicircle of X-ray tubes facing an equal number of image intensifiers acting as detectors [33, 34]. Each tube is exposed in succession to produce an image. With this approach a region of the body can be imaged in a single exposure, but the scanner is prohibitively expensive. A second approach is to use a flying spot X-ray source, produced by focusing a beam of electrons on a series of semicircular anodes surrounding the patient. An overlapping semicircle of detectors completes the circle. A rapid series of exposures produces images through a selected region of the body [34–36]. This system may rev-

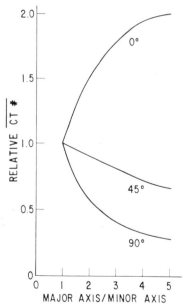

Fig. 13. Dynamic scan artifact for a 1-s bolus moving through an ellipse of varying eccentricity for a scan time of 4.8 s (360°) rotation. The vertical axis is the reconstructed CT number averaged over the ellipse relative to the CT number that would correspond to the time average density of the bolus over the scan time. The bolus was centered at a time corresponding to data collected at 180° of tube rotation. The artifact is shown for three different angles of orientation of the major axis of the ellipse with respect to the angular position of the tube at the start of the scan. [30]

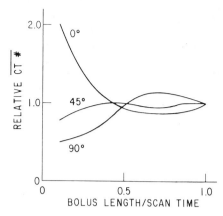

Fig. 14. Variations in relative average CT number (as described in Fig. 13) for various orientations of ellipse and bolus/scan time ratios. As the bolus length increased bolus density decreased so as to maintain a constant time average density. The ellipse eccentricity was 2.0. [30]

olutionize cardiac CT scanning by producing images of the heart unaffected by cardiac motion. Another application is dynamic CT of entire organs, rather than imaging only one or two sections with each CM bolus as must otherwise be done.

F. Pharmacokinetics of Contrast Enhancement

I. Body Compartments

The body can be divided into the *intracellular* and *extracellular* compartments. The iodinated radiographic CM commonly used in urography and angiography are generally considered to remain in the extracellular compartment and not penetrate intact cell membranes [37–40]. A notable exception to this generalization is the hepatocytes, which excrete cholangiographic, cholecystographic, and, to a lesser extent, urographic CM [41].

The cellular compartment also includes the intravascular cells, mainly erythrocytes, leukocytes, and platelets. The extracellular compartment is the domain of urographic CM. With molecular weights ranging from approximately 600 to 1,600, they pass with relative ease through the capillary walls into the *extravascular, extracellular* compartments. These compartments include the interstitial fluid (including lymph), renal tubular fluid and urine, the lumens of the gastrointestinal tract (including the biliary tree), and various glandular lumens. The blood-brain barrier effectively excludes the passage of intravenously injected urographic CM into the extravascular space of neural tissue [42, 43].

II. Diffusion of Contrast Media

During an intravenous injection of a urographic CM the blood concentration rises rapidly [44] and the CM immediately starts to diffuse into the extravascular

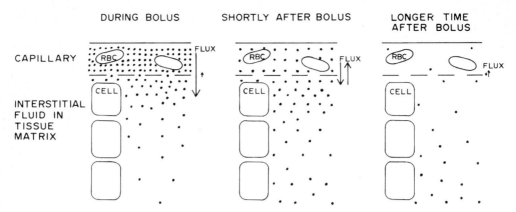

Fig. 15 a–c. Diagrammatic representation of a capillary and its adjoining tissue, with CM represented by *dots*. **a** During the passage of the CM bolus the flux is predominately out of the capillary, although there is a countercurrent water flux into the capillary. **b** Shortly after the bolus, at the time when the CM fluxes into and out of the capillary are equal. At this time the CM concentration more distal to the capillary is lower than that in the capillary. **c** At a longer time after the CM bolus the flux is mainly back into the capillary. At this time the CM concentration is higher in the tissue than in the capillary

space of most tissues [45–48]. This situation is simplified in Fig. 15 a, where the CM (*solid dots*) is shown diffusing across the concentration gradient through clefts or gaps in the capillary wall. Once the contrast molecules are outside the capillary they may diffuse either back into the capillary lumen or, more probably, out into the extravascular fluid space of the tissue in question [49–51]. Diffusion of small molecules within a tissue matrix is rapid [52].

Figure 15 b shows the situation after one or more recirculations of the CM bolus when the flux of the CM out of the capillary equals the flux back into the capillary. From this point onward, provided no further CM is injected, the blood concentration will continue to fall and the flux from the tissue interstitial fluid back into the capillary lumen will exceed the flux in the reverse direction. Both fluxes will gradually decrease with time as the respective driving concentrations fall.

During the early phase of decreasing perivascular concentration (between Fig. 15 b and 15 c) there will still be a further increase in CM concentration in the regions of the tissue more distant from (or less accessible to) the capillaries, although this delayed increase will be negligible in highly vascularized tissues. This delay may result in the vascular and perivascular CM concentrations being lower than the extracellular fluid concentrations elsewhere in the same tissue (Fig. 15 c). In any case, a small concentration gradient across the capillary wall will be necessary to drive the net CM flux out of the extravascular fluid and into the capillary lumen as the remaining CM is gradually excreted.

Contrast media pass so rapidly from the blood to the extravascular space that more than half of a rapidly injected bolus will be extravascular after only a few recirculations (20 s in the rat) [45]. Thus the situation shown in Fig. 15 a, where the CM is predominantly intravasvular, is very short lived. It can be prolonged by repeating the intravenous bolus injection at intervals of approximately ½ min or less.

The *rapidity* with which CM pass into the extravascular space in a given tissue depends on the driving force (concentration gradient) across the capillary wall and the permeability of the capillaries of that particular tissue to the CM in question. Thus, the *amount* of CM which reaches the extravascular space in a given tissue depends upon a rapidly changing blood plasma concentration which is counteracted by the rapidly rising extravascular concentration (Fig. 15a). The CE seen at CT is the sum of the intravascular and extravascular components, which cannot be measured separately from each other by CT. In larger vessels the concentration of iodine in blood can be measured, and the iodine concentration in plasma can be calculated if the hematocrit has been measured (see Sect. F.VII, below) [47].

III. Nonequilibrium Kinetics

The pharmacokinetics of drugs near equilibrium concentrations has been carefully studied [51, 53, 54], but little attention has been given to the nonequilibrium pharmacokinetics of drugs immediately after their administration, as this often has little clinical relevance and is difficult to study. Contrast enhancement, or concentration of CM, is greatest in most body tissues very soon after their intravenous administration [45–48]. By the time the CM concentrations approach quasi-equilibrium, the enhancement in most tissues is only a small fraction of the peak enhancement. This depletion in most tissues is the result of concentration and excretion by the kidney as well as the liver and skin [41, 45, 47, 53, 55]. Since the greatest absolute differences in attenuation between normal and pathologic tissues often (but not always – see Figs. 18, 19) occur at these peak values, equilibrium concentration analysis has little clinical application. Mathematic analysis of rapid time sequence measurements of tissue contrast concentration using dynamic CT after bolus contrast administration has shown some promise for characterizing blood volume and blood flow (see Sect. F.V, below) [56–59].

IV. Dynamic Aspects of Contrast Enhancement

In the *brain* CE is easy to understand. The blood-brain barrier (BBB) in normal brain tissue essentially prevents the CM from diffusing into the extravascular space [42, 43]. Thus CT contrast enhancement in the normal brain is a direct measurement of the vascular contrast alone (concentration in plasma multiplied by plasma volume) and it will fall at a continuously decreasing rate after a bolus contrast injection. In most other tissues the greater part of the CE measured at CT is no longer within the blood vessels but has passed into the extravascular space (Fig. 15b). Only within the first few seconds after the CM bolus reaches the capillaries is the major fraction of contrast within a given tissue still intravascular (Fig. 15a) [60].

Seen in terms of the *whole body* a given dose of rapidly injected intravascularly administered CM will initially mix with the plasma and almost immediately begin

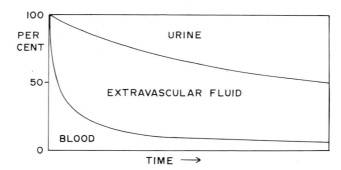

Fig. 16. Diagrammatic representation of relative CM distribution in the body after intravenous bolus injection. Initially entirely in the blood, the CM passes rapidly into the extravascular fluid and is subsequently slowly excreted into the urine

to pass into the various extravascular tissue compartments of most body tissues. Figure 16 shows how the proportion of intravascular contrast falls rapidly as most of it passes into the extravascular tissue space during the first few minutes. Renal excretion, a minor factor at first, soon becomes the major influence, causing CM to shift from the extravascular space back again into the blood and finally to the urine (with a small amount excreted in the feces, sweat, etc.) [55, 61, 62].

The *contrast enhancement of a given tissue* is determined by the total amount (vascular plus extravascular) of iodine in a unit volume. The following three factors all tend to increase the amount of extravascular CM, other variables (plasma concentration) being equal:

1. Highly developed capillary network, with capillaries mostly open
2. Highly permeable capillaries
3. Large extravascular, extracellular fluid volume without barriers to restrict diffusion of CM.

These three factors also increase the rapidity of CM distribution to the extravascular fluid space. Tissues fulfilling these three listed criteria have high CE which reaches peak values nearly as rapidly as the blood, but also falls again nearly as rapidly as blood values [47]. Factors such as:

1. Poorly developed capillary system and/or few capillaries open at any one time
2. Capillary walls of low permeability to CM
3. Relatively small extravascular, extracellular fluid space and/or barriers to contrast diffusion within this space

will all tend to reduce the rapidity and quantity of contrast distribution to the extravascular fluid space.

V. Dynamic Computed Tomography

An intravascular CM bolus generally produces a rise in CE to peak values followed by a fall as the CM bolus passes through the vasculature of the tissue being studied. In most tissues part of the contrast remains in the extravascular fluid space after the bolus has passed through the blood vessels supplying the tissue. With the first recirculation there may be a second, smaller peak in the CE. Measurement of blood vessel CE with rapid sequence CT shows more pronounced enhancement than in other tissues (Fig. 17). The aorta CE exhibits a rapid rise and fall. These data points have been mathematically fitted with a "best-fit" curve using the gamma variate function, which is well suited to fit a set of rising and falling data points [56]. The contrast bolus appears in the portal venous and vena caval circulations as more spread out curves with lower peak enhancement, because the capillary transit time is variable and because some of the CM remains in the extravascular spaces, diffusing slowly back into the capillaries.

Figure 18 shows a series of eight images taken at 3.6 s intervals through a right anterolateral section of the liver following intravenous bolus CE. In this patient with metastatic breast carcinoma the metastasis is initially of lower attenuation than the liver, then attains, in succession, equal, greater, equal, and

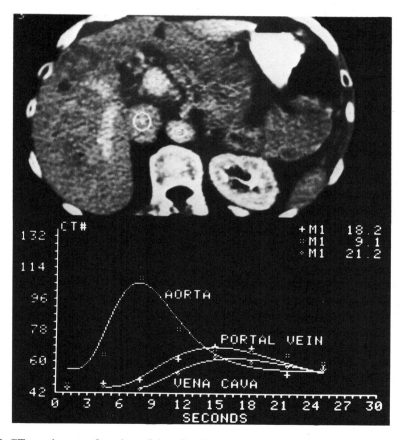

Fig. 17. CT number as a function of time for the aorta, portal vein, and inferior vena cava following a bolus intravenous injection of CM (25 ml, 40 g I/ml)

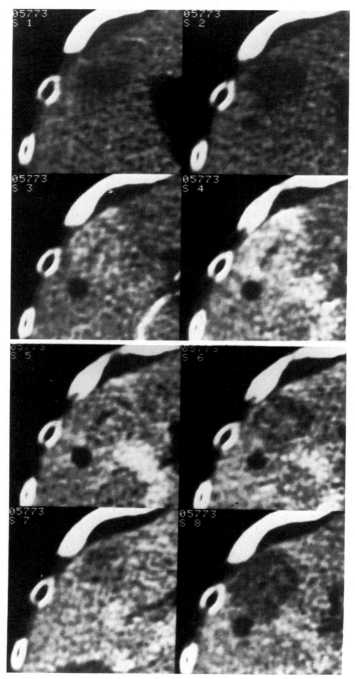

Fig. 18. Right anterior quadrant of the liver in a dynamic CT series (same as Figs. 17, 19) showing a metastasis from breast cancer which is initially hypodense, becoming successively isodense, hyperdense, isodense, and again hypodense [63]

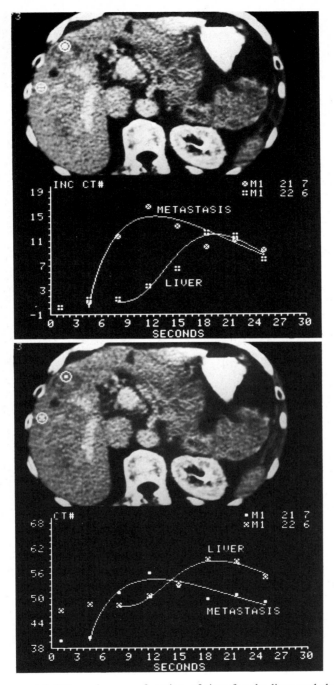

Fig. 19. a Incremental CT number as a function of time for the liver and the metastasis (shown in Fig. 18) following a bolus i.v. injection (see Fig. 17). Note that the initial attenuation values have been set to 0. **b** Absolute CT number of the liver and metastasis shown in **a** [59]

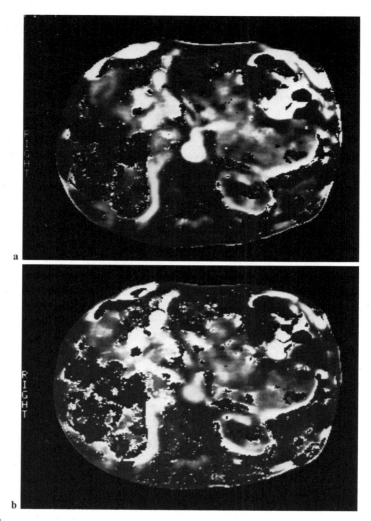

Fig. 20 a, b

Fig. 20 a–d. Function images of the liver in the same case as in Figs. 17–19, calculated from the curves averaged for each pixel point in the dynamic series. **a** Peak enhancement value of the curve. **b** Area under the curve. **c** Area under the curve divided by the dispersion of the data points about the curve. **d** Inverse corrected first moment of the curve [59]

lower attenuation than the surrounding liver as the CM bolus produces maximal attenuation first in the metastasis and then in the liver [63].

These events are depicted graphically in Fig. 19 a, b. Absolute attenuation values (1 CT number = 2 Hounsfield units) for the liver and the lesion are shown in Fig. 19 a, where the lesion initially has lower attenuation and reaches an early peak, temporarily greater than the liver attenuation. The absolute differences in

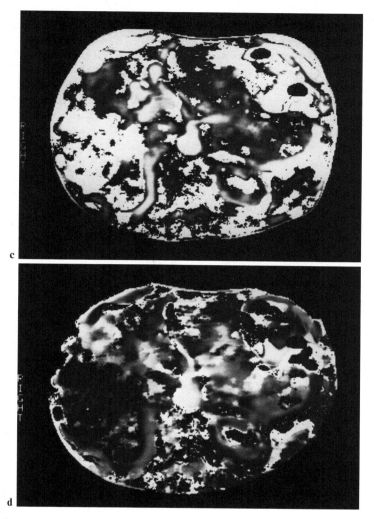

Fig. 20 c,d

attenuation (as well as lesion detectability) are greatest before the arrival of the bolus and at the time of peak liver enhancement. Images were not taken for a longer period because of the difficulty for the patient to hold her breath. Figure 19 b shows the CE for the same points with precontrast attenuation set arbitrarily to zero. Although the difference in enhancement is greatest at the time of peak enhancement of the metastasis, it is clear from Figs. 19 a and 18 that this is not the time of peak detectability of the lesion. Here we see the utility of taking several images during the period of peak CE to find the time of peak lesion detectability [64–66].

VI. Functional Imaging

The curves in Figs. 17 and 19 are made using a best fit to the gamma variate function, which requires a set of data points rising to peak values and then falling, although a curve fit can be approximated in some instances without a falling portion of data points. Such curve fits can be attempted for each pixel point in a series of images taken at a fixed anatomic location during the passage of a contrast bolus in dynamic CT. There are a number of different mathematic parameters which can be calculated for such curves and which can represent such physiologic values as blood flow, blood volume, mean transit time, etc. [57, 59].

Functional images can be created by choosing a single-curve parameter for a given series of images and letting each pixel point represent the value of that parameter over the series of images. Thus we can get functional images such as in Fig. 20a–d, each representing a different parameter of the gamma variate curve fit. Black and white areas represent points which did not produce a curve fit or which produced fitting parameters outside a specified range. These images represent a physiologic means of mathematically analyzing dynamic CT studies to produce information which cannot be appreciated merely by visual inspection of a series of images [57–59, 63, 67].

VII. Distribution Volume

Pharmacologists use this conceptually useful, theoretical tissue space as a means of analyzing the concentration of a drug in body tissues relative to the blood concentration. The distribution volume is the percent volume of a given tissue that a drug could occupy if its concentration in the extravascular tissue fluid were uniform and at equilibrium with the plasma concentration of the same drug [51]. Distribution volume is normally calculated by graphic analysis of blood concentration versus time, but it can be measured directly by taking tissue samples, measuring their drug concentration, and dividing this by the drug concentration of plasma [47]:

$$\text{Distribution volume } [\%] = \frac{\text{tissue CM concentration}}{\text{plasma CM concentration}} \times 100. \tag{8}$$

We know that the tissue CM (iodine) concentration is directly proportional to the CE [10, 68] (attenuation of nonenhanced scan subtracted from attenuation of enhanced scan at an identical location, either a pixel or averaged over a defined volume).

Considering blood as a tissue with plasma as the extracellular space:

$$\frac{\text{Contrast distribution volume in tissue}}{\text{Contrast distribution volume in blood}} = \frac{\dfrac{\text{CE in tissue} \times 100}{\text{CE in plasma}}}{\dfrac{\text{CE in blood} \times 100}{\text{CE in plasma}}}$$

$$= \frac{\text{CE in tissue}}{\text{CE in blood}}. \tag{9}$$

Since the CM is distributed only in the plasma and not within the red blood cells [39]:

$$\text{contrast distribution volume in blood} = 100\% - HCT\% . \tag{10}$$

Substituting (10) into (9) and rearranging [47, 64]:

$$\text{CM distribution volume in tissue} = (100\% - HCT\%)\frac{\text{CE in tissues}}{\text{CE in blood}} . \tag{11}$$

Distribution volume has been shown to correlate positively with growth and negatively with regression of malignant tumors [69].

VIII. Adverse Effects of Contrast Media in Computed Tomography

Intravenous CM have well-known pharmacologic effects in addition to the toxic, idiosyncratic reactions covered in Chap. 11. Since high doses of CM rapidly administered provide high levels of CE, there has been a recent trend to administer increasingly higher doses of CM, up to the range of 1–1.5 g I/kg [70–73]. At these high doses a great deal of attention must be paid to proper hydration [74]. Patients with known risk factors such as diabetes mellitus and renal and cardiac disease [74–76] should be given high doses of CM (in the order of 0.5 g I/kg of higher) only in special circumstances where the expected benefits of the study clearly outweight the known risks. High concentrations of CM can also inhibit platelet function [77].

IX. Intraarterial Contrast Media Administration

Although CT is basically a noninvasive examination technique, selective arterial CM administration offers the distinct advantage of very high CE levels (100–200 HU) at very low total CM doses (0.05–0.10 g I/kg). This has been shown to make possible detection of lesions not seen at CT after intravenous administration of higher iodine doses [63, 78, 79]. The invasive nature of this study has prevented its widespread acceptance. In addition, the scans must be repeated at intervals of 1–5 s to follow the passage of the arterial bolus through arterial, capillary, and venous circulation in a time sequence approaching that of angiography. Few CT scanners are capable of performing scans in rapid sequence and producing images of acceptable quality, and all conventional scanners produce images at only one level at a time. If the patient breathes during an injection or if the appropriate regions are not studied during the arterial bolus administration, smaller lesions could easily remain outside the area studied. A CT scanner which produces a number of images through a region of the body within a very short period (<1 s) and repeats this sequence at frequent intervals [33–36] should make intraarterial injection much more feasible.

X. Intracavitary Contrast Enhancement

Contrast media can be placed within a number of body cavities for improved CT demonstration of normal and pathologic structures. CM can also be excreted into the bladder and into the bile ducts.

The gastrointestinal tract is the most commonly enhanced body cavity, through oral and/or rectal administration. Either water-soluble media or barium sulfate suspensions can be given with equally satisfactory results [80–82]. The intrathecal spaces and the peritoneal cavity can be enhanced to diagnostic advantage [83–87].

XI. Noble Gases

Xenon has a high atomic number, diffuses readily across the blood-brain barrier, and is absorbed preferentially by fat. It can be administered by inhalation as it is rapidly absorbed through the lungs. The brain is ideally suited to CE by xenon as there is virtually complete first-pass uptake. The relative amount of xenon in different portions of the brain thus becomes a measure of the adequacy of circulation, with diminished contrast in regions with impairment [88–90].

XII. Reticuloendothelial System Contrast Enhancement

The Kupffer cells of the liver and the reticular cells of the spleen, in addition to other cells of the reticuloendothelial system, phagocytose foreign particulate matter from the blood. By injecting iodinated CM in the form of fine particulate matter or emulsions, the liver and spleen can be selectively enhanced with very low total body doses of iodine, and the enhancement may persist for periods of from several hours to several days. This topic is discussed in detail in Chap. 13 and will not be covered here.

G. Practical Applications of Contrast Enhancement

I. To Enhance or Not To Enhance?

A basic principle of medical practice is *nil nocere,* a teaching of Hippocrates "above all, do no harm." With a mortality of approximately 1 : 40,000 to 1 : 75,000 [91–95] CM cannot be considered completely harmless. Although intravascular CM unquestionably render many lesions more easily visible at CT, in many situations the principal pathologic findings are visible without CE. For each patient the radiologist should decide whether or not CM should be given during the CT study, and how, how much, when, and by which route it should be given [64]. In many instances the patient's symptoms can be explained on the basis of a noncontrast CT study, and further investigation using CE would not be expected to produce any useful additional information. In other situations the radiologist may decide that a noncontrast CT study, if performed, would yield insufficient information, and the initial CT study is performed after (or during) CM administration. A detailed discussion of all the factors affecting these clinical decisions is beyond the scope of this chapter, but any radiologist performing CT should be aware of the potential dangers of intravascular CM and the fact that careful review of a nonenhanced scan may reveal that a contrast-enhanced CT study is extremely unlikely to provide clinically relevant information. Conversely, a "normal" CT study performed without contrast, on inferior equipment, or with poor technique does not rule out the possibility of detecting clinically significant lesions on a properly performed contrast-enhanced CT study.

II. Basic Problems of Contrast Enhancement

Contrast media are used in CT as one of several diagnostic criteria. CT images are analyzed in terms of normal anatomy versus distorted anatomy, and are evaluated in terms of size, shape, location, homogeneity, and attenuation, with CM primarily affecting the attenuation. CM is used with such widespread acceptance because the attenuation changes are so frequently helpful in diagnosis. Like other imaging modalities, CT does not furnish a histopathologic diagnosis, although it can narrow down the differential diagnostic list. Unfortunately, all imaging modalities, even including histopathology, share the limitation that some pathologic lesions look normal and some normal lesions look pathologic. This overlapping of normal and pathologic appearances is a serious problem in CT, but it can be frequently overcome by biopsy.

Contrast media are not only mildly toxic and cause some patient discomfort, but they are also expensive. It is a matter of great practical concern how much each patient should receive. Although several studies have shown improved diagnosis with greater CM doses [73, 96, 97], at doses in the order of 1 g I/kg the expense and toxicity of the CM may offset the diagnostic advantages of improved CE.

It is unlikely that it will ever be possible to determine in advance the optimal CM dose for a given patient: the optimal dose should be only just enough to allow all pathologic lesions to be visualized, without causing the patient harm. Often this optimal dose does not exist, as in cases when CE cannot improve diagnosis without causing severe toxicity.

Other problems include the difficulty of scanning the correct slice level at the time when CE is maximal. This may be difficult to estimate as the nature of the lesions under study may not always be even suspected. Dynamic CT scanning helps overcome the problem of making an image at the time of greatest CE, but with conventional systems only one slice level can be studied during a CM bolus. Repeating the bolus at several slice levels helps partially to overcome this problem [72, 98]. Scanner performance can be another serious problem.

Computed tomography scanning requires that the radiologist has to make a number of rapid decisions, often on the basis of inadequate information, when using CE.

III. Contrast Enhancement in Cranial Computed Tomography

Contrast enhancement has been an essential part of cranial CT from the very outset [99] and it is used routinely in 78%–86% of cranial CT studies [100]. Fresh hematomas do not enhance, but since their attenuation is greater than normal brain tissue, they cannot be reliably differentiated from an enhancing lesion if the CT study has been performed with CE only. Calcifications within the brain cannot always be reliably differentiated from an enhancing vascular lesion without a precontrast study. If a noncontrast study is required following a contrast only CT examination, this can be performed the following day, as has been found necessary in about 3% of examinations [101]. Such a selective approach eliminates the need for most precontrast brain studies, saving most patients the time and radiation of the noncontrast study, and nearly doubles the limited capacity of available CT equipment.

It has been suggested that high doses of CM may actually enlarge an acute cerebral infarct [102, 103], by damaging marginally viable brain tissue at the borders of the infarction. Intravenous CM should be used with caution in patients suspected of having an ischemic brain lesion, although there has been no confirmation of this reported complication.

1. Detection of Lesions

Enhancement of *normal brain* tissue is greater in the gray matter than in the white matter, but it is otherwise uniform and thus difficult to appreciate against the background of noise in CT images at CM doses (up to approximately 40 g iodine) currently in general use. The relatively low degree of enhancement in the brain is due to the CM being restricted to the blood, which occupies only some 4%–5% of the total brain volume [39]. With high contrast doses and high contrast resolution, this normal enhancement can be quantitated using dynamic CT and differentiated in some cases from the lack of enhancement in a fresh infarct [104–107]. Otherwise, before the onset of edema, fresh infarcts have been difficult or impossible to detect with nondynamic CE [108]. Pituitary microadenomas appear as focal regions of low attenuation with CE [109].

Larger *blood vessels* can be detected with CE; the lower limit of the diameter detectable depends on the iodine concentration in the blood, the spatial and contrast resolution of the scanner, and the orientation of the vessel in the scanning plane (best detectability when parallel [110]). Dynamic CT scanning offers the greatest possibilities for detection of blood vessels [105, 106, 111]. Angiography currently offers a more accurate and effective means of visualizing vascular abnormalities, particularly small aneurysms [112, 113]. Scanning at several levels during peak CE of an extended bolus allows for a decrease in total CM used and improves visualization of the vasculature [114].

Breakdown of the normal blood-brain barrier enables iodinated CM to diffuse into the extravascular fluid space, providing a much greater volume of CM distribution, which accounts for the significant enhancement produced [105, 106]. Diffusion into the extravascular space may be slow, a factor accounting for the greater detectability of some malignant lesions in the brain with delayed CT scans [97]. The ability to detect BBB breakdown remains the most frequent indication for the use of CE in cranial CT, facilitating the detection and differentiation of tumors and infections and resolving hematomas. Detection of brain stem lesions is facilitated with intrathecal CM [115].

2. Differentiation of Cranial Lesions with CT Contrast Enhancement

Several factors are used in the differential diagnosis of cranial lesions, including location, size, shape, homogeneity, and attenuation. CE may affect all or none of these factors, and the degree of change caused by the contrast provides diagnostic clues concerning the probability of a particular diagnosis.

Highly vascular lesions can be most effectively seen with dynamic scanning, but a precontrast scan of a given location is necessary to differentiate vascular lesions and BBB breakdown from calcifications and hematomas [101–107]. The blood-brain barrier, which is normally absent in the anterior pituitary, meninges, and choroid plexus, breaks down or is incomplete in tumors, infections, and trauma, during radiotherapy, and around resolving hematomas [42, 43, 116, 117]. Contrast enhancement of some brain lesions decreases during steroid therapy and after radiotherapy [118–120].

There are a very large number of lesions affecting the brain [121], and completely reliable differentiation cannot be made on the basis of CE alone, although steps have been taken in that direction [122]. The history and physical, laboratory, and other radiologic examinations must all be taken into consideration to determine the relative probabilities of diagnoses in each individual patient.

3. Xenon Enhancement

This is currently in the experimental phase but shows some promise in the evaluation of cerebral blood flow [88–90; V. A. Haughton 1981, personal communication]. The anesthesia and possible cerebral hyperemia produced by inhaling high concentrations of xenon severely limit the maximum useful enhancement obtainable with this agent.

IV. Contrast Enhancement in Body Computed Tomography

1. Maximizing Enhancement

Body CT contrast enhancement is generally greatest during the capillary phase of a CM bolus or shortly thereafter [64, 72, 123]. The only meaningful exception is renal concentration, producing a delayed peak concentration in the collecting system. Since the peak CE values are often short lived, the practical problem facing the radiologist is the following: how can he scan the suspected lesion at the time when CE is greatest?

Dynamic CT can overcome the problem of choosing the moment when CE is greatest by performing a series of scans in rapid succession. If the intravenously injected CM bolus produces maximum enhancement in the chosen tissue during one of the scans, this approach can be considered successful. The two serious limitations are: (a) several scans must be taken at one slice level, giving additional radiation exposure and (b) only one slice level can be studied at maximum enhancement with each CM bolus injection using conventional CT scanners.

Experience with vascular transit time (from antecubital vein injection to maximum CE) for each particular organ can enable the radiologist to obtain near-maximal enhancement from a bolus with only one scan. Repeating smaller boluses and scanning more than one level per bolus are compromises which allow the radiologist to produce a contrast-enhanced study through an entire organ using acceptable CM doses [72, 98, 123].

Dynamic CT – several scans in rapid sequence following a CM bolus – may be criticized as a "shotgun" approach to obtaining a single scan at the time of peak enhancement. As is shown in Fig. 19, peak enhancement may be the time when absolute difference in enhancement between a lesion and the surrounding normal tissue is lowest, and in such cases detectability of small lesions would also be lowest at peak enhancement [63]. Dynamic CT, which may be extended through delayed scans to a period of several minutes, can help to characterize a suspected lesion as well as produce a CT image with the greatest possible contrast resolution [58, 63, 124]. The heterogeneity of single lesions and the overlap of enhancement patterns between widely differing lesions greatly reduces the differential diagnostic value of dynamic CT. It is likely that improvements in equipment, particularly in scanner speed, contrast resolution, and dual-energy imaging, will make dynamic CT a more useful clinical tool.

2. Cardiac Computed Tomography

The principal obstacle for obtaining high-detail images of the heart is cardiac motion, as conventional scanners cannot perform a full scan fast enough to eliminate motion artifacts effectively [33–35]. Working within this severe restriction, a great deal has been accomplished with the use of CE. An additional problem is the relatively long interscan delay time, even with overscan capability.

Vascular anatomy, particularly pathologic, and postoperative alterations have been well demonstrated in a majority of cases. Anomalous vascular structures and aortic aneurysms have been definitively diagnosed in the vast majority of instances, although angiography is still being used for confirmation until radiologists (and surgeons) gain experience and confidence with the method. Dynamic CT has proved especially useful for following the course of dissecting aneurysms [125–127]. A serious drawback is the length of time necessary to scan the entire thoracic and/or abdominal aorta, but this limitation is relative only and is rapidly being overcome by improvements in CT equipment. The noninvasive nature of CT makes it a particularly desirable examination in the critically ill patient.

Coronary artery bypass grafts can be reliably shown to be patent in the immediate postoperative period, when the stress of a repeat coronary angiogram would be highly undesirable. With a specificity and sensitivity of over 90%, this examination, which is performed as a series of dynamic scans through the aortic root, has now gained clinical acceptance [128, 129], although it is underutilized.

Myocardial infarction appears on a dynamic scan first as an area of decreased enhancement (in a region of low baseline attenuation) followed by a period of increased attenuation as the CM slowly diffuses into the nonviable infarct from the borders with normal tissue [130–134]. Infarcts of age exceeding 1 week are more enhanced than normal myocardium [40]. There is still disagreement as to which of these phases provides more reliable diagnosis, although it appears that infarct size can be more reliably measured from the enhanced infarct [132, 133]. All early studies were performed in dogs; anterior and septal acute infarcts are well seen in man, the perfusion deficit phase being most easily identified. Segmental motion abnormalities require either gating with conventional whole body scanners or faster machines. This is the area, therefore, where extremely fast CT scanners can be expected to have great impact. Mural thrombi, cardiac tumors, and pericardial masses can also be evaluated by conventional CT [135, 136].

3. Chest, Lung, and Mediastinal Computed Tomography

The high innate air-tissue contrast differential in the lung makes CE less useful in the lungs than in the solid soft tissues. CE has been shown to be useful in evaluating chest wall lesions, lung abscesses and empyema, pulmonary embolism, and mediastinal structures, particularly tumors [137–144]. Cardiac motion tends to degrade images of the other chest structures as well, but does not degrade images taken during 50 ms [35, 36].

4. Hepatic and Splenic Computed Tomography

The liver receives the greatest part of its blood supply from the portal vein, the heptic artery accounting for less than a quarter of its circulation. Most hepatic malignancies, like tumors elsewhere in the body, take their circulation from the arterial blood. Peak liver enhancement is thus delayed relative to adjacent organs as the CM bolus passes first through the spleen and intestines [79, 145, 146].

The high attenuation of the liver and its great uptake of CM cause it usually to form a background of high attenuation against which most liver tumors are seen as regions of lower attenuation, often with a zone of increased enhancement at the boundary between the liver and the tumor. Although the appearance of cavernous hemangioma is considered to be typical at dynamic scanning, CE with dynamic scanning has not otherwise led to specific differential diagnosis of liver lesions [63, 147–156]. Abscesses not containing gas can be mistaken for tumors [157–160]. Perhaps the most important contribution of CE is in rendering small lesions more visible [9], leading to an improved detection of metastases [152, 153, 161]. In dynamic scanning hepatic arterial enhancement may momentarily make some malignant hepatic lesions relatively hyperdense [63, 145, 162]. Much greater enhancement can be reached with intraarterial contrast injection, although the invasive nature of angiography greatly limits application of this method [63, 79, 162, 163]. Two excellent reviews have recently covered this complex subject [164, 165].

The spleen is more vascular than the liver and normally enhances to a greater degree. The peculiar circulation of the spleen produces a mottled appearance early in a dynamic scan, but this appearance soon becomes homogeneous [166]. CE improves the detection of virtually every abnormality of the spleen [167].

5. Pancreatic Computed Tomography

Although less helpful with slow scanners, CE with rapid i.v. bolus administration has been shown to be of considerable help in defining the extent of normal pancreatic anatomy and some pathologic processes, particularly pancreatitis [123, 168–175]. Since the entire pancreas cannot be scanned without the patient having to breathe once or more between scans with present CT equipment, the development of a very rapid scanner which could image the entire pancreas during the passage of the CM bolus should allow significant improvement in diagnostic accuracy. Such a rapid scanner would enable scanning of the entire organ at peak contrast without leaving some parts of the pancreas unexamined as often happens when patients take breaths of varying depths in between consecutive scans.

6. Renal and Adrenal Computed Tomography

The very high renal enhancement with CT makes possible the detection of very small lesions, as well as detailed investigation of the renal circulation. CE is most useful in diagnosis of adrenal diseases when there is little retroperitoneal fat. Tumors, infection, infarcts, and renovascular hypertension can all be more accurately diagnosed with CE [176–183].

7. Computed Tomography of Abdominal Blood Vessels

Intraarterial CE is generally too great for useful delineation of the arteries, and better images of the arteries can be obtained by arteriography if an intraarterial catheter is used. Optimal delineation of the blood vessels can be obtained following rapid bolus intravenous contrast administration, and the direction of blood flow, collateral circulation, and presence of arteriovenous shunts can often be determined from serial CT scans or dynamic CT studies. Dissecting aneurysms, tumor invasion into veins, and portal venous abnormalities can be detected with a high level of accuracy [72, 125–127, 184–191]. Direct infusion through the inferior vena cava provides precise delineation of this vessel [192, 193]. With abdominal compression, the CM can be visualized in the lumbar veins [194].

8. Computed Tomography of the Pelvic Organs

Contrast enhancement is useful to delineate the extent of pelvic tumors better, including cervical, uterine, ovarian, bladder, prostate and some intestinal tumors, as well as abscesses and vascular lesions [158–160, 195–197].

9. Intracavitary Enhancement

Peroral administration of dilute iodinate- or barium-containing CM to outline the small intestine has become an essential routine in body CT. Retrograde contrast enemas, vaginal tamponade, and even intraperitoneal infusion of CM can be helpful in better delineating pathologic as well as normal structures [81–85, 175, 198–201]. Fat-containing liquids (hyperalimentation fluids are most convenient) are particularly useful for delineating the urinary bladder [202].

V. Choice of Intravascular Contrast Medium

The nonionic CM presently available for experimental or clinical use appear to remain within the vasculature to a slightly greater extent than do the conventional ionic media. There is the possibility that these newer agents may provide greater enhancement per gram iodine injected, although the effect is apparently small [48, 203]. The much greater expense of the nonionic agents will probably be the greatest obstacle to their use.

Cholangiographic agents can be used to give specific enhancement of the hepatocytes and biliary tree. Although they can produce greater liver enhancement per gram iodine injected, the improved enhancement occurs at a considerable increase in CM toxicity, completely negating any specific benefits from selective hepatic uptake and excretion [204].

At present the ionic monomeric CM, diatrizoate, iothalamate, metrizoate, ioxithalamate, and iodamide, appear to be suitable for CT contrast enhancement. A further development to be hoped for in the near future would be a low-cost, low-toxicity intravascular CM which could be given rapidly in large doses without significant side effects. The present nonionic CM, of which metrizamide is the earliest example, are superior in tolerability but cost so much that their use in CT intravascular CE is severely limited. The selective CM (biliary, particulate, emulsions) are still very much in the experimental stage.

Further improvements in CT equipment, particularly in scan speed, contrast resolution, and spatial resolution, are likely to provide greater diagnostic benefit than further improvements in contrast media.

Acknowledgments. This work has been supported in part by financial assistance from the Sigrid Jusélius Foundation, Helsinki, the Emil and Blida Maunola Fund of the Paolo Foundation, Helsinki, and T. A. Bioteknik, Malmö. The manuscript was subsequently revised while P. B. Dean was the recipient of an Eleanor Roosevelt Fellowship of the American Cancer Society administered through the International Union Against Cancer.

References

1. Ter-Pogossian MM (1974) Extraction of the yet unused wealth of information in diagnostic radiology. Radiology 113:515–520
2. Cohen G, DiBianca F (1979) Use of contrast-detail-dose evaluation of image quality in a computed tomographic scanner. J Comput Assist Tomogr 3:189–195
3. Chesler D, Riederer S, Pelc N (1977) Noise due to photon counting statistics in X-ray computed tomography. J Comput Assist Tomogr 1:64–74
4. Brooks RA, DiChiro G (1976) Principles of computer assisted tomography (CAT) in radiographic and radioisotope scanning. Phys Med Biol 21:689–732
5. Joseph PM (1981) Artifacts in computed tomography. In: Newton T, Potts G (eds) Radiology of the skull and brain, vol 5. Mosby, St. Louis, pp 3956–3992
6. Zatz L (1981) General overview of computed tomography – instrumentation. In: Newton T, Potts G (eds) Radiography of the skull and brain, vol 5. Mosby, St. Louis, pp 4025–4057
7. Plewes DB, Dean PB (1979) Detectability of spherical objects by computed tomography. Radiology 133:785–786
8. Plewes DB, Dean PB (1981) The influence of partial volume averaging on sphere detectability in computed tomography. Phys Med Biol 26:913–919
9. Violante MR, Dean PB (1980) Improved detectability of VX2 carcinoma in the rabbit liver with contrast enhancement in computed tomography. Radiology 134:237–239
10. Plewes DB, Violante MR, Morris TW (1980) Intravenous contrast material and tissue enhancement in computed tomography. In: Fullerton GD, Zagzebski JA (eds) Medical physics of CT and ultrasound. American association of physicists in medicine, medical physics monograph no 6. American Institute of Physics, New York, pp 176–220
11. McCullough EC (1975) Photon attenuation in computed tomography. Med Phys 2:307–320
12. Weigle WJ (1973) Photon cross-sections, 0.1 keV to 1 MeV. Atomic data 5:52–111
13. Keller MR, Kessler RM, Brooks RA (1980) Optimum energy for CT iodinated contrast studies. Br J Radiol 53:576–579
14. Seltzer SE (1981) Rare earth contrast agents in hepatic computed tomography. In: Felix R, Kazner E, Wegener OH (eds) Contrast media in computed tomography. Excerpta Medica, Amsterdam, pp 76–84

15. Zilkha E, Ladurner G, Iliff LD, DuBoulay GH, Marshell J (1976) Computed subtraction in regional cerebral blood volume measurements using an EMI scanner. Br J Radiol 49:330–334
16. Zilkha E, Kendall B, Loh L, Hayward R, Radue EW, Ingram GS (1978) Diagnosis of subdural hematoma by computed axial tomography – use of xenon inhalation for contrast enhancement. J Neurol Neurosurg Psychiatry 41:370–373
17. Kelcz F, Hilal SK, Hartwell P, Joseph PM (1978) Computed tomographic measurements of the xenon brain-blood partition coefficient and implications for regional cerebral blood flow: a preliminary report. Radiology 127:385–392
18. Riederer S, Mistretta CA (1977) Selective iodine imaging using K-edge energy in computerized X-ray tomography. Med Phys 4:474–481
19. Zatz LM (1976) The effect of kVp level on EMI values. Radiology 119:683–688
20. Glover GH, Pelc NJ (1980) Nonlinear partial volume artifacts in X-ray computed tomography. Med Phys 7:238–248
21. Hounsfield GN (1973) Computerized transverse axial scanning (tomography): I. Description of system. Br J Radiol 46:1016–1022
22. Brooks RA, DiChiro G (1978) Split detector computed tomography – preliminary report. Radiology 126:255–257
23. Brownell GL (1978) International symposium and course on computed tomography, Miami Beach, March 1978
24. Fenster A (1978) Split xenon detector for tomochemistry in computed tomography. J Comput Assist Tomogr 2:243–252
25. Alvarez R, Seppi E (1979) Workshop on the physics and engineering in computed tomography, Newport Beach, Jan 1979
26. Alvarez R, Macovski A (1976) Energy selective reconstructions in X-ray computerized tomography. Phys Med Biol 21:733–744
27. Kelcz F, Joseph PM, Hilal S (1979) Noise considerations in dual energy CT scanning. Med Phys 6:418–425
28. McCullough EC, Cameron JE (1970) Exposure rates from diagnostic X-ray units. Br J Radiol 43:448–451
29. Holden JE, Ip WR (1978) Continuous time dependence in computed tomography. Med Phys 5:485–490
30. Berninger WH, Redington RW (1981) Dynamic computed tomography. In: Newton TH, Potts DG (eds) Technical aspects of computed tomography. Mosby, St. Louis (Radiology of the skull and brain, vol 5)
31. Hindmarsh T (1975) Elimination of water-soluble contrast media from the subarachnoid space: investigation with computer tomography. Acta Radiol [Suppl 346] 16:45–50
32. Gado MH, Phelps ME, Coleman RE (1975) An extravascular component of contrast enhancement in cranial computed tomography. Radiology 117:589–593
33. Robb RA, Ritman EI, Gilbert BK, Kinsey JH, Harris LD, Wood EH (1979) The DSR: a high-speed three-dimensional X-ray computed tomography system for dynamic spatial reconstruction of the heart and circulation. IEEE Trans Nucl Sci NS-26:2713–2717
34. Boyd DB (1981) Transmission computed tomography. In: Newton TH, Potts DG (eds) Technical aspects of computed tomography. Mosby, St. Louis, pp 4357–4371 (Radiology of the skull and brain, vol 5)
35. Boyd DB, Lipton MJ (1983) Cardiac computed tomography. Proc IEEE 71:298–307
36. Stakun DJ (1983) First clinical results with cine computed tomography scanner. RNM Images 13:14–18
37. Rapoport SI, Levitan H (1974) Neurotoxicity of X-ray contrast media. AJR 122:186–193
38. Gottlob R, Knapp G, Porschinski K, Saghir K (1980) Untersuchungen über den Mechanismus von Kontrastmittelschäden, die Bedeutung der Lipophilia. Fortschr Röntgenstr 132:204–207
39. Phelps ME, Grubb RL Jr, Ter-Pogossian MM (1973) In vivo regional cerebral blood volume by X-ray fluorescence: validation of method. J Appl Physiol 35:741–747

40. Newell JD, Higgins CB, Abraham JL (1982) Uptake of contrast material by the ischemically damaged myocardial cell. Invest Radiol 17:61–65
41. Owman T, Olin T (1978) Biliary excretion of urographic contrast media. Ann Radiol 21:309–314
42. Bradbury M (1979) The concept of a blood-brain barrier. Wiley, Chichester
43. Sage MR (1982) Blood-brain barrier: phenomenon of increasing importance to the clinician. AJR 138:887–898
44. Dean PB, Violante MR, Mahoney JA (1980) Hepatic CT contrast enhancement: effect of dose, length of infusion and time elapsed following infusion. Invest Radiol 15:158–161
45. Dean PB, Kormano M (1977) Intravenous bolus of ^{125}I labeled meglumine diatrizoate. Acta Radiol [Scand] 18:293–304
46. Newhouse JH (1977) Fluid compartment distribution of intravenous iothalamate in the dog. Invest Radiol 12:364–367
47. Dean PB, Kivisaari L, Kormano M (1978) The diagnostic potential of contrast enhancement pharmacokinetics. Invest Radiol 13:533–540
48. Dean PB, Kivisaari L, Kormano M (1983) Contrast enhancement pharmacokinetics of six ionic and nonionic contrast agents. Invest Radiol 18:368–374
49. Axel L (1976) Flow limits of Kedem-Katchalsky equations for fluid flux. Bull Math Biol 38:671–677
50. Homer LD, Weathersby PK (1980) The variance of the distribution of traversal times in a capillary bed. J Theor Biol 87:349–377
51. Gillette JR (1973) The importance of tissue distribution in pharmacokinetics. J Pharmacokinet Biopharm 1:497–520
52. Hogben CAM (1971) Biological membranes and their passage by drugs. In: Brodie BB, Gillette JR, Ackermann HS (eds) Concepts in biochemical pharmacology, part 1. Springer, Berlin Heidelberg New York, pp 1–8 (Handbook of experimental phamacology, vol 28/1)
53. Feldman S (1974) Drug distribution. Med Clin North Am 58:917–926
54. Greenblatt DJ, Koch-Weser J (1975) Clinical pharmacokinetics. N Engl J Med 293:702–705
55. Speck U, Nagel R, Leistenschneider W, Mützel W (1977) Pharmakokinetic und Biotransformation neuer Röntgenkontrastmittel für die Uro- und Angiographie beim Patienten. Fortschr Röntgenstr 127:270–274
56. Axel L (1980) Cerebral blood flow determination by rapid-sequence computed tomography: a theoretical analysis. Radiology 137:679–686
57. Berninger WH, Axel L, Norman D, Napel S, Redington RW (1981) Functional imaging of the brain using computed tomography. Radiology 138:711–716
58. Norman D, Axel L, Berninger WH, Edwards MS, Cann CE, Redington RW, Cox L (1981) Dynamic computed tomography of the brain: techniques, data analysis, and applications. AJNR 2:1–12
59. Axel L, Dean PB, Moss AA, Stansberry D (1984) Functional imaging of the liver: new information from dynamic CT. Invest Radiol 19:23–29
60. Dean PB, Kormano M (1977) Intra-arterial bolus of ^{125}I-labeled meglumine diatrizoate: early extravascular distribution. Acta Radiol [Diagn] 18:293–304
61. Langecker H, Harwart A, Junkmann K (1954) 3,5-Diacetylamino-2,4,6-trijodbenzoesäure als Röntgenkontrastmittel. Arch Exp Pathol Pharmak 222:584–590
62. McChesney EW, Hoppe JO (1957) Studies of the tissue distribution and excretion of sodium diatrizoate in laboratory animals. AJR 78:137–144
63. Moss AA, Dean PB, Axel L, Goldberg HI, Glazer GM, Friedman MA (1982) Dynamic CT of hepatic masses with intravenous and intraarterial contrast material. AJR 138:847–852
64. Dean P (1980) Contrast media in body computed tomography: experimental and theoretical background, present limitations, and proposals for improved diagnostic efficacy. Invest Radiol [Suppl] 15:S164–S170
65. Tschakert H (1980) Zeitlicher Ablauf des Dichteverhaltens von Lebermetastasen nach Kontrastmittelgabe. Fortschr Röntgenstr 133:171–176

66. Young SW, Turner RJ, Castellino RA (1980) A strategy for the contrast enhancement of malignant tumors using dynamic computed tomography and intravascular pharmacokinetics. Radiology 137:137–147
67. Axel L, Moss AA, Berninger W (1981) Dynamic computed tomography demonstration of hepatic arteriovenous fistula. J Comput Assist Tomogr 5:95–98
68. Hatam A, Bergvall U, Lewander R et al. (1975) Contrast medium enhancement with time in computer tomography. Differential diagnosis of intracranial lesions. In: Lindgren E (ed) Computer tomography of brain lesions. Acta Radiol [Suppl] 346:63–81
69. Oppenheimer DA, Young SW, Marmor JB (1983) Work in progress: serial evaluation of tumor volume using computed tomography and contrast kinetics. Radiology 147:495–497
70. Davis JM, Davis KR, Newhouse J, Pfister RC (1979) Expanded high iodine dose in cranial computed tomography: a preliminary report. Radiology 131:373–380
71. Hayman LA, Evans RA, Fahr LM, Hinck VC (1980) Renal consequences of rapid high dose contrast CT. AJR 134:553–555
72. Rossi P (1981) CT contrast enhancement in CT of the great arteries. In: Fuchs WA (ed) Contrast enhancement in body computerized tomography. Thieme, Stuttgart, pp 45–57
73. Raininko R, Majurin ML, Virtama P, Kangasniemi P (1982) Value of high contrast medium dose in brain CT. J Comput Assist Tomogr 6:54–57
74. Cattell WR, Sensi M, Ackrill P, Fry IK (1980) The functional basis for nephrographic patterns in acute tubular necrosis. Invest Radiol [Suppl] 15:S79–S83
75. Golman K, Holtås S (1980) Proteinuria produced by urographic contrast media. Invest Radiol [Suppl] 15:S61–S66
76. Mützel W (1981) Properties of conventional contrast media. In: Felix R, Kazner E, Wegener OH (eds) Contrast media in computed tomography. Excerpta Medica, Amsterdam, pp 19–26
77. Goldstone J, Sandow NH (1976) Inhibition of platelet function by angiographic contrast media. In: Grayson J, Zingg W (eds) Microcirculation, vol 1: blood-vessel interactions, systems in special tissues. Plenum, New York, pp 191–193
78. Prando A, Wallace S, Bernardino ME et al. (1979) Computed tomographic arteriography of the liver. Radiology 130:697–701
79. Freeny PC, Marks WM (1983) Computed tomographic arteriography of the liver. Radiology 148:193–197
80. Ruijs SHJ (1979) A simple procedure for patient preparation in abdominal CT. AJR 133:551–552
81. Megibow AJ, Bosniak MA (1980) Dilute barium as a contrast agent for abdominal CT. AJR 134:1273–1274
82. Kivisaari L, Kormano M (1982) Comparison of diatrizoate and barium sulfate bowel markers in clinical CT. Europ J Radiol 2:33–34
83. Roub LW, Drayer BP, Orr DP, Oh KS (1979) Computed tomographic positive contrast peritoneography. Radiology 131:699–704
84. Dunnick NR, Jones RB, Doppman JL, Speyer J, Myers CE (1979) Intraperitoneal contrast infusion for assessment of intraperitoneal fluid dynamics. AJR 133:221–223
85. Roub LW, Orr DP, Oh KS, Drayer BP, Herbert DL (1980) Early clinical experience with direct peritoneal enhancement for abdominal computed tomography. Comput Tomogr 4:217–224
86. Marc JA, Khan A, Pillari G, Rosenthal A, Baron MG (1980) Positive contrast ventriculography combined with computed tomography: technique and applications. J Comput Assist Tomogr 4:608–613
87. Manelfe C, Chambers EF (1981) Computed tomographic cisternography with water-soluble contrast media: normal and pathologic appearance. In: Felix R, Kazner E, Wegener OH (eds) Contrast media in computed tomography. Excerpta Medica, Amsterdam, pp 107–112
88. Meyer JS, Hayman LA, Yamamoto M, Sakai F, Nakajima S (1980) Local cerebral blood flow measured by CT after stable xenon inhalation. AJNR 1:213–225

89. Haughton VM, Donegan JH, Walsh PR, Syvertsen A, Williams AL (1980) A clinical evaluation of xenon enhancement for computed tomography. Invest Radiol 15:160–163

90. Coin JT, Coin CG (1981) Nontoxic contrast agents for computed tomography. In: Felix R, Kazner E, Wegener OG (eds) Contrast media in computed tomography. Excerpta Medica, Amsterdam, pp 107–112

91. Ansell G (1970) Adverse reactions to contrast agents. Scope of problem. Invest Radiol 5:374–384

92. Fischer HW, Doust VL (1972) An evaluation of pretesting in the problem of serious and fatal reactions to intravenous urography. Radiology 103:497–501

93. Witten DM, Hirsch FD, Hartman GW (1973) Acute reactions to urographic contrast medium. ARJ 119:832–840

94. Ansell G, Tweedie MCK, West CR, Price Evans DA, Couch L (1980) The current status of reactions to intravenous contrast media. Invest Radiol [Suppl] 15:S32–S39

95. Hartman GW, Hattery RR, Witten DM, Williamson B Jr (1982) Mortality during excretory urography: Mayo Clinic experience. AJR 139:919–922

96. Davis JM, Davis KR, Newhouse J et al. (1979) Expanded high iodine dose in computed cranial tomography: a preliminary report. Radiology 131:373–380

97. Hayman LA, Evans RA, Hinck VC (1980) Delayed high iodine dose contrast computed tomography: cranial neoplasms. Radiology 136:677–684

98. Koehler PR, Anderson RE (1961) Computed angiotomography. Radiology 1980:843–845

99. Ambrose J (1973) Computerized transverse axial scanning (tomography): part 2, clinical application. Br J Radiol 46:1023–1047

100. Hughes GMK (1981) National survey of computed tomography unit capacity. Radiology 135:699–703

101. Kricheff II (1981) Discussion. In: Felix R, Kazner E, Wegener OH (eds) Contrast media in computed tomography. Excerpta Medica, Amsterdam, pp 145–146

102. Pullicino P, Kendall BE (1980) Contrast enhancement in ischaemic lesions. I. Relationship to prognosis. Neuroradiology 19:235–239

103. Kendall BE, Pullicino P (1980) Intravascular contrast injection in ischemic lesions. II. Effect on prognosis. Neuroradiology 19:241–243

104. Drayer BP, Rosenbaum AE (1979) Brain edema defined by cranial computed tomography. J Comput Assist Tomogr 3:317–323

105. Traupe H, Heiss W-D, Hoeffken W, Zülch KJ (1980) Perfusion patterns in CT transit studies. Neuroradiology 19:181–191

106. Wing SD, Anderson RE, Osborn AG (1980) Dynamic cranial computed tomography: preliminary results. AJR 134:941–945

107. Inoue Y, Takemoto K, Miyamoto T et al. (1980) Sequential computed tomography scans in actue cerebral infarction. Radiology 135:655–662

108. Skriver EB, Olsen TS (1982) Contrast enhancement of cerebral infarcts. Incidence and clinical value in different states of cerebral infarction. Neuroradiology 23:259–265

109. Chambers EF, Turski PA, LaMasters D, Newton TH (1982) Regions of low density in the contrast-enhanced pituitary gland: normal and pathologic processes. Radiology 144:109–113

110. Asari S, Satoh T, Sakurai M, Yamamoto Y, Sadamoto K (1982) The advantage of coronal scanning in cerebral computed angiotomography for the diagnosis of Moyamoya disease. Radiology 145:709–711

111. Cohen WA, Pinto RS, Kricheff II (1982) Dynamic CT scanning for visualization of the parasellar carotid arteries. AJR 138:905–909

112. Yock DH, Larson DA (1978) Computed tomography of hemorrhage from anterior communicating artery aneurysms, with angiographic correlation. Radiology 134:399–407

113. Numaguchi Y, Kishikawa T, Ikeda J (1980) Prolonged injection angiography for diagnosing intracranial neoplasms. Radiology 136:387–393

114. Wing SD, Anderson RE, Osborn AG (1982) Cranial computed angiotomography. Radiology 143:103–107
115. Mawad ME, Silver AJ, Hilal SK, Ganti SR (1983) Computed tomography of the brain stem with intrathecal metrizamide. Part II: lesions in and around the brain stem. AJR 140:565–571
116. Graeb DA, Steinbok P, Robertson WD (1982) Transient early computed tomographic changes mimicking tumor progression after brain tumor irradiation. Radiology 144:813–817
117. Kieffer SA, Salibi NA, Kim RC, Lee SH, Cacayorin ED, Modesti LM (1982) Multifocal glioblastoma: diagnostic implications. Radiology 143:709–710
118. Lyons BE, Enzmann DR, Britt RH, Obana WG, Placone RC, Yeager AS (1982) Short-term, high-dose corticosteroids in computed tomographic staging of experimental brain abscess. Neuroradiology 23:279–284
119. Brown SB, Brant-Zawadzki M, Efel P, Coleman CN, Enzmann DR (1982) CT of irradiated solid tumor metastases to the brain. Neuroradiology 23:127–131
120. Enzmann DR, Britt RH, Placone RC Jr, Obana W, Lyons B, Yeager AS (1982) The effect of short-term corticosteroid treatment on the CT appearance of experimental brain abscesses. Radiology 145:79–84
121. Zülch KJ (1980) Principles of the new World Health Organization (WHO) classification of brain tumors. Neuroradiology 19:59–66
122. Takeda N, Tanaka R, Nakai O, Ueki K (1982) Dynamics of contrast enhancement in delayed computed tomography of brain tumors: tissue-blood ratio and differential diagnosis. Radiology 142:663–668
123. Baert AL, Wackenheim A, Jeanmart L (1980) Abdominal computer tomography. Springer, Berlin Heidelberg New York
124. Dubois PJ, Drayer BP, Heinz ER, Osborne D, Roberts L, Sage M (1981) Rapid sequence cranial computed tomography for tumor diagnosis. Neuroradiology 21:79–86
125. Godwin JD, Herfkins RL, Skiöldebrand CG, Federle MP, Lipton MJ (1980) Evaluation of dissections and aneurysms of the thoracic aorta by conventional and dynamic CT scanning. Radiology 136:125–133
126. Gross SC, Barr I, Eyler WR, Kaja F, Goldstein S (1980) Computed tomography in dissection of the thoracic aorta. Radiology 136:135–139
127. Lardé D, Belloir C, Vasile N, Frija J, Ferrané J (1980) Computed tomography of aortic dissection. Radiology 136:147–151
128. Lipton MJ, Brundage BH, Doherty PW et al. (1979) Contrast medium-enhanced computed tomography for evaluating ischemic heart disease. Cardiovasc Med 4:1219–1229
129. Brundage BH, Lipton MJ, Herfkens RJ, Berninger WH, Redington RW, Chatterjee K, Carlsson E (1980) Detection of patent coronary by-pass grafts by computed tomography; a preliminary report. Circulation 61:826–831
130. Higgins CB, Sovak M, Schmidt W, Siemers PT (1978) Uptake of contrast materials by experimental acute myocardial infarctions; a preliminary report. Invest Radiol 13:337–339
131. Lipton MJ, Higgins CB (1980) Evaluation of ischemic heart disease by computerized transmission tomography. Radiol Clin North Am 18:557–576
132. Doherty PW, Lipton MJ, Berninger WH, Skiöldebrand CG, Carlsson E, Redington RW (1981) Detection and quantification of myocardial infarction in vivo using transmission computed tomography. Circulation 63:597–606
133. Huber DJ, Lapray J-F, Hessel SJ (1981) In vivo evaluation of experimental myocardial infarcts by ungated computed tomography. AJR 136:469–473
134. Palmer RG, Masuda Y, Carlsson E (1982) Washout curves from myocardial infarctions in dogs, studied by contrast-enhanced computed tomography. Cardiovasc Intervent Radiol 5:221–226
135. Godwin JD, Herfkens RJ, Skiöldebrand CG, Brundage BH, Schiller NB, Lipton MJ (1981) Detection of intraventricular thrombi by computed tomography. Radiology 138:717–721

136. Gross BH, Glazer GM, Francis IR (1983) CT of intracardiac and intrapericardial masses. AJR 140:903–907
137. Gouliamos AD, Carter BL, Emami B (1980) Computed tomography of the chest wall. Radiology 134:433–436
138. Baber CE, Hedlund LW, Oddson TA, Putman CE (1980) Differentiating empyemas and peripheral pulmonary abscesses. Radiology 135:755–758
139. Wegener O-H, Claussen CD (1981) Contrast media in computed tomography of the mediastinum and the lung. In: Felix R, Kazner E, Wegener OH (eds) Contrast media in computed tomography. Excerpta Medica, Amsterdam, pp 214–221
140. Godwin JD, Webb WR, Gamsu G, Ovenfors C-O (1980) Computed tomography of pulmonary embolism. AJR 135:691–695
141. Kormano MJ, Dean PB, Hamlin DJ (1980) Upper extremity contrast medium infusion in computed tomography of upper mediastinal masses. J Comput Assist Tomogr 4:617–620
142. Baron RL, Levitt RG, Sagel SS, White MJ, Roper CL, Marbarger JP (1982) Computed tomography in the preoperative evaluation of bronchogenic carcinoma. Radiology 145:727–732
143. Reinig JW, Stanley JH, Schabel SI (1983) CT evaluation of thickened esophageal walls. AJR 140:931–934
144. Balcar I (1983) Computed tomography of the mediastinum. Postgrad Radiol 3:3–22
145. Itai Y, Moss AA, Goldberg HI (1982) Transient hepatic attenuation difference of lobar or segmental distribution detected by dynamic computed tomography. Radiology 144:835–839
146. Pagani JJ (1983) Intrahepatic vascular territories shown by computed tomography. Radiology 147:173–178
147. Kunstlinger F, Federle MP, Moss AA, Marks W (1980) Computed tomography of hepatocellular carcinoma. AJR 134:431–437
148. Majewski A, Hendrickx P, Brölsch C, Wiese H (1983) Computertomographische Densitometrie primärer Lebertumoren. Fortschr Röntgenstr 138:8–14
149. Itai Y, Furui S, Araki T, Yashiro N, Tasaka A (1980) Computed tomography of cavernous hemangioma of the liver. Radiology 137:149–155
150. Barnett PH, Zerhouni EA, White RL Jr, Siegelman SS (1980) Computed tomography in the diagnosis of cavernous hemangioma of the liver. AJR 134:439–447
151. Itai Y, Araki T, Furui S, Tasaka A (1981) Differential diagnosis of hepatic masses on computed tomography, with particular reference to hepatocellular carcinoma. J Comput Assist Tomogr 5:834–842
152. Hosoki T, Chatani M, Mori S (1982) Dynamic computed tomography of hepatocellular carcinoma. AJR 139:1099–1106
153. Berland LL, Lawson TL, Foley WD, Melrose BL, Chintapalli KN, Taylor AJ (1982) Comparison of pre- and postcontrast CT in hepatic masses. AJR 138:853–858
154. Itai Y, Araki T, Furui S, Yashiro N, Ohtomo K, Iio M (1983) Computed tomography of primary intrahepatic biliary malignancy. Radiology 147:485–490
155. Itai Y, Ohtomo K, Araki T, Furui S, Iio M, Atomi Y (1983) Computed tomography and sonography of cavernous hemangioma of the liver. AJR 141:315–320
156. Burgener FA, Hamlin DJ (1983) Contrast enhancement of focal hepatic lesions in CT: effect of size and histology. AJR 140:297–301
157. Wooten WB, Bernardino ME, Goldstein HM (1978) Computed tomography of necrotic hepatic metastases. AJR 131:839–842
158. Callen PW (1979) Computed tomographic evaluation of abdominal and pelvic abscesses. Radiology 131:171–175
159. Hübener K-H, Schmitt WGH (1979) Die computertomographische Diagnostik von Abszeßbildungen. Fortschr Röntgenstr 130:53–57
160. Feuerbach S, Gullotta U, Reiser M, Ingianni G (1980) Röntgensymptomatik intraabdomineller Abszesse im Computer-Tomogramm. Fortschr Röntgenstr 133:296–298
161. Foley WD, Berland LL, Lawson TL, Smith DF, Thorsen MK (1983) Contrast enhancement technique for dynamic computed tomography scanning. Radiology 147:797–803

162. Matsui O, Kadoya M, Suzuki M, Inoue K, Itoh H, Ida M, Takashima T (1983) Work in progress: dynamic sequential computed tomography during arterial portography in the detection of hepatic neoplasms. Radiology 146:721–727

163. Moss AA (1981) CT contrast enhancement of the liver. In: Fuchs WA (ed) Contrast enhancement in body computerized tomography. Thieme, Stuttgart, pp 95–110

164. Clark RA, Matsui O (1983) CT of liver tumors. Sem Roentgenol 18:149–162

165. Araki T (1983) Diagnosis of liver tumors by dynamic computed tomography. CRC Crit Rev Diag Imag 19:47–87

166. Glazer G, Axel L, Goldberg HI, Moss AA (1981) Dynamic CT of the normal spleen. Am J Roentgenol 137:343–346

167. Federle M, Moss AA (1983) Computed tomography of the spleen. CRC Crit Rev Diag Imag 19:1–16

168. Kivisaari L, Kormano M, Rantakokko V (1979) Contrast enhancement of the pancreas in computed tomography. J Comput Assist Tomogr 3:722–726

169. Hauser H, Battikha JG, Wettstein P (1980) Computed tomography of the dilated main pancreatic duct. J Comput Assist Tomogr 4:53–58

170. Mödder U (1981) Computed tomography of the pancreas with and without contrast media. In: Felix R, Kazner E, Wegener OH (eds) Contrast media in computed tomography. Excerpta Medica, Amsterdam, pp 276–281

171. Baert AL, Marchal G, Wilms G, Usewils R, Ponette E (1981) Contrast enhancement in CT of the pancreas. In: Fuchs WA (ed) Contrast enhancement in body computerized tomography. Thieme, Stuttgart, pp 111–120

172. Itai Y, Moss AA, Ohtomo K (1982) Computed tomography of cystadenoma and cystadenocarcinoma of the pancreas. Radiology 145:419–425

173. Hosoki T (1983) Dynamic CT of pancreatic tumors. AJR 140:959–965

174. Karasawa E, Goldberg HI, Moss AA, Federle MP, London SS (1983) CT pancreatogram in carcinoma of the pancreas and chronic pancreatitis. Radiology 148:489–493

175. Jeffrey RB, Federle MP, Laing FC (1983) Computed tomography of mesenteric involvement in fulminant pancreatitis. Radiology 147:185–188

176. Treugut H, Nyman U, Hildell J (1980) Sequenz-CT: frühe Dichteveränderungen der gesunden Niere nach Kontrastmittelapplikation. Radiologe 20:558–562

177. Heinz ER, Dubois PJ, Drayer BP, Hill R (1980) A preliminary investigation of the role of dynamic computed tomography in renovascular hypertension. J Comput Assist Tomogr 4:63–66

178. Hoffman EP, Mindelzun RE, Anderson RU (1980) Computed tomography in acute pyelonephritis associated with diabetes. Radiology 135:691–695

179. Treugut H, Hübener K-H, Nyman U (1981) Contrast media in computed tomography of the retroperitoneal and pelvic space: kidneys and adrenals. In: Felix R, Kazner E, Wegener OH (eds) Contrast media in computed tomography. Excerpta Medica, Amsterdam, pp 229–236

180. Dunnick NR, Schaner EG, Doppman JL, Strott CA, Gill JR, Javadpour N (1979) Computed tomography in adrenal tumors. AJR 132:43–46

181. Parienty RA, Ducellier R, Pradel J, Lubrano J-M, Coquille F, Richard F (1982) Diagnostic value of CT numbers in pelvocalyceal filling defects. Radiology 145:743–747

182. Glazer GM, Francis IR, Brady TM, Teng SS (1983) Computed tomography of renal infarction: clinical and experimental observations. AJR 140:721–727

183. Gold RP, McClennal BL, Rottenberg RR (1983) CT appearance of acute inflammatory disease of the renal interstitium. AJR 141:343–349

184. Friedmann G, Mödder U, Peters PE (1981) CT evaluation of systemic and portal veins. In: Fuchs WA (ed) Contrast enhancement in body computerized tomography. Thieme, Stuttgart, pp 34–44

185. Faer MJ, Lynch RD, Evans HO, Chin FK (1979) Inferior vena cava duplication: demonstration by computed tomography. Radiology 130:707–709

186. Ishikawa T, Tsukune Y, Ohyama Y, Fujikawa M, Sakuyama K, Fujii M (1980) Venous abnormalities in portal hypertension demonstrated by CT. AJR 134:271–276

187. Vujic I, Rogers CI, LeVeen HH (1980) Computed tomographic detection of portal vein thrombosis. Radiology 135:697–698

188. Young SW, Noon MA, Marincek B (1981) Dynamic computed tomography time-density study of normal human tissue after intravenous contrast administration. Invest Radiol 16:36–39
189. Mark A, Moss AA, Lusby R, Kaiser JA (1982) CT evaluation of complications of abdominal aortic surgery. Radiology 145:409–414
190. Jacobs NM, Godwin JD, Wolfe WG, Moore AV Jr, Breiman RS, Korobkin M (1982) Evaluation of grafted ascending aorta with computed tomography; complications caused by suture dehiscence. Radiology 145:749–753
191. Thorsen MK, San Dretto MA, Lawson TL, Foley WD, Smith DF, Berland LL (1983) Dissecting aortic aneurysms: accuracy of computed tomographic diagnosis. Radiology 148:773–777
192. Pillari G (1979) Computed tomographic cavo-urography: lower extremity contrast infusion simultaneous with computed tomography of the retroperitoneum. Radiology 130:797
193. VanBreda A, Rubin BE, Druy EM (1979) Detection of inferior vena cava abnormalities by computed tomography. J Comput Assist Tomogr 3:164–169
194. Meijenhorst GCH (1982) Computed tomography of the lumbar epidural veins. Radiology 145:687–691
195. Alfidi RJ, Stowe N, Haaga JR, Rao P (1981) Bolus computed angio-tomography of body mass lesions. In: Fuchs WA (ed) Contrast enhancement in body computerized tomography. Thieme, Stuttgart, pp 71–80
196. Husband JE (1981) Contrast media in computed tomography of the pelvic organs. In: Felix R, Kazner E, Wegener OH (eds) Contrast media in computed tomography. Excerpta Medica, Amsterdam, pp 243–248
197. Whitley NO, Shatney CH (1983) Diagnosis of abdominal abscesses in patients with major trauma: the use of computed tomography. Radiology 147:179–183
198. Bernardino ME, Jing BS, Wallace S (1979) Computed diagnosis of mesenteric masses. AJR 132:33–36
199. Levitt RG, Biello DR, Sagel SS et al. (1979) Computed tomography and ^{67}Ga citrate radionuclide imaging for evaluating suspected abdominal masses. AJR 132:529–534
200. Kreel L (1981) Contrast media for gastrointestinal examination with computed tomography. In: Felix R, Kazner E, Wegener OH (eds) Contrast media in computed tomography. Excerpta Medica, Amsterdam, pp 271–274
201. Johnson RJ, Blackledge G, Eddleston B, Crowther D (1983) Abdomino-pelvic computed tomography in the management of ovarian carcinoma. Radiology 146:447–452
202. Sager EM, Talle K, Fosså S, Ous S, Stenwig AE (1983) The role of CT in demonstrating perivesical tumor growth in the preoperative staging of carcinoma of the urinary bladder. Radiology 146:443–446
203. Kormano M (1981) Kinetics of contrast media after bolus injection and infusion. In: Felix R, Kazner E, Wegener OH (eds) Contrast media in computed tomography. Excerpta Medica, Amsterdam, pp 38–45
204. Burgener FA (1981) Contrast agents for body computed tomography. In: Fuchs WA (ed) Contrast enhancement in body computerized tomography. Thieme, Stuttgart, pp 5–19

CHAPTER 11

Adverse Systemic Reactions to Contrast Media

E. C. LASSER

A. General Considerations

Toxic effects resulting from contrast medium (CM) injections can be considered in two major categories: (a) local and (b) systemic. Local toxicity results from injections of high concentrations and/or quantities of CM into a vessel supplying an organ or tissue. Ultimately, the degree of toxicity must be a function of the concentration and the application time of the injected material. Hence, such factors as organic luminal obstructions, functional obstructions, viscosity changes, and other hemodynamic alterations that prolong the application time increase the chemotoxicity of the injected CM. The precise etiology of chemotoxicity is still poorly understood, but it is thought to involve such factors as molecular interference with functional proteins such as enzymes and regulators and/or hyperosmolarity of the CM solution. Underlying the potential of CM to act as general enzyme inhibitors is their ability to bind to proteins. Such binding appears to reflect principally the degree of hydrophobicity of the CM molecules [1–5]. The correlation between the lethal doses of CM in experimental animals and the binding of CM to serum albumins and various enzymes has been established [6]. In a series of studies, all the CM investigated, if present in sufficiently high concentrations, inhibited the enzymes tested [1–3]. The concentrations and total dosages of CM used in intravascular studies are so high that it is not surprising to find downstream from an intravascular injection a concentration of CM sufficient for a 50% inhibition of a given enzyme system in vitro. In addition, following the injection, CM readily enter certain compartments and organs. Thus, extracellular accumulation following a bolus injection of a high dose of a CM can be appreciable, as is the CM concentration in the kidney or in other highly vascularized tissues.

The more hydrophobic the CM molecule, the stronger is its bond to the protein, and the greater is the enzyme inhibition [1]. Hence, one can rank CM in order of binding/inhibiting potency as follows: (a) oral cholecystographic media, (b) intravenous cholangiographic media, (c) all current nonionic triiodinated urographic media, (d) monoionic hexaiodinated molecules, (e) nonionic triiodinated substances, and (f) nonionic hexaiodinated CM.

In addition to adverse effects exerted on enzyme systems, toxicity can result from disturbances of the ionic equilibrium, caused by the ionic character and hyperosmolarity of the contrast solutions. It is likely that these properties can induce cardiac arrythmias, disrupt endothelial cells, break down the blood-brain barrier, and, in some instances, induce acute renal tubular necrosis [3, 7–10]. The chemotoxic effects of the CM on the membranes of mast cells, circulating white blood cells, and platelets result in the release of various mediators [11, 12].

Although systemic toxicity bears a positive statistical correlation to total quantities injected [13], it can result from the introduction of very small quantities of CM into any vessel in the body. Since it is not clear at the present time whether a substantial number of systemic reactions can be attributed to classical immunologic mechanisms, it is probably unwise to refer to them categorically as "allergic" or "hypersensitive" reactions. In the light of present findings, systemic reactions should correctly be labeled as anaphylactoid or idiosyncratic. In this chapter we will concentrate on the current state of knowledge of the pathogenesis of these systemic reactions.

B. Pathogenesis

Current thinking regarding the pathogenesis of idiosyncratic CM reactions can be considered under four major headings: (a) cellular release of mediators (histamine and others), (b) antibody-antigen reactions, (c) psychogenic factors, and (d) involvement of acute activation systems (complement, coagulation, kinins, fibrinolysins). These major headings are not necessarily mutually exclusive, and it is conceivable that some reactions might involve one, all, or any combination of these mechanisms.

It has been known for some years that the in vitro incubation of mast cells, or basophils, with CM results in the direct release of histamine [14–17]. This release can be augmented by the presence of normal human serum, presumably due to the resulting activation of C3 component of the complement system [16, 18]. Correspondingly, it has been appreciated for some time now that contrast injections will result in histamine release in experimental animals and in humans [14, 19–21]. More recently, it has been shown that platelets release serotonin upon incubation with CM [15, 21]. In fact, it has been shown that CM induce complex changes in the interaction between at least three circulating cells: basophils, neutrophils, and platelets [15, 20]. To date, however, no one has shown any direct correlation between the extent of in vivo histamine or serotonin release and the presence or absence of reactions, and/or the severity of reactions. On the other hand, there does appear to be some correlation between the occurrence of reactions and the potential of CM to induce histamine release in vitro [22]. Overall, however, it seems likely that histamine release represents but one, possibly obligatory, component in the chain of events that characterizes untoward reactions to CM.

True hypersensitivity, or contrast allergy, may play a role in some instances of CM reactions. Despite the failure to produce antibodies against CM by appropriate injections of uncoupled CM molecules, antibody-antigen reactions have been described in several clinical instances, and antibodies have been produced in experimental animals by injections of CM covalently coupled to protein carriers [23–25]. The molecular structure of the injectible urographic media does not form an antigenic potential for these molecules. The structure of the cholangiographic media, however, is such that one might anticipate that they could act as divalent antigens. In fact, in the few instances where passive cutaneous transfer studies carried out in humans having a contrast reaction have been positive, the injected material has always had the divalent composition [26]. Anti-CM anti-bodies, however, have been reported in some patients suffering severe reactions from injections of urographic media [24]. Many of these patients had not previously been injected with CM; the reactions were attributed to cross-reacting antibodies, perhaps induced by benzene derivatives found in food additives, pesticides, and herbicides chemically similar to CM. It remains unexplained why the antibodies detected in this group by radioimmunoassay showed approximately the same percentage of binding of labeled media in samples obtained immediately after contrast injection as in samples obtained about 3 weeks later. It might be expected that the antibody binding of radiolabeled CM in the immediate post-reaction period should be considerably diminished by competition with the large quantities of circulating nonlabeled CM molecules.

While the onset of the reaction occurs most commonly within minutes of the completion of the CM injection, on occasion it may be delayed for hours. This, as well as the observation that the systemic reaction occurs more often with greater volumes and concentrations than with smaller ones [13], speaks against an IgE mechanism. On the other hand, the occasional instance of intense acute anaphylaxis occurring after even very small doses of CM suggests a role for IgE in some patients [25][1].

It has been claimed that systemic CM reactions occur on the basis of psychogenic factors [27]. Certainly, the possibility that such factors play a role in some individuals must be seriously considered. Psychogenic factors might engender a reaction through the classical vagovasal mechanisms involving release of circulating mediators. It seems improbable, however, that the psychic trauma of expecting an injection could alone be responsible for the severe anaphylactoid reactions cited in current reports. If such were the case, one would fully expect to see the same incidence of reactions in individuals undergoing intravascular needling for other purposes. There is no evidence to support this. Finally, it should be noted that contrast reactions have been seen in completely obtunded patients and in "sensitized" experimental animals under anesthesia [28].

Accumulated evidence suggests that the so-called activation systems play a major role in CM reactions. Activation of the complement system has been noted to occur after incubation with CM in vitro [29–32]. In vivo activation of the complement system has been noted both in experimental animals [33, 34, 28] and in man [35, 36, 14, 31] following contrast injections. Activation of the coagulation system and elevated fibrinolysins have also been documented [37, 34, 36].

The complement system, coagulation, kinins, and fibrolysins all have components regulated by interaction with the inhibitor of the first component of the complement system, the so-called $C\overline{1}$-esterase inhibitor. The mean concentration of this inhibitor was found to be significantly lower in the prechallenge serum samples of reactors when compared with nonreactors [35]. Particularly low levels were noted in individuals having the most severe reactions. These findings suggest

---

1 Sensitivity against iodide could also account for some contrast reactions. Although the iodine atoms substituted in the benzene rings of the CM molecules are extremely stable, free iodide will be found in each contrast vial as a consequence of the manufacturing process [18]

that any factor that might stress the classical pathway of complement activation, activating C̄1, would result in depletion of the inhibitor, and might predispose patients to contrast reactions. Favoring this notion is the fact that confirmed reactors have a lower mean level of total hemolytic complement than do confirmed nonreactors [35]. In addition, it has been pointed out that individuals with systemic lupus erythematosus (SLE), a disease wherein circulating immune complexes would be expected to stress continuously the classical complement pathway, have a higher incidence of reactions than do individuals without such a history [38].

Additional evidence for a critical role for the C̄1-esterase inhibitor in contrast reactions might be gleaned from experiments with animals pretreated with adrenal corticosteroids. Such animals gained considerable protection against lethal dose range contrast challenge [33], and their levels of C̄1-esterase inhibitor almost doubled as a result of the steroid injections [39]. Elevation of the inhibitor was

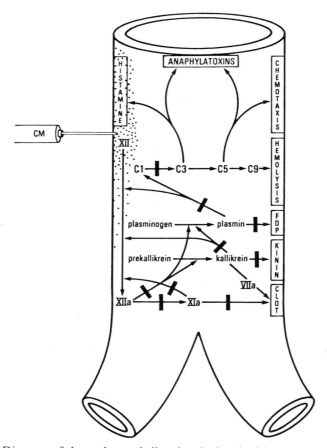

Fig. 1. Diagram of the pathways believed to be involved in contrast activation of acute-phase reactants. Contrast injection produces histamine release and endothelial disruption, exposing factor XII to contact activators. The *black bars* represent the C̄1-esterase inhibitor

thought to have resulted from steroid-induced blunting of a hypothetical, ongoing, low-level activation of factor XII-dependent reactants. These activated reactants combine with, and consume, the C̄I-esterase inhibitor. Supporting the concept of steroid blunting of a circulating endogenous factor is the fact that factor XII levels in the steroid-treated animals were found to be elevated in the prechallenge samples along with the elevated inhibitor levels.

The numerous points of interaction of the C̄I-esterase inhibitor, with the activation systems' components demonstrating that the inhibitor is helping to keep these systems in check, is shown in Fig. 1, which depicts some of the pathways that are believed to be involved in activation of these reactants by CM. As a result of histamine and hypertonicity, injection of CM is thought to disrupt the endothelium directly. Furthermore, disruption of the endothelium exposes circulating plasma elements to the underlying collagen, and to endothelial cell components [40], both known to be factor XII activators. Activation of factor XII results in the sequence of events depicted in Fig. 1. Angioneurotic edema, a common finding in severe reactions, could be produced either directly by bradykinin released via the action of kallikrein on high molecular weight kininogen, or by anaphylatoxins produced by the activation of the C3 and C5 components of the complement system. Activation of C3 would also enhance histamine liberation from mast cells and basophils, thus amplifying the potential for factor XII activation.

C. Pretesting

At the present time there is no test to single out the patients prone to suffer a reaction to injected CM. In some instances, preexisting circumstances can be identified that suggest a heightened potential for an anaphylactoid reaction. For example, individuals with a history of allergy have approximately a fourfold increased likelihood of incurring a reaction [13]. Patients with a previous history of a reaction to CM are approximately ten times more likely to have a subsequent reaction to CM than are individuals without such a history [13]. It is therefore of paramount importance to obtain careful a history and eventually to give special care to the high-risk patients.

In this context, mention should be made of the present status assigned to intravenous pretesting.

Intravascular pretesting, when performed, has usually been carried out with injection of 1 ml of the CM to be used in the study. Numerous authors suggested that this pretesting was without value, and might even be dangerous. It has been reported, however, that pretesting patients with a previous definite history of CM reaction, gave incidence of positive tests as high as 13% [42]. In a series of 375 individuals with positive pretests, a full bolus of CM caused the incidence of total reactions to be 16 times higher than in a series of individuals with a negative pretest or those not tested [43]. Reactions requiring therapy were 15 times more common and fatalities 57 times more common [2]. Significant for the question of in vivo pretesting is the report of positive pretests in 36 patients in 21 (71%) of which between *1 and 5 ml* CM was necessary to elicit the reaction. The remaining 29% de-

---

2 Although statistically significantly different, the validity of the fatality data is open to question due to the small numbers: 2 in 375 versus 11 in 112,000

veloped the reaction with injections of 1 ml CM or less. These findings suggest that the whole subject of in vivo pretesting demands a thorough reevaluation.

It is obvious that any test procedure that might help to identify potential reactors would be of great value. The scheme of the pathophysiologic events depicted in Fig. 1 suggested to us the possibility for the development of an in vitro assay which could predict a CM reaction in patients. Thus, activation of factor XII postulated to occur in vivo can be simulated in vitro. When nonreacting patients are compared with the known reactors to CM [41] there appears to be a difference in the rate at which prekallikrein is converted to kallikrein, following contact activation.

References

1. Lang JH, Lasser EC (1971) Nonspecific inhibition of enzymes by organic contrast media. J Med Chem 14:233–236
2. Lasser EC, Lang JH (1970) Physiologic significance of contrast-protein interactions. I. Study in vitro of some enzyme effects. Invest Radiol 5:514–517
3. Lang JH, Lasser EC (1975) Inhibition of adenosine triphosphatase and carbonic anhydrase by contrast media. Invest Radiol 10:314–316
4. Lasser EC, Lang JH (1970) Contrast-protein interactions. The symposium on contrast media toxicity of the association of University Radiologists, Skytop, May 3–6, 1970. Invest Radiol 5:373–502
5. Lasser EC, Farr RS, Fujimagari T, Tripp WM (1962) The significance of protein-binding of contrast media in roentgen diagnosis. AJR 87:338–360
6. Han SY, Sitten DM (1974) Clinical trial of bilopaque oral cholecystography. Evaluation of time of optimal and peak opacification of the gallbladder. Radiology 112:529–531
7. Simon AL, Shebetai R, Lang JH, Lasser EC (1972) The mechanism of production of ventricular fibrillation in coronary angiography. AJR 114:810–816
8. Golman K (1979) The blood-brain barrier: effects of nonionic contrast media with and without addition of Ca^{2+} and Mg^{2+}. Invest Radiol 14:305–308
9. Ausman JI, Young R, Owens G (1964) Radio-opaque dyes and other agents in the production of endothelial damage. J Surg Res 4:349–355
10. Waldron RL, Bridenbaugh RB, Dempsey EW (1974) Effect of angiographic contrast media at the cellular level in the brain: hypertonic vs. chemical action. AJR 122:469–476
11. Cogen FC, Norman ME, Dunsky E, Hirshfeld J, Zweiman B (1979) Histamine release and complement changes following injection of contrast media in humans. J Allergy Clin Immunol 64:200–303
12. Ring J, Arroyave CM (1979) Alteration of human blood cells and changes in plasma mediators produced by radiographic contrast media. Z Immunitaetsforsch Immunobiol 155:200–211
13. Ansell G, Tweedie MCK, West CR, Evans P, Couch L (1980) The current status of reactions to intravenous contrast media. Material presented at international contrast material symposium, Colorado Springs, May 1979. Invest Radiol 515:32–39
14. Lasser EC, Walters AJ, Lang JH (1974) An experimental basis for histamine release in contrast material reactions. Radiology 110:49
15. Rockoff SD, Brasch R (1971) Contrast media as histamine liberators. III. Histamine release and some associated hemodynamic effects during pulmonary angiography in the dog. Invest Radiol 6:110
16. Rockoff SD, Brasch R (1972) Contrast media as histamine liberators. V. Comparison of in vitro mast cell histamine release by sodium and methylglucamine salts. Invest Radiol 7:177
17. Seidel G, Groppe G, Meyer-Burgdorff HC (1974) Contrast media as histamine liberators in man. Agents Actions 4:143

18. Arroyave CM, Bhat KH, Crown R (1976) Activation of the alternative pathway of the complement system by radiographic contrast media. J Immunol 117:1866
19. Siegle RL, Lieberman P (1976) Measurement of histamine, complement components and immune complexes during patient reactions to iodinated contrast material. Invest Radiol 11:98–101
20. Ring J, Arroyave CM, Fritzler MJ, Tan EM (1978) In vitro histamine and serotonin release by radiographic contrast media (RCM). Complement-dependent and independent release reaction and changes in ultrastructure of human blood cells. Clin Exp Immunol 32:105–118
21. Ring J, Endrich B, Intaglietta M (1978) Histamine release, complement consumption and microvascular changes after radiographic contrast media infusion in rabbits. J Lab Clin Med 92:584
22. Arroyave CM (1980) An in vitro assay for radiographic contrast media idiosyncrasy. Presented at international contrast material symposium, Colorado Springs, May 1979. Invest Radiol 15:21–25
23. Brasch R, Caldwell JL, Fudenberg HH (1976) Antibodies to radiographic contrast agents. Induction and characterization of rabbit antibody. Invest Radiol 2:1–9
24. Brasch RC, Caldwell JL (1976) The allergic theory of radiocontrast agent toxicity: demonstration of antibody activity and sera of patients suffering major radiocontrast agent reactions. Invest Radiol 2:347–356
25. Brasch RC (1980) Allergic reactions to contrast media: accumulated evidence. AJR 134:797–801
26. Wakkers-Garritsen BG, Houwerziji J, Nater JP, Wakkers PJM (1976) IgE-mediated adverse reactivity to a radiographic contrast medium – case report. Ann Allergy 36:122–126
27. Lalli AF (1974) Urographic contrast media reactions and anxiety. Radiology 112:267–271
28. Lasser EC, Sovak M, Lang JH (1976) Development of contrast media idiosyncrasy in the dog. Radiology 119:91–95
29. Kolb WP, Lang JH, Lasser EC (1978) Nonimmunologic complement activation in normal human serum induced by X-ray contrast media. J Immunol 121:1232–1238
30. Till G, Rother U, Gemsa D (1978) Activation of complement by radiographic contrast media. Int Arch Allergy Appl Imunol 56:543–550
31. Arroyave CM, Bhat K, Crown R (1976) Activation of serum complement by contrast media. J Immunol 117:866–869
32. Lang JH, Lasser EC, Kolb WP (1976) Activation of the complement system by X-ray contrast media. Invest Radiol 11:303–308
33. Lasser EC, Lang JH, Sovak M, Kolb WP, Lyon SG, Hamblin AE (1977) Steroids: theoretical and experimental basis for utilization in prevention of contrast media reactions. Radiology 125:1–9
34. Lasser EC, Slivka J, Lang JH, Kolb WP, Lyon SG, Hamblin AE, Nazareno G (1979) Complement and coagulation – causative considerations in contrast catastrophes. AJR 132:171–176
35. Lasser EC, Lang JH, Lyon SG, Hamblin AE (1979) Complement and contrast material reactors. J Allergy Clin Immunol 64:102–112
36. Lasser EC, Lang JH, Lyon SG, Hamblin AE (1980) Changes in complement and coagulation factors in a patient suffering a severe anaphylactoid reaction to injected contrast material: some considerations of pathogenesis. Presented at international contrast material symposium, Colorado Springs, May 1979. Invest Radiol 15:6–12
37. Zeman RK (1977) Disseminated intravascular coagulation following intravenous pyelography. (letter) Invest Radiol 12:203–204
38. Wieners H (1977) Klinisch-immunologische Probleme bei der Kontrastmittelanwendung bei Gammapathien und Erkrankungen des rheumatischen Formenkreises. Symposium on adverse reactions to contrast media, Schering, Berlin, pp 67–69
39. Lasser EC, Lang JH, Lyon SG, Hamblin AE, Howard MM (1981) Glucocorticoid-induced elevations of $C\overline{1}$-esterase inhibitor: a mechanism for protection against lethal dose range contrast challenge in rabbits. Invest Radiol 16:20–23

40. Osterud B (1979) The role of endothelial cells and subendothelial components in the initiation of blood coagulation. Haemostasis 8:324–331
41. Lasser EC, Lang JH, Lyon SG, Hamblin AE, Howard MM (1981) Prekallikrein-kallikrein conversion: conversion rates as a predictor for contrast catastrophes. Radiology 140:11–15
42. Yocum NW, Heller AM, Abels RI (1978) Efficacy of intravenous pretesting and antihistamine prophylaxis in radiocontrast media-sensitive patients. J Allergy Clin Immunol 62:309–313
43. Shehadi WN (1975) Adverse reactions to intravascularly administered contrast media: a comprehensive study based on a prospective study. AJR 124:145–152

CHAPTER 12

Are Contrast Media Mutagenic?

J. A. NELSON

A. Introduction

Radiologists are particularly aware of the importance of genetic damage since it has been known for many years that X-rays can cause sublethal genetic damage in both clinical and experimental settings [1]. Such damage can be expressed clinically as cancer [1], or as a somatic abnormality in the human fetus [2]. Yet, the current picture of mutagenicity is not in particularly sharp focus. Instances of clear-cut carcinogenic mutagens and teratogenic mutagens have been identified in human populations, usually following a tragic underestimation of the potential danger of a chemical or physical agent. Diagnostic radiology has, in the past, learned about such instances the hard way: many early radiologists died of radiation-induced neoplasms, and even today we continue to see, albeit rarely, patients who recieved thorium dioxide and subsequently developed neoplasms induced by that contrast material [3].

The unfortunate past experience with Thorotrast (colloidal thorium dioxide) serves as a reminder that compounds seemingly safe may have demonstrated severe carcinogenic properties only after a long latency. Thorotrast, which had an extremely low acute toxicity, contained a high lineal energy transfer (LET) alpha-emitting thorium. The colloidal suspension which was taken up by the reticuloendothelial system caused, often after many years, tumors in liver, spleen, and lymphatics [3].

The idea that a diagnostic screening technique might cause serious immediate or latent injury in an otherwise healthy patient is particularly abhorrent. The controversy surrounding mammography illustrates the complexity of dealing with a diagnostically useful but potentially carcinogenic diagnostic technique [4]. The very existence of this book proves that efforts are being directed at making contrast media (CM) as safe as possible.

Very little mutagenic research has been performed on modern radiographic CM since there is no clinical evidence suggesting that these compounds are mutagenic. Indeed, cell biologists and biochemists have used these same compounds for density gradient separation of cells and cell components for many years [5].

Classic chromosomal analysis has demonstrated a cytogenetic effect of CM in cultured Chinese Hamster Ovary (CHO) cells [6]. Using this technique, an old CM, iodopyracet, at concentrations of 0.063%–2.0% by volume interrupted the normal process of chromosomal spindle formation much like Colcemid [6]. These results inspired some of the initial thoughts that CM might be mutagenic [7], even though there is no solid evidence for mutagenicity of Colcemid [8].

Based on observation of micronuclei of lymphocytes in patients undergoing angiocardiography with water-soluble radiographic CM, diatrizoate has been implicated to cause chromosome damage [7]. In an effort to separate effects of high radiation doses which some of these patients received, in vitro tests were performed by the same laboratory; these experiments suggest that the CM had effects similar to radiation. Yet, such conclusions were based on a screening technique which consists of counting micronuclei in human lymphocytes. The micronuclei are small extranuclear bits of chromatin seen outside of the nucleus in Wright-stained blood smears. This technique allows simple, rapid scoring of a large number of cells, which is much quicker than routine chromosomal analysis [9], and sensitive to events that occur so rarely that they might be missed by a technique based on counting fewer events [10]. It has been shown, nevertheless, that although the micronucleus technique reflects cell damage due to radiation and other noxious stimuli, factors other than chromosomal breakage can affect the micronucleus frequency, and the technique may be measuring cytotoxic rather than cytogenetic effects [9].

Authors arrived at a tentative conclusion that the changes they observed may lead to delayed effects and that patients receiving CM should be followed to detect early possible pathologic manifestations [11].

Although the relationships between cytotoxicity, genetic damage, mutagenicity, and carcinogenicity are extremely complex, the lay press drew the immediate connection between cytogenetic damage and cancer. This fashion of interpreting preliminary data produced an instant controversy and prompted serious investigation of the phenomenon [1]. It seems obvious that agents which affect spindle formation may produce a cytotoxic rather than a cytogenetic effect. Such drugs, including CM, might cause cell damage resulting in death rather than a mutation to be passed to succeeding generations of cells.

Whether the commonly used diagnostic CM have an adverse nonlethal genetic effect on human cells can only be decided by extremely sensitive and specific tests known for demonstrating genetic damage in living, surviving in vitro cultured cells [12–14]. Even here, caution is warranted: teratogenicity of Thalidomide could not be reproduced uniformly, due to species response variation [15].

B. Methods

Mutagenesis tests which are rapid and relatively inexpensive for screening the mutagenic potential are based on a large, rapidly proliferating population of genetically defined bacteria [13, 14]. Application of such tests ("Ames") for screening environmental chemicals for mutagenic and carcinogenic properties has recently been shown [12]. An extremely readable summary of the theory and techniques involved in bacterial tests is available [14].

The Ames Test is extremely useful in screening chemical mutagens, and appears to identify about 90% of known carcinogens as mutagens [12]. Obviously, some compounds may elude detection by this technique, and Ames points out

1 Thus, the *Chicago Tribune* announced at the time of the 1978 Radiological Society of North America meeting that "Contrast Agent May Cause Cancer"

that some carcinogens may not be detected if they have no direct interaction with nuclear DNA. Thus, although the Ames Test is an excellent, economical screening procedure, further evaluation of suspect chemicals may be in order. AMES also states that "...it is important to view with caution results indicating nonmutagenicity in classes of chemicals for which any test (or any short-term test) has not been validated" [12]. Preliminary reports, however, suggest that the diacetamido derivatives of triiodobenzoic acid are mutagenic by the Ames Test [16]. Since these derivatives are quite similar chemically to the contrast molecules we tested, negative results reported later in this chapter would suggest that the clinical preparations are nonmutagenic members of a class of chemicals which can be mutagenic using the Ames Test technique. Contamination of clinical preparations with significant concentrations of mutagenic derivatives could not be demonstrated.

Although well suited for screening purposes, the bacterial testing has one drawback: since the bacterial nuclei are not organized and also function differently than those of the higher organism cells, the results from bacteria are not necessarily applicable to mammalian cells.

A relatively new and sensitive method which measures chromosomal stability involves the quantitative analysis of sister chromatid exchange (SCE), i.e., the reciprocal interchange of genetic material between the duplicated regions of a chromosome [13]. Occurrence of an SCE requires a DNA four-strand exchange. Because it measures the frequency of breakage and reunion of DNA, it probably provides a reliable index of chromosomal stability. Although the mechanism and biologic significance of SCE is not fully understood, recent evidence suggests that it may be related to mutation rates and malignant transformation in mammalian cells. The current opinion is that the method is the most sensitive indicator for detecting effects of mutagens and carcinogens in eukaryotic chromosomes.

Although the SCE test is extremely sensitive [13], it is relatively inefficient in detecting mutagenic damage caused by low-dose X-rays [17], which is easily demonstrated by the micronucleus technique [9]. For this reason, a negative SCE evaluation is not totally convincing, although recent results suggest a linear SCE dose-response to X-rays [18]. Interestingly enough, under specific experimental conditions which are only remotely related to the clinical situation, diagnostic ultrasound can demonstrate an increase in SCE in human lymphocytes [19]. Thus, it seems imperative that both positive and negative SCE results are interpreted within the broader clinical context.

Further modifications of SCE, including use of the S-9 liver microsome enzyme metabolic activator, have been recently reported [20]. Use of similar modifications in cell cultures, or even use of cultured liver cells themselves [21], offer theoretical possibilities for the study of the mutagenic potential of drugs.

Another in vitro method which is now available is testing for oncogenic transformation of mammalian-cell cultures. This approach might be extremely useful in evaluating mutagenic or carcinogenic potential of radiographic CM. In a recent review article, BOREK points out that these studies must be performed and interpreted with great care and precision because of the complexities inherent in cell transformation studies [21]. The manifestations of malignant-cell transformations in well-defined cell culture lines and the ultimate demonstration of tumorigenicity by in vivo tumor induction make this methodology seem most suitable for providing the final answer regarding diagnostic agents. When this methodology is available, it makes conclusions drawn from less specific methods, such as the micronucleus, SCE, and Ames techniques, less definitive than they might otherwise seem.

In our laboratories, meglumine iothalamate (Conray 60), a mixture of sodium/meglumine diatrizoate (Renografin 76) and sodium iopanoate were tested by the Ames and SCE tests [22].

C. Results

Four standard tester strains of his⁻ *Salmonella typhimurium*, TA 98, TA 100, TA 1535, and TA 1537, were used, and samples were tested in the plate incorporation assay in the presence and absence of a rat liver microsome metabolic activation system, abbreviated as S-9. A known mutagenic chemical control demonstrated sensitivity of the bacterial strains to mutagenic damage on the day of the test. Renografin 76 and Conray 60 were tested from 1.5% to 50% vol concentration, while a 10% w/v solution of iopanoate was tested at 0.5%–5% final concentration because it demonstrated bactericidal activity at concentrations over 5%. The

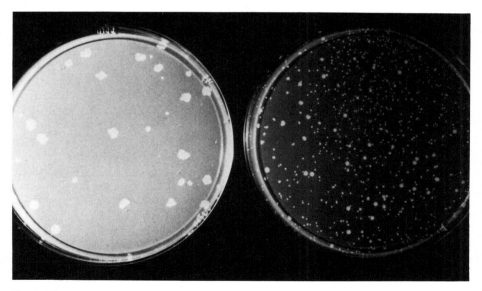

Fig. 1. These two plates characterize the ease with which bacterial mutagenic tests can be scored. Both plates were treated with a mutagenic agent that is mutagenic only when metabolized. The plate on the *left* contained no mammalian microsome preparation (S-9) while that on the *right* did. A count of resulting colonies indicated that the plate on the *left* does not differ from control values, while the one on the *right* contains a quantifiable number of mutant colonies far above control values. In Ames tests of CM both with and without S-9, and with controls for background reversions and response to a known mutagen, no mutagenic properties were indentified

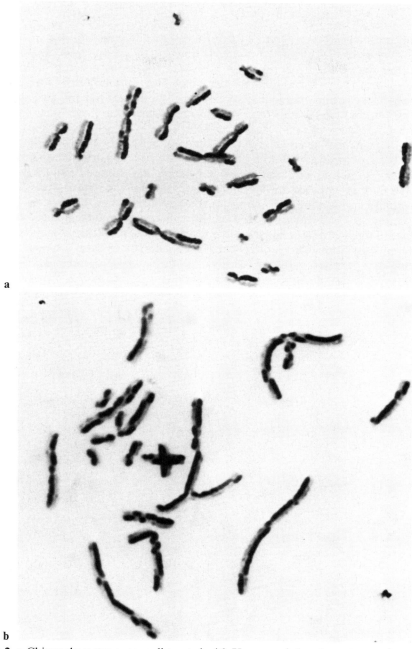

Fig. 2. a Chinese hamster ovary cell treated with X-rays and showing a two to three times increase in SCE, which can be detected by counting the exchange between dark and light chromatids. **b** This CHO cell was treated with a combination of hyperthermia and X-rays, with a resulting much higher SCE rate than seen in **a**. Obviously, any gross chromosomal aberration would be detectable with such a preparation

test was scored by counting the number of his⁻ reversions to his⁺ colonies on the culture media.

Figure 1 shows a typical pair of culture plates, one with and one without a mutation response. Mutagenic criteria included (a) a greater than twofold increase over the spontaneous reversion rate and (b) demonstration of a dose-response curve. Criteria for nonmutagenicity included (a) testing over a wide dose range, (b) testing against all four tester strains, (c) testing in the presence and absence of S-9, and (d) demonstration of no mutagenicity criteria. All three CM tested met the criteria of nonmutagenicity [23].

Sister chromatid exchange in cultured human lymphocytes was studied with Conray 60, Renografin 76, and iopanoic acid at concentrations comparable to those observed in human blood during clinical studies. Figures 2 and 3 demonstrate the final appearance of CHO cells (Fig. 2) and human lymphocytes (Fig. 3) following preparation for SCE scoring [13]. Appropriate controls, with a detectable spontaneous SCE rate, were scored for comparison with treated cells. Multiple tests of these CM have failed to demonstrate evidence of chromosomal damage in human lymphocytes or CHO cells. Figure 4 demonstrates a typical result from one such experiment with Conray 60 at 3% by w/v as compared with control. Figure 5 shows data from another experiment testing both Conray 60 and

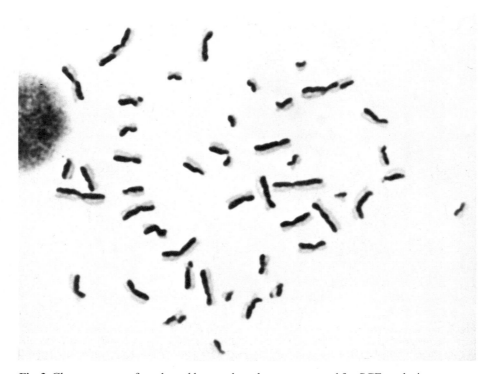

Fig. 3. Chromosomes of a cultured human lymphocyte prepared for SCE analysis

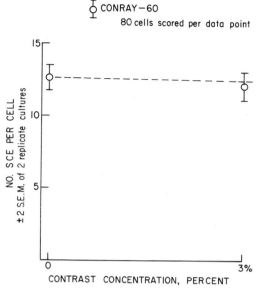

Fig. 4. Data comparing SCE incidence in control CHO cells (*broken line*) and CHO cells treated for 19 h with 3% Conray by weight. There is no significant difference in number of SCEs scored. A control incidence of 11–13 is typical for repeated studies in this laboratory

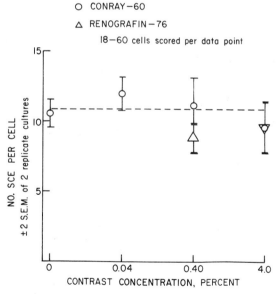

Fig. 5. Results of scoring of a control (*broken line*) and five pooled double cultures of human lymphocytes treated with variable weight concentrations of Conray 60 and Renografin 76. A control value of 11 is quite repetitive from this donor over several months of study in the laboratory. Using Student's *t*-test, no significant difference was noted between control and experimental values

Renografin 76 at varying w/v concentrations. Similar data for iopanoate, at concentrations 20–30 times lower, have been obtained. During SCE scoring, no chromosomal aberrations have been found [22].

D. Discussion

Any chemical or physical agent which causes heritable change in genetic material is termed mutagenic. The basic mechanism of action of most mutagens appears to be damage to nuclear DNA [12]. Such DNA damage can then by expressed in any of several ways, including induction of cancer (carcinogenic mutagen) or somatic birth defects (teratogenic mutagen) [12]. In his recent review of the problem of identifying chemicals causing mutations and cancer, Ames stated: "damage to DNA by environmental mutagens (both natural and man-made) is likely to be a major cause of cancer and genetic birth defects, and may contribute to heart disease, cataracts, and developmental birth defects as well" [12]. The same author, pointing out how complicated the detection of human carcinogenicity by epidemiologic studies can be, noted "the difficulties in connecting cause and effect, the great expense involved, and the fact that people would already have been exposed for decades by the time a particular cause of cancer was identified" [12]. It can be gleaned from the voluminous literature on the subject that there are many pitfalls and inconsistencies in the interpretation of in vitro data and in our ability to translate them from in vitro data to the clinical situation. Yet, using two techniques described above, we have not been able to demonstrate mutagenicity of the commonly used ionic CM. More work is required before radiographic CM can be definitively either indicted or absolved of mutagenicity. So far, no clinical observation suggests CM mutagenicity.

Finally, it should be pointed out that the question of clinically significant mutagenesis remains unclear even in drugs which have been evaluated by nearly all known parameters. Hypoxic-cell sensitizers, such as metronidazole, which are useful in radiotherapy, have been studied by nearly all available techniques. Conflicting in vitro results have been reported [20] and confirmation or denial of carcinogenic properties by small clinical series are statistically difficult, hard to control, and thus relatively unconvincing [24]. It seems clear that no drug should be indicted as a potential clinical mutagen on the basis of only a single type of evaluation. Use of established drugs can be endangered when the lines between theoretical and practical considerations become blurred. The saga of saccharin is an excellent example of the problem that can arise when basic research results are unrealistically translated into public policy [25].

Useful medical treatments [26] and therapeutic medicines [27] have inherent risks which must be considered when risk: benefit decisions are made. Diagnostic agents ideally should be completely inert, but CM elicit some, albeit small, morbidity in the patient population [28]. Since an "acceptable risk" seems nearly impossible to define [29], conclusions of drug-caused cytogenetic damage based on a single nonspecific morphologic assay are hardly warranted [30]. Until a direct correlation between micronuclei induction and in vivo tumorigenicity has been established, such conclusions must be considered to be hypothetical. In the absence of any clinical evidence that CM cause significant cytogenetic damage, the hypothetical nature of such results should be clearly stated and understood.

References

1. Little JB (1966) Environmental hazards: ionizing radiation. N Engl J Med 275:929–938
2. Bushong SC (1976) Pregnancy in diagnostic radiology: radiation control procedures. Appl Radiol 5:63–68
3. Symposium on distribution, retention, and late effects of thorium dioxide. Ann NY Acad Sci 145 (1967)
4. Feig SA (1978) Ionizing radiation and human breast cancer. CRC Crit Rev Diagn Imaging 11:145–166
5. Boyle JA, Seegmiller JE (1971) Preparation and processing of small samples of human material. In: Jakoby WB (ed) Methods in enzymology XXII. Academic, New York, pp 154–160
6. Schmid E, Bauchinger M (1976) The cytogenetic effect of an X-ray contrast medium in Chinese hamster cell cultures. Mutat Res 34:291–298
7. Adams FH, Norman A, Mello RS, Bass D (1977) Effect of radiation and contrast media on chromosomes. Radiology 124:823–826
8. Schmid W (1977) Remarks and data on some methods to monitor the in vivo induction of chromosome aberrations in mammals. In: de la Chapelle A, Sorsa M (eds) Chromosomes today, vol 6. Elsevier, Amsterdam, pp 327–335
9. Heddle JA, Benz RD, Countryman PI (1978) Measurement of chromosomal breakage in cultured cells by the micronucleus technique. In: Evans HJ, Lloyd D (eds) Mutagen-induced chromosome damage in man. Yale University Press, New Haven, pp 191–200
10. Cochran ST, Khodadoust A, Norman A (1980) Cytogenetic effects of contrast material in patients undergoing excretory urography. Radiology 136:43–46
11. Adams FH, Norman A, Bass D, Oku G (1978) Chromosome damage in infants and children after cardiac catheterization and angiocardiography. Pediatrics 62:312–316
12. Ames BN (1979) Identifying environmental chemicals causing mutations and cancer. Science 204:587–593
13. Wolff S (1979) Sister chromatid exchange: the most sensitive mammalian system for determining the effects of mutagenic carcinogens. In: Berg K (ed) Genetic damage in many caused by environmental agents. Academic, New York
14. Devoret R (1979) Bacterial tests for potential carcinogens. Sci Am 241:40–49
15. Scott WJ, Fradkin R, Wilson JG (1977) Non-confirmation of thalidomide induced teratogenesis in rats and mice. Teratology 16:333–336
16. Wheeler LA, Norman A, Riley R (1980) Mutagenicity of diatrizoate and other triiodobenzoic acid derivatives in the Ames *soluronellu*/microsome test. Proc West Pharmacol Soc 23:249–253
17. Painter RB (1980) A replication model for sister chromatid exchange. Mutat Res 70:337–341
18. Livingston GK, Dethlefsen LA (1979) Effects of hyperthermia and x-irradiation on SCE in CHO cells. Radiat Res 77:512–520
19. Liebeskind D, Bases R, Mendez F et al. (1979) Sister chromatid exchanges in human lymphocytes after exposure to diagnostic ultrasound. Science 205:1273–1275
20. Prosser JS, Hesketh LC (1980) Hypoxic-cell sensitizers and sister chromatid exchanges. Br J Radiol 53:376–377
21. Borek C (1979) Malignant transformation in vitro: criteria, biological markers, and application in environmental screening of carcinogens. Radiat Res 79:209–232
22. Nelson JA, Livingston GK, Moon RG (1982) Mutagenic evaluation of radiographic contrast media. Invest Radiol 17:183–185
23. Ames BN, McCann J, Yamasaki E (1975) Methods for detecting carcinogens and mutagens with the salmonella/mammalian microsome mutagenicity test. Mutat Res 31:347–364

24. Beard CM, Noller KL, O'Fallon WM et al. (1979) Lack of evidence for cancer due to use of metronidazole. N Engl J Med 301:519–522
25. Smith RJ (1980) Latest saccharin tests kill FDA proposal. News and comment. Science 208:154–156
26. Singer MM, Wright F, Stanley LK, Roe BB, Hamilton WK (1970) Oxygen toxicity in man. N Engl J Med 283:1473–1477
27. Reimer RR, Hoover R, Fraumeni JF, Young RC (1977) Acute leukemia after alkylating-agent therapy of ovarian cancer. N Engl J Med 297:177–181
28. Baum S, Stein GN, Kmoda KK (1966) Complications of "no arteriography· Radiology 86:835–838
29. Lowrance WW (1976) Of acceptable risk. Kaufmann, Los Altos
30. Weisburger JH, Williams GM (1981) Carcinogen testing: current problems and new approaches. Science 214:401–407

CHAPTER 13

Particulate Suspensions as Contrast Media

M. R. Violante and H. W. Fischer

A. Introduction

Particulate contrast media offer exciting advantages over water-soluble media in several radiologic applications. A truly vascular contrast medium which does not diffuse into the extravascular spaces and is not hyperosmolar would be extremely useful as an intravenous angiographic medium for measuring blood flow and vascular volumes with the novel technologies such as digital fluoroscopy and dynamic computed tomography (CT) scanning. A medium which is less viscous than Ethiodol and does not embolize in the lungs would be advantageous in lymphography. The difference in impedance between solids and liquids means particulate media could potentially be useful as ultrasound contrast media (CM). Paramagnetic compounds in the form of a particulate suspension may be helpful as nuclear magnetic resonance (NMR) contrast media.

Although each of the above-cited applications could potentially be improved by using a particulate CM, much work needs to be done before any of these become a reality. The opacification of liver and spleen in CT is the application where particulate CM will probably first be used. The need for improved visualization of these organs, particularly for earlier detection of liver metastases, and the potential for natural accumulation of a particulate agent by the phagocytic action of the reticuloendothelial (RE) cells of the liver and spleen has led to numerous attempts at developing such a medium. Initially, these agents were intended for use in conventional hepatosplenography, but the dose required was considerable and adverse reactions were substantial [1, 2]. The advent of computed tomography, with its ability to detect minimal density differences, has reduced the dosage necessary for obtaining diagnostically useful contrast enhancement of the liver. The potential for reducing dose-dependent adverse reaction to such agents has generated renewed interest in developing a clinically useful RE-selective agent for the detection of mass lesions of the liver and spleen.

The objective of this chapter is to review those factors important for developing a particulate CM. Because of the extensive efforts in developing a hepatolienographic medium, our knowledge of these requirements is substantially greater than for the other applications mentioned. We will, therefore, discuss RE selective media in considerable detail. Modifications necessary for developing a lymphographic or angiographic medium will be briefly described at the end of the chapter.

I. Definition and Scope

The contrast media discussed in this chapter include water-insoluble media which can be administered intravenously for selective accumulation by the fixed-phagocytic cells of the reticuloendothelial system (RES) located primarily in the liver. Included among this group are media which could be administered in the form of colloids, suspensions of small particles, oil/water emulsions, or contrast encapsulated in liposomes. Although water-soluble cholangiographic media do selectively opacify the liver, the mechanism, and pharmacokinetics of these media are quite different form the media of interest in this chapter and will not be discussed here (see Chap. 7).

The primary purpose of this chapter is to describe and analyze the problems and complexities involved in designing and formulating a CM for accumulation by the RE system. The emphasis in this regard will be on particulate CM since we are most familiar with these media. However, the discussion will be generally valid for any RE selective medium. Since considerable progress has been made in the development of emulsified materials, we will describe the similarities and differences between these media and particulate CM. We will then discuss the usefulness of these media in CT of the liver and spleen. Finally, we will conclude with other potential applications of particulate CM such as in lymphography and angiography.

B. Particulate Contrast Media

The most well-known particulate CM developed to date is Thorotrast, a suspension of thorium dioxide particles in an aqueous medium, used clinically for many years. Although this medium provided excellent radiographic images with very little acute toxicity, the use of Thorotrast had to be discontinued because of its chronic toxicity, primarily induction of fibrosis and possible generation of neoplasms in certain organs resulting from the long retention of this radioactive material [3]. Since then, numerous attempts have been made to simulate the advantages of Thorotrast while overcoming its disadvantages.

We will not present a historical review of these experimental media in this chapter. Rather, we will attempt to describe factors important for a good hepatographic medium, citing appropriate evidence accumulated from studies with these earlier experimental media. These concepts and supporting data will be presented in the following subsections.

We will begin with formulation, covering aspects such as chemical composition, particle size, and suspension stability. This is followed by a discussion on what is known about the interaction of these media with blood components and the implications of these interactions for phagocytosis and toxicity. We then describe, in some detail, those factors important for phagocytosis of the particles by reticuloendothelial cells, particularly the Kupffer cells in the liver.

I. Formulation

Table 1 lists most of the inorganic particulate CM which have been reported to date along with some suspension characteristics of these media. The first column

Table 1. Inorganic particulate contrast media

Radiopaque	Additives	Particle Diameter (μm)	Suspension stability	References
Thorium dioxide (Thorotrast)	Dextrin	0.15	NR	[1, 4, 5]
Thorium dioxide	Gum acacia	NR	NR	[6, 7]
Stannic oxide	Tapioca dextrin Pig gelatin	NR	Settles in days Easily resuspended	[8, 9]
Tantalum pentoxide	Dextrin or gelatin	0.5	Grossly stable Several days Microaggregates	[10]
Barium sulfate	Methylcellulose	≦ 3	Glumps – 10 μm No settling	[11]
Cerium oxide Gadolinium oxide Dysprosium oxide Silver iodide	NR	≦ 2	NR	[12]

NR, not reported

in this table gives the chemical name of the radiopaque component and the second lists the reported additives included in the formulation to provide suspension stability. The third and fourth columns provide the reported range of particle diameters and some indications of suspension stability. Data on these two properties are very meager and not well documented. The range of particle diameters is almost certainly greater than indicated and descriptions of suspension stability are very subjective. The interested reader should consult the appropriate reference for further details on these suspension.

The media reported in this table all provided excellent radiopacification of the liver in animals or patients (Thorotrast). However, most of these inorganic compounds are extremely insoluble and are not metabolized in vivo. These particulate media, therefore, remain in the liver indefinitely and are thus unlikely to be approved for use in humans.

Table 2 contains similar data for particulate CM developed using organic compounds as the radiopaque. Animal studies with most of these media have also demonstrated excellent hepatic radiopacification; somewhat less opacity is obtained with those media having only one or two iodine atoms per molecule. In addition, these compounds are all cleared from the organism, so indefinite retention is not a problem as with the inorganic particulates.

We have again cited, when known, the additives employed for suspension stability and a brief description of stated stability. The particle diameters reported in this table generally pertain to the majority, but not all, of the particles in the suspension. In most cases, the literature reports are not very explicit in describing the actual range of particle sizes contained in the suspension. In general, however, suspensions produced by physical methods – micronizing and grinding – contain a much broader range of particle diameters than is usually obtained with chemical precipitation methods. With suspensions prepared by physical methods, the re-

Table 2. Organic particulate contrast media

Radiopaque	Additives	Particle diameter (μm)	Methods	Suspension	References
Iodipamide ethyl ester	PVP, HSA	0.5–1.5	Precipitation	Easily resuspended	[13]
Iothalamate ethyl ester	PVP, HSA	1–2	Precipitation	Settles in hours	[14, 15]
B 6500, B 13040, B 13630	Gelatin	2–3	Micronized	NR	[16]
Propyliodone	CMC 70, Tween 80 merthiolate	NR	Micronized crystals	NR	[17]
N-Tyrosine-3, 5-diiodo-4-pyridone N-acetate	CMC 70, Tween 80 merthiolate	NR	Micronized crystals	NR	[17]
Tetraiodophthalate derivatives	–	1	Precipitation	Settled in several days; partly resuspendable with shaking	[18]
Tetraiodophenolphthalein	–	2	Wet grinding	NR	[19]

NR, not reported; PVP, polyvinylpyrrolidone; HSA, human serum albumin; CMC, carboxymethylcellulose

ported particle diameters are most likely "maximum" diameters with perhaps a very small minority of larger particles and a substantial fraction of particles of varying, smaller diameters. Chemical precipitation methods, on the other hand, allow for the production of particles of very uniform size. The importance of controlling particle size to within a narrow range will become apparent later in this chapter.

While all of these organic particulate CM have been reported as having some success radiographically, to our knowledge all have been abandoned with the exception of the compounds from our own work, namely, organic esters of water-soluble CM. The reasons for the lack of further development of the other media are not known to us, but may be related to the complexity and difficulties associated with an RE selective agent as is illustrated in the remainder of this chapter.

II. Interactions with Blood Components

As shown in Tables 1 and 2 all of these experimental media were suspensions of particles having diameters less than 3 μm. This upper limit is necessary for the particles to pass through the finest capillaries. Although red blood cells (RBC) are approximately 6–9 μm in diameter, they are known to deform when passing through capillaries. Since the radiopaque particles are generally not deformable the maximum particle diameter must be considerably smaller than 6 μm.

Since capillary diameters of less than 4 μm have been reported [20], particles should have a diameter of 2–3 μm or less to be safe; however, this maximum size must be smaller yet for a number of reasons related to interactions of particles with blood components.

The contact of blood with a foreign surface is well known to elicit reactions with various blood components [21–23] and to activate such important mechanisms as the intrinsic coagulation [24], complement [25], and fibrinolytic [26] systems. We will not attempt to review the considerable literature on this subject but will concentrate on those proteins and blood components which may, or have been shown to, be involved when a particulate medium is injected into the bloodstream.

A number of proteins have been identified or proposed to interact with foreign surfaces. These include: albumin [15, 27–29], acute-phase reactant proteins [30], and globulins [31, 32], including acid glycoprotein and fibronectin [21] among others.

The protein which has been most consistently implicated in reactions with foreign particles is fibrinogen and its degradation products. As early as 1926, fibrinogen was suggested to be transformed to fibrin as a result of injecting a quartz suspension [33]. Fibrin was suggested as the protein associated with carbon particles after injection with India ink [34]. Other particles which cause fibrinogen to be absorbed from plasma include: koalin and graphite [35], latex [36], and iothalamate ethyl ester [15].

Fibrinogen interaction with particles has been implicated in activating platelet aggregation. In a study with India ink, increased dosages of these carbon particles resulted in proportional decreases in blood fibrinogen and the number of platelets [34]. Platelets have been shown to adhere to foreign surfaces only where fibrinogen is deposited and remains on the surface [36, 37]. Latex particles which had absorbed fibrinogen from plasma or from a partially purified fibrinogen preparation stimulated platelet aggregation [35]. Kaolin or graphite particles do not induce platelet aggregation in the absence of proteins, but the addition of fibrinogen solution to the same suspension medium did produce platelet aggregation [38]. These and other studies provide overwhelming evidence that the combination of a foreign surface and fibrinogen can induce platelet aggregation. The significance of these findings is that although particles may be 3 μm or less, in vitro the adherence of fibrinogen and especially platelets to the particles, or the aggregation of platelets themselves, can produce embolic phenomena especially when given in high doses [39].

In addition to platelet activation, fibrinogen has been shown to induce particle:particle aggregation as well. When a stable suspension of iothalamate ethyl ester particles (Fig. 1 a) was mixed with diluted ethylenediaminetetraacetate (ED-TA)-anticoagulated plasma, the particles agglutinated as shown in Fig. 1 b. The severity of aggregation increased for rat, rabbit, dog, and human plasma, respectively [14, 15].

This problem of adverse protein (and/or platelet) interaction causing platelet and/or particle aggregation can be overcome by properly coating the particles prior to introducing them into the bloodstream. With some of the inorganic particulate media, namely Thorotrast and tin oxide, dextrin apparently provided ad-

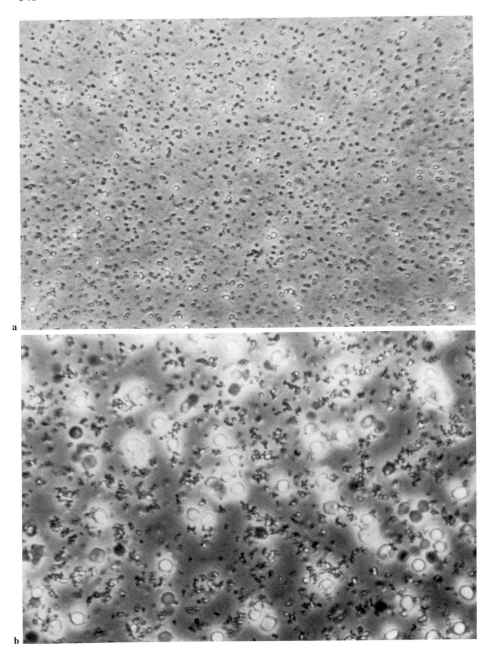

Fig. 1 a–c. Iothalamate ethyl ester particles. × 770. **a** One-micron particles suspended in normal saline. **b** The same particles severely aggregated upon mixing with diluted blood. Aggregates are considerably larger than the red blood cells of 6–9 μm. **c** The same particles, preincupated in serum albumin prior to mixing with blood. Suspension is now stable with no tendency toward particle aggregation. (Adapted from [14])

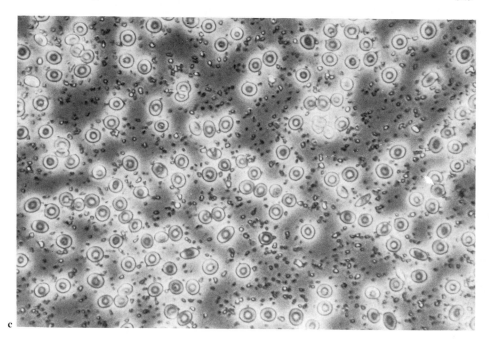

c

equate protection from the interactions described above [9, 40]. In the iothala-mate ethyl ester study referred to earlier, no particle aggregation was observed in the *serum* of those species whose *plasma* did cause particle aggregation. Since gel electrophoresis results indicated substantial albumin (present in both serum and plasma) binding as well as fibrinogen (present in plasma only) binding, we reasoned that preincubation of the iothalamate ethyl ester particles in albumin might prevent the adverse fibrinogen interactions [13]. This is demonstrated in Fig. 1 c, where the same particles as shown in Fig. 1 a, b were now incubated in albumin prior to mixing with the human blood. In contrast to Fig. 1 b, no evidence of particle aggregation is observed. We have since demonstrated this phenomenon with other organic esters and concluded that preincubation with albumin can alter or inhibit adverse interactions of blood components with radiopaque particles (M. R. Violante, unpublished results).

We should clarify that while particle:particle aggregation may be harmful, there is evidence that particle:platelet aggregation may be essential for transport of particles to the RES. Inhibition of platelet aggregation with adenosine diphos-phate (ADP) or its breakdown products has been shown to decrease carbon clear-ance from blood in rats. Conversely, infusion of additional platelets produced in-creased clearance from rat blood. A fairly complex mechanism for RES accumu-lation of carbon particles involving local activation and inhibition of the fibrino-lytic system as well as aggregation and disaggregation of platelets has been pro-posed [26]. The evidence for particle:platelet interactions is very convincing; but the importance and necessity for inducing or avoiding these interactions remains to be determined.

Having discussed problems associated with formulation of particulate suspensions and possible interactions of the particles with blood components, we must next consider those factors which are important for maximizing phagocytosis of these materials especially by the reticuloendothelial cells of the liver and spleen. Among the variables which can affect uptake, we will discuss the importance of: (a) interpreting results in the light of the differences in RES among animal species, (b) particle size, (c) particle surface charge, (d) total administered dose and infusion rate, and (e) so-called blockade of the RES.

III. Phagocytosis

Particulate CM selectively accumulate in the RES, so a much lower dose is needed to provide CT enhancement of liver and spleen than can be obtained with urographic agents, which are broadly distributed throughout the body. Phagocytosis by the Kupffer cells of the liver is, however, affected by a number of factors. In the following discussions, we have attempted to describe what is known about maximizing uptake of particles by the liver.

Efficacy of RE selective media has been reported in rats [41], rabbits [42], dogs [43], monkeys [44], and humans [45, 46]. Since these media are still experimental, differences in the RES among species must be understood to interpret and compare results properly.

1. Reticuloendothelial System – Species Differences

The first important consideration is that phagocytic activity of the RE system is different among animal species. A possible explanation is the relative size of the liver and spleen as a function of body weight. As shown in Table 3, using data taken from the *Handbook of Biological Data* [47], the proportion of body weight of the liver and spleen decreases from mouse to rat, rabbit, dog, monkey, and man, respectively. Since these data were compiled from a variety of sources, the absolute numbers may not be exactly consistent with each other, but the trend from mouse to man is probably real.

Table 3. Proportion of body weight of the liver, spleen, and lungs [47]

Species	Liver (%)	Spleen (%)	Lungs (%)
Mouse	4.6–5.6	NR	1.3–1.7
Rat	3.4	0.3	0.8
Rabbit	2.7–3.2	NR	0.5
Dog	2.9	NR	0.9
Monkey	2.1–3.3	0.7	0.6
Man	2.3–2.8	0.1–0.3	0.7–3.1

NR, not reported

Assuming that the composition of the liver is similar in all species to that found in the rat, namely 2.1% by volume is Kupffer cells [48], then greater contrast enhancement at a given dose per kilogram body weight can be expected for man compared with small animals. This effect should be observable since for humans the same number of particles will be accumulated in a smaller volume (or tissue mass), producing a greater concentration of CM per gram liver tissue, which in turn will produce greater CT enhancement.

In addition, RES activity per cell may be different in the various species. It is reported to be most active in the mouse and to decrease in the rat, pig, rabbit, and man, respectively [49]. This can be at least partly explained by the relative percentage of body weight of the liver in these various species; however, other factors such as relative blood supply, availability of metabolites required for the energy-dependent process of phagocytosis, and other factors may contribute to this difference between species. We must therefore be cautious in extrapolating dose-enhancement results obtained in the various experimental laboratory animals.

Another factor to consider is that the RES is a very complex and diffuse system as indicated in Fig. 2 (from [51]). This schematic illustrates the variety and distribution of cells within the vascular and lymphatic system but does not include cells such as the aveolar macrophages. Even so, the reader can appreciate the complexity of this system and the difficulty in attempting analysis.

As shown, the RES can be divided into mobile and stationary macrophages; the latter classification can be further subdivided into reticular and lining cells. It is this last subgroup facing the bloodstream, which is of primary interest in this chapter as accumulation of contrast in these cells provides the specific organ CT enhancement. We are concerned not only with directing our CM to this particular class of cells but we must also be concerned with the distribution of contrast among the organs within this group.

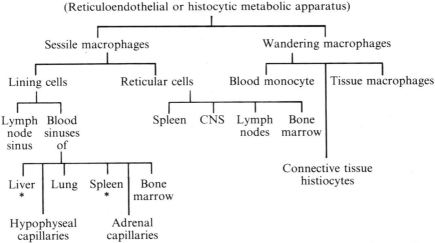

Fig. 2. Slightly modified version of Aschoff's concept of the RES. Liver and spleen (*) are major organs participating in the clearance of particulate matter from the blood. (Adapted from [50])

The exact percentage of each component of this system obviously cannot be measured by surgically removing it and analyzing tissue mass, volume, etc. Rather, investigators have attempted to define the composition of this system by measuring the biodistribution of an intravenously injected particulate tracer. In these studies, more than 90% of the tracer was usually recovered in the liver, spleen, lungs, and bone marrow [34, 51–54], indicating that fixed phagocytic cells lining the blood vessels in these organs either constitute the vast bulk of the RES or have the greatest phagocytic activity.

The distribution of particles among these organs, however, may vary considerably depending upon particle size distribution, surface charge of the particles, dose administered, and status of RE cell activity. Each of these factors can substantially affect the biodistribution of particulates and caution must be exercised in comparing one study with another, since experimental conditions are rarely the same.

2. Particle Size

Variations in the size distribution of injected particles can affect the rate of phagocytosis and the interorgan distribution of the particulates. Colloids of zirconium, columbium, and yttrium, having particles of "relatively large size," were cleared from mouse blood rather rapidly ($t_{1/2} = 30.60$ s) and the uptake of these particles into the liver and spleen exceeded 90% of injected dose. In comparison, the same colloids but of "intermediate particle size" were cleared from blood more slowly (30–80 min) and uptake by bone marrow reportedly exceeded that for liver and spleen in the rabbit, cat, and rat. In the mouse, liver and spleen uptake was still highest but bone marrow uptake was greater than for "large particles" [51]. Unfortunately the lack of good particle size analysis and the relative scarcity of actual distribution data in this paper weakens this conclusion considerably.

In a later paper, similar evidence is presented, indicating that mouse liver and spleen uptake decreased from 90% to 53% of injected dose for "large" and "small" particles, respectively [52], but again actual particle size was not defined. While not known for sure, particle sizes in these studies have been estimated to be a few nanometers for the smaller particles and 100 nm or more for the larger particles [55].

Although no study to our knowledge has carefully documented liver, spleen, lung, and bone marrow uptake as a function of known particle size with all other parameters constant, a number of papers [56–60] offer additional support to the hypothesis that larger particles are cleared from the blood more rapidly and accumulated in liver and spleen more than smaller particles.

3. Particle Surface Charge

The effect of surface charge on particle uptake by liver and spleen is difficult to evaluate because the particle or at least the surface chemical composition must be altered to vary surface charge. It is impossible to isolate truly the effect of one, independent of the other.

One attempt to analyze this parameter involved using 1.3-μm polystyrene latex particles coated with varying mixtures of gum arabic (negative charge) and

Table 4. Effect of particle electrophoretic mobility on blood clearance and organ distribution in the rat. (Adapted from [61])

Ration of PLG-GA in concentrate	Electrophoretic mobility in isotonic Michaelis buffer, pH 7.5 (μm/s/V/cm)	$t_{1/2}$ (min)	Organ distribution in rat 15 min postinjection			Injected dose (%) 72 h postinjection		
			Liver	Spleen	Lung	Liver	Spleen	Lung
GA	−1.10	0.7	92.5	2.7	0.7	95.1	1.9	0.1
10–90	−1.02	1.6	77.8	11.0	7.3	85.2	8.4	0.7
20–80	−0.73	1.5	72.5	6.8	10.6	79.2	10.0	0.7
60–40	+0.36	1.3	68.6	5.0	11.3	82.7	8.2	0.8
80–20	+0.60	1.9	69.0	6.2	14.0	87.7	8.8	0.8
PLG	+1.15	2.3	58.0	8.2	15.2	73.9	14.1	1.1

polylysyl gelatin (positive) [61]. The net surface charge of the particles studied is shown in Table 4. The electrophoretic mobility, a parameter which is a measure of surface charge by analysis of the rate a particle moves in an electric field, varied from −1.10 μm/s per volt per centimeter for particles coated with pure gum arabic (GA) to +1.15 μm/s per volt per centimeter for particles coated with pure polylysyl gelatin (PLG). The values obtained for particles coated with mixtures of these two compounds are shown in Table 4.

The rate of clearance of particles from blood is frequently taken (or mistaken) as a measure of phagocytic activity. The time required for the concentration of particles to decrease to one-half their original concentration, $t_{1/2}$, is also shown in Table 4. The difference in clearance rates between particles coated with pure gum arabic (negative charge) and with pure polylysyl gelatin (positive charge) is very striking, indicating that the negatively charged particles are cleared much more rapidly than positively charged particles. However, while the clearance rate for particles with mixed coatings is intermediate between these two extremes they are all very similar and do not show a trend as would be expected.

The distribution of these charged latex particles among liver, spleen, and lung is also shown in Table 4. At 15 min after injection the liver shows a much higher uptake of negatively charged particles than those with a positive charge. The lungs, however, show exactly the opposite effect, that is, greater accumulation of positively charged particles. The observed variation in splenic uptake was attributed to variations in splenic weight. At 72 h the majority of particles had cleared from the lungs; interestingly, these particles apparently redistributed more to the spleen than to the liver.

The results of this study would seem to imply that negatively charged particles are accumulated in the liver to a greater extent than positively charged particles, which are more apt to be phagocytized in the lungs and spleen. There are several problems with this conclusion, however. When the latex particles were incubated in rat serum, they all became negatively charged, with a mobility corresponding to that of serum albumin. The binding of albumin to these particles is not surprising as discussed in an earlier section. The following speculations might account

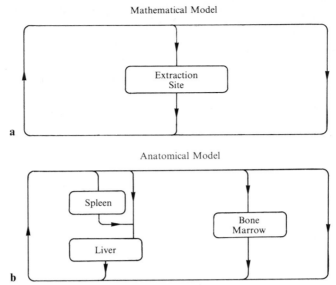

Fig. 3 a, b. Schematic models describing particulate substance clearance from the blood. **a** Simple mathematical model treating all deposition sites as though there was only one extraction site. **b** More complex model reflecting several anatomic deposition sites. (Adapted from [72])

for the observed correlations in clearance rates and organ uptake with charge variations.

1. The rate of albumination may be significantly slower than the rate of phago-cytosis so the initial charge on the particles may predominate.
2. As indicated in the original article and elsewhere [62, 63] the actual spatial arrangement of charges on the surface may be more important than the *net* surface charge as measured by electrophoretic mobility.
3. Proteins other than albumin may bind to the particles, thereby leading to specific recognition by the phagocytic cells. This type of argument is more credible when we consider that liver and spleen cell surfaces are negatively charged [64] and a simple charge attraction model would favor uptake of positively charged particles over those with negative charge which should be repulsed. Since exactly the opposite results are actually observed, it is unlikely that charge alone controls phagocytosis.

4. Dose

Several groups have attempted to quantify the effect of administered dose on clearance of particles from blood [65–71]. Each has developed mathematic expressions to describe observed clearance rates. The major problem with this approach for our purpose is that clearance data do not provide information regarding deposition of particles in a particular organ. For illustration purposes we can consider these mathematic expressions as describing a model as illustrated in Fig. 3 a. These models really make no assumptions about deposition site(s) but effec-

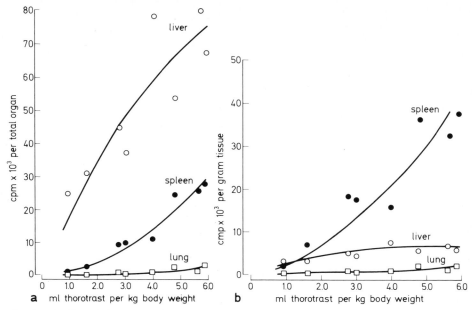

Fig. 4. a Radioactivity of liver, spleen, and lungs per total organ 24 h after intravenous injection of Thorotrast into rats. **b** Radioactivity of liver, spleen, and lungs per gram tissue 24 h after intravenous injection of Thorotrast into rats. (Adapted from [53])

tively describe a system which does not distinguish more than one site. In reality, however, there are several possible sites for particle deposition in vivo as illustrated in Fig. 3 b. Since we are interested in the contrast enhancement of a particular organ (liver), the second model is really more relevant.

At low doses, e.g., those used in radionuclide studies, the difference between these two models is insignificant since the liver is by far the major site of deposition. However, at higher doses such as those needed for contrast enhancement in CT, a substantial fraction of the injected particles will be deposited in the spleen with an additional small but insignificant fraction appearing in the lungs and bone narrow. This was demonstrated in 1967 with Thorotrast in rats. The results are plotted in Fig. 4 to illustrate this point. Twenty-four hours after intravenous injection of increasing doses of Thorotrast, rats were killed and several organs, namely liver, spleen, and lungs, were removed and analyzed for radioactivity. In Fig. 4 a, the radioactivity is found almost exclusively in the liver following low-dose injections of Thorotrast. However, as the dose is increased, not only does the radioactivity found in the liver increase, but a substantial fraction of the radioactivity is now observed in the spleen. When the results are plotted as radioactivity per gram of organ, as in Fig. 4 b, the dose dependence of biodistribution of Thorotrast within the RE system is even more dramatically illustrated. As shown here, at low doses the radioactivity is the same in liver and spleen on a per gram of organ basis; however, as the dose increases, the amount of radioactivity per gram of liver increases only slightly while the radioactivity per gram of spleen increases dramatically. Unfortunately, not all of the radioactivity in this study was in particulate form. Since the Thorotrast suspension used in this study contained dialyzable radioactivity, these should be interpreted as representing relative, not absolute, differences in organ phagocytic activity [53]. Also, the reported particle size (10–25 nm) is extremely small and organ distribution may be quite different for larger particles.

The importance of these data is that unlike nuclear medicine studies in which the small doses of particulates accumulate almost entirely in the liver, the doses required for contrast enhancement in CT are necessarily large so that a significant fraction of the particles will accumulate in organs (primarily spleen) other than the liver. Although specific accumulation in the liver only might be preferable, phagocytic uptake of particles by the spleen should not present any significant problem. On the other hand, administration of these relatively large doses of particulate CM should be made slowly to avoid excessive accumulation in the lungs and other capillary networks. Rapid injections of these materials can lead to aggregation (as described earlier) and lung obstruction, especially if the injection rate exceeds the rate of local clearing mechanisms in this organ.

5. Reticuloendothelial System Blockade

This term has been used to describe the situation wherein the clearance rate of "inert" particles, usually colloidal carbon, from the bloodstream is significantly reduced. This condition has been attributed to satiation of the reticuloendothelial cells, saturation of the phagocytosis mechanism, and/or depletion of opsonins, or serum factors, necessary for phagocytosis to occur [73]. We will not attempt to review this controversial subject in detail; rather, we will stress those factors which could be important for particulate contrast enhancement in CT of the liver.

As indicated earlier, particulate clearance rate from blood is not as important for our purposes as is the site of deposition (liver, spleen, lung, or bone marrow) when the particles are removed from circulation. If the particles are merely taken up more slowly by the Kupffer cells there may be somewhat less enhancement of the liver but this should not be a serious problem. However, if during so-called blockade the particles accumulate in different organs such as the lungs or bone marrow, interference with normal functioning of these organs may create serious adverse reactions or unduly compromise the patient's defense mechanisms.

Mice, intravenously injected with dextran sulfate to create RE blockade, were reinjected with sheep red blood cells labeled with [^{51}Cr] SRBC 3 h later. After another 3 h the animals were killed and the amount of radioactivity in different tissues was determined. The results are shown in Table 5. The importance of these data is that during blockade the [^{51}Cr]SRBC accumulated much more in the spleen and bone marrow compared with controls.

The implication of these results is that if a particulate CM is given to a patient whose functional state of the RE system may be less than normal as a result of disease or RES-depressant therapy (certain drugs or radiation therapy), a substantial portion of CM may accumulate in the spleen and bone marrow, which would be undesirable from the radiologic standpoint and may further compromise the patient's phagocytic capacity.

Table 5. Organ distribution of [^{51}Cr] *SRBC* during *RE* blockade (adapted from [72])

Tissues	Radioactivity (total in organ as % of injected dose) Mean + SEM	
	Controls	Blockaded
Liver	91.1 ± 2.0	12.7 ± 1.3
Spleen	1.1 ± 0.6	31.8 ± 10.1
Bone marrow	NS	39.0

Reticuloendothelial depression or blockade may be related to a specific agent and not a general phenomenon. An example of this is a study where rats were injected with various substances, as shown in Table 6, and clearance rates from plasma were measured to determine whether blockade had occurred. As shown, the clearance rate of gelatin-stabilized radio-CrPO$_4$ or gold was much slower if the rats had been given prior injection of gelatin than was the case with no prior injection, indicating that gelatin had depressed the clearance of gelatin-coated particles. However, when non-gelatin-coated particles were used for the tracer

Table 6. Blockade of the RES by gelatin-stabilized colloids tested 1 h after blockade with gelatin-stabilized radioactive particles and nonstabilized radioactive particles. (Adapted from [74])

No. of animals	Blockading agent stabilized in 2% solution of gelatin	Blockading dose (mg/ 100 g body wt.)	Tracer injection	$T/2$ (min.) tracer dose (mean ± SE)	Edect
10			Gelatin-stabilized Au^{159}	0.92 ± 0.07	
5			Gelatin-stabilized radio-CrPO$_4$	0.94 ± 0.09	
6			Radio-CrPO$_4$ in saline	0.61 ± 0.06	
10	Gelatin[a]	10	Gelatin-stabilized Au^{198}	7.0 ± 0.11	Blockade
4	Carbon	8	Gelatin-stabilized Au^{198}	16.4 ± 0.43	Blockade
8	Gold	4	Gelatin-stabilized Au^{198}	19.2 ± 0.90	Blockade
4	Chromic phosphate	5	Gelatin-stabilized Au^{198}	13.8 ± 0.45	Blockade
5	Gelatin[a]	10	Gelatin-stabilized radio-CrPO$_4$	8.5 ± 0.24	Blockade
5	Carbon	8	Gelatin-stabilized radio-CrPO$_4$	17.1 ± 0.58	Blockade
4	Gold	4	Gelatin-stabilized radio-CrPO$_4$	15.3 ± 0.33	Blockade
4	Chromic phosphate	5	Gelatin-stabilized radio-CrPO$_4$	14.6 ± 0.40	Blockade
5	Gelatin[a]	10	Radio-CrPO$_4$ in saline	0.68 ± 0.07	No blockade
4	Carbon	8	Radio-CrPO$_4$ in saline	0.71 ± 0.09	No blockade
6	gold	4	Radio-CrPO$_4$ in saline	0.65 ± 0.10	No blockade
5	Chromic phosphate	5	Radio-CrPO$_4$ in saline	0.60 ± 0.08	No blockade

[a] Gelatin injected alone as a 5% solution

dose no blockade was observed. These results would indicate that the blockade was specific for gelatin. In addition, the gelatin-coated particles behaved as though they were gelatin, which again emphasizes the importance of particle coating.

In the preceding discussion we have attempted to enumerate and describe some of the factors which could influence phagocytosis of particulate CM when used for hepatic CT enhancement. There are, of course, other factors to consider such as pharmacologic stimulation of the RES and possible factors which have not as yet been identified. Nevertheless, we hope that the reader has acquired an introduction to the problems associated with the development of such a medium and that the interested reader can now pursue further literature search and laboratory investigations into one or more of the areas described above.

In the next section of this chapter we will discuss work conducted with another class of RE selective media, namely oil/water emulsions. These media are very similar to the particulate media in terms of properties and behavior. We will, however, indicate where an important difference does exist between these two types of media.

C. Emulsions

Attempts to use emulsions of radiopaque oily materials in water as RE selective media have historically paralleled efforts with particulate CM. The first use of such a medium in humans was in 1930, involving emulsions of iodized poppyseed oil and brominated olive oil for successful opacification of the liver [75]. This medium was subsequently removed from clinical use after several patients had died presumably from large oil droplets creating emboli in lung capillaries [17]. Since then numerous investigators have tried to develop safer emulsions initially for use in hepatography [76–83] and more recently for CT liver-scanning media [44–46, 84–86]. As with the particulate media, the advent of CT has revitalized efforts in this field. On the assumption that adverse effects with these media are dose dependent, and since doses required for CT are substantially lower than needed for conventional hepatography, adverse side effects may be eliminated or at least minimized to an extent that these media could be clinically useful.

The development of emulsified CM involves basically the same considerations as described in detail for particulate media, including: control of oil droplet size and emulsion stability, interactions of oil droplets with blood components, and uptake, clearance, and possible blockade of the RES. In the following discussion we have attempted to stress those factors which, in our opinion, are of special concern for emulsions compared with particulate RE media.

As shown in Table 7, all emulsions to date have been prepared by some mechanical process of mixing the oil phase with the aqueous phase. As with mechanically prepared suspensions of particulate media, droplets with a relatively broad range of diameters are produced. Since the very large diameter droplets are known to contribute to the toxicity of these media through embolization of the pulmonary capillaries, the upper limit has generally been maintained at 7 μm or less. Since the very small droplets can also contribute to toxicity because of their

Table 7. Emulsified contrast media

Radiopaque component	Additives	Droplet diameter (μm)	Methods	Suspension stability	Ref.
1. Ethiodol[a]	Polysorbate 80, sorbitan momoleate, phosphatidyl, chlorine	0.75–7	Homogenization	Slight flocculent sedimentation after 6 months at 4°–8 °C	[85]
2. Ethiodol[a]	Polyoxyethylene, glyco monostearate, soya, lecithin, glucose, disodium-phosphate	0.1–7	NR	Several weeks	[82]
3. Ethiodol[a]	Dextran 40	(average 1) < 5	Hand homogenization	NR	[83]
4. Ethiodol[a]	Glucose, lecithin, phironic acid	~ 0.3	Chemical	"For long periods"	[80]
5. Ethyl triiodo-stearate	Lecithin, gelatin	~ 1	NR	NR	[77]
6. Lipiodol	Gum acacia	≦ 8–10	Trituration in mortar	NR	[75]

NR, not recorded
[a] Iodinated ester of poppyseed oil (Savage Laboratories, Houston, Texas)

large surface area, which increases the possibility of interactions with blood components, these should also be eliminated from the formulation. The broad range of sizes produced by mechanical homogenization methods generally require further processing to remove droplets of extreme sizes.

Of even greater concern is the difficulty in maintaining emulsion stability; that is, an emulsion which has been carefully formulated to contain oil droplets with a fairly narrow range of diameters can, within days, contain droplets of extreme sizes. This occurs through droplet-droplet interactions resulting in the coalescence of small droplets into larger ones and/or breakdown into even smaller droplets. This is a much more difficult problem for emulsions than for particulate media because of the much lower rigidity and stability of oil droplets compared with solid particles.

Another potential concern with the emulsions is the possibility of deiodination and consequent iodine intoxication. Emulsions, to date, have been prepared using iodinated (or brominated) esters of fatty acids. The iodine atoms in these compounds, bonded to aliphatic carbons, are much less firmly bound than are iodine atoms bonded to aromatic carbon atoms in the commonly used triiodinated benzoic acid derivates. The risk of deiodination occurring is definitely greater with emulsions of iodinated fatty acid esters than with particulates of triiodinated benzoic acid derivatives. Although deiodination is at least of theoretical concern, the extent of this reaction occurring in vivo has not as yet been clearly demonstrated.

Finally, several investigators have reported finding deposits of a brownish pigment in liver cells of animals following intravenous administration of emulsified CM [45] or nutrient emulsions [87]. The exact cause and nature of these deposits have not been well characterized as yet but should be of concern with further development of these media.

Despite the problems cited above, emulsions have been developed which have been recently tested in humans [45, 46]. Since these media have provided the most recent information on RE media in humans, we will discuss these extensively in the following section.

D. Computed Tomography Enhancement

The bulk of this chapter has been devoted to problems encountered in developing a particulate or emulsified contrast medium for selective opacification of the liver and spleen. This we felt was necessary to provide the reader with a thorough understanding of the complexities and potential complications involving its use. With that basis, we are now in a position to describe the usefulness of these media and to illustrate why they may be worth the extensive efforts in their development.

As indicated earlier, the toxicity of these media is such that, at present, they can only be considered for use at low dosage. Therefore, although these media have been used, at least experimentally, in conventional hepatosplenography of animals, we will restrict the following illustrations to those involving contrast enhancement in CT where substantially lower doses are required to obtain useful results. In addition, the bulk of the examples will involve the use of emulsified CM since these media have been used most recently in humans. We can, however, consider the results to be generally valid for both emulsified and particulate CM since both are controlled by similar mechanisms which therefore should lead to similar results.

Most recent emulsions to have been developed for use in CT of the liver consist of formulations involving Ethiodol, the iodinated ester of poppyseed oil and water. To demonstrate the usefulness of emulsion EOE 13 in detecting hepatic tumors, the medium was administered to rhesus monkeys with carcinogen-induced hepatoma. CT scans of the liver taken before contrast injection demonstrated a fairly large tumor nodule in the right lobe of the liver as shown in Fig. 5a. A similar scan taken 30 min after intravenous injection of EOE 13 at the same location not only demonstrated the large nodule more clearly but also that several smaller tumors in the right anterior lobe were visible as shown in Fig. 5b [44]. These images clearly illustrate the selectivity of RE-selective CM for normal hepatic tissue relative to that of tumors. Selective uptake of CM by surrounding parenchyma increases the CT attenuation solely of this tissue, thereby increasing the differential between parenchyma and tumor, making detection of small lesions easier. This study, as well as other experimental animal investigations [42], has

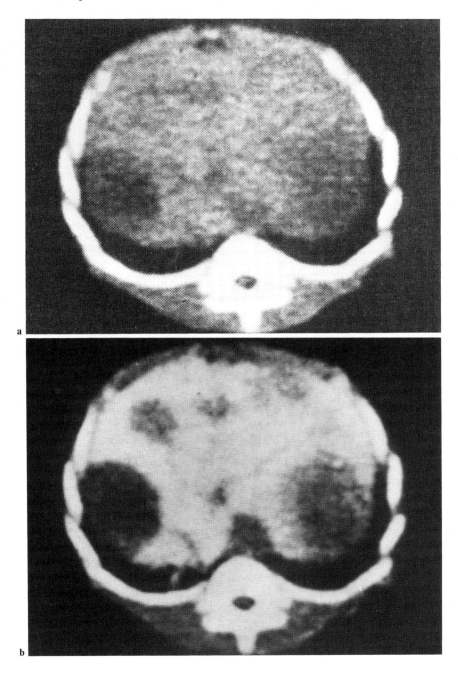

Fig. 5 a, b. Rhesus monkey with carcinogen-induced hepatoma. CT scans of liver before **a** and 30 min after **b** intravenous injection of EOE 13. The large tumors are visible on the preinjection scan, but small tumor nodules in the anterior right lobe are visible only after the injection of EOE 13. (Adapted from [44])

shown such a marked improvement in tumor detectability that at least one medium, emulsion EOE 13, is now being tested in patients [45].

The beneficial effect of using an RE-selective medium in humans is shown in Fig. 6 [45]. In this example, a metastatic sarcoma was barely visible in the right lobe of the liver on CT scanning (Fig. 6a). Injection of water-soluble CM produced almost complete concealment of the lesion as shown in Fig. 6b. Following the infusion of EOE 13 the patient was rescanned; the lesion is now clearly visible in the right lobe of the liver (Fig. 6c). This case is a good example of how water-soluble CM can actually hinder, while an RE-selective medium can improve, detection of a liver lesion.

Emulsion EOE 13 has also been effectively utilized to rule out a possible kidney mass [86]. An example of this is shown in Fig. 7, where the precontrast scan (Fig. 7a) shows a possible mass on the left kidney. Contrast enhancement with a water-soluble medium adds no useful information as the apparent mass is not distinguishable from the kidney as shown in Fig. 7b. However, infusion of emulsion EOE 13 shows clearly that the mass is actually splenic tissue and not a kidney mass (Fig. 7c).

From the above examples it is clear that CM which are selectively accumulated in the reticuloendothelial system can be very useful clinically. What can we say about the behavior of these CM quantitatively? In Fig. 8 we have plotted data following injections of the emulsion AG 60.99 into a rhesus monkey [84]. These data show that as the dose of administered material increases, the attenuation of the liver increases in a linear fashion. The liver of this rhesus monkey registered an attenuation of 78 HU on the precontrast scan. Subsequent injections of 0.1, 0.2, and 0.3 ml emulsion AG 60.99 per kilogram body weight resulted in liver attenuation values of 94, 130, and 150 HU respectively.

The results shown in Fig. 8 demonstrate that the attenuation of the liver parenchyma increases substantially following the infusion of relatively small doses of the emulsion AG 60.99. The real benefit of using such a CM, however, in improving tumor detectability is to increase the differential enhancement of parenchyma relative to that of the mass lesion. These media are particularly effective because reticuloendothelial cells in the hepatic parenchyma accumulate this particulate or emulsified material, but no such uptake has been observed in liver neoplasms [88]. The only contribution to contrast enhancement of the tumor should be from the CM in the blood.

The improvement in the differential enhancement can be appreciated by the results in Fig. 9. In this study [41] rats were injected with iodipamide ethyl ester particles at a dose of 100 mg I/kg body wt. The rats were subsequently killed at appropriate intervals postinfusion and the iodine concentration was determined in several tissues including liver and blood. As shown in this figure, the concentration of CM in the liver increases from 0.5 mg I/g liver tissue at 1 min postinjection to a maximum of 1.38 mg I/g tissue at 30 min postinjection. During this

Fig. 6a–c. Metastatic sarcoma in the right lobe of the human liver. The lesion barely visible on the preinfusion scan **a** is almost completely invisible following water-soluble contrast administration **b**. Improved visualization of lesion and splenic enhancement is evident after infusion of EOE 13 **c**. (Adapted from [45])

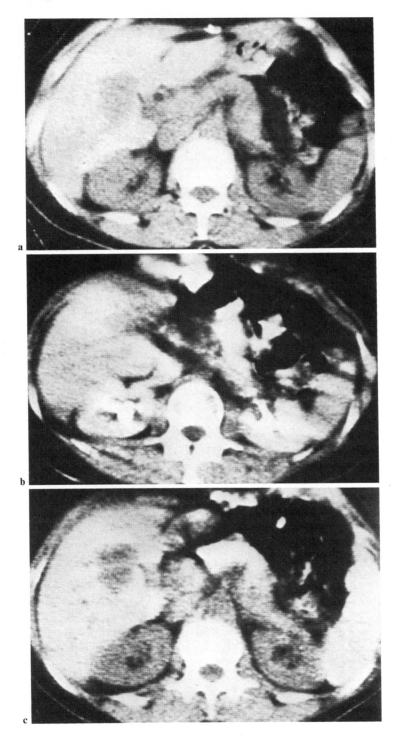

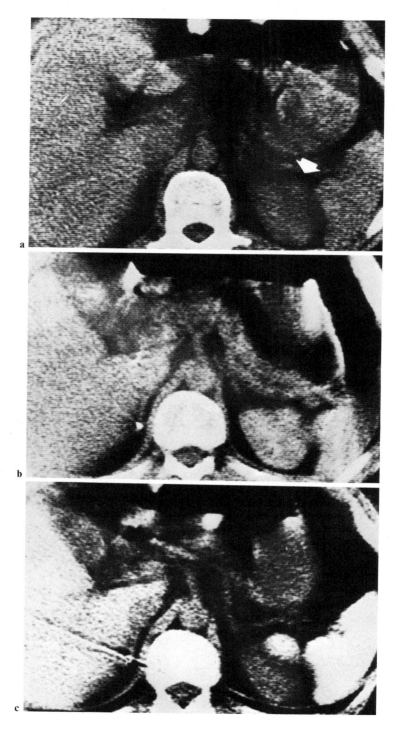

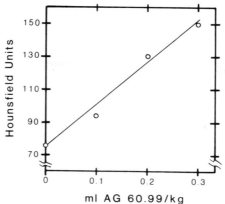

Fig. 8. Attenuation of liver parenchyma after intravenous infusion of Ethiodol emulsion AG 60.99 into rhesus monkeys. (Adapted from [84])

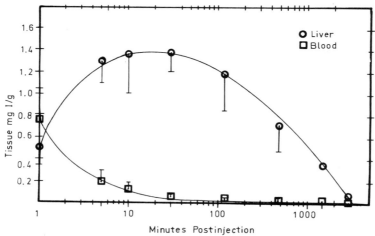

Fig. 9. Concentration of iodipamide ethyl ester (as iodine) particles in liver and blood following intravenous infusion in rats. Marked difference in concentration between liver and blood reflects differential CT enhancement of liver compared with tumor. (Adapted from [41])

same interval concentration of iodine or CM in the blood decreased from 0.76 to 0.06 mg I/g blood. The ratio of contrast in the liver to that in the blood therefore is greater than 20:1 over the period of 30 min to 8 h postinfusion and in fact reaches a maximum of approximately 40:1 at 2 h postinjection. Therefore, these CM are beneficial not only because they increase the attenuation of the hepatic

---

Fig. 7 a–c. Precontrast CT scan **a** demonstrates apparent mass projecting from the upper pole of the left kidney (*arrow*). Following water-soluble CM infusion, no separation of the mass from the kidney can be appreciated **b**. After the injection of EOE 13, the mass shows the same marked enhancement as the spleen, identifying it as splenic tissue while attenuation of the kidney is unchanged **c**. (Adapted from [86])

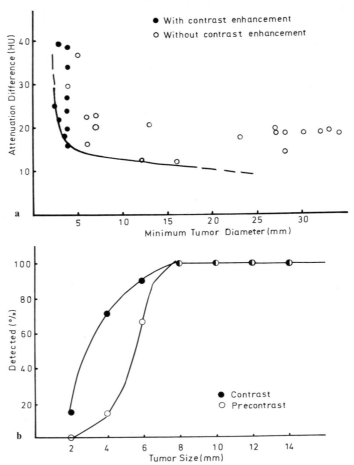

Fig. 10. a Plot of attenuation difference between liver parenchyma and tumor at which a neoplasm of given size became detectable on the CT scan. The *line* in this graph represents a minimum attenuation difference required for tumor detection and is not meant to be a best fit. Note that all but one tumor smaller than the scan width (5 mm) required contrast enhancement of detection. **b** Percentage of tumor detected with CT scanning as a function of tumor size, with and without contrast enhancement. The tumor size was taken as the diameter in the smallest dimension. The detectability of tumors smaller than the section width (5 mm) greatly improved with contrast enhancement. (Adapted from [42])

parenchyma but, more importantly, preferentially increase parenchyma attenuation relative to that of mass lesions, thereby improving detectability.

The value of increasing the attenuation difference for tumor visibility is shown in Fig. 10a, where we have plotted the attenuation difference necessary for tumor visibility as a function of the size of the tumor. In this plot all tumors greater than 5 mm in diameter were readily detectable without any contrast enhancement. This study [42] was conducted on rabbits using a GE 7800 CT scanner with a 5-mm slice width. The rabbit livers were scanned at intervals of 2–13 days following implantation of VX 2 carcinoma cell suspension into the rabbit livers. All tumors which had grown to a diameter greater than that of the slice width (5 mm) were readily detectable without any contrast enhancement. Tumors smaller than this scanning slice width, however, were frequently not detectable without CM. These small tumors required a greater differential enhancement in order to be visible. Thus, tumors were detectable on scans taken following an infusion of iothalamate ethyl ester particles at the increased attenuation difference even though the tumors were not at all visible on the precontrast scans. The curve drawn in this figure does not represent the best fit of the data, but rather an identification of the minimum attenuation difference required to observe a tumor of a given size.

The improved visibility of these small tumors is further demonstrated in Fig. 10 b where the percentage of tumors detected is plotted as a function of minimum tumor size. Again, all tumors greater than the scanning slice width were readily detectable with or without contrast enhancement. However, the tumors smaller than the slice width were much more readily detected following contrast infusion of iothalamate ethyl ester particles than was the case on non-contrast-enhanced scans.

In summary then, CM selectively accumulated in the reticuloendothelial system are of great value to liver CT scanning for the detection of mass lesions in this organ. This beneficial effect of these agents is due primarily to selective accumulation in normal tissue relative to that of the lesion.

The usefulness of RE selective CM may be diminished somewhat as CT instrumentation advances, permitting even more rapid scanning than is possible today. With such improvements it may be possible to observe a first-pass bolus following injection of a water-soluble CM to evaluate differences in vascularity for diagnosis of mass lesions of the liver. To utilize this advantage properly, however, it will first be necessary to detect the lesion, which is less likely to be facilitated by rapid scanning. In our opinion, the need for an RE selective agent to improve detection of liver lesions is a real one and the development of these materials should be pursued.

Before concluding this discussion, we will briefly mention other types of materials which potentially could be utilized as RE-selective CM. Although we will not discuss these in depth, many of the problems already described in this chapter are relevant to these materials as well.

Perfluorocarbons are lipid-soluble compounds which potentially could be developed and utilized as RE-selective media. Two compounds, perfluorohexylbromide and perfluoroctylbromide, have been tested with conventional radiography [89–92] and the former with CT [93]. The compounds have been administered by a variety of routes, including oral, endotracheal, and intraperitoneal, without significant toxicity. In theory, it should be possible to develop emulsions of these CM which could be suitable for intravenous injection. In addition to the problems already described for such emulsions, these compounds should have lower CT attenuation effects since the one bromine per molecule is significantly less radiopaque than the multiple iodines per molecule in compounds currently being evaluated in emulsions.

Another possibility for developing RE-selective CM is to encapsulate radiopaque materials in lipid vesicles (liposomes). Evidence for successful cellular uptake of nonradiopaque vesicles without significant toxicity is accumulating [94–100]. The incorporation of a CM into these vesicles should be possible [101]; however, leakage of contrast by diffusion or vesicle breakdown is a potential concern in addition to the types of problems already cited in this chapter.

The benefits of having an RE-selective CM should be apparent. Although the major emphasis of this chapter has been with the difficulties associated with the development of such agents, we do not believe the problems are insurmountable. Considerable progress has already been made and the lower doses required for CT should provide the incentive for overcoming the remaining complications.

E. Other Potential Applications

The material covered in this chapter has concentrated on the development of a particulate CM for potential use in hepatic CT scanning. We deliberately chose to focus on this particular application because the knowledge available in this field is considerable, albeit incomplete.

Particulate CM have also been evaluated for other applications such as lymphography, angiography, myelography, and ultrasound. Our knowledge and understanding in these areas is, however, much more limited. In this final section, we briefly describe the status of particulate agents in lymphography and angiography, two of the applications where particulates could conceivably be used.

I. Lymphography

The use of particulate materials or colloids in lymphography is based on characteristics similar to their use in hepatosplenography: (a) The particles must be sufficiently small to pass, without difficulty, through the smallest lymphatic vessels and the channels of the lymph nodes; (b) the particles must not interact with the protein and electrolyte components of the lymph to aggregate or clump and form large obstructing particles; and (c) the primary particle must be of sufficiently high iodine or other heavy element content that a reasonable number will afford the radiopacity needed to demonstrate the anatomic structures. These described characteristics are identical to those of a successful hepatosplenographic agent. In addition, the medium must have enough fluidity that introduction through a small-bore needle or catheter is not troublesome. A hepatolienographic agent may be introduced intravenously as a dilute suspension or introduced slowly, allowing the normal phagocytotic process by the RE cells to build up the desired radiopacity of liver and spleen; for lymphography the suspension as injected must be sufficiently radiopaque to visualize the lymph vessels just as an angiographic medium visualizes the vessels upon injection. Thus, a lymphographic medium cannot be a dilute suspension of particles but must have an iodine content of 250–300 mg/ml. Suspensions of particles of iodipamide ethyl ester at 273 mg I/ml are approximately half as viscous as Ethiodol (M. R. Violante, unpublished results). Esters of tetraiodoterephalic acid for direct and indirect lymphography have been patented [16] and described in the literature [102, 103].

The current widely used lymphographic medium is an iodinated ethyl ester of poppyseed oil (Ethiodol). In addition to being highly viscous, Ethiodol has the following disadvantages. The oily globules which are retained in the nodes for long periods produce a granulomatous response in the nodes, while the oily globules which are not retained in the nodes enter the circulation after leaving the lymph system via the thoracic duct and are borne by the blood through the right heart often to embolize in the lung capillaries and arterioles. In the lung, the globules of oil diminish lung diffusion to a degree dependent largely on the number of trapped particles [104]. Rarely, a significant inflammatory reaction occurs in the lung due to the retention of the particles.

A particulate or colloidal lymphographic medium as described above would be one which does not produce the undesirable, deleterious embolization of the lung, and would not hamper the direct injection into the lymph vessel by being highly viscous. In avoiding embolization by limiting the size and aggregation tendency of the particles, the prolonged visualization of the nodes by radiopaque material as occurs with Ethiodol may no longer be obtained. This prolonged visualization, which is an advantage from the clinical viewpoint since it can reduce the need for a repeat lymphogram in the period following the initial lymphogram, occurs because the oily globules are trapped in the interstices of the nodes, where they set up a mild inflammatory reaction and are slowly broken down and removed. A very small particle size may also be disadvantageous because more surface area of the radiopaque material is immediately and rapidly brought into contact with the tissue; if the particle is one which produces an inflammatory response, the response will be heightened. Such increased inflammatory response in the nodes has been noted when emulsions of Ethiodol have been used as lymphographic agents [105].

With these considerations of both advantages and possible disadvantages of radiopaque particulate materials or colloids in mind a thorough evaluation of their usefulness is certainly warranted.

II. Angiography

Potentially, the greatest use of a particulate of colloidal CM could be as an angiographic medium. Although current CM are among the safest drugs injected, toxicity is still encountered [106, 107]. The hyperosmolality of these media is considered to be a major contribution to their toxicity. The relatively recent history of CM research and development consists largely of attempts to produce media of lower osmolality. Dimers and trimers of ionic monomers have been produced [108, 109], with even greater success in reducing osmolality by the recent introduction of nonionic CM such as metrizamide [110].

Theoretical osmolalities of these different types of CM at 370 mg I/ml are as follows:

	mOsm/kg
Ionic Monomer	1,942
Ionic Dimer	1,458
Ionic Trimer	1,296
Nonionic monomer	971
Particulate	290

As shown, each of the newer CM has a lower osmolality than the ionic monomeric media at equivalent iodine concentration. With the nonionics, the actual observed osmolality is even less than theoretical, presumably because of molecular association at these high concentrations. Nevertheless, at the concentrations required for angiography, all of these CM have osmolalities greater than that of blood. This is not true, however, for a particulate CM.

Since particles are, by definition, not in solution, they do not contribute to osmolality. The osmotic properties of a particulate suspension are due entirely to the suspending medium. Therefore, it is possible to suspend the particles, at any desired iodine concentration, in a medium which has an equivalent osmolality to that of blood. Injections of particulate suspensions, therefore, should not induce fluid shifts known to occur with the water-soluble CM. Toxicity resulting from the hyperosmolality of water-soluble media can be eliminated.

The actual chemical composition of CM also contributes to the toxicity of these media. With the ionic CM, the anion is the radiopaque moiety. For satisfactory solubility the cations sodium and methylglucamine have been mainly used. Some favorable use has been made of calcium and magnesium cations but the cationic composition of the radiopaque agent is quite unlike the electrolytic character of the blood, having too much of certain cations – the normally present sodium and the unnatural methylglucamine, and too little of others, while the anionic composition is entirely abnormal. A suspension of particles may be formulated with each and every cation and anion being present in the same concentration as in plasma. Toxicity of angiographic media due to hyperosmolality, abnormal concentrations of normal constituent cations, cations which are not normally present in the blood, or anions which are clearly not normal for blood should be avoidable with a colloidal or particulate CM.

In addition to eliminating the above-described causes of toxicity, a particulate CM would offer the advantage of remaining completely within the vasculature until phagocytosed by RE cells. This property could provide better resolution of vessels in angiography and would certainly be advantageous for intravenous angiography using the newer imaging modalities such as CT and digital fluoroscopy. Unlike water-soluble CM, which are known to diffuse rapidly out of the blood vessels [111, 112], a particulate medium could presumably be formulated to circulate in the bloodstream for some time, making intravenous angiography a truly viable technique.

The characteristics of particulate CM which have been fashioned in the development of a hepatolienographic medium are for the most part essentially the same as those desired for an angiographic medium. The particle must be small enough to pass with ease through the smallest of capillaries, and the particles must not interact with each other or with constituents of the blood to aggregate and form clumps which will embolize. The particles must not break down rapidly within the circulating blood as this would release the radiopaque and other components, causing undesired changes in blood osmolality. Rather, the particulate CM, fashioned solely for angiography, should be slowly solubilized or broken down in the blood into excretable, nontoxic components. A protective coating or other alteration of the particle surface would probably be necessary to prevent phagocytosis while the enzymes of the blood or the solubilizing nature of the blood slowly allow the CM to change into a form which can leave the body. Thus, we would be seeking to avoid rapid phagocytosis which is the opposite of what is desired for hepatolienography. Whether a particulate angiographic medium could be broken down and excreted while it still circulates in the blood at a rate which would not significantly disturb ionic and osmotic balances and yet not be removed rapidly by the phagocytic action of liver and spleen remains to be determined.

The already-developed particulate CM iodipamide ethyl ester, modified to decrease the rate of phagocytosis, would appear promising for certain examinations, such as coronary, carotid, and vertebral arteriography. Injection of only a relatively small amount, 5–15 ml, is necessary for these kinds of arteriography, and solubilization or metabolism should be minimal or nonexistent as the particulate CM transverses the circulation of the heart or brain. A particulate CM might also be used, for example, in pulmonary angiography, left ventriculography, and aortography, but the large doses required for these examinations add substantially to the problems of formulating suitable suspension.

On the other hand, CM which would remain intravascular for an appreciable length of time following intravenous or intraarterial injection would be very valuable in CT scanning or digital fluoroscopy. The current water-soluble media, both ionic and nonionic, very rapidly enter the extravascular space after injection into the circulation. Successive slices in CT scanning reflect the amount of CM both in the vasculature and in the interstitial space in all tissues of the body except the normal brain, where an intact blood-brain barrier does not allow passage of CM into the parenchyma. In the diseased brain, however, water-soluble CM could diffuse through a defective blood-brain barrier. Changes in CT attenuation using water-soluble CM, therefore, cannot be taken as a measure of blood flow. A particulate CM such as IDE, which does not leave the blood vessels, would reflect changes in radiopacity of the blood alone and could be taken as a measure of blood flow. With each successive passage of the particulate matter through the liver some of the particles will be removed, decreasing the CM (and iodine) content of the blood. Too rapid removal of the particulate medium will likely make it unsatisfactory for other than very limited dynamic CT scanning.

We have described three potentially useful applications of particulate CM deliberately stressing the problems and potential complications associated with their development, so that others might contribute to the successful formulation and ultimately clinical application of these new contrast media.

References

1. Thomas SF, Henry GW, Kaplan HS (1953) Hepatolienography: past, present, and future. Radiology 57:669–683
2. Fischer HW (1977) Improvement in radiographic contrast media through the development of colloidal or particulate media: an analysis. J Theor Biol 67:653–670
3. Swarm RL (1971) Colloidal thorium dioxide. In: International encyclopedia of pharmacology and therapeutics. Radioactive agents, section 76. Pergamon
4. Carrigan RH (1967) Manufacture of thorium dioxide suspension (Thorotrast). Ann NY Acad Sci 145:530–531
5. Thomas SF (1962) Hepatolienography ten years later. Radiology 78:435–438

6. Radt P (1929) Eine Methode zur röntgenologischen Kontrastdarstellung von Milz und Leber. Klin Wochenschr 8:2128–2129
7. Oka M (1929) Eine neue Methode zur röntgenologischen Darstellung der Milz. Fortsch Geb Röntgenstr 40:497–501
8. Fischer HW (1957) Colloidal stannic oxide: animal studies on a new hepatolienographic agent. Radiology 68:488–498
9. Fischer HW, Zimmerman GR (1969) Long retention of stannic oxide: lack of tissue reaction in laboratory animals. Arch Pathol 88:259–264
10. Gianturco C, Ruskin B, Steggerda FR, Takeochi T (1972) A feasibility study of splenohepatography with tantalum metal and tantalum pentoxide. Radiology 102:195–196
11. Teplick GJ, Berk JE, Safrin L (1957) Experimental hepatosplenography using barium sulfate. Exp Hepatosplenography 78:328–332
12. Seltzer SE, Adams DF, Davis MA, Hessel SJ, Hurlburt A, Havron A, Hollenberg NK, Abrams HL (1979) Development of selective hepatic contrast agents for CT scanning. Invest Radiol 14:356–357
13. Violante MR, Fischer HW, Mahoney JA (1980) Particulate contrast media. Invest Radiol 15:5329–5334
14. Fischer HW, Barbaric ZL, Violante MR, Stein G, Shapiro ME (1977) Iothalamate ethyl ester as hepatolienographic agent. Invest Radiol 12:96–100
15. Violante MR, Shapiro ME, Fischer HW (1979) Protein binding to iothalamate ethyl ester. Invest Radiol 14:177–179
16. Felder E (1977) Radiopaque esters of tetra-dodoterephthalic acid. US patent 4,044,048
17. Matthews JL (1955) An evaluation of various avenues available for visualization of the liver with X-rays. Doctoral thesis, University Illinois, Department of Physiology
18. Drummel RJ, Madden JD, Thomas SF (1959) New iodine compounds for hepatolienography. J Am Pharm Assoc Sci Ed 48:181–182
19. Zimmon DS, Hadgraft JW (1965) A new method for hepatolienography. Radiology 84:477–482
20. Wiedeman MP (1963) Dimensions of blood vessels from distributing artery to collecting vein. Circ Res 12:375–378
21. Gendreau RM, Jakobsen RJ (1979) Blood-surface interactions: fourier transform infrared studies of protein surface adsorption from flowing blood plasma and serum. J Biomed Mater Res 13:893–906
22. Baier RE (1975) Applied chemistry at protein interfaces. Adv Chem Ser 145:1
23. Leininger RI (1972) Polymers as surgical implants. CRC Crit Rev Bioeng 1:333–381
24. McIntire LV (1980) Dynamic materials testing: biological and clinical applications in network-forming systems. Annu Rev Fluid Mech 12:159–179
25. Pearsall NN, Weiser RS (1970) The macrophage. Lea and Febinger, Philadelphia, pp 62–63
26. Van Aken WG, Vreeken J (1970) The clearance mechanism of the reticuloendothelial system. In: Van Furth R, Davis FA (eds) Mononuclear phagocytes. Blackwell, Philadelphia, pp 382–396
27. Remuzzi G, Mecca G, Marchesi D et al. (1979) Platelet hyperaggregability and the nephrotic syndrome. Thromb Res 16:345–354
28. Grosse-Siestrup G, Olsen DB, Lemm W (1978) A long-term ex vivo shunt for blood compatibility of biomaterials. Trans Soc Biomater 2:102
29. Lee RG, Kim SW (1974) Adsorption of proteins onto hydrophobic polymer surfaces: adsorption isotherms and genetics. J Biomed Mater Res 8:251
30. Cooper EH, Ward AM (1979) Acute phase reactant proteins as aids to monitoring disease. Invest Cell Pathol 2:293–301
31. Watkins RW, Robertson CR (1977) A total internal-reflection technique for the examination of protein adsorption. J Biomed Mater Res 11:215–238
32. Davis BD (1946) Physiological significance of the binding of molecules by plasma proteins. Am Sci 34:611–618
33. Tait J, Elvidge AR (1926) Effect upon platelets and on blood coagulation of injecting foreign particles into the blood stream. J Physiol 62:129–144

34. Biozzi G (1951) Quantitative study of the granulopectic activity of the reticuloendothelial system by intravenous injection of India ink in various animal species. V. Relations between the modifications of blood coagulation in vitro under the effect of intravenous injections of increased doses of India ink and its distribution in the organism. Am Inst Pasteur 81:164–172
35. Pfueller SL, Firkin BG (1978) Role of plasma proteins in the interaction of human platelets with particles. Thromb Res 12:979
36. Vroman L, Adams AL, Klings M et al. (1977) Reactions of formed elements of blood with plasma proteins at interfaces. Ann NY Acad Sci 283:65
37. Zucker MB, Vroman L (1969) Platelet adhesion induced by fibrinogen adsorbed onto glass. Proc Soc Exp Biol Med 131:318
38. Walton KW (1953) Obervations on the effects of a series of dextran sulphates of varying molecular weight on the formed elements of the blood in vitro. Br J Pharmacol 8:340–347
39. Walton KW (1954) Investigation of the toxicity of a series of dextran sulphates of varying molecular weight. Br J Pharmacol 9:1–14
40. Bell E (1953) The origin and nature of granules found in macrophages of the white mouse following intravenous injection of thorotrast. J Cell Comp Physiol 42:125–136
41. Violante MR, Mare K, Fischer HW (1981) Biodistribution of a particulate hepatolienographic CT contrast agent. A study of iodipamide ethyl ester in the rat. Invest Radiol 16:40–45
42. Violante MR, Dean PB (1980) Improved detectability of VX 2 carcinoma in the rabbit liver with contrast enhancement in computed tomography. Radiology 134:237–239
43. Alfidi RJ, Luval-Jeantet M (1976) AG 60.99: a promising contrast agent for computed tomography of the liver and spleen. Radiology 121:491
44. Vermess M, Chatterji DC, Doppman JL et al. (1979) Development and experimental evaluation of a contrast medium for computed tomographic examination of the liver and spleen. J Comput Assist Tomogr 3:25–31
45. Vermess M, Doppman JL, Sugarbaker P et al. (1980) Clinical trials with a new intravenous liposoluble contrast material for computed tomography of the liver and spleen. Radiology 137:217–222
46. Lamarque JL, Bruel JM, Dondelinger R et al. (1979) The use of iodipids in hepatosplenic computed tomography. J Comput Assist Tomogr 3:21–24
47. Spector WS (1956) (ed) Handbook of biological data. Saunders, Philadelphia, p 163
48. Bluin A (1979) Morphometry of liver sinusoidal cells. In: Wisse E, Knook DL (eds) Kupffer cells and other liver sinusoidal cells, 2nd ed. Elsevier, Amsterdam, pp 61–72
49. Beuacerraf B, Biozzi G, Halpern BN et al. (1957) Physiology of phagocytosis of particles by the reticuloendothelial system. In: Halpern BN (ed) Physiopathology of the reticuloendothelial system. Thomas, Springfield, pp 52–79
50. Saba T (1970) Physiology and physiopathology of the reticuloendothelial system. Arch Intern Med 126:1031–1052
51. Dobson EL, Gofman JW, Jones HB, Kelly LS, Walker LA (1949) Studies with colloids containing radioisotopes of yttrium, zerconium, columbium, and lanthanum. II. The controlled selective localization of radioisotopes of yttrium, zerconium, and columbium in the bone marrow, liver, and spleen. J Lab Clin Med 34:305–312
52. Dobson EL, Jones HB (1952) The behavior of intravenously injected particulate material. Acta Med Scand [Suppl] 273:7–71
53. Kabisch WT (1967) Phagocytosis of colloidal thorium dioxide and cobaltic oxide by the reticuloendothelial system of the rat. Ann NY Acad Sci 145:585–594
54. Singer JM, Adlersbert L, Hoenig EM, Ende E, Tchorsch Y (1969) Radiolabeled latex particles in the investigation of phagocytosis in vivo: clearance and histological observations. J Reticuloendothel Soc 6:561–589
55. Nelp WB (1970) Distribution and radiobiological behavior of colloids and macroaggregates. In: Cloutier RJ, Edwards CL, Snyder W (eds) Medical radionuclide: radiation dose and effects. USAEC Symposium Series 20, Springfield
56. Drinker CK, Shaw LA (1921) Quantitative distribution of particulate material (mangenese dioxide) administered intravenously to the cat. J Exp Med 33:77–98
57. Dobson EL (1957) Factors controlling phagocytosis. In: Halpern BN (ed) Physiopathology of the reticuloendothelial system. Thomas, Springfield, pp 80–114

58. Jones HB, Wrobel CJ, Lyons WR (1944) A method of distributing beta-radiation to the reticuloendothelial system and adjacent tissues. J Clin Invest 23:783–788
59. Neukomm S, Lerch P, Jallut O (1957) Physicochemical factors governing the phagocytic function of the RES. In: Halpern BN (ed) Physiopathology of the reticuloendothelial system. Thomas, Springfield, pp 115–127
60. Zilversmit DB, Boyd GA, Brucker M (1952) The effect of particle size on blood clearance and tissue distribution of radioactive gold colloids. J Lab Clin Med 40:255–260
61. Wilkins DJ, Myers PA (1966) Studies on the relationship between the electrophoretic properties of colloids and their blood clearance and organ distribution in the rat. Br J Exp Pathol 47:568–576
62. Curtis ASG (1960) Cell contacts: some physical considerations. Am Nat 94:37–56
63. Steinberg MS (1958) On the chemical bonds between animal cells. A mechanism for type-specific association. Am Nat 92:65–81
64. Ben-or S, Eisenberg S, Doljanski F (1960) Electrophoretic mobilities of normal and regenerating liver cells. Nature 188:1200–1201
65. Benacerraf B, Halpern BN, Biozzi G, Benos SA (1954) Quantitative study of the granulopectic activity of the reticulo-endothelial system. III. The effect of cortisone and nitrogen mustard on the regenerative capacity of the RES after saturation with carbon. Br J Exp Pathol 35:97–106
66. Biozzi G, Benacerraf B, Halpern BN (1953) Quantitative study of the reticulo-endothelial system. II. A study of the granulopectic activity of the RES in relation to the dose of carbon injected. Relationship between the weight of the organs and their activity. Br J Exp Pathol 34:441–457
67. Halpern B (1974) Role of the reticulo-endothelial system in the clearance of macromolecules. In: Jager JM, Houghwinke GJM, Daems WJH (eds) Liposomal therapy in lysosomal disease. Elsevier, Amsterdam, pp 111–123
68. Norman SJ (1974) Kinetics of phagocytosis. II. Analysis of in vivo clearance with demonstration of competitive inhibition between similar and dissimilar foreign particles. Lab Invest 31:161–169
69. Norman SJ (1974) Kinetics of phagocytosis. III. Two colloid reactions, competitive inhibition, and degree of inhibition between similar and dissimilar foreign particles. Lab Invest 31:286–293
70. Ito M, Wagner HN, Scheffel U, Jabbour B (1963) Studies of the reticuloendothelial system. I. Measurement of the phagocytic capacity of the RES in man and dog. J Clin Invest 42:417–426
71. Jacques PJ (1977) Kinetics of test-particle extraction from blood plasma by liver and spleen macrophages. In: Wisse E, Knook DL (eds) Kupffer cells and other liver sinusoidal cells. Elsevier, Amsterdam
72. Bradfield JWB (1977) Reticulo-endothelial blockade: a reassessment. In: Wisse E, Knook DL (eds) Kupffer cells and other liver sinusoidal cells. Elsevier, Amsterdam, pp 365–372
73. Dobson EL, Kelly LS, Finney CR (1967) Kinetics of the phagocytosis of repeated injections of colloidal carbon: blockade, a latent period of stimulation? A question of timing and dose. Adv Exp Med Biol 1:63–73
74. Murray IM, Katz M (1955) Factors affecting the rate of removal of gelatin-stabilized radiogold colloid from the blood. J Lab Clin Med 46:263–269
75. Keith WS, Briggs DR (1930) Roentgen ray visualization of spleen following injection of emulsions of halogenated oils. Proc Soc Exp Biol Med 27:538–540
76. Beckermann F, Popken C (1938) Kontrastdarstellung der Leber und Milz im Röntgenbild mit Jodsolen. Fortschr Röntgenstr 58:519–535
77. Derkwitz R (1938) Kolloidgestaltung und gezielte intravenöse Injection. Fortschr Röntgenstr 58:472–485
78. Olsson O (1944) On hepatosplenography with jodsol. Acta Radiol 22:749–761
79. Berger SM (1956) Angiopac, ethyl di-iodostearate as a hepatosplenographic agent. Preliminary report. AJR 76:39–46
80. Teplick JG, Haskin ME, Skelley J et al. (1964) Experimental studies with a new radiopaque emulsion. Radiology 82:478–485

81. Vermess M, Adamson RH, Doppman JL et al. (1974) Intra-arterial hepatography: experimental evalulation of a new contrast agent. Radiology 110:705–707
82. Laval-Jeantet M, Lamarque JL, Dreux P et al. (1976) Hepatosplenography by intravenous injection of a new iodized oily emulsion. Acta Radiol [Diagn] 17:49–60
83. Baltaxe HA, Katzen B, Alonzo DR et al. (1976) Hepatomography: an experimental technique using an emulsifier. A preliminary study. Radiology 119:27–30
84. Vermess M, Adamson RH, Doppman JL et al. (1977) Computed tomographic demonstration of hepatic tumor with the aid of intravenous iodinated fat emulsion. An experimental study. Radiology 125:711–715
85. Grimes G, Vermess M, Gallelli JF et al. (1979) Formulation and evaluation of ethiodized oil emulsion for intravenous hepatography. J Pharm Sci 68:52–56
86. Vermess M, Inscoe S, Sugarbaker P (1980) Use of liposoluble contrast material to separate left renal and splenic parenchyma on computed tomography. J Comput Assist Tomogr 4:540–542
87. Wretlind A (1964) The pharmacological basis for the use of fat emulsions in intravenous nutrition. Acta Chir Scand [Suppl] 325:31–42
88. McCready R (1972) Scintigraphic studies of space-occupying liver disease. Nuklearmedizin 42:108–127
89. Long DM, Liu M-S, Szanto PS, Alrenga DP, Patel MM, Rios MV, Nyhus LM (1972) Efficacy and toxicity studies with radiopaque perfluorocarbon. Radiology 105:323–332
90. Long DM, Liu M-S, Szanto PS, Alrenga P (1972) Initial observations with an X-ray contrast agent – radiopaque perfluorocarbon. Rev Surg 29:71–76
91. Liu MS, Long DM (1976) Biological disposition of perfluoroctylbromide: tracheal administration in alveolography and bronchography. Invest Radiol 11:479–485
92. Liu MS, Long DM (1977) Perfluoroctylbromide as a diagnostic contrast medium in gastroenterolography. Radiology 122:71–76
93. Enzman D, Young SW (1979) Applications of perfluorinated compounds as contrast agents in computed tomography. J Comput Assist Tomogr 3(4):622–626
94. Paphadjopoulos D, Wilson T, Taber R (1980) Liposomes as vehicles for cellular incorporation of biologically active macromolecules. In Vitro 16(1):49–54
95. Gregoriadis G, Ryman BE (1972) Lysosomal localization of fructofuranosidase-containing liposomes injected into rats. Biochem J 129:123
96. McDougall IR, Dunnick JF, McNamee MG, Kriss JP (1974) Distribution and fate of synthetic lipid vesicles in the mouse: a combined radionuclide and spin label study. Proc Natl Acad Sci USW 71:3487
97. Rahman Y, Wright BJ (1975) Liposomes containing chelating agents. J Cell Biol 65:112
98. Rahman Y, Rosenthal MW, Cerny EA, Moretti ES (1974) Preparation and prolonged tissue retention of liposome-encapsulated chelating agents. J Lab Clin Med 83:640
99. Rahman Y, Cerny EA, Tollaksen SL, Wright BJ, Nance SL, Thomson JF (1974) Liposome-encapsulated actinomycin D: potential in cancer chemotherapy. Proc Soc Exp Biol Med 146:1173
100. Straub SX, Garry RF, Magee WE (1974) Interferon induction by poly (I): poly (C) enclosed in phospholipid particles. Infect Immun 10:783
101. Havron A, Seltzer SE, Davis MA (1980) Liposomes containing diatrizoate: a promising new contrast agent for splenic computed tomography (CT). 66th RSNA, Dallas, Texas, Nov 1980
102. Felder E, Pitre D, Tirone P, Zingales MF (1978) Radiopaque contrast media. XLV experimental lymphography with crystal suspensions. Farmaco 33:302–314
103. Chiappa S, Campani R, Felder E, Ferrari D, Tirone P (1979) Experimental lymphography by intratissue injection of a crystal suspension. In: Malek P, Bartos V, Werssleder H, Witte MH (eds) Proceedings of the VIth international congress, Prague 1977. Thieme, Stuttgart, pp 359–362
104. Gold WM, Yonker J, Anderson S, Nadel JA (1965) Pulmonary function abnormalities after lymphangiography. N Engl J Med 273:519

105. Johansson S, Sternby NH, Theander G, Wehlin L (1966) Iodinated oil emulsion for lymphography. Acta Radiol 4:690
106. Ansell G (1970) Adverse reactions to contrast agents: scope of problem. Invest Radiol 5:374–384
107. Shehadi WH (1975) Adverse reactions to intravascularly administered contrast media: a comprehensive study based on a prospective survey. AJR 124:145–152
108. Bjork L, Erikson J, Ingleman B (1969) Clinical experience with a new type of contrast medium in carotid arteriography. AJR 107:637–640
109. Hilal SK (1970) Trends in preparation of new angiographic contrast media with special emphasis on polymeric derivatives. Invest Radiol 5:458–468
110. Almen T, Wiedeman MP (1968) Application of monomers and polymers to the external surface of the vasculature: effects on microcirculation in the bat wing. Invest Radiol 3:408–413
111. Dean PB, Kivisaari L, Kormano M (1978) The diagnostic potential of contrast enhancement pharmacokinetics. Invest Radiol 13:533–540
112. Newhouse JH (1977) Fluid compartment distribution of intravenous iothalamate in the dog. Invest Radiol 12:364–367

CHAPTER 14

Appendix: Basics of Anesthesia for Experimental Animals

M. Sovak

A. Introduction

Every anesthetic agent will affect not only the nervous system but, to some extent, every organ's physiology. If chronic preparation and awake animals cannot be utilized, an anesthetic for acute experiments must be selected which will not affect the objectives of the experimental protocol. Further, it must be kept in mind that restraint alone can have an adverse effect, and that under general anesthesia most laboratory animals are prone to develop hypothermia. Hypothermia potentiates the depressant effect of most anesthetics on the CNS; even with a light anesthesia, a broad spectrum of heat-loss compensatory mechanisms are activated. Reactive vasoconstriction, increase of peripheral vascular resistance, decrease in cardiac output, etc. can all affect cardiovascular experimentation and introduce artifacts of contrast media into the study. Thus, the importance of preventing hypothermia cannot be overstated. Monitoring of body temperature most conveniently with a rectal thermometer should be, like the use of heat pads, an integral part of the experimental setup.

Consideration should be given to the type of anesthesia: the species, length of the experiment, acute or chronic design should all influence the choice of a proper anesthetic.

There are a number of specialized reviews available [1–8]. The following is a short survey of anesthetic methodology applicable to the day-to-day experimentation.

In order to be able to account for the effects of anesthesia, knowledge of the normal values of heart rate (HR), cardiac output (CO), and blood pressure (BP) in various species is important. In general, heart rate is inversely proportional not only to the size of animal within the same species but also among the various species. For example, a Beagle puppy has a HR of 220 beats/min, while that of a grown Beagle is 80 beats/min. The HR for colibri is about 600 beats/min, while that of an elephant is 35 beats/min.

B. Anesthesia for Cardiovascular Experiments

Cardiac output in mammals decreases with body weight, but its relation to body surface is constant. Surface area can be approximated from weight:

$$\text{Surface area (m}^2) = K \times 2/3 \text{ body weight (kg)}$$

Some K values are: dog, 0.112; pig, 0.09; rabbit, 0.0975.

Table 1. Approximate normal resting values of heart rate (HR), cardiac output (CO), blood pressure (BP), and blood volume (BV) in some nonanesthetized animals

Animal	Body wt. (kg)	HR (beats/min)	CO (liters/min)	Co/wt. (ml/kg/min)	BP (mmHg) Systolic/ diastolic	BV (mg/100 g body wt.)
Dog	19.3	85 (70–130)	2.3	120	95–136/43–66	7.9–10.5
Pig	30	80 (90–90)	4.4	146	110–140/60–80	6.0–8.0
Cat	3.1	120 (110–140)	0.33	110	110–180/	4.5–7.4
Rabbit	2.25	250 (200–300)	0.34	171	95–130/60–90	4.6–7.0
Baboon	22.5	80	2.81	124	140/185	8.1
	500	45–60	46	113	N/A	3.9–7.4

Compiled and calculated from refs. [27–30], and from various handbooks on biological data

Table 2. Average respiratory values in some laboratory animals

Animal	Body wt. (kg)	Respiratory rate (min)	Tidal volume (ml/kg body wt.)	Minute volume (ml/min)
Dog	23.7	18	13.9	5,940
Pig	25	18	16.8	7,560
Rabbit	2.5	85	2.25	510
Cat	2.45	26	5.1	322
Rhesus	2.68	40	7.8	840

Copiled from ref. [31] and [32]

To calculate approximate normal (resting) CO in mammals, the following formula can be applied [9]:

$$CO \text{ (liters/min)} = 2.8795 \times [\text{body surface area } (m^2)]^{1.5054}$$

or:

$$CO \text{ (liters/min)} = 0.1017 \times [\text{body weight (kg)}]^{0.0099}$$

Normal resting values of CO, HR, BP, and blood volume are given in Table 1.

When assisted respiration is used during anesthesia, its rate and magnitude must be correctly set to avoid excessive oxygenation and/or elimination of CO_2, which can lead to profound electrolytic disturbances. A detailed review of ventilation standards for small mammals is available [10]: however, average respiratory parameters in some laboratory animals are presented here in Table 2.

Premedication. The reason for premedication is to provide a smooth introduction to general anesthesia, to restrain the animal momentarily to allow for intubation and/or placement of an intravenous cannula, and to stabilize the responses of the autonomic nervous system to the stress of the general anesthetic.

Phenothiazines. Phenothiazines generally potentiate the barbiturates, thus reducing their dose significantly. Phenothiazines also have a mild anticholinergic effect, suppress vomiting, and act as mild antihistaminics. Although chlorpromazine is the most popular, it should probably be avoided in cardiovascular experiments because of its hypotensive effect mediated by the decrease of peripheral vascular resistance, which reflectorically causes a compensatory increase in CO.

A better choice is promazine hydrochloride, which does not have the pronounced hypotensive effect and significantly reduces the need for barbiturates. If injected 15 min prior to barbiturate anesthesia together with morphine, it reduces the required morphine dose from 1–2 to 0.5 mg/kg and by a synergistic effect prevents the well-known barbiturate tachycardia. Subhuman primates, dogs, or cats need 2–6 mg/kg intramuscularly; pigs, sheep, and goats need 1–2 mg/kg [11].

Butyrophenones. In this group, droperidol is an extremely strong antiemetic which, while producing depression of the CNS, reportedly has little effect on the cardiovascular system. In dogs and pigs, it can be used in doses of 0.2–0.5 mg/kg [12].

Benzodiazepines. Diazepam (Valium) is a muscle relaxant and tranquilizer which does not appreciably affect the cardiovascular system. It can potentiate barbiturate anesthetic activity. As a potent anticonvulsant when given intravenously, it has been used for treatment of animals suffering seizures caused by contrast media.

Steroids. A mixture of steroids alphaxalone and alphadolone is applicable in subhuman primates, cats, dogs, and rodents, but not in rabbits. The advantage of these drugs is their limited effect on CNS activity; however, they depress the blood pressure and increase the heart rate in all species, although the animals usually stabilize within some 15 min after injection [13].

Morphine. By vagal stimulation, morphine induces bradycardia. This effect can be used in premedication to counteract the tachycardia commonly seen with barbiturates. Morphine produces excitation in the feline family even at doses as low as 0.5 mg/kg unless potentiated by phenothiazines. Morphine dosage of 1–2 mg/kg for dogs or pigs given subcutaneously, preferably under the free skin of the posterior neck, is useful as premedication. If used prior to the barbiturate anesthesia, it should be given 30 min prior to the barbiturate injection. Without a combination of phenothiazines it commonly causes vomiting and defecation within 15 min after the administration. Morphine, when combined with pentobarbital, has little place in the experimental protocols that aim at investigation of cardiac reflexes. Such reflexes are known to be depressed by these drugs.

Morphine is not usable for production of experimental bradycardia, which can be achieved more reliably by electrical pacing of the vagal nerve. Morphine is also a histamine releaser and can thus induce hypertension; this effect can be partially counteracted by antihistamines. Practically all effects of morphine can be quickly reversed by *N*-allyl-normorphine at a dose of 5 mg/kg given intravenously.

Pethidine HCl (Demerol). Pethidine is a reliable analgesic in most species except felines. It exerts atropine-like effects on the cardiovascular system. The dosage, i.m. or s.c., is 10 mg/kg for dogs and about 5 mg/kg for subhuman primates.

Ketamine HCl (Ketalar). Ketamine as a premedication drug is useful for producing rapid catalepsis when given intramuscularly. The dose is 1–2 mg/kg for practically all species. The effect, which occurs within 5 min, disappears within half an hour, thus lasting long enough for establishment of an intravenous anesthesia.

Atropine Sulfate. This is probably the best established premedication agent. It is a potent anticholinergic which stabilizes the autonomic nervous system under anesthesia. Atropine depresses vagal heart reflexes and, in general, the activity of the excretory glands. By depressing the output of the salivary and bronchial secretory glands, atropine is particularly useful as adjuvant to inhalation anesthesia. Given in premedication doses, atropine increases the heart rate only minimally while not changing the cardiac output or the systemic blood pressure.

Atropine can be given intramuscularly or subcutaneously some 15 min prior to induction of anesthesia, alone or in combination with ketamine, when restraint is desirable. The dose in subhuman primates, dogs, rats, mice, and guinea pigs is 0.05 mg/kg while pigs and cats need 0.1 mg/kg and rabbits, due to an enzymatic peculiarity, need 0.2 mg/kg.

C. Intravenous Anesthesia

I. Barbiturates

Barbiturate anesthesia, being simple to induce and easy to maintain, is extremely convenient for the investigator. In spite of general belief, barbiturates should not be used automatically in all cardiovascular studies because of their tendency to abolish reflexes, especially the carotid occlusion reflex and reflexes of the spinal cord. Barbiturates depress the potassium levels and have an atropine-like effect on the nervous system. In all laboratory mammals these drugs produce hypertension and tachycardia and often decrease cardiac output. Tachycardia may be especially bothersome since once established it cannot be normalized easily. This effect, however, can be prevented by morphine. It must be remembered that barbiturates are *not* analgesics and that pain of the postoperative recovery is not mitigated by these drugs.

Because of the side effect, the value of studies which investigate a normal cardiophysiological state under barbiturate anesthesia may be severely limited. It was shown that some "normal physiology" cardiovascular data derived from acute experiments using barbiturate anesthesia may be erroneous due to a state of grossly changed physiology [14].

1. Pentobarbital (Nembutal)

Many barbiturates are available, but the majority of cardioradiological experiments can be carried out using this agent. The dose is 25 mg/kg, giving anesthesia lasting 1 h in all species except rabbits, which metabolize barbiturates more rapidly. The drug should be injected slowly intravenously; anesthesia will ensue almost immediately. With supplemental intravenous doses, it can be extended over a period of many hours. Recovery from anesthesia usually takes 24 h. In dogs, pigs, and cats it is often accompanied by vomiting. In rabbits, which are able to release histamine massively, barbiturates even in small doses can produce death.

2. Thiopental (Pentothal)

This is a rapidly acting barbiturate which produces short-term anesthesia, usually of 20- to 45-min duration. It is not suited for long-term procedures since the depth of anesthesia varies and therefore constant monitoring of the anesthesia is necessary. The general pharmacological effects of thiopental are similar to those of pentobarbital, and the drug has no obvious advantage. Thiopental particularly depresses the myocardium.

II. Chloralose

This is a white crystalline powder, poorly soluble in cold water. Only the alpha isomer has a hypnotic effect, while the beta isomer is a convulsant. Alpha-chloralose can be dissolved in water at 70 °C to produce a 1% solution, or in polyethylene glycol-200 to make a 10% solution upon heating to 50 °C. After cooling to 38 °C, it can be given intraperitoneally, intramuscularly, or intravenously. At lower temperatures, chloralose crystals tend to fall out from aqueous solutions. The i.v. dose is 100 mg/kg in all species. It takes approximately 20 min to anesthetize a laboratory mammal; the anesthesia lasts at least 3 h. Pharmacologically, a 1% solution of chloralose in water is superior to the glycol preparation inasmuch as glycol itself has considerable toxicity. the relatively large volume of aqueous solution can be easily managed of several large syringes are prepared prior to the injection. Alpha-chloralose, though not a good anesthetic for chronic experiments because of its hemolytic activity, is useful in acute cardiovascular studies. It does not affect respiration, blood pressure is usually normal, and the drug enhances the reflexes. The initial tachycardia seen in dogs and pigs is in the range of 100 beats/min and usually subsides quickly. The minimal effects of chloralose on hemodynamic parameters make it an anesthetic superior to barbiturates [15].

Since chloralose enhances spinal as well as body receptor reflexes, animals exhibit exaggerated responses to auditory and tactile stimuli though not perceiving pain.

Chloralose can also be used in combination with urethane. A solution of 5% chloralose and 25% urethane can be administered intravenously or intraperitoneally. Usually there is little reason for the use of this combination in acute experiments, except when injection volume must be low.

III. Urethane

This can be used rectally, intramuscularly, or intravenously to produce anesthesia lasting several hours. The dose is 1 g/kg body wt. for intravenous injection and 2 g/kg body wt. for intraperitoneal application. Urethane should definitely not be used in chronic experiments with laboratory animals. It produces some hemolysis and given chronically is known to suppress hematogenesis and be carcinogenic.

IV. Chloral Hydrate

In doses used for intravenous anesthesia (3 g/kg body wt.) depression of respiration and blood pressure result. Arrhythmias and asystole are frequent and hemolysis is not unusual.

V. Ketamine HCl

Mentioned above as a drug useful in temporary restraint, ketamine can also be used for longer anesthesia. Similar to the barbiturates, ketamine increases blood pressure and heart rate. For long anesthesia, ketamine is much safer than the barbiturates and maintains a more stable condition. Spontaneous muscular twitching and/or frank seizures were observed during recovery from longer ketamine anesthesia; this observation should be relevant when epileptogenicity of contrast material, by the vascular or intrathecal route, is studied. Ketamine can be used practically in any species; albeit the dosage varies. In rodents and rabbits, the intramuscular or intraperitoneal dose is 40 mg/kg; in pigs and dogs the dose is 60 mg/kg i.m. or i.p., while 20–25 mg can be given intravenously. In the primates, the intramuscular dose is 25 mg/kg, in cats, 35 mg/kg i.m. In the latter three groups, ketamine is useful for induction, but a stable anesthesia can be achieved with supplementary barbiturates.

D. Volatile Anesthetics

Volatile anesthetics have a very limited application in cardioradiological laboratories. Their administration is difficult, requiring special skills and equipment.

Diethylether. Inexpensive but cannot be used in conjunction with X-ray equipment due to its explosive nature.

Cyclopropane. Likewise explosive. Its possible use is limited to experimental sensitization of myocardium in dog to epinephrine.

Halothane. Nonexplosive and has the advantage of rapid induction and very rapid recovery. To maintain a steady anesthetic state, however, some anesthesiological training is required. Halothane can be used as a supplement to chloralose. However, it depresses HR, CO, and BP.

Other commonly used inhalation anesthetics like *divinylether* (Vinethane), *fluroxine* (Fluoromar), *methoxyflurane* (Pentrane), and *cyclopropane* (Trimethylene) are all unsuitable for cardioradiological experimental use, due to their flammability and/or explosiveness and their tendency to affect the cardiovascular system.

Electroanesthesia. By a sine-wave alternating current [16] this is an established experimental procedure. However, it has no application in cardiophysiological research because of its effect on the autonomic nervous system. Respiratory rate, HR, and BP are always affected, and at times evoked muscular contractions make simultaneous use of physiological recording apparatus impossible.

Muscle Relaxants. In cardiovascular experimentation involving surgery, it is not usually necessary to achieve deeper muscular relaxation than that obtained by general anesthesia. Should the need occur, *succinylcholine chloride, d-tubocurarine* (Tubarine), or *gallamine* (Flaxadil) can be used.

Succinylcholine causes depolarization of the muscle end-plate without destroying acetylcholine. A single i.v. dose in dogs, cats, rabbits, and pigs is about

0.1 mg/kg body wt. Infrahuman primates and calves are more sensitive. There may be a large dose variation even in the same species. The duration of relaxation is limited to 5–10 min, after which additional injections are needed. This, however, leads to a steadily increasing dosage which may end in a persisting nonpolarizing blockade.

Curare alkaloids and *gallamine* interfere with the depolarization of the muscle end-plates, thus producing a neuromuscular block. Effects of both drugs can be counteracted with neostigmine or prostigmine.

d-Tubocurarine in larger doses increases arterial pressure, by ganglionic blocking. It is a potent releaser of histamine, both in dogs and cats. It has an atropine like effect and in cardiac experiments can replace atropine. The usual i.v. dose for dogs, cats, monkeys, and pigs is 0.5 mg/kg body wt., while in subhuman primates and rodents, which are more sensitive, an i.v. dose of about 0.25 mg/kg body wt. is required.

Gallamine (Flaxadil) is used at an i.v. dosage of 0.25 mg/kg body wt. for dogs, pigs, calves, and rabbits to produce relaxation not accompanied by atropine-like effects. Gallamine is not metabolized and is excreted quantitatively into the urine.

E. Short-term Reversible Hypotension

Arteriotomy, conduction block anesthesia, and ganglioplegia all have major drawbacks. Hypotension without tachyphylaxis caused by direct action on the arterial muscles can be induced in laboratory mammals by i.v. sodium nitroprusside (2 µg/kg body wt. in dog) or Trimethophan, by an i.v. infusion of 1 : 10,000 solution. (One-time dose in dog is 0.04 mg/kg body wt. [17–19].)

F. Blood Transfusion

In acute experiments, rabbits, pigs, or dogs can be transfused with homologous blood. Although there are 8 known main blood groups in rabbit, 14 in pig and 7 in dog [20], appreciable agglutination does not occur within the same species. Massive infusion of homologous blood may produce a histamine-release type reaction with urticaria, preventable by antihistamines or steroids [21].

G. Euthanasia

Experimental anesthetized animals are most economically euthanized by rapid intravenous injection of a concentrated solution of potassium chloride to cause myocardial paresis. Another possibility is the injection of a large amount of air intravenously or via cardiac puncture (15 ml for rabbits and up to 150 ml for dogs or pigs). Euthanasia with barbiturates is needlessly expensive for use in animals already under general anesthesia, but can be used to kill conscious animals.

The most convenient animals for experimentation with contrast media involving radiography are dogs, pigs, and rabbits; specific basic aspects of their anesthesia are summarized in the following sections.

I. Anesthesia in Dogs

No special restraint is needed for most dogs; in aggressive animals, prompt control can be achieved with intramuscular ketamine. Phenothiazine derivatives can be used for premedication. Promazine reduces the dose of barbiturates. Morphine is useful in cardiovascular experiments when given at least 15 min prior to injections of barbiturates; not only does it reduce the barbiturate dose, but also effectively counteracts the barbiturate tachycardia. In dogs, however, rapid intravenous injections must be avoided; they are known to elicit convulsions. Morphine is best given subcutaneously into the posterior neck region (1–2 mg/kg).

Atropine is rapidly excreted from the canine circulation; in cardiovascular studies which may depend on the anticholinergic effect of atropine, supplemental doses after the first 2 h may be required.

Pethidine has an effect in dogs similar to morphine, but of shorter duration.

Intravenous barbiturates are used extensively and, in general, what has been said in this chapter applies. In addition, it should be kept in mind that in dogs simultaneously given chloramphenicol bentobarbitol anesthesia is potentiated, and that bentobarbitol produces considerable respiratory and metabolic acidosis. Leukopenia with a maximum of 1½ h p.i. has also been observed. Barbiturates depress the respiratory activity in dogs, and assisted respiration is thus recommended.

Thiopental is a useful barbiturate in dogs, except for puppies, which cannot catabolize the drug efficiently.

Alphachloralose, as previously mentioned, is an extremely useful agent since it does not depress most of the reflexes, including barrel reflexes.

From the inhalational agents, halothane is probably the best suited for cardiovascular experiments, due to its relatively moderate effects; a mixture of N_2O and O_2 is necessary with halothane. Anesthesia in dogs has been reviewed extensively [4, 11].

II. Anesthesia in Pigs

Unlike dogs, an unrestrained pig may react to a simple venipuncture in a most aggressive manner. Thus, if a restraining cage is not available, it is necessary to grasp the animals limbs from behind and tie them with a rope. The head must be immobilized and it is good practice either to place a tape around the pig's snout or to insert a gag, since pigs do bite. Also, their vocal response to these procedures is notorious and should be taken into account if the laboratory is in the proximity of clinical facilities. In veterinary practice, tranquilizers are routinely used, but neither is this desirable nor should it be necessary in pharmacological experiments.

Inhalation anesthesia has the same drawbacks, which make it a second choice in practically all laboratory animals. The inhalation anesthesia level in pigs can greatly change from minute to minute; the fatter the pig, the more difficult it is to regulate the depth of the anesthesia. If a volatile anesthetic must be used, it should be preceded by an i.v. short-acting barbiturate (Thiopental) in doses of 15 mg/kg. Therefore, unless there is a special reason for using inhalation anesthesia, intravenous barbiturates of chloralose are preferable.

The inducing dose of *pentobarbital* is 30 mg/kg for animals up to 50 kg, 20 mg/kg for animals between 50 and 100 kg, and 10 mg/kg for animals between 100 and 300 kg. The dosage of chloralose is 10 ml 1% solution/kg body wt. for the body weight range up to 100 kg. Between 200 and 300 kg, the dose is reduced to 5 ml/kg body wt. The anesthetic is slowly injected, preferably into one of the ear veins. In younger pigs, the external jugular vein can also be conveniently punctured; the limb veins are often inaccessible. Similar to the dog, pentobarbital produces tachycardia and hypertension. This can be avoided by premedication with morphine, subcutaneously injected into the posterior neck region in a dose of 1 mg/kg, 15 min before injecting the barbiturate.

Contrary to popular myth, the pig's skin is *not* like that of the human. It is much less vascular and lacks sweat glands. Thus, its contribution to thermoregulation is minimal. Since pigs do not sweat, their temperature is regulated mostly by breathing. When using a respirator, the breathing frequency should be regulated with extreme care to prevent the undercooling or overheating of the animal (see Table 2).

III. Anesthesia in Rabbits

Anesthesiological methods applicable to the rabbit have been described in detail [22–24]. The reactivity of rabbits to anesthetic agents varies widely because of the unpredictability of the individual response, anesthesia with any agent must be induced slowly, and the proper dosage must be determined only by observation of the drug's effects. A fatal outcome of anesthesia can most often be ascribed to the depression of the rabbit's respiratory center and/or to a sudden release of histamine.

A useful indicator of anesthesia depth is the toe reflex (limb flexion) produced by pinching between the toes of the hindfoot. The size of the eye pupil is misleading. Rabbits are prone to develop laryngospasm and therefore should be intubated prior to surgery. In acute experiments a simple tracheotomy is sufficient; in chronic experiments a catheter must be used for intubation. This is difficult because of the size of the rabbit tongue, which, even when completely extended, obscures the larynx to direct inspection. A pediatric laryngoscope is helpful.

What may be a limitation to cardiovascular studies is the large amount of enzyme atropine esterase in a rabbit's liver, making this animal react unpredictably to atropine. Rabbits require larger doses of atropine than any other animal [25].

Volatile anesthetics can be, in principle, used in rabbits, but with the exception of halothane they are flammable and should not be used together with X-ray equipment. Moreover, the safety margin of all volatile agents in rabbits is relatively low and their use in cardiophysiological experimentation is limited due to their depressing effect on the cardiac muscle.

Barbiturates can be used although rabbit reaction to this group of anesthetics varies. Long-acting barbiturates (i.e., *phenobarbital* or *barbital*) anesthetize rabbits for many hours. The effect of *pentobarbital* (Nembutal) in doses of 25–35 mg/kg normally does not exceed an hour. Half of the dose should be administered slowly, over several minutes, into the marginal ear vein, which has been dilated prior to injection by rubbing the ear with warm water or ethanol. The remainder of the dose is given only after respiration is stabilized and the toe reflex only partially diminished. *Phenobarbital* can be injected intraperitoneally in a dose of 100 mg/kg and it may be combined with pentobarbital. For very short anesthesia (15–20 min), *thiopental* can be used in doses of 50 mg/kg. The drug, however, can depress respiration, which is the major cause of accidental death during experiments. Barbiturates produce tachycardia and some decrease of cardiac output.

Long-term anesthesia in rabbits can be achieved with *urethane*. Urethane can be given intraperitoneally in a dose of 1.6 g/kg body wt., taking effect after approximately 1 h. Urethane is not suited for chronic experiments because after several hours it tends to produce pulmonary edema with hemolysis [23].

Alpha-chloralose in a dose of 10 ml of 1% solution/kg body wt. is the drug of choice in cardiovascular experiments conducted in rabbits since it has minimal effects on myocardial performance (see Sect. C.II).

Muscle-relaxing drugs can be used in rabbits properly intubated and provided with respiratory assistance.

d-Tubocurarine is used for longer experiments and is given intravenously in a dose of 1½ mg/kg body wt. *Gallamine-triethiodide* in an i.v. dose varying from 0.15 to 0.25 mg/kg body wt. produces short relaxation.

Under restraint, rabbits are prone to develop a *catalyptic state* accompanied by anesthesia. The technique is to flip the rabbit very rapidly on to its back, stretch the neck, and tie down the legs. Then, gentle stroking of the abdomen and a monotonous sound induce relaxation, bradypnea, miosis (with open eyelids), and insensitivity to painful stimuli for a varying period [26]. If properly practiced, this method can anesthetize the animal for hours; nevertheless, it is at best applicable only to minor surgical procedures.

References

1. Barnes CD, Etherington LG (1973) Drug dosage in laboratory animals, 2nd edn. University of California Press, Berkeley
2. Goodman LS, Gilman A (1980) Pharmacological basis of therapeutics, 6th edn. Macmillan, New York
3. Comparative anesthesia in laboratory animals (1969) Planned by the Committee for the Preparation of a Technical Guide for Comparative Anesthesia in Laboratory Animals. Fed Proc 28:1369–1586
4. Lumb WV, Jones EW (1973) Veterinary anesthesia. Lee and Febiger, Philadelphia
5. Melby EC, Altman NH (eds) (1974) Handbook of laboratory animal science. CRC, Cleveland
6. Russell RJ, David TD (1977) A guide to the type and amount of tranquilizers, anesthetics, analgesics, and euthanasia agents for laboratory animals. Naval Medical Research Institute, Bethesda, p 36
7. Soma LR (ed) (1971) Textbook of veterinary anesthesia. Williams and Wilkins, Baltimore
8. Jones LM, Booth NH, McDonald LE (eds) (1977) Veterinary pharmacology and therapeutics, 4th edn. Iowa State University Press, Ames
9. Patterson JL Jr, Goetz RH, Doyle JT, Warren JV, Gauer OH, Said SI (1965) Cardiorespiratory dynamics in the ox and giraffe with comparative observations on man and other mammals. Ann NY Acad Sci 127:393–413
10. Kleinman LK, Radford EP Jr (1964) Ventilation standards for small mammals. J Appl Physiol 19:260–362
11. Green CJ (1979) Animal anesthesia. Laboratory Animals, London

12. Edmonds-Seal J, Prys-Roberts C (1970) Pharmacology of drugs used in neuroleptanalgesia. Br J Anaesth 42:207–216
13. Child KJ, Currie JP, Davis B, Dodds MG, Pearce DR, Twissell DJ (1971) The pharmacological properties in animals of CT-1341, a new steroid anesthetic agent. Br J Anaesth 43:2–13
14. Priano LL, Traber DL, Wilson RD (1969) Barbiturate anesthesia: an abnormal physiological situation. J Pharmacol Exp Ther 165:126–135
15. Shabetai R, Fowler NO, Hurlburt O (1963) Hemodynamic studies of dogs under pentobarbital and morphine chloralose anesthesia. J Surg Res 3:263–267
16. Herin RA (1968) Electroanesthesia in the dog: comparative study of electric wave forms. Am J Vet Res 29:601–607
17. Page IH, Corcoran AC, Dustan HP, Koppanyi T (1955) Cardiovascular actions of sodium nitroprusside in animals and hypertensive patients. Circulation 11:188–198
18. Mannheimer WH (1969) Induced hypotension. Fed Proc 29:1463–1468
19. Little DM (1956) "Controlled hypotension" in anesthesia and surgery. Thomas, Springfield
20. Swisher SN, Young LE, Trabold N (1962) In vitro and in vivo studies of the behavior of canine erythrocyte-isoantibody systems. Ann NY Acad Sci 97:15–25
21. Dow IW, Dickson JF, Hamer NAJ, Cadboys HG (1960) Anaphylactoid shock due to homologous blood exchange in the dog. J Thorac Cardiovasc Surg 30:449–456
22. Murdock HR Jr (1969) Anesthesia in the rabbit. Fed Proc 28:1510–1516
23. Long HW (1957) Anesthesia in rabbits. J Anim Tech Assoc 8:58
24. Cass JS (1971) Laboratory animals; an annotated bibliography of informational resources covering medicine-science (including husbandry)-technology, 3rd comp. Hafner, New York
25. Godeaux J, Tonnesen M (1949) Investigations into atropine metabolism in the animal organism. Acta Pharmacol Toxicol 5:95–109
26. Gruber RP, Amato JJ (1970) Hypnosis for rabbit surgery. Lab Anim Care 20:741–742
27. Altman PL, Dittmer DS (eds) (1964) Biology data book, 2nd edn. Federation of American Societies for Experimental Biology, Bethesda
28. Sisson S, Grossman JD (1962) Anatomy of the domestic animals, 4th edn. Saunders, Philadelphia
29. American Physiological Society (1963) In: Dow P, Hamilton FW (eds) Circulation. American Physiological Society, Washington DC (Handbook of physiology, sect 2, vol 2)
30. Burke JD (1954) Blood volume in mammals. Physiol Zool 27:1–21

Subject Index

Abrodil 307, 308
  toxicity 310
Acetrizoate 129, 237
Adverse reactions 153, 310, 317, 507, 569
  see also toxicity
  anaphylactoid reactions 527
  antibody-antigen reactions 526
  cerebral infarct 510
  cholecystographic CM, oral 406
  Dimer-X 311
  enzyme inhibition 525
  extravasation 465
  general considerations 525
  glomerular damage 154, 155
  GTS (Gilles de la Tourette Syndrome) 301
  headaches, postmyelographic 305
  hypersensitivity 465
  intrathecal CM 311
  iocarmate, ionic dimer (Dimer-X) 311
  iodipamide 406
  meglumine iothalamate 311
  oil embolism 465
  oily CM 465
  pantopaque myelography 309
  pathogenesis 526–529
  pretesting patients 529
  protein binding 525
  tubular damage 157
  urographic CM 130, 158
  vascular pain 7, 10, 303
AG 60.99 562
AG-52-315 472
AH interval 203
Alphafurine 2G 464
Alphaxolone-alphadolone 343
Ames test 534, 535
Aminoglycerol 7
2,3-Aminopropanediol 7
Amipaque 218, 233
Anaphylactoid reactions 19, 527
Anesthesia
  administration 428
  alphaxolone-alphadolone 343
  atropine sulfate 580

barbiturates 343, 425, 580, 581
benzodiazepines 579
butyrophenones 579
cardiac output 577
chloral hydrate 343, 581
chloralose 581
α-chloralose 343
chlorpromazine 425
cyclopropane 344
d-tubocurarine 344
diethyl ether 425
diphenylether 344
dogs 430, 584
electroanesthesia 344
ether 344
experimental animals 577–586
fluoroxine 344
for cardiovascular experiments 577
gallamine 344
halothane 344
heart rate 577
hypotension, reversible 583
hypothermia 577
in rabbits 585
injectable 342–344
intravenous 580–582
Ketamine HCl 582
Ketamine HCl (Ketalar) 579
lidocaine 425
methoxyfluorane 344
morphine 426, 579
muscle relaxants 344
Pentobarbital (Nembutal) 580
pethidine HCl (Demerol) 579
phenothiazines 578
pigs 262, 584
premedication 342, 578
promazine hydrochloride 426
rabbits 586
rats 428
secobarbital sodium 426
stages 424
steroids 579
succinyl choline 344
thimylal sodium 426

Anesthesia
  Thiopental (Pentothal) 581
  thipental sodium 426
  urethane 581
  volatile 344, 582, 583
Angio Conray 200, 228, 229, 232
Angiografin 60 232
Angiographic CM
  cardiovascular effects 228
  circulatory reflexes 228
Angiography, CNS 297
  CM currently in use in 298
  effects of ionic CM 298
  iohexol 303
  iopamidol 303
  ioxaglate, Hexabrix 302
  meglumine iothalamate 302
  meglumine metrizoate (Isopaque
    Cerebral) 302
  metrizamide 302, 303
  monovalent dimer 302
  nonionic monomers 302
Angiography, cranial
  bradycardia 299
  dimer-X 299
  experimental designs 299
  GTS (Gilles de la Tourette Syndrome)
    301
  hemodynamic effects of CM 300
  hyperosmolality 299
  ionic CM 297
  ionic dimers 300
  ionic monomers, toxicological
    comparisons of 300
  iopamidol 299
  metrizamide 299
  pain 301
  receptors located in the carotid
    circulation 299
  vasomotor brain center 299
Angiography, spinal cord
  Brown-Séquard syndrome 302
  chemotoxicity of CM 301
  experimental spinal cord trauma 301
  paraplegias 302
  vasoactive substances 302
Angiotensin II 211
Anilide-containing cholecystopaque
  structure 111–113
  toxicity 111–113
Animal models 344, 394, 470
  aneurysms 348
  aortic stenosis 285
  aortic valve insufficiency 285
  arachnoiditis 315
  arteriosclerosis (AS) 276–279
  atherosclerosis 348

aversion conditioning 322, 325
avian atherosclerosis 349
breakdown of the BBB 349
cardiac hypertrophy 281
cardiovascular effects of CM, dogs 199
cardiovascular pathological states 276–
  287
cerebral infarction 349
cerebral vasospasm 349
chronic catheterization of monkey SAS
  325
chronic congestive heart failure 281
cisterna magna infusion 322
coarctation 282
comparison with iohexal 325
congenital cardiac defects 282
congenital heart disease 282
contrast ventriculography 198
diencephalon injection in a rat 324
ductus arteriosus 283
endocardial fibroelastosis 281
endocarditis 283
endomyocardial fibrosis 281
experimental spinal cord trauma 301
field potentials from the pyramidal cell
  layers 325
heart block 281
heart valves diseases 283
hepatoma, rhesus monkey 561
infrahuman primates 260
infundibular pulmonic stenosis 285
intracisternal injection 322
intracisternal injection in
  nonanesthetized rabbits 325
investigative lymphangiography 471
left ventricular hypertrophy (LVH) 282
lumbar puncture 350
lymphatic regeneration 471
lymphaticovenous communications
  471
lymphedema 471
lymphopathies, obstructive 471
lymphostasis 471
Macaca cynomolgus 325
Macaca fascicularis 349
mitral stenosis 283
mitral valve insufficiency 283
myocardial infarction 279, 280
newborn models, contrast
  ventriculography 198
percutaneous thrombosis 348
perfusion pulmonary hypertension 282
pericarditis, experimental 280
poststenotic dilation 282
pulmonary air embolism 286
pulmonary embolism 285
pulmonary stenosis 285

pulmonary valves 285
pulmonic artery stenosis 285
reticuloendothelial system 550
sclerosis of aorta 348
septal defects 282
spinal cord trauma 349
suboccipital puncture 350
thromboembolism 349
thrombosis 286
tricuspid valve 285
ulcerations 349
ventricular fibrilation, experimental
    280
ventricular sampling 351
Wolff-Parkinson-White syndrome 281
Antibiotics, effect of
enterohepatic circulation 390
fasting 390
Antibody-antigen reactions 526
Antidiuretic hormone (ADH) 145
Aortic stenosis
animal models 285
Aortic valve insufficiency
animal models 285
Arachnoiditis 305, 309, 310, 315
detection 354
experimental 354
hyperosmolal solutions 354
pulsations 354
Arfonade 469
Aroylamino acids
toxicity 47
urinary excretion 47
Arrhythmias 207
Arteriography, coronary
coronary vascular resistance 239
Arteriography, spinal cord 297
Arteriosclerosis (AS)
animal models 276–279
Assays for CM
alkaline ashing 161
combustion 161
computed tomography 162
high-pressure liquid chromatography
    162
neutron activation 161
radioactive labeling 162
UV spectrophotometry 161
X-ray fluorescence 162
Assays for contrast media
radiographic densitometry 160
Asystole 229
Atrial contraction rate
meglumine diatrizoate 207
meglumine iothalamate 207
sodium meglumine calcium metrizoate
    207

Attenuation of X-rays 132–149
ratio-3 CM 142
AV node, effect of CM on
experimental model 257
Aversion conditioning 355, 356

B 6500, B 13040, B 13630 546
Barbiturates 343
Pentobarbital (Nembutal) 580
Thiopental (Pentothal) 581
Barium sulfate 545
Baroreceptor reflex 200
Benzamides/-2-glycose derivatives
solubility 64
toxicity 64
Benzamides/1-glucamine derivatives
solubility 65
toxicity 65
Benzamides/alkanol derivatives
solubility 67
toxicity 67
Benzamides/heptitol derivatives
solubility 66
toxicity 66
Benzoate esters 103
carbonates/thiolcarbonates 106
ethyl iothalamate 106
iophendylate 106
Benzopyrones 469
lymphostatic edema 469
Benzyl amines 48
Benzyl-containing cholecystopaques
structure 109
toxicity 109
Beta-adrenergic blockade 219
Bezold-Jarisch reflex 201, 230, 231
Bile, electrolyte composition
iodoxamate 402
SC 2644 402
taurocholate 402
Bile flow
caiman 377
clearance (Cl) 380
colchicine 380
cytochalasin B 380
guinea pig 377
half-life analysis 380
man 377
phalloidin 380
rates of bile flow 377
volume of distribution (V_d) 380
Bile salts
quantitation 458
Biliary CM 367–408
biliary concentration 400, 401
biliary excretion 394, 395, 397, 398
biotransformation 393, 394

Biliary CM
  choleresis 398, 400
  choleretic increments in dogs 399
  CM reabsorption by gallbladder 404
  concentration in bile 398
  enterohepatic circulation 404, 405
  first-pass effect 391
  gallbladder 403
  hepatotoxicity 406
  laboratory techniques 419
  maximum biliary excretion rates 397
  nephrotoxicity 406
  nonvisualization 404
  RCK-136 399
  renal excretion 405
  toxicity 406
  transport in blood 391
Biliary concentration
  basal bile flow influence 400, 401
  maximum 400, 401
Biliary excretion 394, 396, 398
  enhancement by taurocholate 395, 397
  gallbladder function 403
Biliary physiology 374–380
  bile composition 374
  canalicular bile formation 378
  choleresis 378
  ductular bile flow 378
  hepatocyte cytoskeleton and bile flow
    379
Biligrafin 384
Bilirubin analysis 456, 457
Bilopaque 384
Biological data 378, 397
Biological values, normal
  blood presure 578
  blood volume 578
  cardiac output 578
  heart rate 578
  liver, spleen, lungs (weight) 550
  respiratory values, average 578
Biotransformation of CM
  glucuronide conjugate 393
Bis compounds 38
  iocarmate 51
  iocarmic acid 51
  iodipamide 51
  ioglycamate 51
  iosefamate 51
  structure 51
  toxicity 40, 41
Bis compounds (amide coupler)
  osmolality 69, 70
  solubility 69
  toxicity 69–71
Bis-compounds 42, 72
  iodoaroylamino acids 46

ioxaglic acid 45
„monoacid dimers" 45
  solubility 46
  toxicity 46
  triiodobenzoic acids 46
Bis-hydroxyethylester of 2,3,5,6-tetra-
  iodoterephthalic acid 472
Blood brain barrier (BBB)
  colloidal iron 347
  horseradish peroxidase 347
  lanthanum hydroxide 347
Blood pool CM 5
Blood rheology
  effects of CM 344
Blood transfusion 583
Blood-brain barrier (BBB) 499, 510
  damage 346
  damage by CM 300
  ionic CM 300
  site of 346
  Trypan blue 300
Blood-organ barrier 26
Bradycardia 200–202, 230
  CM potencies, relative 229
  osmolality 229
  sodium content 229
Bromine compounds, aromatic 17
BSP, glutathione conjugate (BSP-GSH)
  398

C-29
  solubility problems 322
C545 206
Calcium disodium edetate 27
Cannulation
  chronic preparations 437
  for biliary CM 434
  of dog bile duct 436–442
  of rat bile duct 434
  Thomas cannula 437
Carbamate coupler 91
Carbamates 95
  solubility 61
  toxicity 61
Carbon-iodine bond 17
  deiodination 27
Carboxymethylcellulose 104
Cardiac hypertrophy
  animal models 281
Cardiografin 229
Cardioradiographic visualization,
  experimental 259, 260
  blood flow patterns 260
  carbon dioxide 259
  gelatin droplets 260
  intravascular clots 259

tantalum powder 259
Thorotrast 259
Cardiovascular catheterization 272–276
Cardiovascular CM 236
  asystole 229
  bradycardia 229, 230
  C-29 223
  carotid circulation 237
  cerebral blood flow 237
  clinical evaluation 227, 228
  conductance 240
  coronary circulation 238–240
  diatrizoate 223
  electrophysiologic effects 224
  endothelial injury 237
  general circulation 231
  hyperosmolality 226, 233
  hypertension 230
  hypotension 229, 230
  inotropic effect 224
  intracarotid injection 229, 230
  intracoronary administration 222
  iopamidol 222, 223
  ioxaglate 222
  isopaque 370 222
  limb circulation 231
  magnesium ions 232
  mesenteric blood flow 236
  metrizamide 222
  microcirculation 240, 242
  myocardial contractile effects 226
  myocardial subcellular structure, effect
    on 240
  P286 223
  P297 222
  pain 233
  potassium, intracellular 240
  reflex circulatory effects 230
  reflex or neurally mediated circulatory
    effects 228–243
  renal arteriography 234
  renal circulation 233–236
  renal vascular resistance 234
  saralasin 235
  sodium shift 240
  splanchnic circulation 236, 237
  tachycardia 230
  toxicity 227, 242
  vascular effects 231
  vascular endothelium 240–243
  vasoconstriction 232–234
  vasodilatation 231, 233, 234, 237, 238
  vasodilation 232
  ventricular arrhythmias 226
Cardiovascular effects of CM 193–243
  aortic root injection 196
  C-29 223
  coronary sinus ionic calcium 219
  diatrizoate 223
  electrophysiologic effects 199–210,
    224–226
  experimental model 195, 196
  failing myocardium 224
  hemodynamic effects 210–213
  inotropic effects 219, 224
  intracoronary administration 223
  ionic CM 225
  iopamidol 223
  ioxaglate 223
  ischemic myocardium 224
  myocardial contractile effects 226
  myocardial effects 213–228
  nonionic CM 225
  osmolality 225
  P286 223
  site of injection 196–199
  sodium content 225
  ventricular arrhythmias 226
Cardiovascular radiology, experimental
  259
  animal models 276
  arteriosclerosis (AS) 276
  cardiovascular catheterization 272–276
  contrast media 253–259
  laboratory equipment 267
  planning experimental protocols 260
Cardiovascular system, CM in 193–243
Carotid circulation 237
  autonomic blockade 299
  nicotine 230
  reflexes 228
Cationic CM 49
  diiodofumaric acid 49
  iodomethanesulfonamides 49
  tetraiodoterephthalic acid 49, 50
  trisiodomethylacetamide 49
Central nervous system (CNS)
  angiographic CM 296
  nuclear magnetic resonance (NMR)
    tomography 296
Cerebral blood flow
  cushing reflex 299
  measurement by proton state changes
    347
Cerebral blood flow (CBF)
  effects of CM 298
Cerebrospinal fluid (CSF)
  flow 353
  formation 353
  kinetics, effect of CM on 354
  leukocyte count 354
  pressure 354
  total volume 353
Cerium oxide 545

Charge 15
Chelating agents 206
    depleting calcium ion in the heart 27
Chemical structure 75, 384
    bis-arabinos-2-yl ether 320
    bis-glucose-3-yl ether 320
    bis-glycolyl bridge 324
    cost 322
    diiodotriglucosylbenzene 320
    hindered glycolytic bond 320
    iocetamic acid 385
    iodipamide 386
    iodoxamate 386
    ioglycamide 386
    iopanoic acid 385
    iopronic acid 385
    iosulamide 386
    iosumetic acid 385
    iotrol 324
    iotroxamide 386
    ipodatic acid 385
    malonyl bridge 324
    methylene group toxicology 320
    nonionic CM 74, 75
    steric variability 324
    sugar derivative 320
    tyropanoic acid 385
    DL-2-98 320
Chemistry 23
    biological requirements 23
Chemoreceptor reflex 198
Chloral hydrate 343, 581
Chloralose 581
α-chloralose 343
Cholangiographic CM 383, 384
    iodipamide 386
    iodoxamate 386
    ioglycamide 386
    iosulamide 386
    iotroxamide 386
Cholebrine 386
Cholecystographic CM
    albumin binding 391
    anilide-containing 111–113
    benzyl-containing 109
    biliary excretion 394, 396
    BSP 396
    ether-containing 108
    first-pass effect 391
    intravenous 391, 394
    iopanoate 396
    iopanoic acid 383
    oral 107–109, 111–113, 391
    solubility 386
    structure 107
    Telepaque 383
    transport in blood 391

Cholecystographic CM, oral 406
    Bilopaque 384
    chemical structure 385
    intestinal absorption 387–390
    iocetamic acid 385
    iopanoic acid 284, 385
    iopronic acid 385
    iosumetic acid 385
    ipodatic acid 385
    partition ratio 387
    physicochemical properties 384
    sodium iodipamide (Biligrafin) 384
    solubility 384, 387
    tyropanoic acid 385
Cholecystopaques, intravenous
    aroylaminoacyl-aminobenzoic acids 42
    iodipamide 42
    structures 42
Cholecystopaques
    amino acids 392
    bile salts 392
    BSP 392
    extraction ratio 381
    half-life analysis 380
    hepatic clearance 380, 381
    hepatic extraction 382
    hepatic uptake 392
    intrinsic clearance 381
    ouabain 392
    pharmacokinetic principles 380–383
    preferential hepatic excretion 392
    steroid hormones 392
    structure 114
Cholegrafin 384
Choleresis 376, 398, 400
    secretin-induced 378, 379
Chromatography
    high pressure (HPLC) 454
    reversed phase (RPLC) 455
    thin layer 454
Chronic congestive heart failure
    animal models 281
Cinemicroangiography, high speed 241
Clearance
    evaluation of 175
CM concentration 133
    cortical nephrogram 134
    medullary nephrogram 134
    pyelogram 134
CM pharmacokinetics
    contrast distribution volume in blood
        506
    contrast distribution volume in tissue
        506
    distribution volume 506
CM reactions 525
    antibody-antigen reactions 526

cellular release of mediators 526
factor XII activators 529
histamine release 526
involvement of acute activation
    systems 527
iodide sensitivity 527
kallikrein 530
lupus erythematosus 528
prekallikrein 530
psychogenic factors 527
role for the C1-esterase inhibitor 528
serotonin release 526
CNS angiography 296, 297
  CM currently in use in 298
  effects of ionic CM 298
CNS electrophysiology
  CNS electroactivity, measurement 356
Coarctation
  animal models 282
Colcemid 533
Colloidal carbon 556
Complement system 527
Compound 593
  cost 322
Computed tomography
  abdominal blood vessels 514
  chest, lung, and mediastinal 513
  choice of intravascular CM 514
  cholangiographic CM 514
  contrast enhancement 511
  dual-energy CT 490
  hepatic and splenic 513
  iodine noise 490
  ionic monomeric CM 515
  metastases, detection 513
  multiple energy methods 486
  nonionic CM 514
  pancreatic 513
  pelvic organs 514
  renal and adrenal 514
  subtraction 486
Computed tomography, dual energy
  cerium 492
  high atomic number absorbers 490
Computed tomography, dual energy
  alternatives 487
Computed tomography, dynamic 500–
  505
Computed tomography (CT)
  and CM, adverse reactions 507
  artifacts 493, 495
  attenuation values 504
  cardiac 512
  cardiac CT scanning 497
  computed tomography, dual energy
    492

contract enhancement (CE) 479, 484,
    556, 560
contrast enhancement, iodine 482
contrast enhancement,
    pharmacokinetics 497
cranial, CE 509
density resolution 480
dynamic CT 500
dynamic scanners survey 494
dynamic scanning 492, 510
enhanced infarct 512
equipment 492
flow phantom, simulations 495
fresh hematomas 509
functional imaging 506
image manipulation 485–492
imaging properties 479
intraarterial CM 507
iodine noise determination 489
lesions, detection 510
liver and spleen 560
maximum specific enhancement 485
myocardial infarction 512
partial volume artifact 481
particulate CM 556, 560
principles 479–481
segmented reconstruction 492, 493
specific iodine enhancement 484
very high speed scanners 496
Congenital cardiac defects
  animal models 282
Congenital heart disease
  animal models 282
Conray 400 206, 232
Conray 60 200, 229, 232, 237, 301
  Ames and SCE tests (results) 536–540
Conray 60 (methylglucamine
    iothalamate) 232
Contrast enhancement 497, 562
  abdominal blood vessels 514
  blood-brain barrier 499, 511
  body cavities 507
  cardiac 512
  cerebral infarct 510
  chest, lung, and mediastinal 513
  choice of intravascular CM 514
  cholangiographic CM 514
  computed tomography (CT) 509–515
  CT number (HU) versus iodine
    concentration 483
  distribution volume 506
  dynamic aspects of 499
  dynamic CT 500, 501
  emulsified CM 560
  fresh hematomas 509
  hepatic and splenic 513
  high atomic number absorbers 484

Contrast enhancement
  intraarterial CM   507
  intracavitary   514
  iodine, characteristics   482
  iodine, specific enhancement   483
  lesions, detection   510
  maximizing enhancement   511
  metastases, detection   513
  myocardial infarction   512
  nonequilibrium kinetics   499
  nonionic CM   514
  of the brain   499
  optimum beam energies   483
  pancreatic   513
  particulate CM   556
  pelvic organs   514
  practical applications   508–515
  problems   509
  renal and adrenal   514
  reticuloendothelial system   508
  whole body   499, 500
  xenon   508, 511
Contrast enhancement, pharmacokinetics
  body compartments   497
  diffusion of CM   497–499
Contrast media (CM)
  absorption from CSF   353
  Ames and SCE tests (results)   536–540
  basic properties   9
  biliary   367
  biological half-life in CSF   353
  biological requirements   23
  biological safety   28
  blood pool   5
  central nervous system   295
  cerebral infarct   510
  chemistry   23, 55
  computed tomography (CT)   479, 509–
    515
  cytogenetic effect   533
  2-[^{18}F]-2-deoxy-D-glucose   295
  formulation   94
  Gd3$^+$/DTPA/bismeglumine complexes
    296
  intestinal absorption   388
  iodoantipyrine   295
  isomers   95
  manufacturing costs   92
  mutagenicity   533
  osmolality   25
  osmolality, theoretical   569
  particulate suspensions   543–571
  perfluorocarbons   6
  physicochemical properties   24
  radiopaque cations   6
  solubility   24
  stability   26

  stereochemical aspects   95
  strontium bromide   296
  ultrasound   6
  viscosity   25
  xenon   295
Coronary angiography
  Bezold-Jarisch reflex   230
  reflex circulatory effects   230
Coronary arteriography
  coronary vascular resistance   239
Coronary artery disease
  CM stress test   212, 213
Coronary artery stenosis
  coronary flow reserve   239
Coronary circulation   238
Cortical nephrogram   127, 134, 138
Coumarin   469
Coupler groups
  amide   55
  carbamate   56
  ester   56
  glycoside   56
  hydrolysis   83
  peptide   56
  reversed amide   55
  stability   83
  toxicity   56
  ureide   56
Cranial angiography (CA)
  bradycardia   299
  damage to the blood-brain barrier   300
  dimer-X   299
  GTS (Gilles de la Tourette Syndrome)
    301
  experimental designs   299
  hemodynamic effects of CM   300
  hyperosmolality   299
  hypotension   299
  ionic CM   297
  ionic dimers   300
  ionic monomers, toxicological
    comparisons of   300
  iopamidol   299
  metrizamide   299
  pain   301
  receptors located in the carotid
    circulation   299
  vasomotor brain center   299
Cushing reflex   299
Cyanoacrylates (tissue adhesive)
  carbonyl iron   348
  percutaneous thrombosis   348
Cytogenetic effect of CM   533

Decarboxylation   27
Decomposition   80

Dehydration 146
  diuretics 145
Deiodination 80
  calcium disodium edetate 27
2-[^{18}F]-2-deoxy-D-glucose 295
2-[^{14}C]-deoxy-D-glucose (DG) 347
Design principles 1, 27, 547, 570
  aminoalkanol substitutes 16
  anaphylactoid reactions 19
  biological safety 28
  charge 15, 16
  chemotoxicity 12, 14
  cost 19, 31
  coupler groups 56
  couples groups 55
  crowding effect 14
  emulsified CM 558
  hyperosmolality 26
  hypertonicity 4
  iodine masking 14
  isomerism 15
  lymphographic CM 468
  nonionic CM 18, 54, 77
  osmolality 25
  particulate CM 558
  physicochemical properties 24
  pi electron withdrawal 13, 14
  polyhydroxyalkylamides 16
  solubility 12, 24, 77
  stability 16, 26
  sugar residue 16
  toxicity 18
  triiodoaniline 16
  viscosity 14, 25
Dextrose, hyperosmolal solutions 200
DG(2-[^{14}C]-deoxy-D-glucose) 347
Diastereoisomers 99
Diatrizoate 129, 130, 138, 201, 237, 298
  chromosome damage 534
Diiodofumaric acid 49
Dimer-X 299, 312
  experimental studies 311
Dimers (bis-compounds)
  monovalent 6
Dimethiodal sodium 129
Diskography 304
Disodium edetate 206
Diuresis, osmotic 141–145
  ratio-1.5 CM 141
  ratio-3 CM 141
DL-Threitol 75
Dogs 263–267
  breeds 263
  cardiac conduction system 265
  coronary vessels 266
  ECG 265
  heart, lymphatic system 267

heart, radiographic anatomy 264
heart valves 265
pericardium 264
thoracic cavity 264
thoracotomy 264
Dose 145
Ductus arteriosus
  animal models 283
Dysprosium oxide 545

EEG, experimental
  average amplitude 359
  CM epileptogenicity 358
  desynchronization 358
  effects of anesthesia 359
  evaluation of CM toxicity 360
  evoked response 360
  frequency spectrum analysis 359, 360
  synchronization 358
  with unanesthetized animals 359
  Xylocaine 359
Electrocorticogram (ECoG) 356
Electroencephalogram (EEG) 356
Electroencephalogram (EEG),
  experimental 357–360
Electrophysiologic cardiac effects
  arrhythmias 204–208
  baroreceptor reflex 200
  bradycardia 200–202
  conduction disturbances 204
  diatrizoate 201
  ECG-toxicity index 208
  electrocardiographic changes 208–210
  impulse conduction 202
  impulse generation 200
  infusion rate 200
  intracoronary cholinergic reflex 201
  ionic CM 204, 208, 209
  metrizamide 201
  osmolality 200
  sinus arrest 200
  vectorcardiographic changes 208
  ventricular fibrillation 205
Emulsified CM
  adverse reactions 560
  AG 60.99 562
  contrast enhancement 560
  deiodination, risk 559
  design principles 558
  stability 559
  toxicity 560
Endocardial fibroelastosis
  animal models 281
Endocarditis
  animal models 283
Endomyocardial fibrosis
  animal models 281

Enterohepatic circulation   404
    antibiotic treatment   405
    biliary CM   405
EOE 13   560, 562
Epidurography, lumbar   304
Epileptogenicity   322
Erythrocytes
    effects of ionic CM   298
Ester coupler   91
Esters
    solubility   62
    toxicity   62
Ether-containing cholecystopaques
    structure   108
    toxicity   108
Ethiodol   464, 560, 568
    adverse reactions   569
Ethiodol (Lipiodol Ultrafluide)
    clearance   465
    injection rates   465
    viscosity   465
Ethyliodo-phenylundecylate
    (iodophenylate)
    advantages and disadvantages   308
Experimental animals   358, 471, 585
    anesthesia   577–586
    anesthesia, administration   428
    animal models   470
    bile flow rate   424
    bile flow rates, ratio animals/man   424
    bile production, endogenous rates   424
    biological data   378, 397, 421
    biological values, normal   550, 578
    blood transfusion   583
    cannulation, dog bile duct   436–442
    cannulation, rat bile duct   434–436
    choice of   349
    euthanasia   583
    holding and restraint   426
    in vivo animal preparation   434–442
    investigative lymphangiology   470
    management   420, 421
    pigs   348
    respiratory values, average   578
    reticuloendothelial system   550
    serum constituents   422, 423
    urographic CM, mice   150
    urography, rabbits   148, 149
    venipuncture, dogs   429
Experimental animals, choice of
    calves   261
    cats   261
    dogs   263–267
    for EEG   359
    infrahuman primates   260
    miniature pigs   263
    pigs   262, 263
    rabbits   261

Experimental CM   473
    Iotasul   472
    nonionic dimer   472
    perfluorocarbons   472
Experimental model   257
    coronary arteriography   258
    regional ischemia   258
    regional myocardial contractile
        function   258
Experimental neuroradiology see
    Neuroradiology, experimental
Experimental urography   148

Femoral artery
    blood flow   232
    Conray 60   232
    isolated hind limb circulation   232
Field emission X-ray apparatus   270
First-pass effect   391
Fluorescent excitation analysis (FEA)
    absorption edge   453
    advantages, with biological tissues   454
    detector   453
    iodine analysis   453, 454
Frank-Starling effect   198

Gadolinium oxide   545
Gallbladder function   403
    CM reabsorption   404
Gd3$^+$/DTPA/bismeglumine complexes
    296
    glomerular damage   156
    tubular damage   156
Glomerular filtration   140
Gluconanilides
    solubility   57
    toxicity   57
Glycoside coupler   92
Glycosides and glucose derivatives
    solubility   63
    toxicity   63

H-reflex   360
Half-life analysis   380
Headaches, postmyelographic
    hydration   305
    prophylaxis   305
    tiapride   305
Heart block
    animal models   281
Heart valves diseases
    animal models   283
Hemodynamic cardiac effects
    CM stress test   212, 213
    ventriculography   210–213
Hemodynamic response   198
Hepatic physiology   374–380
    bile composition   347

bile formation 376–379
  bile salt-independent fraction 377
  canalicular bile flow 376
  cellular anatomy 368–373
  choleresis, bile-salt-associated 376
  choleretic 377
  classic liver lobule 368, 369
  erythritol clearance 377
  gallbladder anatomy 373
  liver anatomy 367
  liver blood flow 367
  mannitol clearance 377
  micelles 376
Hepatic uptake, cholecystopaques
  albumin binding 392
Hepatotoxicity
  iodipamide 407
Hexabrix
  see ioxaglate
High-performance or high-pressure liquid
  chromatography (HPLC) 454
  partition coefficients 99
Hydergine 469
Hydrolysis 27
Hydrolytic esters
  stability 105
  toxicity 105
Hydrophilicity 12
Hydrophobicity 12
  enzyme inhibition 525
  ionic equilibirium, disturbances 525
Hydrophobicity/philicity
  enzyme kinetics 13
  partition 13
  ring (pi) electrons 13
  toxicity 13
Hydroxyalkyltetraiodoterephthalates 104
Hypaque 229
Hypaque 50 200, 229, 237
Hypaque 75 232
Hypaque 75M 200
Hypaque 76 206
Hypaque 85 228
Hypaque M-75 231, 238, 239
Hypaque M-90 237, 241
Hyperosmolality
  arachnoiditis 26
  blood-organ barrier 26
Hypertension 230
Hypertonicity (Hyperosmolality)
  bis-compounds 51
  polymers 51
  reduction of 51
Hypocalcemia 206
Hypotension 229, 230
Hypotension, reversible
  sodium nitroprusside 583
  trimethophan 583

In vitro liver preparations 442–451
  Hanks-HEPES buffer 450
  isolated liver perfusion, rat 442
  liver homogenate preparation 450
  perfusion apparatus 444
  perfusion medium 442–444
  subcellular fractionation of liver 450
Infundibular pulmonic stenosis
  animal models 285
Inorganic colloids 5
Inotropic effects 219, 220
Intestinal absorption 388
  maximum rates 389
  passive permeability coefficient 389
Intracarotid injection 228, 229
  ionic CM 229
Intracoronary cholinergic reflex 201
Intracoronary injection 197
Intrathecal CM
  Abrodil 308, 310
  CM neuroleptic drug interaction 306
  design principles 306
  diiodotriglucosylbenzene 320
  Dimer-X 312
  double contrast techniques 304
  ethyl iopodate 308
  hyperosmolality 314
  iocarmate, ionic dimer (Dimer-X) 311
  iodo-methane-sulfonic acid (Abrodil)
    307
  ionic dimer P-193 318
  ionic monomers P-94, P-115, and P-
    182 318
  iopamidol 321, 324
  iotrol 306, 324
  Lipiodol 307
  meglumine iothalamate 311
  Methiodal 310
  metrizamide 312, 313
  MP-1013 320
  MP-328 323
  Myelografin 312
  N-(3-acetamido-5-N-methyl acetamino-
    2,4,6-triidobenzoyl)-2-amino-2-de-
    oxy-D-glucitol 313
  neurotoxicity 324
  nonionic dimer P-308 319
  nonionic dimers 323
  P-297 (ioglunide) 319
  Pantopaque arachnoiditis 304
  PhDZ59B 312
  polymerized diiodothyrosine 308
  pyrogens 320
  2,3,5,6-tetraiodohydroquinone-diethyl
    ether 308
  Thorotrast 307
  trimer P-291 318
  DL-2-98 320

Intrathecal visualization 306–320
    oily CM 307
Investigative lymphangiology 470
Iobenzamic acid
    structure 114
Iocarmate 207
Iocetamic acid 387
    chemical structure 114, 385
Iodamine 130
Iodecol 10
    carotid angiography in rabbits 303
    critical threshold 303
    vascular pain 303
Iodinated aromatic alcohols
    lethal dose 103
Iodine
    wet chemical assay 457
Iodine, plasma concentration 135–138
    dose 135
    injection rate 135
    ratio-1.5 CM 135
    ratio-3 CM 135
    volume distribution 136, 137
Iodine, urine concentration 138–146
    cortical nephrograms 138
    diuresis, osmotic 138
    dose 138, 139
    excretion mechanisms 139
    injection rate 138, 139
    medullary nephrogram 138
    pyelogram 138
Iodine analysis
    fluorescent excitation analysis (FEA)
        452
    X-ray energy spectrometry 452
Iodiophenylundecenoic acid ester
        (iophendylate) 102
Iodipamide
    adverse reactions 406
    chemical structure 386
Iodipamide ethyl ester 546, 571
    differential CT enhancement 565
Iodoantipyrine 295
Iodoaroylamino acids 46
Iodomethamate 129
Iodomethanesulfonamides 49
Iodopyracet 129
Iodoxamate 402
    chemical structure 386
Ioglicinate 298
Ioglucol (MP-6026) 74
Ioglucomide (MP-8000) 74
Ioglunide (P-297) 7
    elimination 319
    gluconic acid 319
    neurotoxicity 319

Ioglycamide
    chemical structure 386
Iogulamide (MP-10013) 75
Iohexol 7, 131
    i.v. LD_{50} in mice 323
    i.v. LD_{50} in rats 323
    iohexol and metrizamide 323
    neurotoxicity 323
    osmolality 322
    synthesis 86, 88
Ionic CM 31, 50
    amide side chains 32
    aroylamino acids 47
    benzyl amines 48
    bis compounds 32, 38, 40, 41, 42, 45,
        46
    cationic CM 49
    diiodofumaric acid 49
    dimers 32
    ECG toxicity 208
    electrocardiographic effects 209
    endothelial damage 241
    iodination 31
    iodoaroylacylbenzoates 44
    iodoaroylamino acids 46
    iodomethanesulfonamides 49
    mesenteric blood flow 236
    „monoacid dimers" 46
    polymeric X-ray CM 52, 53
    purification 31
    radiopaque cations 48
    structural types 32
    substituted triiodobenzoic acids 33,
        35–37, 39
    synthesis 31
    tetraiodoterephthalic acid 49, 50
    toxicity 47
    triiodobenzoic acids 46
    triiodobenzylamines 47
    trimers 32
    tris compounds 42–44
    trisiodomethylacetamide 49
Ionic dimers
    dimer-X 312
    P-193 318
    PhDZ59B 312
Ionic monomers 318
    P-115 318
    P-182 318
    P-94 318
Iopamidol 74, 131, 222, 229
    cardiovascular responses 321
    deiodination 322
    hemodynamic changes 199
    metabolism 322
    serinol 7

synthesis 86
toxicity, systemic 321
Iopanoate 396
  biliary excretion 397
  rate of biliary excretion 395
Iopanoate glucuronide
  enterohepatic circulation 390
Iopanoic acid 383, 384, 387
  biologic half-life of 391
  chemical structure 385
  enterohepatic circulation 390
  rate of biliary excretion 395
  structure 114
Iophenoxic acid
  biologic half-life of 391
Iopromide 7, 75
Iopronic acid
  chemical structure 114, 385
Ioserinate 318
Iosulamide
  chemical structure 386
Iosumetic acid
  chemical structure 385
Iotasul 10
  indirect lymphography 472
Iothalamate 130, 298
Iothalamate ethyl ester 546
Iotrol 75, 324
  adverse reactions 325
  arthrographic 11
  synthesis 88
Iotroxamide
  chemical structure 386
Ioxaglate 131
Ioxaglate, Hexabrix 302
Ioxaglate (P286) 222
Ioxaglic acid 6
  synthesis 45
Ioxithalamate 130, 138
Iozomate 207
Ipodate 387
Ipodatic acid
  chemical structure 385
Ipodic acid (ipodate)
  chemical structure 114
Ischemia, myocardial 224
  CM effects 215
Isolated hepatocytes
  preparation 448
Isolated rabbit heart 30
Isomerism
  geometrical 97
  optical 97
Isopaque 224
Isopaque 370 218, 220, 222
Isopaque 379 206

Isopaque 60 232
Isopaque Coronar 227, 228
Isophthalamides
  solubility 68
  toxicity 68

Kallikrein 530
Ketamine 342
Ketamine HCl 582
2-Ketogulonamides
  solubility 58
  toxicity 58

Laboratory equipment
  amplifiers 271
  automatic injectors 270
  biplane X-ray apparatus 269
  cardiovascular CM research 269–271
  cine analysis 269
  cinefluorographic equipment 268
  computed tomography 270
  correlation systems 269
  dynamic scanners, survey 494
  electromagnetic flowmeters 172
  electromagnetic tape recorder 271
  field emission X-ray apparatus 270
  layout 267
  magnification radiography 269, 270
  oscilloscopes 271
  physiological recording equipment 271
  recorders 271
  video recording systems 268
  X-ray equipment 267
Laboratory techniques 30, 169, 348
  alkaline ashing 161
  Ames test 534, 535
  anesthesia 159, 424–426
  anesthesia, administration 428
  animal holding and restraint 426–428
  assays for CM 161–163
  aversion conditioning 355, 356
  bile salts analysis 458, 459
  biliary CM study 419–459
  bilirubin analysis 456, 457
  blood transfusion 583
  cannulation, dog bile duct 436–442
  cannulation, rat bile duct 434–436
  cannulation, veins 431–434
  cardiovascular catheterization 272–276
  carotid angiography in rabbits 303
  cell cultures, mammalian 535
  chemotoxicity of CM 301
  chromatography 454–456
  combustion 161
  computed tomography 162
  determining CM clearance 166

Laboratory techniques
  diencephalic injection ED_{50} in rats 324
  dye dilution 173, 233
  electrophysiological methods 356
  euthanasia 583
  experimental spinal cord trauma 301
  fluorescent excitation analysis (FEA)
    452–454
  for studying renal pharmacodynamics
    171
  hepatic physiology 377
  high-performance or high-pressure
    liquid chromatography (HPLC) 99,
    162, 454
  in vitro liver preparation 442–451
  in vivo animal preparation 434–442
  inert gas technique 175
  infusion of CM 166
  intracisternal LD_{50} in rats 324
  intraperitoneal injection 427
  investigative uroradiology 158–180
  iodine analysis 452
  iodine determination 457
  isolated hepatocytes, preparation 448,
    449
  isolated liver perfusion, rat 442
  microsphere technique 175
  mutagenesis tests 534
  mutagenicity tests 535
  neural deficit scores 324
  neurovascular 344
  neutron activation 161
  partition coefficients 99
  planimetry 163
  radioactive labeling 162
  renal function tests 176
  renal microradiography 179
  SCE test 535
  single-injection technique 166
  spectrophotometry 451
  T-tube chronic fistula 441
  thin-layer chromatography (TLC) 454
  Thomas cannula 437, 438
  tubular micropuncture and
    microperfusion 170
  ureteral catheterization 164
  UV spectrophotometry 161
  venipuncture 428
  Walton-Brodie strain gauge 216
  X-ray fluorescence 162
Left coronary arterial injection
  glucose 202
  ionic CM 202
  Isopaque 370 202
  mannitol 202
  metrizamide 202
  polyvinyl pyrilidone 202

  Renografin-76 202
  sodium chloride 202
  sucrose 202
Left ventricular hypertrophy (LVH)
  animal models 282
Lethal dose 30, 254
Lethal dose, animals
  death causes 151
Lipiodol 102
  iodiophenylundecenoic acid ester
    (iophendylate) 102
Lipiodol Ultrafluide (Ethiodol)
  clearance 465
  injection rates 465
  viscosity 465
Liposomes 567
  brominated liposomes 6
Lumbar epidurography 304
LV contractile state
  meglumine sodium diatrizoate 219
  metrizamide 219
Lymph 468
  composition 466
  flow 467
Lymph nodes
  retention of CM 465
Lymphangiography
  benzopyrones 469
  coumarin 469
  hyaluronidase, use of 469
  hydergine 469
  lymphatic kinetics, pharmacological
    manipulation 469
  trimethaphen camphosulfonate 469
  troxerutin 469
  L-arginine 469
Lymphatic kinetics
  benzopyrones 469
  coumarin 469
  hydergine 469
  pharmacological manipulations 469
  trimethaphen camphosulfonate 469
  troxerutin 469
  L-arginine 469
Lymphatic physiology 466
Lymphodynamics
  autorhythmicity 467
  lymph flow 467
Lymphographic CM
  bis-hydroxyethylester of 2,3,5,6-tetra-
    iodoterephthalic acid 472
  chlorophyll 463
  design principles 468
  Ethiodol 464, 568
  hyaluronidase, use of 469
  Lipiodol 463
  nonionic dimer 472

particulate CM   464, 468
perfluorocarbons   472
Thorotrast   463
toxicity   471
transport into lymph capillaries   468
tumor dissemination   463
Urografin   464
water-soluble CM   464
Lymphography   568
  alphafurine 2G   464
  bis-hydroxyethyl ester of 2,3,5,6-tetra-
    iodoterephthalic acid   472
  Ethiodol   464
  experimental   464, 470
  experimental CM   471–473
  extravasation   465
  faradic current   470
  hypersensitivity   465
  in various species   471
  indirect   471
  laboratory techniques   470, 471
  lymphatic kinetics, pharmacological
    manipulation   469, 470
  methods   464
  nonionic dimer   472
  oil embolism   465, 466
  oily CM   464, 465
  particulate CM   464
  perfluorocarbons   472, 473
  perfluorooctyl and perflurohexyl
    bromides   473
  Urografin   464
  Venalot   470
  water-soluble CM   464
Lymphography, experimental
  Ethiodol, with ether   464
  oily CM   464
  particulate CM   464
  water-soluble CM   464

Magnesium ions   232
Medullary nephrogram   127, 134, 138
Meglumine   220
Meglumine diatrizoate   205
Meglumine iothalamate   205, 302
Meglumine metrizoate   205
Meglumine metrizoate (Isopaque
  Cerebral)   302
Meglumine sodium calcium metrizoate
  219
Meglumine sodium diatrizoate   220, 236
Methiodal
  toxicity   310
Metrizamide   7, 74, 131, 148, 200, 201,
  206, 222, 224, 225, 229, 233, 236, 239,
  312
  adverse reactions   317

cervical myelography   318
CNS penetration   316
depressive effect on the motor centers
  314
EMG   314
epileptogenic potential   313
epimerization   83
excretion   315
headache   317
meningeal irritation   317
neuroleptic drugs   314
psychoorganic syndromes   317
subacute reactions   315
synthesis   85
toxicity of   313
volume distributions   315
Metrizoate   130, 138, 148, 298, 303
Microcirculation   240
  endothelial damage   241, 242
  measurement of flow dynamics   345
  monomeric CM   241
  submucosal injection   241
  syllectograme   345
  topical application   241
Mitral stenosis
  animal models   283
Mitral valve insufficiency
  animal models   283
Monoacid dimers   46
Monomeric ionic CM
  legs, blood flow and venous tone   232
Monovalent dimer   302
MP-238   18
MP-328   323
MP-7011   75
MP-7012   75
Multiple energy methods
  in computed tomography   486
Mutagenicity
  Ames test   535
  chromosomes   538
  criteria   538
  review of the problem   540
  SCE test   535
Mutagenicity of CM
  Colcemid   533
  Thorotrast   533
Myelografin   312
Myelographic CM
  toxicity   305
Myelography
  headaches   304, 322
  headaches, prophylaxis   305
  hydration   305
  intrathecal corticoids   305
  ioglunide   305
  iohexol   305

Myelography
  iopamidol 305
  late arachnoiditis 305
  meningism 305
  metrizamide 305, 318
  postlumbar puncture syndrome 305
  tiapride 305
Myocardial depression 216
  calcium ions, addition 214
  ionic CM 214, 221
  monomeric ionic CM 214
  nonionic CM 214
  with metrizamide 217
Myocardial effects of CM
  cation composition of ionic CM 216
  hypertonicity 216
  intracoronary administration 216
  ionic and nonionic CM 214, 215, 217
  isolated heart and isolated cardiac
    tissue 213–216
  myocardial depression 214, 216, 217
  viscosity 216
Myocardial function in dogs
  experimental model 255
Myocardial infarction
  animal models 279, 280

N-Tyrosine-3,5-diiodo-4-pyridone N-
  acetate 546
N-(3-acetamido-5-N-methyl acetamino-
  2,4,6-triiodobenzoyl)-2-amino-2-deoxy-D-
  glucitol 313
Nephrogram 128, 138
  cortical 127
  medullary 127
Nephrotoxicity
  glomerular damage 154, 155
  tubular damage 157
  vascular damage 153
Nerve roots, intradural
  monosynaptic reflex 361
Neural conductivity
  effects of CM 360
  evaluation of CM toxicity 360
  H-reflex 360
Neuroleptic drugs
  interaction with metrizamide 314
Neuroradiology, experimental 354
  anesthesia 341–343
  animal models 348, 349
  assessment of cerebral hemodynamics
    346
  aversion conditioning 355, 356
  avian atherosclerosis 349
  basic methods 341
  blood-brain barrier (BBB) 346
  breakdown of the BBB 349

  cerebral hemodynamics 345
  cerebral infarction 349
  cerebral vasospasm 349
  choice of animal models 349–350
  chronic cannulation of SAS 352
  CM effects in cerebral angiography
    345
  electrophysiological methods 356
  impedance plethysmography 345
  interventional vascular neuroradiology
    348
  laboratory techniques 344
  light plethysmography 345
  lumbar puncture 350
  Macaca fascicularis 349–350
  Macaca mulatta 350
  mapping the local cerebral metabolic
    rate 347
  microcirculation 345
  neuroradiology, interventional
    vascular 348
  NMR tomography 347
  organ perfusion 345
  pericerebral injection 352
  pig posterior lumbar SAS 350
  positron computed tomography 347
  premedication 342
  serum complement system 347
  spinal cord trauma 349
  subarachnoid space 349
  suboccipital puncture 350
  thermography 346
  thromboembolism 349
  tissue adhesive (cyanoacrylates) 348
  toxicity screening of experimental
    compounds 355
  ulcerations 349
  ultrasonic techniques 346
  ventricular sampling 351
  volatile anesthetics 344
Neurotoxicity 30, 324
Nicotine 230
Nonionic CM 54, 55, 302
  benzamides/-2-glycose derivatives 64
  benzamides/1-glucamine derivatives 65
  benzamides/alkanol derivatives 67
  benzamides/heptitol derivatives 66
  benzoate esters 103
  bis compounds (amide coupler) 69–71
  bis compounds 72
  C-29 322
  carbamates 61
  chemical structure 8, 74, 75
  compound 593 322
  cost 322
  design principles 77
  dl-threitol 75

esters   62
formulation   76
gluconanilides   57
glycosides and glucose derivatives   63
iodomethane sulfonamides   73
ioglucol (MP-6026)   74
ioglucomide (MP-8000)   74
iogulamide (MP-10013)   75
iopamidol   74
iopromide   75
iotrol   75
isophthalamides   68
2-ketogulonamides   58
metrizamide   55, 74
MP 328   323
MP-7011   75
MP-7012   75
oily CM   102
osmolality   78, 79
P-297   75
peptides   60
physical properties   321
reversed amides   59
reversed amide couplers   89
solubility   76
stability   79
structural types   56
synthesis   85, 89
toxicity   18, 56
ureides   61
viscosity   77
water-insoluble   101
Nonionic dimers   472
iodecol   10
iotasul   10
iotrol   11
isoosmolarity   323
P-308   319
renal excretion   11
Nonionic monomers   7
P-232 and P-236   318
Nuclear magnetic resonance (NMR)
tomography
central nervous system (CNS)   296

Oil embolism   465
Oily CM   102, 464, 465
toxicity   471
Oragrafin   386
Osmolality   7, 50, 141, 225, 235, 303, 569
angiography   570
design principles   570
ionic CM   25
molecular aggregates   78
particulate CM   570
ratio-3 CM   142

second generation nonionic monomers
7
toxicity   570
urine   171
Osmotic diuresis   143

P-297   75
P-297 (ioglunide)
elimination   319
gluconic acid   319
neurotoxicity   319
stability   319
P286 (ioxaglate)   222
P297   222
Pain
osmotic pressure   233
Pantopaque   310
advantages and disadvantages   308
adverse reactions   309
removal of   306
Particulate CM   5, 558
advantages over water-soluble CM   543
adverse reactions   569
albumin preincubation   549
angiography   569
clearance rates   553–554
clearance rates, effect of dose   554–556
computed tomography   560
deiodination, risk   559
design principles   547, 570
dextrin   547
fibrinogen interaction   547
for CT (liver and spleen)   543
for ultrasound   543
inorganic   544, 545
interactions with blood components
546–550
iodipamide ethyl ester   571
latex particles   553
liposome-encapsulated CM   567
liver attenuation values   562
liver lesion, detection   562
lymphography   568
organ uptake   554
organic   545, 546
osmolality, theoretical   569
particle aggregation   547, 549
particle diameter   545, 546
particle size   552
perfluorocarbons   567
phagocytosis   550
platelet activation   547
potential applications   568
RE-selective   543
RES uptake   553
reticuloendothelial system   550

Particulate CM
  stability 545, 559
  surface charge 552, 553
  Thorotrast 544
Particulate suspensions 543–571
Peptide coupler 90
Peptides 60
  solubility 60
  toxicity 60
Perfluoroalkyl halides
  perfluorohexylbromide 106
  perfluorohydrocarbons 106
  perfluorooctylbromide 106
Perfluorocarbons 6, 472
  excretion 473
Perfluoroctylbromide 106, 310
Perfluorohexylbromide 106
Perfluorohydrocarbons 106
Perfused rabbit heart 254
Perfusion pulmonary hypertension
  animal models 282
Pericarditis, experimental
  animal models 280
Pharmacokinetics 497
Pharmacological evaluation
  intact heart 254
  lethal dose 254
  perfused rabbit heart 254
  systemic toxicity 254
PhDZ59B 312
Phlebography, spinal cord 297
Pigs
  acute catheterization 263
  anesthesia 262
  azygoz vein 262
  chest configuration 262
  chronic catheters implantation 263
  ductus arteriosus 262
Polyhydroxylated acylamides 72
Polymeric X-ray CM
  range mol. wt. 52, 53
  solubility 52, 53
  toxicity 52, 53
Poststenotic dilation
  animal models 282
Prekallikrein 530
Pretesting
  intravascular 529
Propyliodone 546
Protein binding
  CM 525
Proteinuria 176
Pulmonary air embolism
  animal models 286
Pulmonary embolism
  animal models 285

Pulmonary stenosis
  animal models 285
Pulmonary valves
  animal models 285
Pulmonic artery stenosis
  animal models 285
Pyelogram 127, 128, 134, 138, 145

Radiculosaccography 304
Radiographic CM 254
Radiopaque anions
  dimeric, monovalent 2
  monomeric, monovalent 2
  monomeric, trivalent 2
Radiopaque cations 2
  cartilage binding 48
  structure 48
Ratio-1.5 CM 130, 131, 141, 147, 158
Ratio-3 CM 131, 141, 147
  advantages 158
RCK-136 399
Renal circulation 233–236
Renal excretion
  intravenous biliary CM 405
  iodipamide 405
  iopanoic acid 405
  ipodate 405
  tyropanoate 405
Renal failure 146
Renal function tests 176
Renal histology 178
Renal microradiography 179
Renal pharmacodynamics
  ability to concentrate urine 171
Renografin 60 229, 237, 301
Renografin 75 231, 237
Renografin 76 200, 201, 206, 207, 220,
    221, 224, 225, 228, 237–241
  Ames and SCE tests (results) 536–540
  Saralasin 235
Renografin-M-60 301
Renovist 232, 241
Reticulo-endothelial selective CM 544
Reticuloendothelial system (RES) 508
  blockade 556, 557
  CM concentration 551
  CM uptake 552
  composition 552
  phagocytosis 551
Reticuloendothelial-selective CM
  contrast enhancement 562
  emulsions 558
  liposome-encapsulated CM 567
  perfluorocarbon 567
Reversed amides
  solubility 59
  toxicity 59

SA node, effect of CM on
  experimental model 257
Saline, hyperosmolal 200
Saralasin 235
SC 2644 402
SCE test 535
Septal defects
  animal models 282
Serinol 7
  synthesis 87
Side chains
  acetamido 34
  acylamidomethyl 34
  acylmethyl/acyl series 38
  acyl/acyl series 34
  amyl 34
  carbamyl 34
  carbamyl/acyl series 38
Silver iodide 545
Sinoatrial node
  dextrose, hyperosmolal solution 200
  metrizamide 200
  Renografin-76 200
  saline, hyperosmolal 200
Sinus arrest 200
Sodium acetrizoate 70 229
Sodium calcium metrizoate 220
Sodium citrate 206
Sodium content 225
Sodium diatrizoate 232
Sodium iodipamide 233, 384
Sodium iopanoate
  Ames and SCE tests (results) 536–540
Sodium iothalamate 232
Sodium nitroprusside 583
  Trimethophan 583
Sodium tyropanoate (Bilopaque) 384
Solubility 76, 384
  ether functions (methoxy 1,2-
    dihydroxypropoxy) 24
  hydroxyalkyl functions 24
  hydroxyl groups 24
  nonionic CM 77
  relative polarities 386
Spectrophotometry 451
Spinal cord arteriography (SCA) 297
Spinal cord phlebography (SCP) 297
Spinal cord trauma
  experimental 301
Spinal subarachnoid space (SAS)
  techniques of entry into 304
Splanchnic circulation 236, 237
Stability 26, 79
  aromatic bromine compounds 17
  carbon-iodine bond 17
  decarboxylation 27
  decomposition 80

deiodination 27, 80
epimerization 80
hydrolysis 27
hydrolysis, glycosides 85
hydrolysis, ureide and carbamate
  couplers 85
hydrolysis of the peptide coupler 84
hydrolysis of reversed amides 84
lactomization 83
mechanisms of decomposition 16
meglumine iothalamate 81
routes of decomposition 28
sodium iothalamate 82
stability studies 27
Stannic oxide 545
Stereochemical aspects
  isomerism 95
Strontium bromide 296
Structural types 32, 34
  carbamyl/acyl series 38
Structure
  radiopaque cations 48
Subarachnoid space
  methods of access 350
Subarachnoid space (SAS), spinal
  anatomy 352–353
  velocity of CM absorption 353
Substituted triiodobenzoic acids
  acylmethyl/acyl series 39
  acyl/acyl series 35
  carbamyl/acyl series 36, 37
  solubility 33, 35–37, 39
  toxicity 33, 35–37, 39
Subtraction
  in computed tomography 486
Synthesis
  bis-compounds 88, 90
  carbamate coupler 91
  carbamates 95
  ester coupler 91, 96
  glycoside coupler 92
  nonionic CM 85
  peptide coupler 90
  reversed amide couplers 89
  ureide coupler 90
Systemic toxicity 30

T-tube chronic fistula 441
Tachycardia 230
Tantalum pentoxide 545
Taurocholate 402
Telepaque 383
Tetraiodophenolphthalein 546
Tetraiodophthalate derivatives 546
Tetraiodoterephthalic acid 49, 50
  toxicity 104
Thalamic stereotaxy 352

Thin-layer chromatography (TLC) 454
Thomas cannula 437, 440
  surgical preparation of 438
Thorium dioxide 545
Thorotrast 5, 259, 297, 533, 545
  kinetics 555
  toxicity 307
D,L threitol 69
Thrombosis
  animal models 286
Tin oxide 5
Tissue adhesive (cyanoacrylates)
  carbonyl iron 348
  percutaneous thrombosis 348
Toxicity 30, 303, 471, 570
  see also adverse reaction
  cardiovascular CM 221, 227
  chelating agents 221
  cholecystographic CM, oral 406
  enzyme inhibition 525
  general considerations 525
  glomerular damage 156
  iodinated aromatic alcohols 103
  iodipamide 406
  ionic equilibrium, disturbances 525
  local 525
  lung edema 151
  of intravenous CM 151
  osmolality 131
  pharmacological evaluation 254
  preclinical pharmacology 29
  protein binding 525
  ratio-1.5 CM 130
  red blood cell changes 151
  systemic 525
  tubular damage 156
  urographic CM 130
Toxicology
  preclinical pharmacology 29
Toxicology evaluation 29
Tricuspid valve
  animal models 285
Triiodo-trimesic acid 13
Triiodobenzoic acids 46
Triiodobenzylamines 47
Trimers 318
Tris-compounds 43
  iodoaroylacylbenzoates 44
Trisiodomethylacetamide 49
Troxerutin 469
Tyropanoate 387, 390
Tyropanoic acid
  chemical structure 114, 385

Ureide coupler 90
Ureides

solubility 61
  toxicity 61
Urethane 581
Urinary enzymes 177
  activities measured 180
  main localization sites of 178
Urografin 228, 464
Urografin 45 232
Urografin 60 232, 233
Urografin 75 232
Urografin-76 240
Urographic CM 127
  adverse reactions 153, 158
  diatrizoate 138
  distribution volume 138
  glomerular damage 154–156
  injection rate 150
  ioxithalamate 138
  lethal dose, intravenous 150
  metrizoate 138
  nephrotoxicity 153
  osmolality 130, 131
  physical properties 135
  toxicity 149, 150
  tubular damage 156
  viscosity 135, 136
  volume distribution 136, 137
Urography
  experimental 148, 164
Urography, infusion 138
Urokon 229
Urokon 70 238, 241
Urokon sodium 70 237
Uroradiology, experimental 158–180
  anesthesia 159
  choice of species 159
Uroradiology, experimental procedures
  anesthesia 160
  assays for contrast media 160
  surgical procedures 160
Uroselektan 128, 129

Vascoray 215
Vascular endothelium 240–243
Vascular pain 303
  critical threshold 10
  intraarterial anesthetics 7
  iohexol 10
  iopamidol 10
  iopromide 10
  ioxaglate 10
  osmolality 7
Venalot 470
Ventricular arrhythmias
  diatrizoate 205
  meglumine diatrizoate 205

Ventricular fibrillation
  chelating agents 206
  fibrillation threshold 206
  frequency 207
  hypocalcemia 206
  sodium ions 207
Ventricular fibrillation, experimental
  animal models 280
Viscosity 77
  ionic CM 25

Wolff-Parkinson-White syndrome
  animal models 281

X-ray attenuation
  ratio-1.5 CM 147
  ratio-3 CM 147
^{133}Xe 298
Xenon 295, 508
Xylocaine
  ketamine potentiation 359

Handbook of Experimental Pharmacology

Continuation of
"Handbuch der
experimentellen
Pharmakologie"

Editorial Board
G. V. R. Born, A. Farah,
H. Herken, A. D. Welch

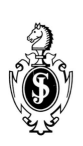

Springer-Verlag
Berlin
Heidelberg
New York
Tokyo

Volume 25
**Bradykinin, Kallidin and
Kallikrein**

Volume 26
**Vergleichende Pharmako-
logie von Überträgersub-
stanzen in tiersystema-
tischer Darstellung**

Volume 27
Anticoagulantinen

Volume 28: Part 1
**Concepts in Biochemical
Pharmacology I**

Part 3
**Concepts in Biochemical
Pharmacology III**

Volume 29
Oral wirksame Antidiabetika

Volume 30
**Modern Inhalation
Anesthetics**

Volume 32: Part 2
Insulin II

Volume 34
**Secretin, Cholecystokinin
Pancreozymin and Gastrin**

Volume 35: Part 1
Androgene I

Part 2
**Androgens II and Antiandro-
gens/Androgene II und
Antiandrogene**

Volume 36
**Uranium – Plutonium –
Transplutonic Elements**

Volume 37
Angiotensin

Volume 38: Part 1
**Antineoplastic and
Immunosuppressive
Agents I**

Part 2
**Antineoplastic and
Immunosuppressive
Agents II**

Volume 39
Antihypertensive Agents

Volume 40
Organic Nitrates

Volume 41
Hypolipidemic Agents

Volume 42
Neuromuscular Junction

Volume 43
**Anabolic-Androgenic
Steroids**

Volume 44
Heme and Hemoproteins

Volume 45: Part 1
Drug Addiction I

Part 2
Drug Addiction II

Volume 46
**Fibrinolytics and
Antifibronolytics**

Volume 47
Kinetics of Drug Action

Volume 48
Arthropod Venoms

Volume 49
**Ergot Alkaloids and Related
Compounds**

Volume 50: Part 1
Inflammation

Part 2
Anti-Inflammatory Drugs

Volume 51
Uric Acid

Handbook of Experimental Pharmacology

Continuation of
"Handbuch der
experimentellen
Pharmakologie"

Editorial Board
G. V. R. Born, A. Farah,
H. Herken, A. D. Welch

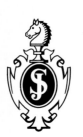

Springer-Verlag
Berlin
Heidelberg
New York
Tokyo

Volume 52
Snake Venoms

Volume 53
Pharmacology of Gang-lionic Transmission

Volume 54: Part 1
Adrenergic Activators and Inhibitors I

Part 2
Adrenergic Activators and Inhibitors II

Volume 55
Psychotropic Agents

Part 1
Antipsychotics and Antidepressants

Part 2
Anxiolytics, Gerontopsycho-pharmacological Agents and Psychomotor Stimulants

Part 3
Alcohol and Psychotomime-tics, Psychotropic Effects of Central Acting Drugs

Volume 56, Part 1 + 2
Cardiac Glycosides

Volume 57
Tissue Growth Factors

Volume 58
Cyclic Nucleotides

Part 1: **Biochemistry**

Part 2: **Physiology and Pharmacology**

Volume 59
Mediators and Drugs in Gastrointestinal Motility

Part 1: **Morphological Basis and Neurophysiological Control**

Part 2: **Endogenous and Exogenous Agents**

Volume 60
Pyretics and Antipyretics

Volume 61
Chemotherapy of Viral Infections

Volume 62
Aminoglycoside Antibiotics

Volume 63
Allergic Reactions to Drugs

Volume 64
Inhibition of Folate Metabolism in Chemotherapy

Volume 65
Teratogenesis and Reproductive Toxicology

Volume 66
Part 1: **Glucagon I**
Part 2: **Glucagon II**

Volume 67
Part 1
Antibiotics Containing the Beta-Lactam Structure I

Part 2
Antibiotics Containing the Beta-Lactam Structure II

Volume 68, Part 1 + 2
Antimalarial Drugs

Volume 69
Pharmacology of the Eye

Volume 70
Pharmacology of Intestinal Permeation

Volume 71
Interferons and Their Applications

Volume 72
Antitumor Drug Resistance